# INGENIX®

## 2008 Coders' Desk Reference for Procedures

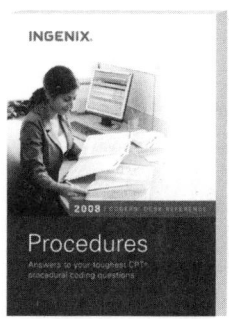

ISBN: 978-1-60151-011-2
Item Number: 5596
Available: December 2007
Price: $134.95

## SAVE 15%
when you order at www.shopingenix.com and enter source code FOBW8 in the lower right-hand corner of the home page.

## Master CPT® Components and Code with Confidence.

Now with significant changes included for 2008, this desk reference will help you master the components and details behind CPT® codes for better coding success. Reduce the number of errors in code selection, improve understanding of the clinical meanings behind codes and check billing and coding information for Medicare.

← **Know the differences between similar CPT® codes**

← **Code more accurately from the operative reports**

← **Train new coders and medical staff**

## Key Features and Benefits

The **Coders' Desk Reference for Procedures** provides coders, medical staff, payers and health care professionals with a comprehensive and informative guide to a wide variety of commonly asked questions and definitions for CPT® codes.

- **Ingenix Edge—More than 7,000 lay descriptions for 2008 CPT® codes.** A one-stop resource, providing lay descriptions for surgery, laboratory/pathology, radiology and medicine codes.

- **Ingenix Edge—Anatomical illustrations for coding.** Understand the body sites described in operative reports and code more confidently.

- **Ingenix Edge—Modifier definitions, narrative descriptions and rules for use.** Reduce research time and improve accuracy by assigning and documenting modifiers and E/M codes appropriately.

- **Ingenix Edge—Surgical terms chapter.** Define the components of surgical

procedures, and break the terms into components.

- **Ingenix Edge—Procedure eponym crosswalk.** Eponyms are defined and linked to codes in this alpha-ordered chapter.

- **Ingenix Edge—Reimbursement terms glossary.** Understand the peculiar terms used by payers.

- **Ingenix Edge—Abbreviations, acronyms, symbols, prefixes and suffixes.** Learn how best to understand and use these valuable tools.

CPT is a registered trademark of the American Medical Association.

**Ingenix | Intelligence for Health Care | Call toll-free 1.800.INGI**

*Also available from your medical bookstore or distributor.*

FOBA8

# INGENIX®

## Four simple ways to place an order.

### Call
1.800.ingenix (464.3649), option 1. Mention source code FOBA8 when ordering.

### Mail
PO Box 27116
Salt Lake City, UT 84127-0116
With payment and/or purchase order.

### Fax
801.982.4033
With credit card information and/or purchase order.

### Click
www.shopingenix.com
*Save 15% when you order online today—use source code FOBW8.*

**ingenix e smart**
ShopIngenix.com frequent buyer program

GET REWARDS FOR SHOPPING ONLINE!
To find out more, visit www.shopingenix.com

eSmart program available only to Ingenix customers who are not part of Medallion, Gold Medallion or Partner Accounts programs. You must be registered at ShopIngenix.com to have your online purchases tracked for rewards purposes. Shipping charges and taxes still apply and cannot be used for rewards. Offer valid online only.

## 100% Money Back Guarantee
If our merchandise* ever fails to meet your expectations, please contact our Customer Service Department toll-free at 1.800.ingenix (464.3649), option 1 for an immediate response.

*Software: Credit will be granted for unopened packages only.

## Customer Service Hours
7:00 am - 5:00 pm Mountain Time
9:00 am - 7:00 pm Eastern Time

## Shipping and Handling

| no. of items | fee |
|---|---|
| 1 | $10.95 |
| 2-4 | $12.95 |
| 5-7 | $14.95 |
| 8-10 | $19.95 |
| 11+ | Call |

# Order Form

## Information

Customer No. _____ Contact No. _____

Source Code _____

Contact Name _____

Title _____ Specialty _____

Company _____

Street Address _____

City _____ State _____ Zip _____
NO PO BOXES, PLEASE

Telephone ( ) _____ Fax ( ) _____
IN CASE WE HAVE QUESTIONS ABOUT YOUR ORDER

E-mail _____ @ _____
REQUIRED FOR ORDER CONFIRMATION AND SELECT PRODUCT DELIVERY.

Ingenix respects your right to privacy. We will not sell or rent your e-mail address or fax number to anyone outside Ingenix and its business partners. If you would like to remove your name from Ingenix promotion, please call 1.800.ingenix (464.3649), option 1.

## Product

| Item No. | Qty | Description | Price | Total |
|---|---|---|---|---|
| | | | | |
| | | | | |
| | | | | |
| | | | | |
| | | | | |
| | | | | |
| | | | | |
| | | | | |
| | | | | |
| | | | | |
| | | | | |

Subtotal _____

UT, VA, TN, OH, CT, IA, MD, MN, NC & NJ residents, please add applicable  Sales tax _____

(See chart on the left)  Shipping & handling charges _____
*All foreign orders, please call for shipping costs*

Total _____

## Payment

○ Please bill my credit card  ○ MasterCard  ○ VISA  ○ Amex  ○ Discover

Card No. | | | | | | | | | | | | | | | |  Expires | |
MONTH  YEAR

Signature _____

○ Check enclosed, made payable to: Ingenix, Inc.  ○ Please bill my office

Purchase Order No. _____
ATTACH COPY OF PURCHASE ORDER

FOBA8

**INGENIX**®

# HCPCS Level II
# Professional

2008

## Acknowledgments

Mike Goleman, *Product Manager*

Michael E. Desposito, *Vice President, Coding & Referential*

Lynn Speirs, *Senior Director, Editorial/Desktop Publishing*

Karen Schmidt, BSN, *Technical Director*

Stacy Perry, *Manager, Desktop Publishing*

Sherry Faass, *Project Manager*

Wendy Gabbert, CPC, CPC-H, *Clinical/Technical Editor*

Steven Espinosa, *Clinical/Technical Editor*

Jean Parkinson, *Editor*

## Technical Editors

### Wendy Gabbert, CPC, CPC-H
### Clinical/Technical Editor

Ms. Gabbert has more than 25 years of experience in the health care field. She has extensive background in CPT/HCPCS and ICD-9-CM coding. She served several years as a coding consultant. Her areas of expertise include physician and hospital CPT coding assessments, chargemaster reviews, and the Outpatient Prospective Payment System (OPPS). She is a member of the American Academy of Professional Coders (AAPC).

### Steven Espinosa
### Clinical/Technical Editor

Mr. Espinosa has over 15 years of experience in the health care industry. His areas of expertise include patient billing, CPT/HCPCS coding, the outpatient prospective payment system (OPPS), and chargemaster development and maintenance. He recently served as a health care consultant conducting chart-to-claim audits with emphasis on documentation and coding. He has developed and executed numerous multidisciplinary education plans. Mr. Espinosa earned his Bachelor of Arts in Health Information Management from St. Regis University. He is an active member of the American Academy of Professional Coders.

# Introduction

## ORGANIZATION OF HCPCS

The Ingenix 2008 *HCPCS Level II* book contains mandated changes and new codes for use as of January 1, 2008. Deleted codes have also been indicated and cross-referenced to active codes when possible. New codes have been added to the appropriate sections, eliminating the time-consuming step of looking in two places for a code. However, keep in mind that the information in this book is a reproduction of the 2008 HCPCS; additional information on coverage issues may have been provided to Medicare contractors after publication. All contractors periodically update their systems and records throughout the year. If this book does not agree with your contractor, it is either because of a mid-year update or correction or a specific local or regional coverage policy.

To make this year's HCPCS book even more useful, we have included codes noted in addendum B of the 2008 Outpatient Prospective Payment System (OPPS) update as published in the *Federal Register* and from transmittals through 2007 that include codes not discussed in other Centers for Medicare and Medicaid Services (CMS) documents. The sources for these codes are often noted in blue beneath the description.

### Index

Because HCPCS is organized by code number rather than by service or supply name, the index enables the coder to locate any code without looking through individual ranges of codes. Just look up the medical or surgical supply, service, orthotic, prosthetic, or generic or brand name drug in question to find the appropriate codes. This index also refers to many of the brand names by which these items are known.

### Table of Drugs

The brand names of drugs listed are examples only and may not include all products available for that type of drug. Our table of drugs lists HCPCS codes from any available sections including A codes, C codes, J codes, S codes, and Q codes under brand and generic drug names with amount, route of administration, and code numbers. While we try to make the table comprehensive, it is not all-inclusive.

### Color-coded Coverage Instructions

The Ingenix HCPCS Level II codebook provides colored symbols for each coverage and reimbursement instruction. A legend to these symbols is provided on the bottom of each two-page spread.

## HOW TO USE INGENIX HCPCS LEVEL II BOOK

### Blue Color Bar—Special Coverage Instructions

A blue bar for "special coverage instructions" over a code means that special coverage instructions apply to that code. These special instructions are also typically given in the form of Medicare Pub.100 reference numbers. The appendixes provide the full text of the cited Medicare Pub.100 references.

**A4211**    Supplies for self-administered injections

### Yellow Color Bar—Contractor Discretion

Issues that are left to "contractor discretion" are covered with a yellow bar. Contact the contractor for specific coverage information on those codes.

**A4248**    Chlorhexidine containing antiseptic, 1 ml

### Red Color Bar—Not Covered by or Invalid for Medicare

Codes that are not covered by or are invalid for Medicare are covered by a red bar. The pertinent Medicare internet-only manuals (Pub. 100) reference numbers are also given explaining why a particular code is not covered. These numbers refer to the appendixes, where we have listed the Medicare references.

**A4232**    Syringe with needle for external insulin pump, sterile, 3cc

The Ingenix HCPCS Level II codes follow the AMA CPT code book conventions to indicate new, revised, and deleted codes.

- A black circle (●) precedes a new code.
- A black triangle (▲) precedes a code with revised terminology or rules.
- A circle (○) precedes a reissued code.
- Codes deleted from the 2008 active codes appear with a strike-out.

| | | |
|---|---|---|
| ● | A4650 | Implantable radiation dosimeter, each |
| ▲ | A5105 | Urinary suspensory with leg bag, with or without tube, each |
| ○ | D2970 | Temporary crown (fractured tooth) |
| | ~~J7319~~ | ~~Hyaluronan (sodium hyaluronate) or derivatives; intra-articular injection, per injection~~ |

See code(s) Q4083-Q4086

### ☑ Quantity Alert

Many codes in HCPCS report quantities that may not coincide with quantities available in the marketplace. For instance, a HCPCS code for an ostomy pouch with skin barrier reports each pouch, but the product is generally sold in a package of 10; "10" must be indicated in the quantity box on the CMS claim form to ensure proper reimbursement. This symbol indicates that care should be taken to verify quantities in this code.

☑    **A4207**    Syringe with needle, sterile 2 cc, each

♀ **Female Only**

This icon identifies procedures that should only be reported for female patients.

A4280    Adhesive skin support attachment for use with external breast prosthesis, each ♀

♂ **Male Only**

This icon identifies procedures that should only be reported for male patients.

A4326    Male external catheter specialty type with integral collection chamber, any type, each ♂

**A Age Edit**

This icon denotes codes intended for use with a specific age group, such as neonate, newborn, pediatric, and adult. Carefully review the code description to ensure that the code you report most appropriately reflects the patient's age.

D8010    Limited orthodontic treatment of the primary dentition A

**M Maternity**

This icon identifies procedures that by definition should only be used for maternity patients generally between 12 and 55 years of age.

H1001    Prenatal care, at-risk enhanced service; antepartum management M

**A2-Z3 ASC Payment Indicators**

Codes designated as being paid by ASC groupings that were effective at the time of printing are denoted by the group number.

G0105    Colorectal cancer screening; colonoscopy on individual at high risk A2

**& DMEPOS**

Use this icon to identify when to consult the CMS durable medical equipment, prosthetics, orthotics, and supplies (DMEPOS) for payment of this durable medical item.

A4600    Sleeve for intermittent limb compression device, replacement only, each &

⊘ **Skilled Nursing Facility (SNF)**

Use this icon to identify certain items and services excluded from SNF consolidated billing. These items may be billed directly to the Medicare contractor by the provider or supplier of the service or item.

A4653    Peritoneal dialysis catheter anchoring device, belt, each ⊘

Drugs commonly reported with a code are listed underneath by brand or generic name.

J7310 Ganciclovir, 4.5 mg, long-acting implant

Use this code for Vitasert.

CMS does not use consistent terminology when a code for a specific procedure is not listed. The code description may include any of the following terms: unlisted, not otherwise classified (NOC), unspecified, unclassified, other, and miscellaneous. If you are sure there is no code for the service or supply provided or used, be sure to provide adequate documentation to the payer. Check with the payer for more information.

A0999    Unlisted ambulance service

## OPPS Status Indicators

Ⓐ-Ⓨ OPPS status indicators

Status indicators identify how individual HCPCS Level II codes are paid or not paid under the OPPS. The same status indicator is assigned to all the codes within an ambulatory payment classification (APC). Consult the payer or resource to learn which CPT codes fall within various APCs. Status indicators for HCPCS and their definitions follow:

Ⓐ Indicates services that are paid under some other method such as the DMEPOS fee schedule or the physician fee schedule

Ⓑ Indicates codes not allowed or paid under OPPS

Ⓒ Indicates inpatient services that are not paid under the OPPS

Ⓔ Indicates services for which payment is not allowed under the OPPS (In some instances, the service is not covered by Medicare. In other instances, Medicare does not use the code in question but does use another code to describe the service)

Ⓕ Indicates corneal tissue acquisition costs, certain certified registered nurse anesthetist (CRNA) services, and hepatitis B vaccines that are paid at reasonable cost

Ⓖ Indicates a current drug or biological for which payment is made under the transitional pass-through provisions

Ⓗ Indicates either a device paid under pass-through provisions or brachytherapy sources and radiopharmaceuticals that are paid at reasonable cost

Ⓚ Indicates non-pass-through drugs and biologicals

Ⓛ Indicates influenza or pneumococcal pneumonia vaccine paid as of reasonable cost with no deductible or coinsurance

Ⓜ Indicates that this code should not be reported by hospitals to their fiscal intermediary

Ⓝ Indicates services that are incidental with payment packaged into another service or APC group

Ⓟ Indicates services paid only in partial hospitalization programs

Ⓢ Indicates significant procedures for which payment is allowed under the hospital OPPS but to which the multiple procedure reduction does not apply

Ⓣ Indicates surgical services for which payment is allowed under the hospital OPPS (Services with this payment indicator are the only ones to which the multiple procedure payment reduction applies)

Ⓥ Indicates visits for which payment is allowed under the hospital OPPS

Ⓧ Indicates ancillary services for which payment is allowed under the hospital OPPS

Ⓨ Indicates nonimplantable durable medical equipment (DME) that is billed by providers other than home health agencies to the DMERC

| | | |
|---|---|---|
| Ⓐ | A4321 | Therapeutic agent for urinary catheter irrigation |
| Ⓑ | Q4005 | Cast supplies, long arm cast, adult (11 years +), plaster |
| Ⓒ | G0341 | Percutaneous islet cell transplant, includes portal vein catheterization and infusion |
| Ⓔ | A0021 | Ambulance service, outside state per mile, transport (Medicaid only) |
| Ⓕ | V2785 | Processing, preserving and transporting corneal tissue |
| Ⓖ | J0129 | Injection, abatacept, 10 mg |
| Ⓗ | C1821 | Interspinous process distraction device (implantable) |
| Ⓚ | J7501 | Azathioprine, parenteral, 100 mg |
| Ⓜ | G0333 | Dispense fee initial 30 day |
| Ⓝ | A4220 | Refill kit for implantable infusion pump |
| Ⓟ | G0129 | Occupational therapy requiring the skills of a qualified occupational therapist, furnished as a component of a partial hospitalization treatment program, per day |
| Ⓢ | G0251 | Linear accelerator based stereotactic radiosurgery, delivery including collimator changes and custom plugging, fractionated treatment, all lesions, per session, maximum five sessions per course of treatment |
| Ⓣ | C9724 | Endoscopic full-thickness plication in the gastric cardia using endoscopic plication system (EPS); includes endoscopy |
| Ⓥ | G0101 | Cervical or vaginal cancer screening; pelvic and clinical breast examination |
| Ⓧ | Q0035 | Cardiokymography |
| Ⓨ | A4222 | Infusion supplies for external drug infusion pump, per cassette or bag (list drugs separately) |

## ASC Payment Indicators

**A2–Z3** **ASC Payment Indicators**
This icon identifies the new ASC status payment indicators, effective January 1, 2008. They indicate how the ASC payment rate was derived and/or how the procedure, item, or service is treated under the revised ASC payment system. For more information about these new indicators and how they affect billing, consult Ingenix's *Outpatient Billing Editor*.

**A2** Surgical procedure on proposed ASC list in calendar year (CY) 2007; payment based on OPPS relative payment weight.

**F4** Corneal tissue acquisition; paid at reasonable cost.

**G2** Non-office-based surgical procedure added in CY 2008 or later; payment based on outpatient prospective payment system (OPPS) relative payment weight.

**H2** Brachytherapy source paid separately when provided integral to a surgical procedure on ASC list; payment contractor-priced.

**H8** Device-intensive procedure on ASC list in CY 2007; paid at adjusted rate.

**J7** OPPS pass-through device paid separately when provided integral to a surgical procedure on ASC list; payment contractor-priced.

**J8** Device-intensive procedure added to ASC list in CY 2008 or later; paid at adjusted rate.

**K2** Drugs and biologicals paid separately when provided integral to a surgical procedure on ASC list; payment based on OPPS rate.

**K7** Unclassified drugs and biologicals; payment contractor-priced.

**L6** New technology intraocular lens (NTIOL); special payment.

**N1** Packaged procedure/item; no separate payment made.

**P2** Office-based surgical procedure added to ASC list in CY 2008 or later with Medicare physician fee schedule (MPFS) nonfacility practice expense (PE) RVUs; payment based on OPPS relative payment weight.

**P3** Office-based surgical procedure added to ASC list in CY 2008 or later with MPFS nonfacility PE RVUs; payment based on MPFS nonfacility PE RVUs.

**R2** Office-based surgical procedure added to ASC list in CY 2008 or later without MPFS nonfacility PE RVUs; payment based on OPPS relative payment weight.

**Z2** Radiology service paid separately when provided integral to a surgical procedure on ASC list; payment based on OPPS relative payment weight.

**Z3** Radiology service paid separately when provided integral to a surgical procedure on ASC list; payment based on MPFS nonfacility PE RVUs

| | | |
|---|---|---|
| **A2** | G0105 | Coloerectal cancer screening; colonoscopy on individual at high risk **A2** ⊘ |
| **F4** | V2785 | Processing, preserving and transporting corneal tissue **F4** |
| **G2** | C9716 | Creations of thermal anal lesions by radiofrequency energy **G2** |
| **H2** | A9527 | Iodine I-125, sodium iodide solution, therapeutic per millicurie **H2** |
| **J7** | L8690 | Auditory osseointegrated device, includes all internal and external components **J7** |
| **K2** | J0128 | Injection, abarelix, 10 mg **K2** |
| **K7** | C9399 | Unclassified drugs or biologicals **K7** |

**MED:** This notation precedes an instruction pertaining to this code in the CMS Publication 100 (Pub 100) electronic manual or in a National Coverage Determination (NCD). These CMS sources, formerly called the Medicare Carriers Manual (MCM) and Coverage Issues Manual (CIM), present the rules for submitting these services to the federal government or its contractors and are included in the appendix of this book.

A4300    **Implantable access catheter, (e.g., venous, arterial, epidural subarachnoid, or peritoneal, etc.) external access**

MED: 100-2, 15, 120

**AHA:** American Hospital Association Coding Clinic for HCPCS citations help you find expanded information about specific codes and their usage.

A4290    **Sacral nerve stimulation test lead, each**

AHA: 1Q, '02, 9

**Current as of 11/21/2007**

You may subscribe to an email service to receive special reports when information in this book changes. Contact Customer Service at 1.800.INGENIX (464.3649), option 1.

## ABOUT HCPCS CODES

Ingenix does not develop or maintain HCPCS Level II codes. The federal government does.

Any supplier or manufacturer can submit a request for coding modification to the HCPCS Level II national codes. A document explaining the HCPCS modification process, as well as a detailed format for submitting a recommendation for a modification to HCPCS Level II codes, is available on the HCPCS website at www.cms.hhs.gov/medhcpcsgeninfo/01_overview.asp. Besides the information requested in this format, a requestor should also submit any additional descriptive material, including the manufacturer's product literature and information that is believed would be helpful in furthering CMS's understanding of the medical features of the item for which a coding modification is being recommended. The HCPCS coding review process is an ongoing, continuous process.

Requests for coding modifications should be sent to the following address:

Alpha-Numeric HCPCS Coordinator
Center for Medicare Management
Centers for Medicare and Medicaid Services
C5-08-27
7500 Security Boulevard
Baltimore, MD 21244-1850

## HOW TO USE HCPCS LEVEL II

Coders should keep in mind, however, that the insurance companies and government do not base payment solely on what was done for the patient. They need to know why the services were performed. In addition to using the HCPCS coding system for procedures and supplies, coders must also use the ICD-9-CM coding system to denote the diagnosis. This book will not discuss ICD-9-CM codes, which can be found in a current ICD-9-CM code book for diagnosis codes. To locate a HCPCS Level II code, follow these steps:

1.  Identify the services or procedures that the patient received.

    Example:

    Patient administered PSA exam.

2.  Look up the appropriate term in the index.

    Example:

    Screening

    prostate

    Coding Tip: Coders who are unable to find the procedure or service in the index can look in the table of contents for the type of procedure or device to narrow the code choices. Also, coders should remember to check the unlisted procedure guidelines for additional choices.

3.  Assign a tentative code.

    Example:

    Code G0103

    Coding Tip: To the right of the terminology, there may be a single code or multiple codes, a cross-reference, or an indication that the code has been deleted. Tentatively assign all codes listed.

4.  Locate the code or codes in the appropriate section. When multiple codes are listed in the index, be sure to read the narrative of all codes listed to find the appropriate code based on the service performed.

    Example:

    > **G0103** **Prostate cancer screening; prostate specific antigen test (PSA)**

5.  Check for color bars, symbols, notes, and references.

    Example:

    > Ⓐ  **G0103** **Prostate cancer screening; prostate specific antigen test (PSA)**  ♂
    >
    > **MED:** 100-3, 210.1; 100-4, 18, 50

6.  Review the appendixes for the reference definitions and other guidelines for coverage issues that apply.

7.  Determine whether any modifiers should be used.

8.  Assign the code.

    Example:

    The code assigned is G0103.

## CODING STANDARDS

### Levels of Use

Coders may find that the same procedure is coded at two or even three levels. Which code is correct? There are certain rules to follow if this should occur.

When both a CPT and a HCPCS Level II code have virtually identical narratives for a procedure or service, the CPT code should be used. If, however, the narratives are not identical (e.g., the CPT code narrative is generic, whereas the HCPCS Level II code is specific), the Level II code should be used.

Be sure to check for a national code when a CPT code description contains an instruction to include additional information, such as describing a specific medication. For example, when billing Medicare or Medicaid for supplies, avoid using CPT code 99070 Supplies and materials (except spectacles), provided by the physician over and above those usually included with the office visit or other services rendered (list drugs, trays, supplies, or materials provided). There are many HCPCS Level II codes that specify supplies in more detail.

### Special Reports

Submit a special report with the claim when a new, unusual, or variable procedure is provided or a modifier is used. Include the following information:

*   A copy of the appropriate report (e.g., operative, x-ray), explaining the nature, extent, and need for the procedure

*   Documentation of the medical necessity of the procedure

*   Documentation of the time and effort necessary to perform the procedure

**Arm**
  sling
    deluxe, A4565
      mesh cradle, A4565
    universal
      arm, A4565
      elevator, A4565
    wheelchair, E0973
**Arrestin**, J3250
**Arrow, power wheelchair**, K0014
**Arsenic trioxide**, J9017
**Arthrocentesis, dental**, D7870
**Arthroereisis**
  subtalar, S2117
**Arthroplasty, dental**, D7865
**Arthroscopy**
  dental, D7872-D7877
  knee
    harvest of cartilage, S2112
    removal loose body, FB, G0289
  shoulder
    with capsulorrhaphy, S2300
**Arthrotomy, dental**, D7860
**Artifcial**
  kidney machines and accessories
    (see also Dialysis), E1510-
    E1699
  larynx, L8500
  saliva, A9155
**Asparaginase**, J9020
**Aspart insulin**, S5551
**Aspiration, bone marrow**, G0364
**Assertive community treatment**,
  H0039-H0040
**Assessment**
  alcohol and/or substance, G0396-
    G0397
  audiologic, V5008-V5020
  family, H1011
  geriatric, S0250
  mental health, H0031
  speech, V5362-V5364
**Assisted living**, T2030-T2031
**Assistive listening device**, V5268-
  V5274
  alerting device, V5269
  cochlear implant assistive device,
    V5273
  TDD, V5272
  telephone amplifier, V5268
  television caption decoder, V5271
**Asthma**
  education, S9441
**Astramorph**, J2275
**Atgam**, J7504
**Ativan**, J2060
**Atropine**
  inhalation solution
    concentrated, J7635
    unit dose, J7636
  sulfate, J0460
**Attends, adult diapers**, A4335
**Audiologic assessment**, V5008-V5020
**Audiometry**, S0618
**Auditory osseointegrated device**,
  L8690
  replacement external processor,
    L8691
**Augmentation**
  sinus, D7951
**Auricular prosthesis**, D5914, D5927
**Aurothioglucose**, J2910
**Autoclix lancet device**, A4258
**Auto-Glide folding walker**, E0143
**Autolance lancet device**, A4258
**Autolet lancet device**, A4258
**Autolet Lite lancet device**, A4258
**Autolet Mark II lancet device**, A4258
**Autoplex T**, J7198
**Avastin**, J9035
**Avonex**, J1825
**Azacitidine**, J9025
**Azathioprine**, J7500
  parenteral, J7501
**Azithromycin**
  injection, J0456

**Azithromycin** — continued
  oral, Q0144
**Aztreonam**, S0073

## B

**Babysitter, child of parents in treat-**
  **ment**, T1009
**Back supports**, L0430-L0710
**Baclofen**, J0475, J0476
  intrathecal, J0475-J0476
**Bacterial sensitivity study**, P7001
**Bactocill**, J2700
**Bag**
  drainage, A4357
  irrigation supply, A4398
  spacer, for metered dose inhaler,
    A4627
  urinary, A4358, A5112
**BAL in oil**, J0470
**Balken, fracture frame**, E0946
**Bandage**
  adhesive, A6413
  compression
    high, A6452
    light, A6448-A6450
    medium, A6451
  conforming, A6442-A6447
  Orthoflex elastic plastic bandages,
    A4580
  padding, A6441
  self-adherent, A6413, A6453-A6455
  Specialist Plaster bandages, A4580
**Banflex**, J2360
**Bariatric**
  bed, E0302-E0304
  brief/diaper, T4543
  surgery, S2083
**Barium enema**, G0106
  cancer screening, G0120
**Barrier**
  with flange, A4373
  4 x 4, A4372
  adhesion, C1765
**Baseball finger splint**, A4570
**Basiliximab**, J0480
**Bath chair**, E0240
**Bathtub**
  chair, E0240
  heat unit, E0249
  stool or bench, E0245
  transfer bench, E0247, E0248
  transfer rail, E0246
  wall rail, E0241, E0242
**Battery**, L7360, L7364
  blood glucose monitor, A4233-A4236
  charger, L7362, L7366, L8695,
    L8699, Q0495
  cochlear implant device
    alkaline, L8622
    lithium, L8623-L8624
    zinc, L8621
  hearing device, V5266
  lithium, A4601, L7367
    charger, L7368
  replacement
    ear pulse generator, A4638
    external defibrillator, K0607
    external infusion pump, K0601-
      K0605
  six volt battery, L7360
  TENS, A4630
  twelve volt bettery, L7364
  ventilator, A4611-A4613
  ventricular assist device, Q0496,
    Q0503
  wheelchair, E2397, K0733
**Bayer chemical reagent strips, box of**
  **100 glucose/ketone urine test**
  **strips**, A4250
**BCG live, intravesical**, J9031
**BCW 600, manual wheelchair**, K0007
**BCW Power, power wheelchair**, K0014
**BCW recliner, manual wheelchair**,
  K0007
**B-D alcohol swabs, box**, A4245

**B-D disposable insulin syringes, up to**
  **1 cc, per syringe**, A4206
**B-D lancets, per box of 100**, A4258
**Bebax, foot orthosis**, L3160
**Becaplermin gel**, S0157
**Bed**
  accessory, E0315
  air fluidized, E0194
  cradle, any type, E0280
  drainage bag, bottle, A4357, A5102
  extra size for bariatric patients,
    E0302-E0304
  hospital, E0250-E0270
    full electric, home care, without
      mattress, E0297
    manual, without mattress, E0293
    pediatric, E0328-E0329
    safety enclosure frame/canopy,
      E0316
    semi-electric, without mattress,
      E0295
  pan, E0275, E0276
    Moore, E0275
  rail, E0305, E0310
  safety enclosure frame/canopy, hos-
    pital bed, E0316
**Behavioral health**, H0002-H0030
  day treatment, H2013
  per hour, H2012
**Behavior management, dental care**,
  D9920
**Bell-Horn**
  prosthetic shrinker, L8440-L8465
**Belt**
  adapter, A4421
  extremity, E0945
  Little Ones Sur-Fit pediatric, A4367
  ostomy, A4367
  pelvic, E0944
  ventricular assist device, Q0499
  wheelchair, E0978, K0098
**Bena-D (10, 50)**, J1200
**Benadryl**, J1200
**Benahist (10, 50)**, J1200
**Ben-Allergin-50**, J1200
**Bench, bathtub** (see also Bathtub),
  E0245
**Benesch boot**, L3212-L3214
**Benoject (-10, -50)**, J1200
**Bentyl**, J0500
**Benztropine**, J0515
**Berkeley shell, foot orthosis**, L3000
**Berubigen**, J3420
**Betadine**, A4246
  swabs/wipes, A4247
**Betalin 12**, J3420
**Betameth**, J0704
**Betamethasone**, J7622-J7624
  acetate and betamethasone sodium
    phosphate, J0702
  sodium phosphate, J0704
**Betaseron**, J1830
**Bethanechol chloride**, J0520
**Bevacizumab**, J9035
**Bicarbonate concentration for**
  **hemodialysis**, A4706-A4707
**Bicillin, Bicillin C-R, Bicillin C-R**
  **900/300, and Bicillin L-A**,
  J0530-J0580
**BiCNU**, J9050
**Bifocal, glass or plastic**, V2200-V2299
**Bilirubin (phototherapy) light**, E0202
**Binder**
  extremity, nonelastic, A4465
**Biofeedback device**, E0746
**Bio Flote alternating air pressure**
  **pump, pad system**, E0181,
  E0182
**Biologic materials, dental**, D4265
**Biologics, unclassified**, J3590
**Biopsy**
  bone marrow with aspiration, G0364
  hard tissue, dental, D7285
  soft tissue, dental, D7286
  transepithelial brush, D7288
    concentrated, J7628

**Biopsy** — continued
  transepithelial brush — continued
    unit dose, J7629
**Biperiden lactate**, J0190
**Birth control pills**, S4993
**Birthing classes**, S9436-S9439, S9442
**Bite disposable jaw locks**, E0700
**Bitewing radiographs**, D0270-D0277
**Bitewings**, D0272-D0274, D0277
**Bivalirudin**, J0583
**Bleaching, dental**
  external, per arch, D9972
  external, per tooth, D9973
  internal, per tooth, D9974
**Blenoxane**, J9040
**Bleomycin sulfate**, J9040
**Blood**
  Congo red, P2029
  fecal occult test, G0394
  glucose monitor, A4258, E0607
    with integrated lancing system,
      E2101
    with voice synthesizer, E2100
    disposable, A9275
  glucose test strips, A4253
  ketone test strips, A4252
  leak detector, dialysis, E1560
  leukocyte poor, P9016
  mucoprotein, P2038
  pressure equipment, A4660, A4663,
    A4670
  pump, dialysis, E1620
  split unit, P9011
  strips
    blood glucose test or reagent
      strips, A4253
    blood ketone test or reagent strip,
      A4252
  supply, P9010-P9022
  testing supplies, A4770
  transfusion, home, S9538
  tubing, A4750, A4755
    leukocytes reduced, P9051-P9056
      CMV-negative, P9051, P9053,
        P9055
**Bock Dynamic, foot prosthesis**, L5972
**Bock, Otto** — see Otto Bock
**Body jacket**
  scoliosis, L1300, L1310
**Body sock**, L0984
**Body wrap**
  foam positioners, E0191
  therapeutic overlay, E0199
**Bond or cement, ostomy, skin**, A4364
**Bone replacement graft, dental**, D7953
**Bone tissue excision, dental**, D7471-
  D7490
**Boot**
  pelvic, E0944
  surgical, ambulatory, L3260
  walking
    nonpneumatic, L4386
    pneumatic, L4360
**Bortezomib**, J9041
**Boston type spinal orthosis**, L1200
**Botulinum toxin**
  type A, J0585
  type B, J0587
**Brachytherapy**
  cesium 131, C2642-C2643
  gold 198, C1716
  iodine 125, A9527
  iridium 192
    high dose, C1717
    nonhigh dose, C1719
  needle, C1715
  nonhigh dose rate iridium 192,
    C1719
  nonstranded
    NOS, C2699
    cesium-131, C2643
    gold-198, C1716
    iodine-125, C2634, C2639
    iridium-192, C1717, C1719
    palladium-103, C2635-C2636,
      C2641

**Levonorgestrel, contraceptive implants and supplies**, J7302, J7306
**Levorphanol tartrate**, J1960
**Librium**, J1990
**Lice infestation treatment**, A9180
**Lidocaine HCl for intravenous infusion**, J2001
**Lifescan lancets, box of 100**, A4259
**Lifestand manual wheelchair**, K0009
**Lifestyle modification program, coronary heart disease**, S0340-S0342
**Lift**
  combination, E0637
  patient, and seat, E0621-E0635
    Hoyer
      Home Care, E0621
      Partner All-Purpose, hydraulic, E0630
      Partner Power Multifunction, E0625
  shoe, L3300-L3334
  standing frame system, E0638
**Lift-Aid patient lifts**, E0621
**Light box**, E0203
**Lincocin**, J2010
**Lincomycin HCl**, J2010
**Lioresal**, J0475
**Liquaemin sodium**, J1644
**Lispro insulin**, S5551
**Lithium battery for blood glucose monitor**, A4233-A4236
**Lithotripsy, gallstones**, S9034
**Little Ones**
  drainable pouch, A5063
  mini-pouch, A5054
  one-piece custom drainable pouch, A5061
  one-piece custom urostomy pouch, A5071
  pediatric belt, A4367
  pediatric urine collector, A4335
  urostomy pouch, transparent, A5073
**Lively, knee-ankle-foot orthosis**, L2038
**LMD, 10%**, J7100
**Lobectomy, lung, donor**, S2061
**Localized osteitis, dry socket**, D9110, D9930
**Lodging**
  NOS, S9976
  recipient, escort nonemergency transport, A0180, A0200
  transplant-related, S9975
**Lomustine**, S0178
**Lonalac powder, enteral nutrition**, B4150
**Lorazepam**, J2060
**Lovenox**, J1650
**Lower limb, prosthesis, addition**, L5968
**Low osmolar contrast**
  100-199 mgs iodine, Q9965
  200-299 mgs iodine, Q9966
  300-399 mgs iodine, Q9967
  400 or greater mgs iodine, Q9951
**Low vision**
  rehabilitation service, G9041-G9044
**LPN services**, T1003
**Lubricant**, A4332, A4402
**Lufyllin**, J1180
**Lumbar**
  orthosis, L0625-L0627
  pad, L1030, L1040
  sacral orthosis (LSO), L0628-L0640
**Luminal sodium**, J2560
**Lunelle**, J1056
**Lung volume reduction surgery services**, G0302-G0305
**Lupron**, J9218
  depot, J1950
**Lutrepulse**, J1620
**LVRS services**, G0302-G0305
**Lymphedema therapy**, S8950
**Lymphocyte immune globulin**, J7504, J7511

## M

**Madamist II medication compressor/nebulizer**, E0570
**Magnacal, enteral nutrition**, B4152
**Magnesium sulphate**, J3475
**Magnetic**
  resonance angiography, C8901-C8914, C8918-C8920
  resonance imaging, low field, S8042
  source imaging, S8035
**Maintenance contract, ESRD**, A4890
**Malar bone, fracture repair**, D7650, D7750, D7760
**Malibu cervical turtleneck safety collar**, L0150
**Malocclusion correction**, D8010-D8999
**Mammography**, G0202-G0206
**Management**
  disease, S0316-S0317
**Mandible, fracture**, D7630-D7640, D7730-D7740
**Mannitol**, J2150
**Mapping**
  topographic brain, S8040
  vessels, G0365
**Marker**
  tissue, A4648, C1879
**Marmine**, J1240
**Maryland bridge (resin-bonded fixed prosthesis)**
  pontic, D6210-D6252
  retainer/abutment, D6545
**Mask**
  burn compression, A6513
  CPAP, A7027
  oxygen, A4620
  surgical, for dialysis, A4928
**Mastectomy**
  bra, L8002
  camisole, S8460
  form, L8020
  prosthesis, L8000-L8039, L8600
  sleeve, L8010
**Masterbrace 3**, L2999
**Masterfoot Walking Cast Sole**, L3649
**Masterhinge Adjustabrace 3**, L2999
**Masterhinge Elbow Brace 3**, L3999
**Masterhinge Hip Hinge 3**, L2999
**Masterhinge Shoulder Brace 3**, L3999
**Mattress**
  air pressure, E0186, E0197
  alternating pressure, E0277
    pad, Bio Flote, E0181
    pad, KoalaKair, E0181
  AquaPedic Sectional, E0196
  decubitus care, E0196
  dry pressure, E0184
  flotation, E0184
  gel pressure, E0196
  hospital bed, E0271, E0272
    non-powered, pressure reducing, E0373
  Iris Preventix pressure relief/reduction, E0184
  Overlay, E0371-E0372
  pressure reducing, E0181
  TenderFlor II, E0187
  TenderGel II, E0196
  water pressure, E0187, E0198
    powered, pressure reducing, E0277
**Maxilla, fracture**, D7610-D7620, D7710-D7720
**Maxillofacial dental procedures**, D5911-D5999
**MCP, multi-axial rotation unit**, L5986
**MCT Oil, enteral nutrition**, B4155
**Meals**
  adults in treatment, T1010
  per diem NOS, S9977
**Mecasermin**, J2170
**Mechanical**
  hand, L6708-L6709
  hook, L6706-L6707
**Mechlorethamine HCl**, J9230

**Medialization material for vocal cord**, C1878
**Medical and surgical supplies**, A4206-A6404
**Medical conference**, S0220-S0221
**Medical food**, S9435
**Medical records copying fee**, S9981-S9982
**Medicare "welcome"**
  ECG, G0366-G0368
  physical, G0344
**Medi-Jector injection device**, A4210
**MediSense 2 Pen blood glucose monitor**, E0607
**Medralone**
  40, J1030
  80, J1040
**Medrol**, J7509
**Medroxyprogesterone acetate**, J1055
  with estradiol cypionate, J1056
**Mefoxin**, J0694
**Megestrol acetate**, S0179
**Melphalan HCl**, J9245
  oral, J8600
**Menotropins**, S0122
**Mental health**
  assessment, H0031
  hospitalization, H0035
  peer services, H0038
  self-help, H0038
  service plan, H0032
  services, NOS, H0046
  supportive treatment, H0026-H0037
**Mepergan**, J2180
**Meperidine**, J2175
  and promethazine, J2180
**Mepivacaine HCl**, J0670
**Mercaptopurine**, S0108
**Meritene, enteral nutrition**, B4150
  powder, B4150
**Meropenem**, J2185
**Mesh**, C1781
**Mesna**, J9209
**Mesnex**, J9209
**Metabolism error, food supplement**, S9434
**Metacarpophalangeal joint prosthesis**, L8630
**Metaraminol bitartrate**, J0380
**Metatarsal joint, prosthetic implant**, L8641
**Metatarsal neuroma injection**, S2135
**Meter, bath conductivity, dialysis**, E1550
**Methacholine chloride**, J7674
**Methadone**, J1230
  oral, S0109
**Methergine**, J2210
**Methocarbamol**, J2800
**Methotrexate, oral**, J8610
  sodium, J9250, J9260
**Methyldopate HCl**, J0210
**Methylene blue injection**, A9535
**Methylergonovine maleate**, J2210
**Methylprednisolone**
  acetate, J1020-J1040
  oral, J7509
  sodium succinate, J2920, J2930
**Metoclopramide HCl**, J2765
**Metronidazole**, S0030
**Meunster Suspension, socket prosthesis**, L6110
**Miacalcin**, J0630
**Micafungin sodium**, J2248
**Microabrasion, enamel**, D9970
**Microbiology test**, P7001
**Microcapillary tube**, A4651
  sealant, A4652
**Micro-Fine**
  disposable insulin syringes, up to 1 cc, per syringe, A4206
  lancets, box of 100, A4259
**Microlipids, enteral nutrition**, B4155
**Microspirometer**, S8190
**Midazolam HCl**, J2250
**Mileage, ambulance**, A0380, A0390

**Milk, breast**
  processing, T2101
**Milrinone lactate**, J2260
**Milwaukee spinal orthosis**, L1000
**Minerva, spinal orthosis**, L0700, L0710
**Mini-bus, nonemergency transportation**, A0120
**Minimed**
  3 cc syringe, A4232
  506 insulin pump, E0784
  insulin infusion set with bent needle wings, each, A4231
  Sof-Set 24" insulin infusion set, each, A4230
**Minoxidil**, S0139
**Mitomycin**, J9280-J9291
**Mitoxantrone HCl**, J9293
**Mobilite hospital beds**, E0293, E0295, E0297
**Moducal, enteral nutrition**, B4155
**Moisture exchanger for use with invasive mechanical ventilation**, A4483
**Moisturizer, skin**, A6250
**Monarc-M**, J7190
**Monitor**
  apnea, E0618
  blood glucose, E0607
    Accu-Check, E0607
    Tracer II, E0607
  blood pressure, A4670
  device, A9279
  ECG, S0345-S0347
  pacemaker, E0610, E0615
  ventilator, E0450
**Monitoring**
  electrocardiographic, S0345-S0347
**Monoclonal antibodies**, J7505
**Monoject disposable insulin syringes, up to 1 cc, per syringe**, A4206
**Monojector lancet device**, A4258
**Morcellator**, C1782
**Morphine sulfate**, J2270, J2271, S0093
  sterile, preservative-free, J2275
**Moulage, facial**, D5911-D5912
**Mouth exam, athletic**, D9941
**Mouthpiece (for respiratory equipment)**, A4617
**Moxifloxacin**, J2280
**M-Prednisol-40**, J1030
  -80, J1040
**MRI**
  contrast material, A9576-A9579, Q9954
  low field, S8042
**Mucoprotein, blood**, P2038
**Multifetal pregnancy reduction, ultrasound guidance**, S8055
**Multiple post collar, cervical**, L0180-L0200
**Multipositional patient support system**, E0636
**Muscular dystrophy, genetic test**, S3853
**Muse**, J0275
**Mutamycin**, J9280
**Mycophenolate mofetil**, J7517
**Mycophenolic acid**, J7518
**Mylotarg**, J9300
**Myochrysine**, J1600
**Myolin**, J2360
**Myotonic muscular dystrophy, genetic test**, S3853
**Myringotomy**, S2225

## N

**Nabilone, oral**, J8650
**Nafcillin sodium**, S0032
**Nail trim**, G0127, S0390
**Nalbuphine HCl**, J2300
**Naloxone HCl**, J2310
**Naltrexone depot injection**, J2315
**Nandrobolic L.A.**, J2321
**Nandrolone**
  decanoate, J2320-J2322
**Narcan**, J2310

## TRANSPORTATION SERVICES INCLUDING AMBULANCE
## A0000-A0999

This code range includes ground and air ambulance, nonemergency transportation (taxi, bus, automobile, wheelchair van), and ancillary transportation-related fees.

HCPCS Level II codes for ambulance services must be reported with modifiers that indicate pick-up origins and destinations. The modifier describing the arrangement (QM, QN) is listed first. The modifiers describing the origin and destination are listed second. Origin and destination modifiers are created by combining two alpha characters from the following list. Each alpha character, with the exception of X, represents either an origin or a destination. Each pair of alpha characters creates one modifier. The first position represents the origin and the second the destination. The modifiers most commonly used are:

**D** Diagnostic or therapeutic site other than "P" or "H"

**E** Residential, domiciliary, custodial facility (nursing home, not skilled nursing facility)

**G** Hospital-based dialysis facility (hospital or hospital-related)

**H** Hospital

**I** Site of transfer (for example, airport or helicopter pad) between types of ambulance

**J** Nonhospital-based dialysis facility

**N** Skilled nursing facility (SNF)

**P** Physician's office (includes HMO nonhospital facility, clinic, etc.)

**R** Residence

**S** Scene of accident or acute event

**X** Intermediate stop at physician's office enroute to the hospital (includes HMO nonhospital facility, clinic, etc.)

Note: Modifier X can only be used as a designation code in the second position of a modifier.

See S0215. For Medicaid, see T codes and T modifiers.

| | | |
|---|---|---|
| E | A0021 | Ambulance service, outside state per mile, transport (Medicaid only) |
| E | A0080 | Nonemergency transportation, per mile — vehicle provided by volunteer (individual or organization), with no vested interest |
| E | A0090 | Nonemergency transportation, per mile — vehicle provided by individual (family member, self, neighbor) with vested interest |
| E | A0100 | Nonemergency transportation; taxi |
| E | A0110 | Nonemergency transportation and bus, intra- or interstate carrier |
| E | A0120 | Nonemergency transportation: mini-bus, mountain area transports, or other transportation systems |
| E | A0130 | Nonemergency transportation: wheelchair van |
| E | A0140 | Nonemergency transportation and air travel (private or commercial), intra- or interstate |
| E | A0160 | Nonemergency transportation: per mile — caseworker or social worker |
| E | A0170 | Transportation ancillary: parking fees, tolls, other |
| E | A0180 | Nonemergency transportation: ancillary: lodging — recipient |
| E | A0190 | Nonemergency transportation: ancillary: meals — recipient |
| E | A0200 | Nonemergency transportation: ancillary: lodging — escort |
| E | A0210 | Nonemergency transportation: ancillary: meals — escort |

| | | | |
|---|---|---|---|
| E | | A0225 | Ambulance service, neonatal transport, base rate, emergency transport, one way |
| | | | MED: 100-4,1,10.1.4.1 |
| E | ☑ | A0380 | BLS mileage (per mile) |
| | | | See code(s): A0425 |
| | | | MED: 100-2,6,10; 100-4,1,10.1.4.1 |
| A | | A0382 | BLS routine disposable supplies |
| A | | A0384 | BLS specialized service disposable supplies; defibrillation (used by ALS ambulances and BLS ambulances in jurisdictions where defibrillation is permitted in BLS ambulances) |
| E | ☑ | A0390 | ALS mileage (per mile) |
| | | | See code(s): A0425 |
| | | | MED: 100-4,1,10.1.4.1 |
| A | | A0392 | ALS specialized service disposable supplies; defibrillation (to be used only in jurisdictions where defibrillation cannot be performed in BLS ambulances) |
| A | | A0394 | ALS specialized service disposable supplies; IV drug therapy |
| A | | A0396 | ALS specialized service disposable supplies; esophageal intubation |
| A | | A0398 | ALS routine disposable supplies |

## WAITING TIME TABLE

| | Units | | Time |
|---|---|---|---|
| 1 | 1/2 | to | 1 hr. |
| 2 | 1 | to | 1 1/2 hrs. |
| 3 | 1 1/2 | to | 2 hrs. |
| 4 | 2 | to | 2 1/2 hrs. |
| 5 | 2 1/2 | to | 3 hrs. |
| 6 | 3 | to | 3 1/2 hrs. |
| 7 | 3 1/2 | to | 4 hrs. |
| 8 | 4 | to | 4 1/2 hrs. |
| 9 | 4 1/2 | to | 5 hrs. |
| 10 | 5 | to | 5 1/2 hrs. |

| | | | |
|---|---|---|---|
| A | ☑ | A0420 | Ambulance waiting time (ALS or BLS), one-half (1/2) hour increments ⊘ |
| A | | A0422 | Ambulance (ALS or BLS) oxygen and oxygen supplies, life sustaining situation ⊘ |
| A | | A0424 | Extra ambulance attendant, ground (ALS or BLS) or air (fixed or rotary winged); (requires medical review) ⊘ **Pertinent documentation to evaluate medical appropriateness should be included when this code is reported.** |
| A | ☑ | A0425 | Ground mileage, per statute mile |
| | | | MED: 100-2,6,10; 100-2,10,20; 100-4,1,10.1.4.1 |
| A | | A0426 | Ambulance service, advanced life support, nonemergency transport, level 1 (ALS 1) |
| | | | MED: 100-2,6,10; 100-2,10,20; 100-4,1,10.1.4.1 |
| A | | A0427 | Ambulance service, advanced life support, emergency transport, level 1 (ALS 1 — emergency) |
| | | | MED: 100-2,6,10; 100-2,10,20; 100-4,1,10.1.4.1 |
| A | | A0428 | Ambulance service, basic life support, nonemergency transport (BLS) |
| | | | MED: 100-2,6,10; 100-2,10,20; 100-4,1,10.1.4.1 |
| A | | A0429 | Ambulance service, basic life support, emergency transport (BLS — emergency) |
| | | | MED: 100-2,6,10; 100-2,10,20; 100-4,1,10.1.4.1 |

| Special Coverage Instructions | Noncovered by Medicare | Carrier Discretion | ☑ Quantity Alert | ● New Code | ○ Recycled/Reinstated | ▲ Revised Code |

**2008 HCPCS** | A2-Z3 ASC Payment Indicators | **MED:** Pub 100/NCD References | ⅍ DMEPOS Paid | ⊘ SNF Excluded | PQ PQRI | **A Codes — 1**

[A]  **A0430**  Ambulance service, conventional air services, transport, one way (fixed wing)
MED: 100-2,6,10; 100-2,10,20; 100-4,1,10.1.4.1

[A]  **A0431**  Ambulance service, conventional air services, transport, one way (rotary wing)
MED: 100-2,6,10; 100-2,10,20; 100-4,1,10.1.4.1

[A]  **A0432**  Paramedic intercept (PI), rural area, transport furnished by a volunteer ambulance company which is prohibited by state law from billing third-party payers
MED: 100-2,10,20

[A]  **A0433**  Advanced life support, level 2 (ALS 2)
MED: 100-2,10,20

[A]  **A0434**  Specialty care transport (SCT)
MED: 100-2,10,20

[A] ☑  **A0435**  Fixed wing air mileage, per statute mile
MED: 100-2,10,20

[A] ☑  **A0436**  Rotary wing air mileage, per statute mile
MED: 100-2,10,20

[E] ☑  **A0888**  Noncovered ambulance mileage, per mile (e.g., for miles traveled beyond closest appropriate facility)
MED: 100-2,10,20

[E]  **A0998**  Ambulance response and treatment, no transport

[A]  **A0999**  Unlisted ambulance service ⊘
Determine if an alternative HCPCS Level II or a CPT code better describes the service being reported. This code should be used only if a more specific code is unavailable.
MED: 100-2,10,20; 100-4,1,10.1.4.1

## MEDICAL AND SURGICAL SUPPLIES A4000-A8999

This section covers a wide variety of medical, surgical, and some durable medical equipment (DME) related supplies and accessories. DME-related supplies, accessories, maintenance, and repair required to ensure the proper functioning of this equipment is generally covered by Medicare under the prosthetic devices provision.

## MISCELLANEOUS SUPPLIES

These codes are to be filed with the Medicare local contractor, unless otherwise noted (if incident to a physicians' services, not separately billable) unless they represent incidental services or supplies which are referred to the DME Medicare Administrative Contractor (DME MAC).

▲ [E] ☑  **A4206**  Syringe with needle, sterile, 1 cc or less, each

[E] ☑  **A4207**  Syringe with needle, sterile 2 cc, each

[E] ☑  **A4208**  Syringe with needle, sterile 3 cc, each

[E] ☑  **A4209**  Syringe with needle, sterile 5 cc or greater, each

[E] ☑  **A4210**  Needle-free injection device, each
Sometimes covered by commercial payers with preauthorization and physician letter stating need (e.g., for insulin injection in young children).
MED: 100-3,280.1

[E]  **A4211**  Supplies for self-administered injections
When a drug that is usually injected by the patient (e.g., insulin or calcitonin) is injected by the physician, it is excluded from Medicare coverage unless administered in an emergency situation (e.g., diabetic coma).
MED: 100-2,15,50

[B]  **A4212**  Noncoring needle or stylet with or without catheter

[E] ☑  **A4213**  Syringe, sterile, 20 cc or greater, each

[E] ☑  **A4215**  Needle, sterile, any size, each

[A] ☑  **A4216**  Sterile water, saline and/or dextrose, diluent/flush, 10 ml  ♿
MED: 100-2,15,50

[A] ☑  **A4217**  Sterile water/saline, 500 ml  ♿
MED: 100-2,15,50

[N] ☑  **A4218**  Sterile saline or water, metered dose dispenser, 10 ml  [N]
MED: 100-4,4,230.1

[N]  **A4220**  Refill kit for implantable infusion pump  [N]
Implantable infusion pumps are covered by Medicare for 5-FUdR therapy for unresected liver or colorectal cancer and for opioid drug therapy for intractable pain. They are not covered by Medicare for heparin therapy for thromboembolic disease. Report drugs separately.
MED: 100-3,280.14

[Y]  **A4221**  Supplies for maintenance of drug infusion catheter, per week (list drug separately)  ♿

[Y]  **A4222**  Infusion supplies for external drug infusion pump, per cassette or bag (list drugs separately)  ♿

[E] ☑  **A4223**  Infusion supplies not used with external infusion pump, per cassette or bag (list drugs separately)

[Y] ☑  **A4230**  Infusion set for external insulin pump, nonneedle cannula type
Covered by some commercial payers as ongoing supply to preauthorized pump.
MED: 100-3,280.14

[Y] ☑  **A4231**  Infusion set for external insulin pump, needle type
Covered by some commercial payers as ongoing supply to preauthorized pump.
MED: 100-3,280.14

[E] ☑  **A4232**  Syringe with needle for external insulin pump, sterile, 3 cc
Covered by some commercial payers as ongoing supply to preauthorized pump.
MED: 100-3,280.14

[Y] ☑  **A4233**  Replacement battery, alkaline (other than J cell), for use with medically necessary home blood glucose monitor owned by patient, each

[Y] ☑  **A4234**  Replacement battery, alkaline, J cell, for use with medically necessary home blood glucose monitor owned by patient, each

[Y] ☑  **A4235**  Replacement battery, lithium, for use with medically necessary home blood glucose monitor owned by patient, each

[Y] ☑  **A4236**  Replacement battery, silver oxide, for use with medically necessary home blood glucose monitor owned by patient, each

[E] ☑  **A4244**  Alcohol or peroxide, per pint

[E] ☑  **A4245**  Alcohol wipes, per box

[E] ☑  **A4246**  Betadine or pHisoHex solution, per pint

[E] ☑  **A4247**  Betadine or iodine swabs/wipes, per box

[N] ☑  **A4248**  Chlorhexidine containing antiseptic, 1 ml  [N]

---

Special Coverage Instructions    Noncovered by Medicare    Carrier Discretion    ☑ Quantity Alert   ● New Code   ○ Recycled/Reinstated   ▲ Revised Code

**2 — A Codes**      [A] Age Edit      [M] Maternity Edit   ♀ Female Only   ♂ Male Only   [A]-[Y] OPPS Status Indicators      **2008 HCPCS**

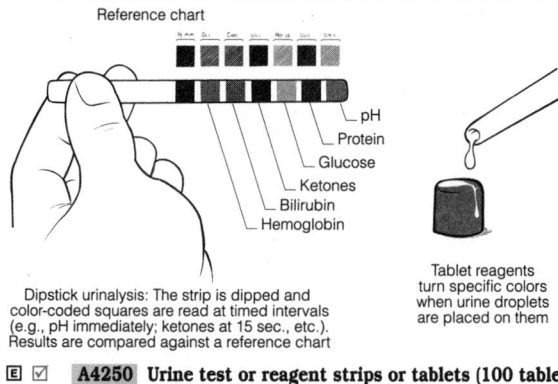

Reference chart

pH
Protein
Glucose
Ketones
Bilirubin
Hemoglobin

Dipstick urinalysis: The strip is dipped and color-coded squares are read at timed intervals (e.g., pH immediately; ketones at 15 sec., etc.). Results are compared against a reference chart

Tablet reagents turn specific colors when urine droplets are placed on them

E ☑ **A4250** Urine test or reagent strips or tablets (100 tablets or strips)

MED: 100-2,15,110

● E ☑ **A4252** Blood ketone test or reagent strip, each

Y ☑ **A4253** Blood glucose test or reagent strips for home blood glucose monitor, per 50 strips     ⅋
Medicare covers glucose strips for diabetic patients using home glucose monitoring devices prescribed by their physicians.

MED: 100-3,40.2

Y ☑ **A4255** Platforms for home blood glucose monitor, 50 per box     ⅋
Some Medicare contractors cover monitor platforms for diabetic patients using home glucose monitoring devices prescribed by their physicians. Some commercial payers also provide this coverage to noninsulin dependent diabetics.

MED: 100-3,40.2

Y **A4256** Normal, low, and high calibrator solution/chips     ⅋
Some Medicare contractors cover calibration solutions or chips for diabetic patients using home glucose monitoring devices prescribed by their physicians. Some commercial payers also provide this coverage to noninsulin dependent diabetics.

MED: 100-3,40.2

Y ☑ **A4257** Replacement lens shield cartridge for use with laser skin piercing device, each     ⅋

Y ☑ **A4258** Spring-powered device for lancet, each     ⅋
Some Medicare contractors cover lancing devices for diabetic patients using home glucose monitoring devices prescribed by their physicians. Medicare jurisdiction: DME regional contractor. Some commercial payers also provide this coverage to noninsulin dependent diabetics.

MED: 100-3,40.2

Y ☑ **A4259** Lancets, per box of 100     ⅋
Medicare covers lancets for diabetic patients using home glucose monitoring devices prescribed by their physicians. Medicare jurisdiction: DME regional contractor. Some commercial payers also provide this coverage to noninsulin dependent diabetics.

MED: 100-3,40.2

E **A4261** Cervical cap for contraceptive use     ♀

N ☑ **A4262** Temporary, absorbable lacrimal duct implant, each     N1
Always report concurrent to the implant procedure.

N ☑ **A4263** Permanent, long-term, nondissolvable lacrimal duct implant, each     N1
Always report concurrent to the implant procedure.

Y ☑ **A4265** Paraffin, per pound     ⅋

MED: 100-3,280.1

E **A4266** Diaphragm for contraceptive use     ♀

E ☑ **A4267** Contraceptive supply, condom, male, each

E ☑ **A4268** Contraceptive supply, condom, female, each     ♀

E ☑ **A4269** Contraceptive supply, spermicide (e.g., foam, gel), each     A

N ☑ **A4270** Disposable endoscope sheath, each     N1

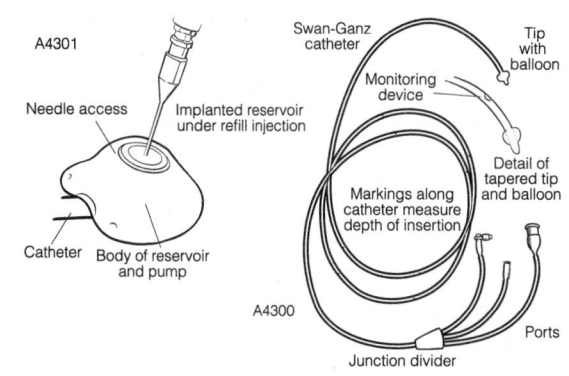

Two part prosthesis

Adhesive skin support (A4280)

Any of several breast prostheses fits over skin support

A ☑ **A4280** Adhesive skin support attachment for use with external breast prosthesis, each     A ♀ ⅋

E **A4281** Tubing for breast pump, replacement     M ♀

E **A4282** Adapter for breast pump, replacement     M ♀

E **A4283** Cap for breast pump bottle, replacement     M ♀

E **A4284** Breast shield and splash protector for use with breast pump, replacement     M ♀

E **A4285** Polycarbonate bottle for use with breast pump, replacement     M ♀

E **A4286** Locking ring for breast pump, replacement     M ♀

B ☑ **A4290** Sacral nerve stimulation test lead, each

AHA: 1Q,'02,9

## VASCULAR CATHETERS

A4301

Swan-Ganz catheter

Tip with balloon

Needle access

Implanted reservoir under refill injection

Monitoring device

Detail of tapered tip and balloon

Markings along catheter measure depth of insertion

Catheter

Body of reservoir and pump

A4300

Junction divider

Ports

A4301

N **A4300** Implantable access catheter, (e.g., venous, arterial, epidural subarachnoid, or peritoneal, etc.) external access     N1

MED: 100-2,15,120

N **A4301** Implantable access total catheter, port/reservoir (e.g., venous, arterial, epidural, subarachnoid, peritoneal, etc.)     N1

N ☑ **A4305** Disposable drug delivery system, flow rate of 50 ml or greater per hour     N1

N **A4306** Disposable drug delivery system, flow rate of less than 50 ml per hour     N1

## INCONTINENCE APPLIANCES AND CARE SUPPLIES

Covered by Medicare when the medical record indicates incontinence is permanent, or of long and indefinite duration.

Special Coverage Instructions     Noncovered by Medicare     Carrier Discretion     ☑ Quantity Alert     ● New Code     ○ Recycled/Reinstated     ▲ Revised Code

**2008 HCPCS**     A2–Z3 ASC Payment Indicators     **MED:** Pub 100/NCD References     ⅋ DMEPOS Paid     Ⓢ SNF Excluded     PQ PQRI     **A Codes — 3**

**Medical and Surgical Supplies**

**A4310 — A4363**

[A] **A4310** Insertion tray without drainage bag and without catheter (accessories only) &
MED: 100-2,15,120

[A] **A4311** Insertion tray without drainage bag with indwelling catheter, Foley type, two-way latex with coating (Teflon, silicone, silicone elastomer or hydrophilic, etc.) &
MED: 100-2,15,120

[A] **A4312** Insertion tray without drainage bag with indwelling catheter, Foley type, two-way, all silicone &
MED: 100-2,15,120

[A] **A4313** Insertion tray without drainage bag with indwelling catheter, Foley type, three-way, for continuous irrigation &
MED: 100-2,15,120

[A] **A4314** Insertion tray with drainage bag with indwelling catheter, Foley type, two-way latex with coating (Teflon, silicone, silicone elastomer or hydrophilic, etc.) &
MED: 100-2,15,120

[A] **A4315** Insertion tray with drainage bag with indwelling catheter, Foley type, two-way, all silicone &
MED: 100-2,15,120

[A] **A4316** Insertion tray with drainage bag with indwelling catheter, Foley type, three-way, for continuous irrigation &
MED: 100-2,15,120

[A] **A4320** Irrigation tray with bulb or piston syringe, any purpose &
MED: 100-2,15,120

[A] **A4321** Therapeutic agent for urinary catheter irrigation &
MED: 100-2,15,120

[A] ☑ **A4322** Irrigation syringe, bulb or piston, each &
MED: 100-2,15,120

[A] ☑ **A4326** Male external catheter with integral collection chamber, any type, each ♂&
MED: 100-2,15,120

[A] ☑ **A4327** Female external urinary collection device; meatal cup, each ♀&
MED: 100-2,15,120

[A] ☑ **A4328** Female external urinary collection device; pouch, each ♀&
MED: 100-2,15,120

[A] ☑ **A4330** Perianal fecal collection pouch with adhesive, each &
MED: 100-2,15,120

[A] ☑ **A4331** Extension drainage tubing, any type, any length, with connector/adaptor, for use with urinary leg bag or urostomy pouch, each &
MED: 100-2,15,120

[A] ☑ **A4332** Lubricant, individual sterile packet, each &
MED: 100-2,15,120

[A] ☑ **A4333** Urinary catheter anchoring device, adhesive skin attachment, each &
MED: 100-2,15,120

[A] ☑ **A4334** Urinary catheter anchoring device, leg strap, each &
MED: 100-2,15,120

[A] **A4335** Incontinence supply; miscellaneous
MED: 100-2,15,120

[A] ☑ **A4338** Indwelling catheter; Foley type, two-way latex with coating (Teflon, silicone, silicone elastomer, or hydrophilic, etc.), each &
MED: 100-2,15,120

[A] ☑ **A4340** Indwelling catheter; specialty type, (e.g., Coude, mushroom, wing, etc.), each &
MED: 100-2,15,120

[A] ☑ **A4344** Indwelling catheter, Foley type, two-way, all silicone, each &
MED: 100-2,15,120

Left ureter　Urachus　Peritoneum　Left ureter
Ureteral orifice　Normal anatomy anterior view　Pubic bone　Urogenital diaphragm
Urethra　Urethral sphincter　Spongiosal muscles　Foley-style indwelling catheter (A4344-A4346)　Side view
Multiple port indwelling catheters allow for irrigation and drainage

[A] ☑ **A4346** Indwelling catheter; Foley type, three-way for continuous irrigation, each &
MED: 100-2,15,120

[A] ☑ **A4349** Male external catheter, with or without adhesive, disposable, each ♂
MED: 100-2,15,120

[A] ☑ **A4351** Intermittent urinary catheter; straight tip, with or without coating (Teflon, silicone, silicone elastomer, or hydrophilic, etc.), each &
MED: 100-2,15,120

[A] ☑ **A4352** Intermittent urinary catheter; Coude (curved) tip, with or without coating (Teflon, silicone, silicone elastomeric, or hydrophilic, etc.), each &
MED: 100-2,15,120

[A] **A4353** Intermittent urinary catheter, with insertion supplies &
MED: 100-2,15,120

[A] **A4354** Insertion tray with drainage bag but without catheter &
MED: 100-2,15,120

[A] ☑ **A4355** Irrigation tubing set for continuous bladder irrigation through a three-way indwelling Foley catheter, each &
MED: 100-2,15,120

## EXTERNAL URINARY SUPPLIES

[A] ☑ **A4356** External urethral clamp or compression device (not to be used for catheter clamp), each &
MED: 100-2,15,120

[A] ☑ **A4357** Bedside drainage bag, day or night, with or without anti-reflux device, with or without tube, each &
MED: 100-2,15,120

[A] ☑ **A4358** Urinary drainage bag, leg or abdomen, vinyl, with or without tube, with straps, each &
MED: 100-2,15,120

## OSTOMY SUPPLIES

[A] ☑ **A4361** Ostomy faceplate, each &
MED: 100-2,15,120

[A] ☑ **A4362** Skin barrier; solid, 4 x 4 or equivalent; each &
See code(s) A4461 or A4463

[A] **A4363** Ostomy clamp, any type, replacement only, each &

---

| Special Coverage Instructions | Noncovered by Medicare | Carrier Discretion | ☑ Quantity Alert | ● New Code | ○ Recycled/Reinstated | ▲ Revised Code |

**4 — A Codes**　　[A] Age Edit　　[M] Maternity Edit　　♀ Female Only　　♂ Male Only　　[A]-[Y] OPPS Status Indicators　　**2008 HCPCS**

A ☑ **A4364** Adhesive, liquid, or equal, any type, per oz. &
MED: 100-2,15,120

A ☑ **A4365** Adhesive remover wipes, any type, per 50 &
MED: 100-2,15,120

A ☑ **A4366** Ostomy vent, any type, each &

A ☑ **A4367** Ostomy belt, each &
MED: 100-2,15,120

A ☑ **A4368** Ostomy filter, any type, each &

A ☑ **A4369** Ostomy skin barrier, liquid (spray, brush, etc.), per oz. &
MED: 100-2,15,120

A ☑ **A4371** Ostomy skin barrier, powder, per oz. &
MED: 100-2,15,120

A ☑ **A4372** Ostomy skin barrier, solid 4 x 4 or equivalent, standard wear, with built-in convexity, each &
MED: 100-2,15,120

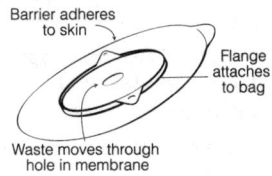

Barrier adheres to skin
Flange attaches to bag
Waste moves through hole in membrane

Faceplate flange and skin barrier combination (A4373)

A ☑ **A4373** Ostomy skin barrier, with flange (solid, flexible or accordion), with built-in convexity, any size, each &
MED: 100-2,15,120

A ☑ **A4375** Ostomy pouch, drainable, with faceplate attached, plastic, each &
MED: 100-2,15,120

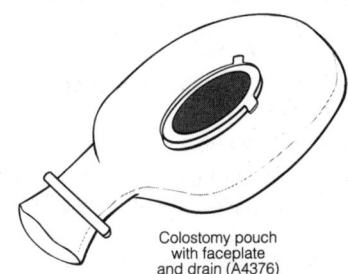

Colostomy pouch with faceplate and drain (A4376)

A ☑ **A4376** Ostomy pouch, drainable, with faceplate attached, rubber, each &
MED: 100-2,15,120

A ☑ **A4377** Ostomy pouch, drainable, for use on faceplate, plastic, each &
MED: 100-2,15,120

A ☑ **A4378** Ostomy pouch, drainable, for use on faceplate, rubber, each &
MED: 100-2,15,120

A ☑ **A4379** Ostomy pouch, urinary, with faceplate attached, plastic, each &
MED: 100-2,15,120

A ☑ **A4380** Ostomy pouch, urinary, with faceplate attached, rubber, each &
MED: 100-2,15,120

A ☑ **A4381** Ostomy pouch, urinary, for use on faceplate, plastic, each &
MED: 100-2,15,120

A ☑ **A4382** Ostomy pouch, urinary, for use on faceplate, heavy plastic, each &
MED: 100-2,15,120

A ☑ **A4383** Ostomy pouch, urinary, for use on faceplate, rubber, each &
MED: 100-2,15,120

A ☑ **A4384** Ostomy faceplate equivalent, silicone ring, each &
MED: 100-2,15,120

A ☑ **A4385** Ostomy skin barrier, solid 4 x 4 or equivalent, extended wear, without built-in convexity, each &
MED: 100-2,15,120

A ☑ **A4387** Ostomy pouch, closed, with barrier attached, with built-in convexity (one piece), each &
MED: 100-2,15,120

A ☑ **A4388** Ostomy pouch, drainable, with extended wear barrier attached, (one piece), each &
MED: 100-2,15,120

A ☑ **A4389** Ostomy pouch, drainable, with barrier attached, with built-in convexity (one piece), each &
MED: 100-2,15,120

A ☑ **A4390** Ostomy pouch, drainable, with extended wear barrier attached, with built-in convexity (one piece), each &
MED: 100-2,15,120

A ☑ **A4391** Ostomy pouch, urinary, with extended wear barrier attached (one piece), each &
MED: 100-2,15,120

A ☑ **A4392** Ostomy pouch, urinary, with standard wear barrier attached, with built-in convexity (one piece), each &
MED: 100-2,15,120

A ☑ **A4393** Ostomy pouch, urinary, with extended wear barrier attached, with built-in convexity (one piece), each &
MED: 100-2,15,120

A ☑ **A4394** Ostomy deodorant, with or without lubricant, for use in ostomy pouch, per fluid ounce &
MED: 100-2,15,120

A ☑ **A4395** Ostomy deodorant for use in ostomy pouch, solid, per tablet &
MED: 100-2,15,120

A **A4396** Ostomy belt with peristomal hernia support &
MED: 100-2,15,120

A ☑ **A4397** Irrigation supply; sleeve, each &
MED: 100-2,15,120

A ☑ **A4398** Ostomy irrigation supply; bag, each &
MED: 100-2,15,120

A **A4399** Ostomy irrigation supply; cone/catheter, including brush &
MED: 100-2,15,120

A **A4400** Ostomy irrigation set &
MED: 100-2,15,120

A ☑ **A4402** Lubricant, per oz. &
MED: 100-2,15,120

A ☑ **A4404** Ostomy ring, each &
MED: 100-2,15,120

A ☑ **A4405** Ostomy skin barrier, nonpectin-based, paste, per oz. &
MED: 100-2,15,120

A ☑ **A4406** Ostomy skin barrier, pectin-based, paste, per oz. &
MED: 100-2,15,120

---

Special Coverage Instructions    Noncovered by Medicare    Carrier Discretion    ☑ Quantity Alert    ● New Code    ○ Recycled/Reinstated    ▲ Revised Code

**Medical and Surgical Supplies**

**A4407 — A4490**

A ☑ **A4407** Ostomy skin barrier, with flange (solid, flexible, or accordion), extended wear, with built-in convexity, 4 x 4 in. or smaller, each &
MED: 100-2,15,120

A ☑ **A4408** Ostomy skin barrier, with flange (solid, flexible or accordion), extended wear, with built-in convexity, larger than 4 x 4 in., each &
MED: 100-2,15,120

A ☑ **A4409** Ostomy skin barrier, with flange (solid, flexible or accordion), extended wear, without built-in convexity, 4 x 4 in. or smaller, each &
MED: 100-2,15,120

A ☑ **A4410** Ostomy skin barrier, with flange (solid, flexible or accordion), extended wear, without built-in convexity, larger than 4 x 4 in., each &
MED: 100-2,15,120

A ☑ **A4411** Ostomy skin barrier, solid 4 x 4 or equivalent, extended wear, with built-in convexity, each

A ☑ **A4412** Ostomy pouch, drainable, high output, for use on a barrier with flange (2 piece system), without filter, each &
MED: 100-2,15,120

A ☑ **A4413** Ostomy pouch, drainable, high output, for use on a barrier with flange (two piece system), with filter, each &
MED: 100-2,15,120

A ☑ **A4414** Ostomy skin barrier, with flange (solid, flexible or accordion), without built-in convexity, 4 x 4 in. or smaller, each &
MED: 100-2,15,120

A ☑ **A4415** Ostomy skin barrier, with flange (solid, flexible or accordion), without built-in convexity, larger than 4 x 4 in., each &
MED: 100-2,15,120

A ☑ **A4416** Ostomy pouch, closed, with barrier attached, with filter (one piece), each &

A ☑ **A4417** Ostomy pouch, closed, with barrier attached, with built-in convexity, with filter (one piece), each &

A ☑ **A4418** Ostomy pouch, closed; without barrier attached, with filter (one piece), each &

A ☑ **A4419** Ostomy pouch, closed; for use on barrier with nonlocking flange, with filter (two piece), each &

A ☑ **A4420** Ostomy pouch, closed; for use on barrier with locking flange (two piece), each &

E **A4421** Ostomy supply; miscellaneous
Determine if an alternative HCPCS Level II or a CPT code better describes the service being reported. This code should be used only if a more specific code is unavailable.
MED: 100-2,15,120

A ☑ **A4422** Ostomy absorbent material (sheet/pad/crystal packet) for use in ostomy pouch to thicken liquid stomal output, each &
MED: 100-2,15,120

A ☑ **A4423** Ostomy pouch, closed; for use on barrier with locking flange, with filter (two piece), each &

A ☑ **A4424** Ostomy pouch, drainable, with barrier attached, with filter (one piece), each &

A ☑ **A4425** Ostomy pouch, drainable; for use on barrier with nonlocking flange, with filter (two piece system), each &

A ☑ **A4426** Ostomy pouch, drainable; for use on barrier with locking flange (two piece system), each &

A ☑ **A4427** Ostomy pouch, drainable; for use on barrier with locking flange, with filter (two piece system), each &

A ☑ **A4428** Ostomy pouch, urinary, with extended wear barrier attached, with faucet-type tap with valve (one piece), each &

A ☑ **A4429** Ostomy pouch, urinary, with barrier attached, with built-in convexity, with faucet-type tap with valve (one piece), each &

A ☑ **A4430** Ostomy pouch, urinary, with extended wear barrier attached, with built-in convexity, with faucet-type tap with valve (one piece), each &

A ☑ **A4431** Ostomy pouch, urinary; with barrier attached, with faucet-type tap with valve (one piece), each &

A ☑ **A4432** Ostomy pouch, urinary; for use on barrier with nonlocking flange, with faucet-type tap with valve (two piece), each &

A ☑ **A4433** Ostomy pouch, urinary; for use on barrier with locking flange (two piece), each &

A ☑ **A4434** Ostomy pouch, urinary; for use on barrier with locking flange, with faucet-type tap with valve (two piece), each &

## ADDITIONAL MISCELLANEOUS SUPPLIES

A ☑ **A4450** Tape, nonwaterproof, per 18 sq. in. &
See also code A4452.
MED: 100-2,15,120

A ☑ **A4452** Tape, waterproof, per 18 sq. in. &
See also code A4450.
MED: 100-2,15,120

A ☑ **A4455** Adhesive remover or solvent (for tape, cement or other adhesive), per oz. &
MED: 100-2,15,120

E **A4458** Enema bag with tubing, reusable

A ☑ **A4461** Surgical dressing holder, nonreusable, each

A ☑ **A4463** Surgical dressing holder, reusable, each

A **A4465** Nonelastic binder for extremity

A **A4470** Gravlee jet washer
The Gravlee jet washer is a sterile, disposable, diagnostic device used to detect endometrial cancer. It is covered only in patients exhibiting clinical symptoms or signs suggestive of endometrial disease. Medicare jurisdiction: local contractor.
MED: 100-2,16,90; 100-3,230.5

A **A4480** VABRA aspirator ♀
The VABRA aspirator is a sterile, disposable, vacuum aspirator which collects uterine tissue so that it can be studied to detect endometrial carcinoma. The use of this device is indicated where the patient exhibits clinical symptoms or signs suggestive of endometrial disease, such as irregular or heavy vaginal bleeding.
MED: 100-2,16,90; 100-3,230.6

A ☑ **A4481** Tracheostoma filter, any type, any size, each &
MED: 100-2,15,120

A **A4483** Moisture exchanger, disposable, for use with invasive mechanical ventilation &
MED: 100-2,15,120

E ☑ **A4490** Surgical stockings above knee length, each
MED: 100-2,15,100; 100-2,15,110; 100-3,280.1

---

| Special Coverage Instructions | Noncovered by Medicare | Carrier Discretion | ☑ Quantity Alert | ● New Code | ○ Recycled/Reinstated | ▲ Revised Code |

**6 — A Codes**   A Age Edit   M Maternity Edit   ♀ Female Only   ♂ Male Only   A-Y OPPS Status Indicators   **2008 HCPCS**

E ☑ **A4495** Surgical stockings thigh length, each
MED: 100-2,15,100; 100-2,15,110; 100-3,280.1

E ☑ **A4500** Surgical stocking below knee length, each
MED: 100-2,15,100; 100-2,15,110; 100-3,280.1

E ☑ **A4510** Surgical stocking full-length, each
MED: 100-2,15,100; 100-2,15,110; 100-3,280.1

E ☑ **A4520** Incontinence garment, any type, (e.g., brief, diaper), each
MED: 100-3,280.1

B **A4550** Surgical trays

E ☑ **A4554** Disposable underpads, all sizes
MED: 100-2,15,120; 100-3,280.1

Y ☑ **A4556** Electrodes (e.g., apnea monitor), per pair &

Y ☑ **A4557** Lead wires (e.g., apnea monitor), per pair &

Y ☑ **A4558** Conductive gel or paste, for use with electrical device (e.g., TENS, NMES), per oz. &

Y ☑ **A4559** Coupling gel or paste, for use with ultrasound device, per oz. &

N **A4561** Pessary, rubber, any type A♀&
Medicare Jurisdiction: DME Regional contractor.

N **A4562** Pessary, nonrubber, any type A♀&
Medicare jurisdiction: DME regional contractor.

A **A4565** Slings
Dressings applied by a physician are included as part of the professional service. Surgical dressings obtained by the patient to perform homecare as prescribed by the physician are covered.

E **A4570** Splint
Dressings applied by a physician are included as part of the professional service.
MED: 100-2,6,10; 100-2,15,100; 100-4,4,240

E **A4575** Topical hyperbaric oxygen chamber, disposable
MED: 100-3,20.29

E **A4580** Cast supplies (e.g., plaster)
See Q4001-Q4048.
MED: 100-2,6,10; 100-2,15,100; 100-4,4,240

E **A4590** Special casting material (e.g., fiberglass)
See Q4001-Q4048.
MED: 100-2,6,10; 100-2,15,100; 100-4,4,240

Y **A4595** Electrical stimulator supplies, 2 lead, per month, (e.g., TENS, NMES) &
MED: 100-3,160.13

Y ☑ **A4600** Sleeve for intermittent limb compression device, replacement only, each &

Y **A4601** Lithium ion battery for nonprosthetic use, replacement &

Y **A4604** Tubing with integrated heating element for use with positive airway pressure device

Y ☑ **A4605** Tracheal suction catheter, closed system, each

A **A4606** Oxygen probe for use with oximeter device, replacement

Y ☑ **A4608** Transtracheal oxygen catheter, each &
Medicare jurisdiction: DME Medicare Administrative Contractor (DME MAC).

## SUPPLIES FOR OXYGEN AND RELATED RESPIRATORY EQUIPMENT

Y **A4611** Battery, heavy duty; replacement for patient-owned ventilator &
Medicare jurisdiction: DME Medicare Administrative Contractor (DME MAC).

Y **A4612** Battery cables; replacement for patient-owned ventilator &
Medicare jurisdiction: DME Medicare Administrative Contractor (DME MAC).

Y ☑ **A4613** Battery charger; replacement for patient-owned ventilator &
Medicare jurisdiction: DME Medicare Administrative Contractor (DME MAC).

N **A4614** Peak expiratory flow rate meter, hand held &

Y **A4615** Cannula, nasal &
MED: 100-3,160.6; 100-4,20,100.2

Y ☑ **A4616** Tubing (oxygen), per foot &
MED: 100-3,160.6; 100-4,20,100.2

Y **A4617** Mouthpiece &
MED: 100-3,160.6; 100-4,20,100.2

Y **A4618** Breathing circuits &
MED: 100-3,160.6; 100-4,20,100.2

Y **A4619** Face tent &
MED: 100-3,160.6; 100-4,20,100.2

Y **A4620** Variable concentration mask &
MED: 100-3,160.6; 100-4,20,100.2

A **A4623** Tracheostomy, inner cannula &
MED: 100-2,15,120; 100-3,20.9

Y ☑ **A4624** Tracheal suction catheter, any type other than closed system, each &

A **A4625** Tracheostomy care kit for new tracheostomy &
MED: 100-2,15,120

A ☑ **A4626** Tracheostomy cleaning brush, each &
MED: 100-2,15,120

E **A4627** Spacer, bag or reservoir, with or without mask, for use with metered dose inhaler
MED: 100-2,15,110

Y ☑ **A4628** Oropharyngeal suction catheter, each &

A **A4629** Tracheostomy care kit for established tracheostomy &
MED: 100-2,15,120

## SUPPLIES FOR OTHER DURABLE MEDICAL EQUIPMENT

Y ☑ **A4630** Replacement batteries, medically necessary, transcutaneous electrical stimulator, owned by patient &
MED: 100-3,160.7

Y ☑ **A4633** Replacement bulb/lamp for ultraviolet light therapy system, each &

A **A4634** Replacement bulb for therapeutic light box, tabletop model

Y ☑ **A4635** Underarm pad, crutch, replacement, each &
Medicare jurisdiction: DME Medicare Administrative Contractor (DME MAC).
MED: 100-3,280.1

▨ Special Coverage Instructions ▨ Noncovered by Medicare ▨ Carrier Discretion ☑ Quantity Alert ● New Code ○ Recycled/Reinstated ▲ Revised Code

**2008 HCPCS** A2-Z3 ASC Payment Indicators **MED:** Pub 100/NCD References & DMEPOS Paid ⊘ SNF Excluded PQ PQRI **A Codes — 7**

**Medical and Surgical Supplies**

**A4636 — A4736**

Y ☑ **A4636** Replacement, handgrip, cane, crutch, or walker, each   ♿
Medicare jurisdiction: DME Medicare Administrative Contractor (DME MAC).
MED: 100-3,280.1

Y ☑ **A4637** Replacement, tip, cane, crutch, walker, each   ♿
Medicare jurisdiction: DME Medicare Administrative Contractor (DME MAC).
MED: 100-3,280.1

Y ☑ **A4638** Replacement battery for patient-owned ear pulse generator, each   ♿

Y ☑ **A4639** Replacement pad for infrared heating pad system, each   ♿

Y **A4640** Replacement pad for use with medically necessary alternating pressure pad owned by patient   ♿
Medicare jurisdiction: DME Medicare Administrative Contractor (DME MAC).
MED: 100-3,280.1; 100-8,5,5.2.3

## SUPPLIES FOR RADIOLOGIC PROCEDURES

N **A4641** Radiopharmaceutical, diagnostic, not otherwise classified
MED: 100-4,13,60.3; 100-4,13,60.3.1

N ☑ **A4642** Indium In-111 satumomab pendetide, diagnostic, per study dose, up to 6 millicuries
Use this code for Oncoscint.
MED: 100-4,4,20.5; 100-4,4,230.1

## MISCELLANEOUS SUPPLIES

● N ☑ **A4648** Tissue marker, implantable, any type, each   N1

A **A4649** Surgical supply; miscellaneous
Determine if an alternative HCPCS Level II or a CPT code better describes the service being reported. This code should be used only if a more specific code is unavailable.

● N ☑ **A4650** Implantable radiation dosimeter, each   N1

A ☑ **A4651** Calibrated microcapillary tube, each   ⊘
MED: 100-4,3,40.3

A **A4652** Microcapillary tube sealant   ⊘
MED: 100-4,3,40.3

## DIALYSIS SUPPLIES

A ☑ **A4653** Peritoneal dialysis catheter anchoring device, belt, each   ⊘
MED: 100-4,3,40.3

A ☑ **A4657** Syringe, with or without needle, each   ⊘
MED: 100-4,3,40.3

A **A4660** Sphygmomanometer/blood pressure apparatus with cuff and stethoscope   ⊘
MED: 100-4,3,40.3

A **A4663** Blood pressure cuff only   ⊘
MED: 100-4,3,40.3

E **A4670** Automatic blood pressure monitor   ⊘
MED: 100-3,20.19; 100-4,3,40.3

B ☑ **A4671** Disposable cycler set used with cycler dialysis machine, each   ⊘
MED: 100-4,3,40.3

B ☑ **A4672** Drainage extension line, sterile, for dialysis, each   ⊘
MED: 100-4,3,40.3

B **A4673** Extension line with easy lock connectors, used with dialysis   ⊘
MED: 100-4,3,40.3

B ☑ **A4674** Chemicals/antiseptics solution used to clean/sterilize dialysis equipment, per 8 oz.   ⊘
MED: 100-4,3,40.3

A ☑ **A4680** Activated carbon filter for hemodialysis, each   ⊘
MED: 100-3,230.7; 100-4,3,40.3

A ☑ **A4690** Dialyzer (artificial kidneys), all types, all sizes, for hemodialysis, each   ⊘
MED: 100-4,3,40.3

A ☑ **A4706** Bicarbonate concentrate, solution, for hemodialysis, per gallon   ⊘
MED: 100-4,3,40.3

A ☑ **A4707** Bicarbonate concentrate, powder, for hemodialysis, per packet   ⊘
MED: 100-4,3,40.3

A ☑ **A4708** Acetate concentrate solution, for hemodialysis, per gallon   ⊘
MED: 100-4,3,40.3

A ☑ **A4709** Acid concentrate, solution, for hemodialysis, per gallon   ⊘
MED: 100-4,3,40.3

A ☑ **A4714** Treated water (deionized, distilled, or reverse osmosis) for peritoneal dialysis, per gallon   ⊘
MED: 100-3,230.7; 100-4,3,40.3

A **A4719** Y set tubing for peritoneal dialysis   ⊘
MED: 100-4,3,40.3

A ☑ **A4720** Dialysate solution, any concentration of dextrose, fluid volume greater than 249 cc, but less than or equal to 999 cc, for peritoneal dialysis   ⊘
MED: 100-4,3,40.3

A ☑ **A4721** Dialysate solution, any concentration of dextrose, fluid volume greater than 999 cc, but less than or equal to 1999 cc, for peritoneal dialysis   ⊘
MED: 100-4,3,40.3

A ☑ **A4722** Dialysate solution, any concentration of dextrose, fluid volume greater than 1999 cc, but less than or equal to 2999 cc, for peritoneal dialysis   ⊘
MED: 100-4,3,40.3

A ☑ **A4723** Dialysate solution, any concentration of dextrose, fluid volume greater than 2999 cc, but less than or equal to 3999 cc, for peritoneal dialysis   ⊘
MED: 100-4,3,40.3

A ☑ **A4724** Dialysate solution, any concentration of dextrose, fluid volume greater than 3999 cc, but less than or equal to 4999 cc, for peritoneal dialysis   ⊘
MED: 100-4,3,40.3

A ☑ **A4725** Dialysate solution, any concentration of dextrose, fluid volume greater than 4999 cc, but less than or equal to 5999 cc, for peritoneal dialysis   ⊘
MED: 100-4,3,40.3

A ☑ **A4726** Dialysate solution, any concentration of dextrose, fluid volume greater than 5999 cc   ⊘
MED: 100-4,3,40.3

B ☑ **A4728** Dialysate solution, nondextrose containing, 500 ml   ⊘
MED: 100-4,3,40.3

A ☑ **A4730** Fistula cannulation set for hemodialysis, each   ⊘
MED: 100-4,3,40.3

A ☑ **A4736** Topical anesthetic, for dialysis, per gm   ⊘
MED: 100-4,3,40.3

Special Coverage Instructions    Noncovered by Medicare    Carrier Discretion    ☑ Quantity Alert    ● New Code    ○ Recycled/Reinstated    ▲ Revised Code

**8 — A Codes**    A Age Edit    M Maternity Edit    ♀ Female Only    ♂ Male Only    A-Y OPPS Status Indicators    **2008 HCPCS**

**[A]** ☑ A4737 Injectable anesthetic, for dialysis, per 10 ml ⊘
MED: 100-4,3,40.3

**[A]** A4740 Shunt accessory, for hemodialysis, any type, each ⊘
MED: 100-4,3,40.3

**[A]** ☑ A4750 Blood tubing, arterial or venous, for hemodialysis, each ⊘
MED: 100-4,3,40.3

**[A]** ☑ A4755 Blood tubing, arterial and venous combined, for hemodialysis, each ⊘
MED: 100-4,3,40.3

**[A]** ☑ A4760 Dialysate solution test kit, for peritoneal dialysis, any type, each ⊘
MED: 100-4,3,40.3

**[A]** ☑ A4765 Dialysate concentrate, powder, additive for peritoneal dialysis, per packet ⊘
MED: 100-4,3,40.3

**[A]** ☑ A4766 Dialysate concentrate, solution, additive for peritoneal dialysis, per 10 ml ⊘
MED: 100-4,3,40.3

**[A]** ☑ A4770 Blood collection tube, vacuum, for dialysis, per 50 ⊘
MED: 100-4,3,40.3

**[A]** ☑ A4771 Serum clotting time tube, for dialysis, per 50 ⊘
MED: 100-4,3,40.3

**[A]** ☑ A4772 Blood glucose test strips, for dialysis, per 50 ⊘
MED: 100-4,3,40.3

**[A]** ☑ A4773 Occult blood test strips, for dialysis, per 50 ⊘
MED: 100-4,3,40.3

**[A]** ☑ A4774 Ammonia test strips, for dialysis, per 50 ⊘
MED: 100-4,3,40.3

**[A]** ☑ A4802 Protamine sulfate, for hemodialysis, per 50 mg ⊘
MED: 100-4,3,40.3

**[A]** ☑ A4860 Disposable catheter tips for peritoneal dialysis, per 10 ⊘
MED: 100-4,3,40.3

**[A]** A4870 Plumbing and/or electrical work for home hemodialysis equipment ⊘
MED: 100-4,3,40.3

**[A]** A4890 Contracts, repair and maintenance, for hemodialysis equipment ⊘
MED: 100-2,15,110.2; 100-4,3,40.3

**[A]** ☑ A4911 Drain bag/bottle, for dialysis, each ⊘

**[A]** A4913 Miscellaneous dialysis supplies, not otherwise specified ⊘
Pertinent documentation to evaluate medical appropriateness should be included when this code is reported. Determine if an alternative HCPCS Level II or a CPT code better describes the service being reported. This code should be used only if a more specific code is unavailable.

**[A]** ☑ A4918 Venous pressure clamp, for hemodialysis, each ⊘

**[A]** ☑ A4927 Gloves, nonsterile, per 100 ⊘

**[A]** ☑ A4928 Surgical mask, per 20 ⊘

**[A]** ☑ A4929 Tourniquet for dialysis, each ⊘

**[A]** ☑ A4930 Gloves, sterile, per pair ⊘

**[A]** ☑ A4931 Oral thermometer, reusable, any type, each ⊘

**[E]** ☑ A4932 Rectal thermometer, reusable, any type, each

## ADDITIONAL OSTOMY SUPPLIES

**[A]** ☑ A5051 Ostomy pouch, closed; with barrier attached (one piece), each ♿
MED: 100-2,15,120

**[A]** ☑ A5052 Ostomy pouch, closed; without barrier attached (one piece), each ♿
MED: 100-2,15,120

**[A]** ☑ A5053 Ostomy pouch, closed; for use on faceplate, each ♿
MED: 100-2,15,120

**[A]** ☑ A5054 Ostomy pouch, closed; for use on barrier with flange (two piece), each ♿
MED: 100-2,15,120

**[A]** A5055 Stoma cap ♿
MED: 100-2,15,120

**[A]** ☑ A5061 Ostomy pouch, drainable; with barrier attached, (one piece), each ♿
MED: 100-2,15,120

**[A]** ☑ A5062 Ostomy pouch, drainable; without barrier attached (one piece), each ♿
MED: 100-2,15,120

**[A]** ☑ A5063 Ostomy pouch, drainable; for use on barrier with flange (two piece system), each ♿
MED: 100-2,15,120

**[A]** ☑ A5071 Ostomy pouch, urinary; with barrier attached (one piece), each ♿
MED: 100-2,15,120

**[A]** ☑ A5072 Ostomy pouch, urinary; without barrier attached (one piece), each ♿
MED: 100-2,15,120

**[A]** ☑ A5073 Ostomy pouch, urinary; for use on barrier with flange (two piece), each ♿
MED: 100-2,15,120

**[A]** A5081 Continent device; plug for continent stoma ♿
MED: 100-2,15,120

**[A]** A5082 Continent device; catheter for continent stoma ♿
MED: 100-2,15,120

● **[A]** A5083 Continent device, stoma absorptive cover for continent stoma

**[A]** A5093 Ostomy accessory; convex insert ♿
MED: 100-2,15,120

## ADDITIONAL INCONTINENCE APPLIANCES/SUPPLIES

**[A]** ☑ A5102 Bedside drainage bottle, with or without tubing, rigid or expandable, each ♿
MED: 100-2,15,120

▲ **[A]** ☑ A5105 Urinary suspensory with leg bag, with or without tube, each ♿
MED: 100-2,15,120

**[A]** A5112 Urinary leg bag; latex ♿
MED: 100-2,15,120

**[A]** ☑ A5113 Leg strap; latex, replacement only, per set ♿
MED: 100-2,15,120

**[A]** ☑ A5114 Leg strap; foam or fabric, replacement only, per set ♿
MED: 100-2,15,120

## SUPPLIES FOR EITHER INCONTINENCE OR OSTOMY APPLIANCES

For additional skin barrier codes see codes A4405-A4415.

Special Coverage Instructions    Noncovered by Medicare    Carrier Discretion    ☑ Quantity Alert    ● New Code    ○ Recycled/Reinstated    ▲ Revised Code

**2008 HCPCS**   A2-Z3 ASC Payment Indicators    **MED:** Pub 100/NCD References    ♿ DMEPOS Paid    ⊘ SNF Excluded    PQ PQRI    **A Codes — 9**

Ⓐ ☑ **A5120** Skin barrier, wipes or swabs, each
MED: 100-2,15,120

Ⓐ ☑ **A5121** Skin barrier; solid, 6 x 6 or equivalent, each  ♿
MED: 100-2,15,120

Ⓐ ☑ **A5122** Skin barrier; solid, 8 x 8 or equivalent, each  ♿
MED: 100-2,15,120

Ⓐ **A5126** Adhesive or nonadhesive; disk or foam pad  ♿
MED: 100-2,15,120

Ⓐ ☑ **A5131** Appliance cleaner, incontinence and ostomy appliances, per 16 oz.  ♿
MED: 100-2,15,120

Ⓐ **A5200** Percutaneous catheter/tube anchoring device, adhesive skin attachment  ♿
MED: 100-2,15,120

## DIABETIC SHOES, FITTING, AND MODIFICATIONS

According to Medicare, documentation from the prescribing physician must certify the diabetic patient has one of the following conditions: peripheral neuropathy with evidence of callus formation; history of preulcerative calluses; history of ulceration; foot deformity; previous amputation; or poor circulation. The footwear must be fitted and furnished by a podiatrist, pedorthist, orthotist, or prosthetist.

Ⓨ ☑ **A5500** For diabetics only, fitting (including follow-up), custom preparation and supply of off-the-shelf depth-inlay shoe manufactured to accommodate multi-density insert(s), per shoe
MED: 100-2,15,140

Ⓨ ☑ **A5501** For diabetics only, fitting (including follow-up), custom preparation and supply of shoe molded from cast(s) of patient's foot (custom molded shoe), per shoe
MED: 100-2,15,140

Ⓨ ☑ **A5503** For diabetics only, modification (including fitting) of off-the-shelf depth-inlay shoe or custom molded shoe with roller or rigid rocker bottom, per shoe
MED: 100-2,15,140

Ⓨ ☑ **A5504** For diabetics only, modification (including fitting) of off-the-shelf depth-inlay shoe or custom molded shoe with wedge(s), per shoe
MED: 100-2,15,140

Ⓨ ☑ **A5505** For diabetics only, modification (including fitting) of off-the-shelf depth-inlay shoe or custom molded shoe with metatarsal bar, per shoe
MED: 100-2,15,140

Ⓨ ☑ **A5506** For diabetics only, modification (including fitting) of off-the-shelf depth-inlay shoe or custom molded shoe with off-set heel(s), per shoe
MED: 100-2,15,140

Ⓨ ☑ **A5507** For diabetics only, not otherwise specified modification (including fitting) of off-the-shelf depth-inlay shoe or custom molded shoe, per shoe
MED: 100-2,15,140

Ⓨ ☑ **A5508** For diabetics only, deluxe feature of off-the-shelf depth-inlay shoe or custom molded shoe, per shoe
MED: 100-2,15,140

Ⓔ ☑ **A5510** For diabetics only, direct formed, compression molded to patient's foot without external heat source, multiple-density insert(s) prefabricated, per shoe
MED: 100-2,15,140

Ⓨ ☑ **A5512** For diabetics only, multiple density insert, direct formed, molded to foot after external heat source of 230 degrees Fahrenheit or higher, total contact with patient's foot, including arch, base layer minimum of 1/4 inch material of shore a 35 durometer or 3/16 inch material of shore a 40 durometer (or higher), prefabricated, each  ♿

Ⓨ ☑ **A5513** For diabetics only, multiple density insert, custom molded from model of patient's foot, total contact with patient's foot, including arch, base layer minimum of 3/16 inch material of shore a 35 durometer or higher, includes arch filler and other shaping material, custom fabricated, each  ♿

## DRESSINGS

Medicare claims for A6010-A6024 and A6154-A6404 fall under the jurisdiction of the local contractor if the supply or accessory is used for an implanted prosthetic device (e.g., pleural catheter) or implanted DME (e.g., infusion pump). Medicare claims for other uses of A6021-A6404 fall under the jurisdiction of the DME Medicare Administrative Contractor (DME MAC). The jurisdiction for Medicare claims containing all other codes falls to the DME MAC, unless otherwise noted.

Ⓔ **A6000** Noncontact wound-warming wound cover for use with the noncontact wound-warming device and warming card
MED: 100-2,16,20

Ⓐ ☑ **A6010** Collagen based wound filler, dry form, per gram of collagen  ♿
MED: 100-2,15,100

Ⓐ ☑ **A6011** Collagen based wound filler, gel/paste, per gram of collagen  ♿
MED: 100-2,15,100

Ⓐ ☑ **A6021** Collagen dressing, pad size 16 sq. in. or less, each  ♿
MED: 100-2,15,100; 100-4,4,240

Ⓐ ☑ **A6022** Collagen dressing, pad size more than 16 sq. in. but less than or equal to 48 sq. in., each  ♿
MED: 100-2,15,100; 100-4,4,240

Ⓐ ☑ **A6023** Collagen dressing, pad size more than 48 square inches, each  ♿
MED: 100-2,15,100; 100-4,4,240

Ⓐ ☑ **A6024** Collagen dressing wound filler, per 6 in.  ♿
MED: 100-2,15,100; 100-4,4,240

Ⓔ ☑ **A6025** Gel sheet for dermal or epidermal application, (e.g., silicone, hydrogel, other), each

Ⓐ ☑ **A6154** Wound pouch, each  ♿
MED: 100-2,15,100

Ⓐ ☑ **A6196** Alginate or other fiber gelling dressing, wound cover, pad size 16 sq. in. or less, each dressing  ♿
MED: 100-2,15,100; 100-4,4,240

Ⓐ ☑ **A6197** Alginate or other fiber gelling dressing, wound cover, pad size more than 16 sq. in. but less than or equal to 48 sq. in., each dressing  ♿
MED: 100-2,15,100; 100-4,4,240

Ⓐ ☑ **A6198** Alginate or other fiber gelling dressing, wound cover, pad size more than 48 sq. in., each dressing
MED: 100-2,15,100; 100-4,4,240

Ⓐ ☑ **A6199** Alginate or other fiber gelling dressing, wound filler, per 6 in.  ♿
MED: 100-2,15,100; 100-4,4,240

Ⓔ ☑ **A6200** Composite dressing, pad size 16 sq. in. or less, without adhesive border, each dressing  ♿
MED: 100-2,15,100; 100-4,4,240

Ⓔ ☑ **A6201** Composite dressing, pad size more than 16 sq. in. but less than or equal to 48 sq. in., without adhesive border, each dressing  ♿
MED: 100-2,15,100; 100-4,4,240

Ⓔ ☑ **A6202** Composite dressing, pad size more than 48 sq. in., without adhesive border, each dressing  ♿
MED: 100-2,15,100; 100-4,4,240

---

A ☑ **A6203** Composite dressing, pad size 16 sq. in. or less, with any size adhesive border, each dressing
MED: 100-2,15,100; 100-4,4,240

A ☑ **A6204** Composite dressing, pad size more than 16 sq. in. but less than or equal to 48 sq. in., with any size adhesive border, each dressing
MED: 100-2,15,100; 100-4,4,240

A ☑ **A6205** Composite dressing, pad size more than 48 sq. in., with any size adhesive border, each dressing
MED: 100-2,15,100; 100-4,4,240

A ☑ **A6206** Contact layer, 16 sq. in. or less, each dressing
MED: 100-2,15,100; 100-4,4,240

A ☑ **A6207** Contact layer, more than 16 sq. in. but less than or equal to 48 sq. in., each dressing
MED: 100-2,15,100; 100-4,4,240

A ☑ **A6208** Contact layer, more than 48 sq. in., each dressing
MED: 100-2,15,100; 100-4,4,240

A ☑ **A6209** Foam dressing, wound cover, pad size 16 sq. in. or less, without adhesive border, each dressing
MED: 100-2,15,100; 100-4,4,240

A ☑ **A6210** Foam dressing, wound cover, pad size more than 16 sq. in. but less than or equal to 48 sq. in., without adhesive border, each dressing
MED: 100-2,15,100; 100-4,4,240

A ☑ **A6211** Foam dressing, wound cover, pad size more then 48 sq. in., without adhesive border, each dressing
MED: 100-2,15,100; 100-4,4,240

A ☑ **A6212** Foam dressing, wound cover, pad size 16 sq. in. or less, with any size adhesive border, each dressing
MED: 100-2,15,100; 100-4,4,240

A ☑ **A6213** Foam dressing, wound cover, pad size more than 16 sq. in. but less than or equal to 48 sq. in., with any size adhesive border, each dressing
MED: 100-2,15,100; 100-4,4,240

A ☑ **A6214** Foam dressing, wound cover, pad size more than 48 sq. in., with any size adhesive border, each dressing
MED: 100-2,15,100; 100-4,4,240

A ☑ **A6215** Foam dressing, wound filler, per gm
MED: 100-2,15,100; 100-4,4,240

A ☑ **A6216** Gauze, nonimpregnated, nonsterile, pad size 16 sq. in. or less, without adhesive border, each dressing
MED: 100-2,15,100; 100-4,4,240

A ☑ **A6217** Gauze, nonimpregnated, nonsterile, pad size more than 16 sq. in. but less than or equal to 48 sq. in., without adhesive border, each dressing
MED: 100-2,15,100; 100-4,4,240

A ☑ **A6218** Gauze, nonimpregnated, nonsterile, pad size more than 48 sq. in., without adhesive border, each dressing
MED: 100-2,15,100; 100-4,4,240

A ☑ **A6219** Gauze, nonimpregnated, pad size 16 sq. in. or less, with any size adhesive border, each dressing
MED: 100-2,15,100; 100-4,4,240

A ☑ **A6220** Gauze, nonimpregnated, pad size more than 16 sq. in. but less than or equal to 48 sq. in., with any size adhesive border, each dressing
MED: 100-2,15,100; 100-4,4,240

A ☑ **A6221** Gauze, nonimpregnated, pad size more than 48 sq. in., with any size adhesive border, each dressing
MED: 100-2,15,100; 100-4,4,240

A ☑ **A6222** Gauze, impregnated with other than water, normal saline, or hydrogel, pad size 16 sq. in. or less, without adhesive border, each dressing
MED: 100-2,15,100; 100-4,4,240

A ☑ **A6223** Gauze, impregnated with other than water, normal saline, or hydrogel, pad size more than 16 sq. in. but less than or equal to 48 sq. in., without adhesive border, each dressing
MED: 100-2,15,100; 100-4,4,240

A ☑ **A6224** Gauze, impregnated with other than water, normal saline, or hydrogel, pad size more than 48 sq. in., without adhesive border, each dressing
MED: 100-2,15,100; 100-4,4,240

A ☑ **A6228** Gauze, impregnated, water or normal saline, pad size 16 sq. in. or less, without adhesive border, each dressing
MED: 100-2,15,100; 100-4,4,240

A ☑ **A6229** Gauze, impregnated, water or normal saline, pad size more than 16 sq. in. but less than or equal to 48 sq. in., without adhesive border, each dressing
MED: 100-2,15,100; 100-4,4,240

A ☑ **A6230** Gauze, impregnated, water or normal saline, pad size more than 48 sq. in., without adhesive border, each dressing
MED: 100-2,15,100; 100-4,4,240

A ☑ **A6231** Gauze, impregnated, hydrogel, for direct wound contact, pad size 16 sq. in. or less, each dressing
MED: 100-2,15,100; 100-4,4,240

A ☑ **A6232** Gauze, impregnated, hydrogel, for direct wound contact, pad size greater than 16 sq. in., but less than or equal to 48 sq. in., each dressing
MED: 100-2,15,100; 100-4,4,240

A ☑ **A6233** Gauze, impregnated, hydrogel for direct wound contact, pad size more than 48 sq. in., each dressing
MED: 100-2,15,100; 100-4,4,240

A ☑ **A6234** Hydrocolloid dressing, wound cover, pad size 16 sq. in. or less, without adhesive border, each dressing
MED: 100-2,15,100; 100-4,4,240

A ☑ **A6235** Hydrocolloid dressing, wound cover, pad size more than 16 sq. in. but less than or equal to 48 sq. in., without adhesive border, each dressing
MED: 100-2,15,100; 100-4,4,240

A ☑ **A6236** Hydrocolloid dressing, wound cover, pad size more than 48 sq. in., without adhesive border, each dressing
MED: 100-2,15,100; 100-4,4,240

A ☑ **A6237** Hydrocolloid dressing, wound cover, pad size 16 sq. in. or less, with any size adhesive border, each dressing
MED: 100-2,15,100; 100-4,4,240

A ☑ **A6238** Hydrocolloid dressing, wound cover, pad size more than 16 sq. in. but less than or equal to 48 sq. in., with any size adhesive border, each dressing
MED: 100-2,15,100; 100-4,4,240

A ☑ **A6239** Hydrocolloid dressing, wound cover, pad size more than 48 sq. in., with any size adhesive border, each dressing
MED: 100-2,15,100; 100-4,4,240

A ☑ **A6240** Hydrocolloid dressing, wound filler, paste, per fl. oz.
MED: 100-2,15,100; 100-4,4,240

A ☑ **A6241** Hydrocolloid dressing, wound filler, dry form, per gm
MED: 100-2,15,100; 100-4,4,240

Special Coverage Instructions    Noncovered by Medicare    Carrier Discretion    ☑ Quantity Alert    ● New Code    ○ Recycled/Reinstated    ▲ Revised Code

**2008 HCPCS**    A2-Z3 ASC Payment Indicators    **MED:** Pub 100/NCD References    & DMEPOS Paid    ○ SNF Excluded    PQ PQRI    **A Codes — 11**

**Medical and Surgical Supplies**

**A6242 — A6413**

Ⓐ ☑ **A6242** Hydrogel dressing, wound cover, pad size 16 sq. in. or less, without adhesive border, each dressing ♿
MED: 100-2,15,100; 100-4,4,240

Ⓐ ☑ **A6243** Hydrogel dressing, wound cover, pad size more than 16 sq. in. but less than or equal to 48 sq. in., without adhesive border, each dressing ♿
MED: 100-2,15,100; 100-4,4,240

Ⓐ ☑ **A6244** Hydrogel dressing, wound cover, pad size more than 48 sq. in., without adhesive border, each dressing ♿
MED: 100-2,15,100; 100-4,4,240

Ⓐ ☑ **A6245** Hydrogel dressing, wound cover, pad size 16 sq. in. or less, with any size adhesive border, each dressing ♿
MED: 100-2,15,100; 100-4,4,240

Ⓐ ☑ **A6246** Hydrogel dressing, wound cover, pad size more than 16 sq. in. but less than or equal to 48 sq. in., with any size adhesive border, each dressing ♿
MED: 100-2,15,100; 100-4,4,240

Ⓐ ☑ **A6247** Hydrogel dressing, wound cover, pad size more than 48 sq. in., with any size adhesive border, each dressing ♿
MED: 100-2,15,100; 100-4,4,240

Ⓐ ☑ **A6248** Hydrogel dressing, wound filler, gel, per fl. oz. ♿
MED: 100-2,15,100; 100-4,4,240

Ⓐ **A6250** Skin sealants, protectants, moisturizers, ointments, any type, any size
Surgical dressings applied by a physician are included as part of the professional service. Surgical dressings obtained by the patient to perform homecare as prescribed by the physician are covered.
MED: 100-2,15,100; 100-4,4,240

Ⓐ ☑ **A6251** Specialty absorptive dressing, wound cover, pad size 16 sq. in. or less, without adhesive border, each dressing ♿
MED: 100-2,15,100; 100-4,4,240

Ⓐ ☑ **A6252** Specialty absorptive dressing, wound cover, pad size more than 16 sq. in. but less than or equal to 48 sq. in., without adhesive border, each dressing ♿
MED: 100-2,15,100; 100-4,4,240

Ⓐ ☑ **A6253** Specialty absorptive dressing, wound cover, pad size more than 48 sq. in., without adhesive border, each dressing ♿
MED: 100-2,15,100; 100-4,4,240

Ⓐ ☑ **A6254** Specialty absorptive dressing, wound cover, pad size 16 sq. in. or less, with any size adhesive border, each dressing ♿
MED: 100-2,15,100; 100-4,4,240

Ⓐ ☑ **A6255** Specialty absorptive dressing, wound cover, pad size more than 16 sq. in. but less than or equal to 48 sq. in., with any size adhesive border, each dressing ♿
MED: 100-2,15,100; 100-4,4,240

Ⓐ ☑ **A6256** Specialty absorptive dressing, wound cover, pad size more than 48 sq. in., with any size adhesive border, each dressing ♿
MED: 100-2,15,100; 100-4,4,240

Ⓐ ☑ **A6257** Transparent film, 16 sq. in. or less, each dressing ♿
Surgical dressings applied by a physician are included as part of the professional service. Surgical dressings obtained by the patient to perform homecare as prescribed by the physician are covered. Use this code for Polyskin, Tegaderm, and Tegaderm HP.
MED: 100-2,15,100; 100-4,4,240

Ⓐ ☑ **A6258** Transparent film, more than 16 sq. in. but less than or equal to 48 sq. in., each dressing ♿
Surgical dressings applied by a physician are included as part of the professional service. Surgical dressings obtained by the patient to perform homecare as prescribed by the physician are covered.
MED: 100-2,15,100; 100-4,4,240

Ⓐ ☑ **A6259** Transparent film, more than 48 sq. in., each dressing ♿
Surgical dressings applied by a physician are included as part of the professional service. Surgical dressings obtained by the patient to perform homecare as prescribed by the physician are covered.
MED: 100-2,15,100; 100-4,4,240

Ⓐ **A6260** Wound cleansers, any type, any size
Surgical dressings applied by a physician are included as part of the professional service. Surgical dressings obtained by the patient to perform homecare as prescribed by the physician are covered.
MED: 100-2,15,100; 100-4,4,240

Ⓐ ☑ **A6261** Wound filler, gel/paste, per fl. oz., not elsewhere classified
Surgical dressings applied by a physician are included as part of the professional service. Surgical dressings obtained by the patient to perform homecare as prescribed by the physician are covered.
MED: 100-2,15,100; 100-4,4,240

Ⓐ ☑ **A6262** Wound filler, dry form, per gm, not elsewhere classified
MED: 100-2,15,100; 100-4,4,240

Ⓐ ☑ **A6266** Gauze, impregnated, other than water, normal saline, or zinc paste, any width, per linear yd. ♿
Surgical dressings applied by a physician are included as part of the professional service. Surgical dressings obtained by the patient to perform homecare as prescribed by the physician are covered.
MED: 100-2,15,100; 100-4,4,240

Ⓐ ☑ **A6402** Gauze, nonimpregnated, sterile, pad size 16 sq. in. or less, without adhesive border, each dressing ♿
Surgical dressings applied by a physician are included as part of the professional service. Surgical dressings obtained by the patient to perform homecare as prescribed by the physician are covered.
MED: 100-2,15,100; 100-4,4,240

Ⓐ ☑ **A6403** Gauze, nonimpregnated, sterile, pad size more than 16 sq. in. but less than or equal to 48 sq. in., without adhesive border, each dressing ♿
Surgical dressings applied by a physician are included as part of the professional service. Surgical dressings obtained by the patient to perform homecare as prescribed by the physician are covered.
MED: 100-2,15,100; 100-4,4,240

Ⓐ ☑ **A6404** Gauze, nonimpregnated, sterile, pad size more than 48 sq. in., without adhesive border, each dressing
MED: 100-2,15,100; 100-4,4,240

Ⓐ ☑ **A6407** Packing strips, nonimpregnated, up to 2 in. in width, per linear yd. ♿

Ⓐ ☑ **A6410** Eye pad, sterile, each ♿
MED: 100-2,15,100

Ⓐ ☑ **A6411** Eye pad, non-sterile, each ♿
MED: 100-2,15,100

Ⓔ ☑ **A6412** Eye patch, occlusive, each

● Ⓔ ☑ **A6413** Adhesive bandage, first aid type, any size, each

---

■ Special Coverage Instructions    ■ Noncovered by Medicare    ■ Carrier Discretion    ☑ Quantity Alert    ● New Code    ○ Recycled/Reinstated    ▲ Revised Code

**12 — A Codes**    Ⓐ Age Edit    Ⓜ Maternity Edit    ♀ Female Only    ♂ Male Only    Ⓐ-Ⓨ OPPS Status Indicators    **2008 HCPCS**

Ⓐ ☑ A6441 Padding bandage, nonelastic, nonwoven/nonknitted, width greater than or equal to 3 in. and less than 5 in., per yd.

Ⓐ ☑ A6442 Conforming bandage, nonelastic, knitted/woven, nonsterile, width less than 3 in., per yd. &

Ⓐ ☑ A6443 Conforming bandage, nonelastic, knitted/woven, nonsterile, width greater than or equal to 3 in. and less than 5 in., per yd.

Ⓐ ☑ A6444 Conforming bandage, nonelastic, knitted/woven, nonsterile, width greater than or equal to 5 in., per yd. &

Ⓐ ☑ A6445 Conforming bandage, nonelastic, knitted/woven, sterile, width less than 3 in., per yd. &

Ⓐ ☑ A6446 Conforming bandage, nonelastic, knitted/woven, sterile, width greater than or equal to 3 in. and less than 5 in., per yd.

Ⓐ ☑ A6447 Conforming bandage, nonelastic, knitted/woven, sterile, width greater than or equal to 5 in., per yd. &

Ⓐ ☑ A6448 Light compression bandage, elastic, knitted/woven, width less than 3 in., per yd. &

Ⓐ ☑ A6449 Light compression bandage, elastic, knitted/woven, width greater than or equal to three in. and less than five in., per yd. &

Ⓐ ☑ A6450 Light compression bandage, elastic, knitted/woven, width greater than or equal to 5 inches, per yard &

Ⓐ ☑ A6451 Moderate compression bandage, elastic, knitted/woven, load resistance of 1.25 to 1.34 foot pounds at 50% maximum stretch, width greater than or equal to 3 in. and less than 5 in., per yd. &

Ⓐ ☑ A6452 High compression bandage, elastic, knitted/woven, load resistance greater than or equal to 1.35 foot pounds at 50% maximum stretch, width greater than or equal to three in. and less than five in., per yd.

Ⓐ ☑ A6453 Self-adherent bandage, elastic, nonknitted/nonwoven, width less than three in., per yd.

Ⓐ ☑ A6454 Self-adherent bandage, elastic, nonknitted/nonwoven, width greater than or equal to 3 in. and less than 5 in., per yard &

Ⓐ ☑ A6455 Self-adherent bandage, elastic, nonknitted/nonwoven, width greater than or equal to 5 in., per yd. &

Ⓐ ☑ A6456 Zinc paste impregnated bandage, nonelastic, knitted/woven, width greater than or equal to 3 in. and less than 5 in., per yd. &

Ⓐ A6457 Tubular dressing with or without elastic, any width, per linear yard

Ⓐ A6501 Compression burn garment, bodysuit (head to foot), custom fabricated &
MED: 100-2,15,100

Ⓐ A6502 Compression burn garment, chin strap, custom fabricated &
MED: 100-2,15,100

Ⓐ A6503 Compression burn garment, facial hood, custom fabricated &
MED: 100-2,15,100

Ⓐ A6504 Compression burn garment, glove to wrist, custom fabricated &
MED: 100-2,15,100

Ⓐ A6505 Compression burn garment, glove to elbow, custom fabricated &
MED: 100-2,15,100

Ⓐ A6506 Compression burn garment, glove to axilla, custom fabricated &
MED: 100-2,15,100

Ⓐ A6507 Compression burn garment, foot to knee length, custom fabricated &
MED: 100-2,15,100

Ⓐ A6508 Compression burn garment, foot to thigh length, custom fabricated &
MED: 100-2,15,100

Ⓐ A6509 Compression burn garment, upper trunk to waist including arm openings (vest), custom fabricated &
MED: 100-2,15,100

Ⓐ A6510 Compression burn garment, trunk, including arms down to leg openings (leotard), custom fabricated &
MED: 100-2,15,100

Ⓐ A6511 Compression burn garment, lower trunk including leg openings (panty), custom fabricated &
MED: 100-2,15,100

Ⓐ A6512 Compression burn garment, not otherwise classified
MED: 100-2,15,100

Ⓑ A6513 Compression burn mask, face and/or neck, plastic or equal, custom fabricated

Ⓔ ☑ A6530 Gradient compression stocking, below knee, 18-30 mm Hg, each

Ⓐ ☑ A6531 Gradient compression stocking, below knee, 30-40 mm Hg, each
MED: 100-2,15,100

Ⓐ ☑ A6532 Gradient compression stocking, below knee, 40-50 mm Hg, each
MED: 100-2,15,100

Ⓔ ☑ A6533 Gradient compression stocking, thigh length, 18-30 mm Hg, each
MED: 100-2,15,130

Ⓔ ☑ A6534 Gradient compression stocking, thigh length, 30-40 mm Hg, each
MED: 100-2,15,130

Ⓔ ☑ A6535 Gradient compression stocking, thigh length, 40-50 mm Hg, each
MED: 100-2,15,130

Ⓔ ☑ A6536 Gradient compression stocking, full length/chap style, 18-30 mm Hg, each
MED: 100-2,15,130

Ⓔ ☑ A6537 Gradient compression stocking, full length/chap style, 30-40 mm Hg, each
MED: 100-2,15,130

Ⓔ ☑ A6538 Gradient compression stocking, full length/chap style, 40-50 mm Hg, each
MED: 100-2,15,130

Ⓔ ☑ A6539 Gradient compression stocking, waist length, 18-30 mm Hg, each
MED: 100-2,15,130

Ⓔ ☑ A6540 Gradient compression stocking, waist length, 30-40 mm Hg, each
MED: 100-2,15,130

Ⓔ ☑ A6541 Gradient compression stocking, waist length, 40-50 mm Hg, each
MED: 100-2,15,130

Ⓔ ☑ A6542 Gradient compression stocking, custom made
MED: 100-2,15,130

Ⓔ A6543 Gradient compression stocking, lymphedema
MED: 100-2,15,130

---

▨ Special Coverage Instructions    Noncovered by Medicare    Carrier Discretion    ☑ Quantity Alert    ● New Code    ○ Recycled/Reinstated    ▲ Revised Code

[E]  A6544  Gradient compression stocking, garter belt
MED: 100-2,15,130

[E]  A6549  Gradient compression stocking, not otherwise specified
MED: 100-2,15,130

[Y] ☑  A6550  Wound care set, for negative pressure wound therapy electrical pump, includes all supplies and accessories  &

## MISCELLANEOUS SUPPLIES

[Y] ☑  A7000  Canister, disposable, used with suction pump, each  &

[Y] ☑  A7001  Canister, nondisposable, used with suction pump, each  &

[Y] ☑  A7002  Tubing, used with suction pump, each  &

[Y]  A7003  Administration set, with small volume nonfiltered pneumatic nebulizer, disposable

[Y]  A7004  Small volume nonfiltered pneumatic nebulizer, disposable  &

[Y]  A7005  Administration set, with small volume nonfiltered pneumatic nebulizer, nondisposable

[Y]  A7006  Administration set, with small volume filtered pneumatic nebulizer

[Y]  A7007  Large volume nebulizer, disposable, unfilled, used with aerosol compressor  &

[Y]  A7008  Large volume nebulizer, disposable, prefilled, used with aerosol compressor  &

[Y]  A7009  Reservoir bottle, nondisposable, used with large volume ultrasonic nebulizer  &

[Y] ☑  A7010  Corrugated tubing, disposable, used with large volume nebulizer, 100 ft.  &

[Y] ☑  A7011  Corrugated tubing, nondisposable, used with large volume nebulizer, 10 ft.

[Y]  A7012  Water collection device, used with large volume nebulizer  &

[Y]  A7013  Filter, disposable, used with aerosol compressor  &

[Y]  A7014  Filter, nondisposable, used with aerosol compressor or ultrasonic generator  &

[Y]  A7015  Aerosol mask, used with DME nebulizer  &

[Y]  A7016  Dome and mouthpiece, used with small volume ultrasonic nebulizer  &

[Y]  A7017  Nebulizer, durable, glass or autoclavable plastic, bottle type, not used with oxygen  &
MED: 100-3,280.1

[Y] ☑  A7018  Water, distilled, used with large volume nebulizer, 1000 ml  &

[Y] ☑  A7025  High frequency chest wall oscillation system vest, replacement for use with patient owned equipment, each  &

[Y] ☑  A7026  High frequency chest wall oscillation system hose, replacement for use with patient owned equipment, each  &

● [Y] ☑  A7027  Combination oral/nasal mask, used with continuous positive airway pressure device, each

● [Y] ☑  A7028  Oral cushion for combination oral/nasal mask, replacement only, each

● [Y] ☑  A7029  Nasal pillows for combination oral/nasal mask, replacement only, pair

[Y] ☑  A7030  Full face mask used with positive airway pressure device, each  &

[Y] ☑  A7031  Face mask interface, replacement for full face mask, each  &

[Y] ☑  A7032  Cushion for use on nasal mask interface, replacement only, each  &

[Y] ☑  A7033  Pillow for use on nasal cannula type interface, replacement only, pair  &

[Y]  A7034  Nasal interface (mask or cannula type) used with positive airway pressure device, with or without head strap

[Y]  A7035  Headgear used with positive airway pressure device  &

[Y]  A7036  Chinstrap used with positive airway pressure device  &

[Y]  A7037  Tubing used with positive airway pressure device  &

[Y]  A7038  Filter, disposable, used with positive airway pressure device  &

[Y]  A7039  Filter, nondisposable, used with positive airway pressure device  &

[A]  A7040  One way chest drain valve

[A]  A7041  Water seal drainage container and tubing for use with implanted chest tube

[A] ☑  A7042  Implanted pleural catheter, each  &

[A]  A7043  Vacuum drainage bottle and tubing for use with implanted catheter  &

[Y] ☑  A7044  Oral interface used with positive airway pressure device, each  &

[Y]  A7045  Exhalation port with or without swivel used with accessories for positive airway devices, replacement only
MED: 100-3,230.17

[Y] ☑  A7046  Water chamber for humidifier, used with positive airway pressure device, replacement, each  &
MED: 100-3,230.17

[A] ☑  A7501  Tracheostoma valve, including diaphragm, each  &
MED: 100-2,15,120

[A] ☑  A7502  Replacement diaphragm/faceplate for tracheostoma valve, each  &
MED: 100-2,15,120

[A] ☑  A7503  Filter holder or filter cap, reusable, for use in a tracheostoma heat and moisture exchange system, each  &
MED: 100-2,15,120

[A] ☑  A7504  Filter for use in a tracheostoma heat and moisture exchange system, each  &
MED: 100-2,15,120

[A] ☑  A7505  Housing, reusable without adhesive, for use in a heat and moisture exchange system and/or with a tracheostoma valve, each  &
MED: 100-2,15,120

[A] ☑  A7506  Adhesive disc for use in a heat and moisture exchange system and/or with tracheostoma valve, any type each  &
MED: 100-2,15,120

[A] ☑  A7507  Filter holder and integrated filter without adhesive, for use in a tracheostoma heat and moisture exchange system, each  &
MED: 100-2,15,120

[A] ☑  A7508  Housing and integrated adhesive, for use in a tracheostoma heat and moisture exchange system and/or with a tracheostoma valve, each  &
MED: 100-2,15,120

---

Special Coverage Instructions      Noncovered by Medicare      Carrier Discretion      ☑ Quantity Alert      ● New Code      ○ Recycled/Reinstated      ▲ Revised Code

**A** ☑ **A7509** Filter holder and integrated filter housing, and adhesive, for use as a tracheostoma heat and moisture exchange system, each ♿
MED: 100-2,15,120

**A** ☑ **A7520** Tracheostomy/laryngectomy tube, noncuffed, polyvinylchloride (PVC), silicone or equal, each ♿
MED: 100-2,1,40

**A** ☑ **A7521** Tracheostomy/laryngectomy tube, cuffed, polyvinylchloride (PVC), silicone or equal, each ♿
MED: 100-2,1,40

**A** ☑ **A7522** Tracheostomy/laryngectomy tube, stainless steel or equal (sterilizable and reusable), each ♿
MED: 100-2,1,40

**A** ☑ **A7523** Tracheostomy shower protector, each

**A** ☑ **A7524** Tracheostoma stent/stud/button, each ♿

**A** ☑ **A7525** Tracheostomy mask, each ♿

**A** ☑ **A7526** Tracheostomy tube collar/holder, each ♿

**A** ☑ **A7527** Tracheostomy/laryngectomy tube plug/stop, each ♿

**Y** **A8000** Helmet, protective, soft, prefabricated, includes all components and accessories ♿

**Y** **A8001** Helmet, protective, hard, prefabricated, includes all components and accessories ♿

**Y** **A8002** Helmet, protective, soft, custom fabricated, includes all components and accessories ♿

**Y** **A8003** Helmet, protective, hard, custom fabricated, includes all components and accessories ♿

**Y** **A8004** Soft interface for helmet, replacement only ♿

## ADMINISTRATIVE, MISCELLANEOUS & INVESTIGATIONAL A9000-A9999

This section of codes reports items such as nonprescription drugs, noncovered items/services, exercise equipment and, most notably, radiopharmaceutical diagnostic imaging agents.

**B** **A9150** Nonprescription drug
MED: 100-2,15,50

**E** ☑ **A9152** Single vitamin/mineral/trace element, oral, per dose, not otherwise specified

**E** ☑ **A9153** Multiple vitamins, with or without minerals and trace elements, oral, per dose, not otherwise specified

● **B** **A9155** Artificial saliva, 30 ml

**E** **A9180** Pediculosis (lice infestation) treatment, topical, for administration by patient/caretaker

**E** **A9270** Noncovered item or service
MED: 100-2,16,20

● **E** ☑ **A9274** External ambulatory insulin delivery system, disposable, each, includes all supplies and accessories

**E** **A9275** Home glucose disposable monitor, includes test strips

● **E** ☑ **A9276** Sensor; invasive (e.g., subcutaneous), disposable, for use with interstitial continuous glucose monitoring system, 1 unit = 1 day supply

● **E** **A9277** Transmitter; external, for use with interstitial continuous glucose monitoring system

● **E** **A9278** Receiver (monitor); external, for use with interstitial continuous glucose monitoring system

**E** **A9279** Monitoring feature/device, stand-alone or integrated, any type, includes all accessories, components and electronics, not otherwise classified

**E** **A9280** Alert or alarm device, not otherwise classified

**E** ☑ **A9281** Reaching/grabbing device, any type, any length, each

**E** ☑ **A9282** Wig, any type, each

● **E** ☑ **A9283** Foot pressure off loading/supportive device, any type, each

**E** **A9300** Exercise equipment
MED: 100-2,15,110.1; 100-3,280.1

## RADIOPHARMACEUTICALS

**N** ☑ **A9500** Technetium Tc-99m sestamibi, diagnostic, per study dose, up to 40 millicuries
Use this code for Cardiolite.
MED: 100-4,4,20.5; 100-4,4,230.1; 100-4,12,70; 100-4,13,20; 100-4,13,90

● **N** ☑ **A9501** Technetium Tc-99m teboroxime, diagnostic, per study dose

**N** ☑ **A9502** Technetium Tc-99m tetrofosmin, diagnostic, per study dose, up to 40 millicuries
Use this code for Myoview.
MED: 100-4,4,230.1; 100-4,12,70; 100-4,13,20; 100-4,13,90

**N** ☑ **A9503** Technetium Tc-99m medronate, diagnostic, per study dose, up to 30 millicuries
Use this code for CIS-MDP, Draximage MDP-10, Draximage MDP-25, MDP-Bracco, Technetium Tc-99m MPI-MDP
MED: 100-4,4,230.1; 100-4,12,70; 100-4,13,20; 100-4,13,90
AHA: 2Q,'02,9

**N** ☑ **A9504** Technetium Tc-99m apcitide, diagnostic, per study dose, up to 20 millicuries
Use this code for Acutect
MED: 100-4,4,230.1; 100-4,12,70; 100-4,13,20; 100-4,13,90
AHA: 2Q,'02,9; 4Q,'01,5

**N** ☑ **A9505** Thallium Tl-201 thallous chloride, diagnostic, per millicurie
Use this code for MIBG, Thallous Chloride USP.
MED: 100-4,4,230.1; 100-4,12,70; 100-4,13,20; 100-4,13,90
AHA: 2Q,'02,9

**N** ☑ **A9507** Indium In-111 capromab pendetide, diagnostic, per study dose, up to 10 millicuries
Use this code for Prostascint.
MED: 100-4,4,230.1; 100-4,12,70; 100-4,13,20; 100-4,13,90

**N** ☑ **A9508** Iodine I-131 iobenguane sulfate, diagnostic, per 0.5 millicurie
Use this code for MIBG.
MED: 100-4,4,230.1
AHA: 2Q,'02,9

● **N** ☑ **A9509** Iodine I-123 sodium iodide, diagnostic, per millicurie

**N** ☑ **A9510** Technetium Tc-99m disofenin, diagnostic, per study dose, up to 15 millicuries
Use this code for Hepatolite.
MED: 100-4,4,230.1

**N** ☑ **A9512** Technetium Tc-99m pertechnetate, diagnostic, per millicurie
Use this code for Technelite, Ultra-Technelow.
MED: 100-4,4,230.1

▲ **N** ☑ **A9516** Iodine I-123 sodium iodide, diagnostic, per 100 microcuries, up to 999 microcuries
MED: 100-4,4,230.1

---

Special Coverage Instructions   Noncovered by Medicare   Carrier Discretion   ☑ Quantity Alert   ● New Code   ○ Recycled/Reinstated   ▲ Revised Code

**2008 HCPCS**   A2-Z3 ASC Payment Indicators   **MED:** Pub 100/NCD References   ♿ DMEPOS Paid   ⊘ SNF Excluded   PQ PQRI   **A Codes — 15**

К ☑ **A9517** Iodine I-131 sodium iodide capsule(s), therapeutic, per millicurie
MED: 100-4,4,230.1

N ☑ **A9521** Technetium Tc-99m exametazime, diagnostic, per study dose, up to 25 millicuries
**Use this code for Ceretec.**
MED: 100-4,4,230.1

N ☑ **A9524** Iodine I-131 iodinated serum albumin, diagnostic, per 5 microcuries
MED: 100-4,4,230.1; 100-4,12,70; 100-4,13,20; 100-4,13,90

N ☑ **A9526** Nitrogen N-13 ammonia, diagnostic, per study dose, up to 40 millicuries
MED: 100-3,220.6; 100-4,4,230.1; 100-4,13,60.3; 100-4,13,60.3.1; 100-4,13,60.3.2

К ☑ **A9527** Iodine I-125, sodium iodide solution, therapeutic, per millicurie                                   H2

N ☑ **A9528** Iodine I-131 sodium iodide capsule(s), diagnostic, per millicurie
MED: 100-4,4,230.1

N ☑ **A9529** Iodine I-131 sodium iodide solution, diagnostic, per millicurie
MED: 100-4,4,230.1

К ☑ **A9530** Iodine I-131 sodium iodide solution, therapeutic, per millicurie                                   ⊘
MED: 100-4,4,230.1

N ☑ **A9531** Iodine I-131 sodium iodide, diagnostic, per microcurie (up to 100 microcuries)
MED: 100-4,4,230.1

N ☑ **A9532** Iodine I-125 serum albumin, diagnostic, per 5 microcuries
MED: 100-4,4,230.1

N ☑ **A9535** Injection, methylene blue, 1 ml                            N1

N ☑ **A9536** Technetium Tc-99m depreotide, diagnostic, per study dose, up to 35 millicuries
MED: 100-4,4,230.1

N ☑ **A9537** Technetium Tc-99m mebrofenin, diagnostic, per study dose, up to 15 millicuries
MED: 100-4,4,230.1

N ☑ **A9538** Technetium Tc-99m pyrophosphate, diagnostic, per study dose, up to 25 millicuries
**Use this code for CIS-PYRO, Phosphostec, Technescan Pyp Kit**
MED: 100-4,4,230.1

N ☑ **A9539** Technetium Tc-99m pentetate, diagnostic, per study dose, up to 25 millicuries
**Use this code for AN-DTPA, DTPA, Magnavist, MPI-DTPA Kit-Chelate, MPI Indium DTPA IN-111, Pentate Calcium Trisodium, Pentate Zinc Trisodium**
MED: 100-4,4,230.1

N ☑ **A9540** Technetium Tc-99m macroaggregated albumin, diagnostic, per study dose, up to 10 millicuries
MED: 100-4,4,230.1

N ☑ **A9541** Technetium Tc-99m sulfur colloid, diagnostic, per study dose, up to 20 millicuries
MED: 100-4,4,230.1

N ☑ **A9542** Indium In-111 ibritumomab tiuxetan, diagnostic, per study dose, up to 5 millicuries                            ⊘
**Use this code for Zevalin.**
MED: 100-4,4,230.1

К ☑ **A9543** Yttrium Y-90 ibritumomab tiuxetan, therapeutic, per treatment dose, up to 40 millicuries               ⊘
MED: 100-4,4,230.1

N ☑ **A9544** Iodine I-131 tositumomab, diagnostic, per study dose                            ⊘

К ☑ **A9545** Iodine I-131 tositumomab, therapeutic, per treatment dose                            ⊘
**Use this code for Bexxar.**

N ☑ **A9546** Cobalt Co-57/58, cyanocobalamin, diagnostic, per study dose, up to 1 microcurie

N ☑ **A9547** Indium In-111 oxyquinoline, diagnostic, per 0.5 millicurie
MED: 100-4,4,230.1

N ☑ **A9548** Indium In-111 pentetate, diagnostic, per 0.5 millicurie
MED: 100-4,4,230.1

N ☑ **A9550** Technetium Tc-99m sodium gluceptate, diagnostic, per study dose, up to 25 millicurie
MED: 100-4,4,230.1

N ☑ **A9551** Technetium Tc-99m succimer, diagnostic, per study dose, up to 10 millicuries
**Use this code for MPI-DMSA Kidney Reagent.**
MED: 100-4,4,230.1

N ☑ **A9552** Fluorodeoxyglucose F-18 FDG, diagnostic, per study dose, up to 45 millicuries
MED: 100-4,4,230.1

N ☑ **A9553** Chromium Cr-51 sodium chromate, diagnostic, per study dose, up to 250 microcuries
**Use this code for Chromitope Sodium.**
MED: 100-4,4,230.1

N ☑ **A9554** Iodine I-125 sodium iothalamate, diagnostic, per study dose, up to 10 microcuries
**Use this code for Glofil-125.**
MED: 100-4,4,230.1

N ☑ **A9555** Rubidium Rb-82, diagnostic, per study dose, up to 60 millicuries
**Use this code for Cardiogen 82.**
MED: 100-4,4,230.1

N ☑ **A9556** Gallium Ga-67 citrate, diagnostic, per millicurie
**Use this code for Ganite.**
MED: 100-4,4,230.1

N ☑ **A9557** Technetium Tc-99m bicisate, diagnostic, per study dose, up to 25 millicuries
**Use this code for Neurolite.**
MED: 100-4,4,230.1

N ☑ **A9558** Xenon Xe-133 gas, diagnostic, per 10 millicuries
MED: 100-4,4,230.1

N ☑ **A9559** Cobalt Co-57 cyanocobalamin, oral, diagnostic, per study dose, up to 1 microcurie
MED: 100-4,4,230.1

N ☑ **A9560** Technetium Tc-99m labeled red blood cells, diagnostic, per study dose, up to 30 millicuries
MED: 100-4,4,230.1

N ☑ **A9561** Technetium Tc-99m oxidronate, diagnostic, per study dose, up to 30 millicuries
**Use this code for TechneScan.**
MED: 100-4,4,230.1

N ☑ **A9562** Technetium Tc-99m mertiatide, diagnostic, per study dose, up to 15 millicuries
**Use this code for TechneScan MAG-3.**
MED: 100-4,4,230.1

К ☑ **A9563** Sodium phosphate P-32, therapeutic, per millicurie
MED: 100-4,4,230.1

---

Special Coverage Instructions    Noncovered by Medicare    Carrier Discretion    ☑ Quantity Alert    ● New Code    ○ Recycled/Reinstated    ▲ Revised Code

**16 — A Codes**    Age Edit    Maternity Edit    ♀ Female Only    ♂ Male Only    A-Y OPPS Status Indicators    **2008 HCPCS**

K ☑ **A9564** Chromic phosphate P-32 suspension, therapeutic, per millicurie
Use this code for Phosphocol (P32).
MED: 100-4,4,230.1

~~**A9565** Indium In-111 pentetreotide, diagnostic, per millicurie~~
See A9572.
MED: 100-4,4,230.1

N ☑ **A9566** Technetium Tc-99m fanolesomab, diagnostic, per study dose, up to 25 millicuries
MED: 100-4,4,230.1

N ☑ **A9567** Technetium Tc-99m pentetate, diagnostic, aerosol, per study dose, up to 75 millicuries
Use this code for AN-DTPA, DTPA, Magnavist, MPI-DTPA Kit-Chelate, MPI Indium DTPA IN-111, Pentate Calcium Trisodium, Pentate Zinc Trisodium.

N ☑ **A9568** Technetium Tc-99m arcitumomab, diagnostic, per study dose, up to 45 millicuries
Use this code for CEA Scan.

● N ☑ **A9569** Technetium Tc-99m exametazime labeled autologous white blood cells, diagnostic, per study dose
Use this code for Ceretec.

● N ☑ **A9570** Indium In-111 labeled autologous white blood cells, diagnostic, per study dose

● N ☑ **A9571** Indium In-111 labeled autologous platelets, diagnostic, per study dose

● N ☑ **A9572** Indium In-111 pentetreotide, diagnostic, per study dose, up to 6 millicuries
Use this code for Ostreoscan.

● N ☑ **A9576** Injection, gadoteridol, (ProHance multipack), per ml

● N ☑ **A9577** Injection, gadobenate dimeglumine (MultiHance), per ml

● N ☑ **A9578** Injection, gadobenate dimeglumine (MultiHance multipack), per ml

● N ☑ **A9579** Injection, gadolinium based magnetic resonance contrast agent, not otherwise specified, per ml
Use this code for Omniscan.

K ☑ **A9600** Strontium Sr-89 chloride, therapeutic, per millicurie

Use this code for Metastron.
MED: 100-4,4,230.1
AHA: 2Q,'02,9

K ☑ **A9605** Samarium Sm-153 lexidronamm, therapeutic, per 50 millicuries
Use this code for Quadramet.
MED: 100-4,4,20.5; 100-4,4,230.1
AHA: 2Q,'02,9

N **A9698** Nonradioactive contrast imaging material, not otherwise classified, per study N1
MED: 100-4,12,70; 100-4,13,20; 100-4,13,90

N **A9699** Radiopharmaceutical, therapeutic, not otherwise classified

B **A9700** Supply of injectable contrast material for use in echocardiography, per study
MED: 100-4,12,30.4
AHA: 4Q,'01,5

## MISCELLANEOUS

Y **A9900** Miscellaneous DME supply, accessory, and/or service component of another HCPCS code ⅙
Medicare jurisdiction: local contractor if implanted DME; DME MAC.

A **A9901** DME delivery, set up, and/or dispensing service component of another HCPCS code

Y **A9999** Miscellaneous DME supply or accessory, not otherwise specified

---

Special Coverage Instructions    Noncovered by Medicare    Carrier Discretion    ☑ Quantity Alert    ● New Code    ○ Recycled/Reinstated    ▲ Revised Code

**2008 HCPCS**    A2-Z3 ASC Payment Indicators    **MED:** Pub 100/NCD References    ⅙ DMEPOS Paid    ⊘ SNF Excluded    P0 PQRI    **A Codes — 17**

## ENTERAL AND PARENTERAL THERAPY B4000-B9999

This section includes codes for supplies, formulae, nutritional solutions, and infusion pumps.

## ENTERAL FORMULAE AND ENTERAL MEDICAL SUPPLIES

Certification of medical necessity is required for coverage. Submit a revision to the certification of medical necessity if the patient's daily volume changes by more than one liter; if there is a change in infusion method; or if there is a change from premix to home mix or parenteral to enteral therapy.

▲ Y ☑ **B4034** Enteral feeding supply kit; syringe fed, per day
MED: 100-2,15,120; 100-3,180.2; 100-4,20,100.2.2; 100-4,20,160.1

Y ☑ **B4035** Enteral feeding supply kit; pump fed, per day
MED: 100-2,15,120; 100-3,180.2; 100-4,20,100.2.2; 100-4,20,160.1

Y ☑ **B4036** Enteral feeding supply kit; gravity fed, per day
MED: 100-2,15,120; 100-3,180.2; 100-4,20,100.2.2; 100-4,20,160.1

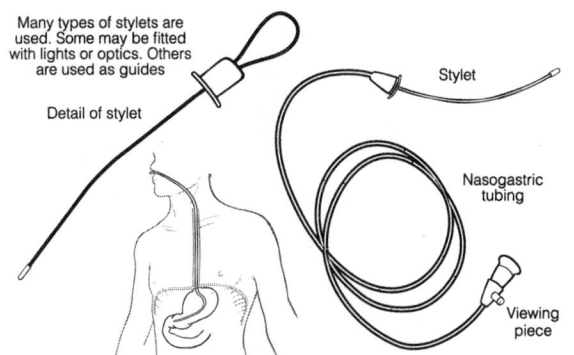

Many types of stylets are used. Some may be fitted with lights or optics. Others are used as guides

Detail of stylet

Stylet

Nasogastric tubing

Viewing piece

Y **B4081** Nasogastric tubing with stylet
MED: 100-2,15,120; 100-3,180.2; 100-4,20,100.2.2; 100-4,20,160.1

Y **B4082** Nasogastric tubing without stylet
MED: 100-2,15,120; 100-3,180.2; 100-4,20,100.2.2; 100-4,20,160.1

Y **B4083** Stomach tube — Levine type
MED: 100-2,15,120; 100-3,180.2; 100-4,20,100.2.2

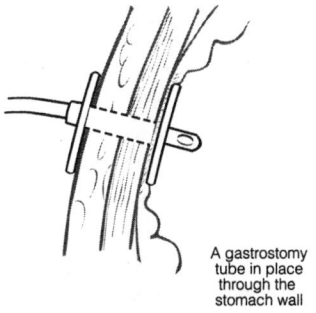

A gastrostomy tube in place through the stomach wall

~~B4086~~ ~~Gastrostomy/jejunostomy tube, any material, any type, (standard or low profile), each~~
See B4087-B4088.

● A ☑ **B4087** Gastrostomy/jejunostomy tube, standard, any material, any type, each

● A ☑ **B4088** Gastrostomy/jejunostomy tube, low-profile, any material, any type, each

E ☑ **B4100** Food thickener, administered orally, per oz.

Y ☑ **B4102** Enteral formula, for adults, used to replace fluids and electrolytes (e.g., clear liquids), 500 ml = 1 unit
MED: 100-3,180.2; 100-4,20,160.1

Y ☑ **B4103** Enteral formula, for pediatrics, used to replace fluids and electrolytes (e.g., clear liquids), 500 ml = 1 unit
MED: 100-3,180.2; 100-4,20,160.1

E **B4104** Additive for enteral formula (e.g., fiber)
MED: 100-3,180.2; 100-4,20,160.1

Y ☑ **B4149** Enteral formula, manufactured blenderized natural foods with intact nutrients, includes proteins, fats, carbohydrates, vitamins and minerals, may include fiber, administered through an enteral feeding tube, 100 calories = 1 unit
MED: 100-2,15,120; 100-3,180.2; 100-4,20,100.2.2; 100-4,20,160.1

Y ☑ **B4150** Enteral formula, nutritionally complete with intact nutrients, includes proteins, fats, carbohydrates, vitamins and minerals, may include fiber, administered through an enteral feeding tube, 100 calories = 1 unit
Use this code for Enrich, Ensure, Ensure HN, Ensure Powder, Isocal, Lonalac Powder, Meritene, Meritene Powder, Osmolite, Osmolite HN, Portagen Powder, Sustacal, Renu, Sustagen Powder, Travasorb.
MED: 100-2,15,120; 100-3,180.2; 100-4,20,100.2.2; 100-4,20,160.1

Y ☑ **B4152** Enteral formula, nutritionally complete, calorically dense (equal to or greater than 1.5 kcal/ml) with intact nutrients, includes proteins, fats, carbohydrates, vitamins and minerals, may include fiber, administered through an enteral feeding tube, 100 calories = 1 unit
Use this code for Magnacal, Isocal HCN, Sustacal HC, Ensure Plus, Ensure Plus HN.
MED: 100-2,15,120; 100-3,180.2; 100-4,20,100.2.2; 100-4,20,160.1

Y ☑ **B4153** Enteral formula, nutritionally complete, hydrolyzed proteins (amino acids and peptide chain), includes fats, carbohydrates, vitamins and minerals, may include fiber, administered through an enteral feeding tube, 100 calories = 1 unit
Use this code for Criticare HN, Vivonex t.e.n. (Total Enteral Nutrition), Vivonex HN, Vital (Vital HN), Travasorb HN, Isotein HN, Precision HN, Precision Isotonic.
MED: 100-2,15,120; 100-3,180.2; 100-4,20,100.2.2; 100-4,20,160.1

Y ☑ **B4154** Enteral formula, nutritionally complete, for special metabolic needs, excludes inherited disease of metabolism, includes altered composition of proteins, fats, carbohydrates, vitamins and/or minerals, may include fiber, administered through an enteral feeding tube, 100 calories = 1 unit
Use this code for Hepatic-aid, Travasorb Hepatic, Travasorb MCT, Travasorb Renal, Traum-aid, Tramacal, Aminaid.
MED: 100-2,15,120; 100-3,180.2; 100-4,20,100.2.2; 100-4,20,160.1

Y ☑ **B4155** Enteral formula, nutritionally incomplete/modular nutrients, includes specific nutrients, carbohydrates (e.g., glucose polymers), proteins/amino acids (e.g., glutamine, arginine), fat (e.g., medium chain triglycerides) or combination, administered through an enteral feeding tube, 100 calories = 1 unit
Use this code for Propac, Gerval Protein, Promix, Casec, Moducal, Controlyte, Polycose Liquid or Powder, Sumacal, Microlipids, MCT Oil, Nutri-source.
MED: 100-2,15,120; 100-3,180.2; 100-4,20,100.2.2; 100-4,20,160.1

Y ☑ **B4157** Enteral formula, nutritionally complete, for special metabolic needs for inherited disease of metabolism, includes proteins, fats, carbohydrates, vitamins and minerals, may include fiber, administered through an enteral feeding tube, 100 calories = 1 unit
MED: 100-3,180.2; 100-4,20,160.1

Special Coverage Instructions    Noncovered by Medicare    Carrier Discretion    ☑ Quantity Alert    ● New Code    ○ Recycled/Reinstated    ▲ Revised Code

**2008 HCPCS**    A2-Z3 ASC Payment Indicators    **MED:** Pub 100/NCD References    ♿ DMEPOS Paid    ⊘ SNF Excluded    PQ PQRI    **B Codes — 19**

Enteral and Parenteral Therapy

B4034 — B4157

Ⓨ ☑ **B4158** Enteral formula, for pediatrics, nutritionally complete with intact nutrients, includes proteins, fats, carbohydrates, vitamins and minerals, may include fiber and/or iron, administered through an enteral feeding tube, 100 calories = 1 unit &

MED: 100-3,180.2; 100-4,20,160.1

Ⓧ ☑ **B4159** Enteral formula, for pediatrics, nutritionally complete soy based with intact nutrients, includes proteins, fats, carbohydrates, vitamins and minerals, may include fiber and/or iron, administered through an enteral feeding tube, 100 calories = 1 unit

MED: 100-3,180.2; 100-4,20,160.1

Ⓨ ☑ **B4160** Enteral formula, for pediatrics, nutritionally complete calorically dense (equal to or greater than 0.7 kcal/ml) with intact nutrients, includes proteins, fats, carbohydrates, vitamins and minerals, may include fiber, administered through an enteral feeding tube, 100 calories = 1 unit &

MED: 100-3,180.2; 100-4,20,160.1

Ⓨ ☑ **B4161** Enteral formula, for pediatrics, hydrolyzed/amino acids and peptide chain proteins, includes fats, carbohydrates, vitamins and minerals, may include fiber, administered through an enteral feeding tube, 100 calories = 1 unit &

MED: 100-3,180.2; 100-4,20,160.1

Ⓨ ☑ **B4162** Enteral formula, for pediatrics, special metabolic needs for inherited disease of metabolism, includes proteins, fats, carbohydrates, vitamins and minerals, may include fiber, administered through an enteral feeding tube, 100 calories = 1 unit &

MED: 100-3,180.2; 100-4,20,160.1

## PARENTERAL NUTRITION SOLUTIONS AND SUPPLIES

Ⓨ ☑ **B4164** Parenteral nutrition solution: carbohydrates (dextrose), 50% or less (500 ml = 1 unit) — homemix &

MED: 100-2,15,120; 100-3,180.2; 100-4,3,10.4; 100-4,20,100.2.2

Ⓨ ☑ **B4168** Parenteral nutrition solution; amino acid, 3.5%, (500 ml = 1 unit) — home mix &

MED: 100-2,15,120; 100-3,180.2; 100-4,3,10.4; 100-4,20,100.2.2

Ⓨ ☑ **B4172** Parenteral nutrition solution; amino acid, 5.5% through 7%, (500 ml = 1 unit) — home mix &

MED: 100-2,15,120; 100-3,180.2; 100-4,3,10.4; 100-4,20,100.2.2

Ⓨ ☑ **B4176** Parenteral nutrition solution; amino acid, 7% through 8.5%, (500 ml = 1 unit) — home mix &

MED: 100-2,15,120; 100-3,180.2; 100-4,3,10.4; 100-4,20,100.2.2

Ⓨ ☑ **B4178** Parenteral nutrition solution; amino acid, greater than 8.5% (500 ml = 1 unit) — home mix &

MED: 100-2,15,120; 100-3,180.2; 100-4,3,10.4; 100-4,20,100.2.2

Ⓨ ☑ **B4180** Parenteral nutrition solution; carbohydrates (dextrose), greater than 50% (500 ml = 1 unit) — home mix &

MED: 100-2,15,120; 100-3,180.2; 100-4,3,10.4; 100-4,20,100.2.2

Ⓑ ☑ **B4185** Parenteral nutrition solution, per 10 grams lipids

Ⓨ ☑ **B4189** Parenteral nutrition solution; compounded amino acid and carbohydrates with electrolytes, trace elements, and vitamins, including preparation, any strength, 10 to 51 grams of protein — premix &

MED: 100-2,15,120; 100-3,180.2; 100-4,3,10.4; 100-4,20,100.2.2

Ⓨ ☑ **B4193** Parenteral nutrition solution; compounded amino acid and carbohydrates with electrolytes, trace elements, and vitamins, including preparation, any strength, 52 to 73 grams of protein — premix &

MED: 100-2,15,120; 100-3,180.2; 100-4,3,10.4; 100-4,20,100.2.2

Ⓨ ☑ **B4197** Parenteral nutrition solution; compounded amino acid and carbohydrates with electrolytes, trace elements and vitamins, including preparation, any strength, 74 to 100 grams of protein — premix &

MED: 100-2,15,120; 100-3,180.2; 100-4,3,10.4; 100-4,20,100.2.2

Ⓨ ☑ **B4199** Parenteral nutrition solution; compounded amino acid and carbohydrates with electrolytes, trace elements and vitamins, including preparation, any strength, over 100 grams of protein — premix &

MED: 100-2,15,120; 100-3,180.2; 100-4,3,10.4; 100-4,20,100.2.2

Ⓨ **B4216** Parenteral nutrition; additives (vitamins, trace elements, heparin, electrolytes) — home mix, per day &

MED: 100-2,15,120; 100-3,180.2; 100-4,3,10.4; 100-4,20,100.2.2

Ⓨ **B4220** Parenteral nutrition supply kit; premix, per day &

MED: 100-2,15,120; 100-3,180.2; 100-4,3,10.4; 100-4,20,100.2.2

Ⓨ **B4222** Parenteral nutrition supply kit; home mix, per day &

MED: 100-2,15,120; 100-3,180.2; 100-4,3,10.4; 100-4,20,100.2.2

Ⓨ **B4224** Parenteral nutrition administration kit, per day &

MED: 100-2,15,120; 100-3,180.2; 100-4,3,10.4; 100-4,20,100.2.2

Ⓨ **B5000** Parenteral nutrition solution; compounded amino acid and carbohydrates with electrolytes, trace elements, and vitamins, including preparation, any strength, renal — Amirosyn RF, NephrAmine, RenAmine — premix &
Use this code for Amirosyn-RF, NephrAmine, RenAmin.

MED: 100-2,15,120; 100-3,180.2; 100-4,3,10.4; 100-4,20,100.2.2

Ⓨ **B5100** Parenteral nutrition solution; compounded amino acid and carbohydrates with electrolytes, trace elements, and vitamins, including preparation, any strength, hepatic — FreAmine HBC, HepatAmine — premix &
Use this code for FreAmine HBC, HepatAmine.

MED: 100-2,15,120; 100-3,180.2; 100-4,3,10.4; 100-4,20,100.2.2

Ⓨ **B5200** Parenteral nutrition solution; compounded amino acid and carbohydrates with electrolytes, trace elements, and vitamins, including preparation, any strength, stress — branch chain amino acids — premix &

MED: 100-2,15,120; 100-3,180.2; 100-4,3,10.4; 100-4,20,100.2.2

## ENTERAL AND PARENTERAL PUMPS

Submit documentation of the need for the infusion pump. Medicare will reimburse for the simplest model that meets the patient's needs.

Ⓨ **B9000** Enteral nutrition infusion pump — without alarm &

MED: 100-2,15,120; 100-3,180.2; 100-4,20,100.2.2

Ⓨ **B9002** Enteral nutrition infusion pump — with alarm &

MED: 100-2,15,120; 100-3,180.2; 100-4,20,100.2.2

Ⓨ **B9004** Parenteral nutrition infusion pump, portable &

MED: 100-2,15,120; 100-3,180.2; 100-4,3,10.4; 100-4,20,100.2.2

Ⓨ **B9006** Parenteral nutrition infusion pump, stationary &

MED: 100-2,15,120; 100-3,180.2; 100-4,3,10.4; 100-4,20,100.2.2

Ⓨ **B9998** NOC for enteral supplies &

MED: 100-2,15,120; 100-3,180.2; 100-4,3,10.4; 100-4,20,100.2.2

Ⓨ **B9999** NOC for parenteral supplies &
Determine if an alternative HCPCS Level II or a CPT code better describes the service being reported. This code should be used only if a more specific code is unavailable.

MED: 100-2,15,120; 100-3,180.2; 100-4,3,10.4; 100-4,20,100.2.2

Special Coverage Instructions ▫ Noncovered by Medicare ▫ Carrier Discretion ☑ Quantity Alert ● New Code ○ Recycled/Reinstated ▲ Revised Code

**20 — B Codes** Ⓐ Age Edit Ⓜ Maternity Edit ♀ Female Only ♂ Male Only Ⓐ-Ⓨ OPPS Status Indicators **2008 HCPCS**

## OUTPATIENT PPS C1000-C9999

This section reports drugs, biologicals, and devices codes that must be used by OPPS hospitals. Non-OPPS hospitals, Critical Access Hospitals (CAHs), Indian Health Service Hospitals (HIS), hospitals located in American Samoa, Guam, Saipan, or the Virgin Islands, and Maryland waiver hospitals may report these codes at their discretion.  The codes can only be reported for facility (technical) services. The C series of HCPCS may include device catagories, new technology procedures, and drugs, biologicals and radiopharmaceuticals that do not have other HCPCS codes assigned. Some of these items and services are eligible for transitional pass-through payments for OPPS hospitals, have separate APC payments, or are items that are packag Hospitals are encouraged to report all appropriate C codes regardless of payment status.

[S] ☑ **C1300** Hyperbaric oxygen under pressure, full body chamber, per 30 minute interval
MED: 100-4,32,30.1

[N] **C1713** Anchor/screw for opposing bone-to-bone or soft tissue-to-bone (implantable) [N1]
MED: 100-4,4,61.1
AHA: 3Q,'02,5; 1Q,'01,5

[N] **C1714** Catheter, transluminal atherectomy, directional [N1]
MED: 100-4,4,61.1; 100-4,4,61.2
AHA: 4Q,'03,8; 3Q,'02,5; 1Q,'01,5

[N] **C1715** Brachytherapy needle [N1] ⊘
MED: 100-4,4,61.1
AHA: 3Q,'02,5; 1Q,'01,5

▲ [K] ☑ **C1716** Brachytherapy source, nonstranded, gold-198, per source [H2] ⊘
MED: 100-4,4,61.1
AHA: 3Q,'02,5; 1Q,'01,5

▲ [K] ☑ **C1717** Brachytherapy source, nonstranded, high dose rate iridium-192, per source [H2] ⊘
MED: 100-4,4,61.1
AHA: 3Q,'02,5; 1Q,'01,5

~~C1718 Brachytherapy source, iodine-125, per source~~
See code(s) C2638-C2639.

AHA: 1Q,'04,2; 3Q,'02,5; 1Q,'01,5

▲ [K] ☑ **C1719** Brachytherapy source, nonstranded, nonhigh dose rate iridium-192, per source [H2] ⊘
MED: 100-4,4,61.1
AHA: 3Q,'02,5; 1Q,'01,5

~~C1720 Brachytherapy source, palladium-103, per source~~
See code(s) C2640-C2641.

AHA: 1Q,'04,2; 3Q,'02,5; 1Q,'01,5

[N] **C1721** Cardioverter-defibrillator, dual chamber (implantable) [N1]
MED: 100-4,4,61.1; 100-4,4,61.2
AHA: 3Q,'02,5; 1Q,'01,5

[N] **C1722** Cardioverter-defibrillator, single chamber (implantable) [N1]
MED: 100-4,4,61.1; 100-4,4,61.2
AHA: 3Q,'02,5; 1Q,'01,5

[N] **C1724** Catheter, transluminal atherectomy, rotational [N1]
MED: 100-4,4,61.1; 100-4,4,61.2
AHA: 4Q,'03,8; 3Q,'02,5; 1Q,'01,5

[N] **C1725** Catheter, transluminal angioplasty, nonlaser (may include guidance, infusion/perfusion capability) [N1]
MED: 100-4,4,61.1; 100-4,4,61.2
AHA: 4Q,'03,8; 3Q,'02,5; 1Q,'01,5

[N] **C1726** Catheter, balloon dilatation, nonvascular [N1]
MED: 100-4,4,61.1
AHA: 3Q,'02,5; 1Q,'01,5

[N] **C1727** Catheter, balloon tissue dissector, nonvascular (insertable) [N1]
MED: 100-4,4,61.1
AHA: 3Q,'02,5; 1Q,'01,5

○ [N] **C1728** Catheter, brachytherapy seed administration [N1] ⊘
MED: 100-4,4,61.1
AHA: 3Q,'02,5; 1Q,'01,5

[N] **C1729** Catheter, drainage [N1]
MED: 100-4,4,61.1
AHA: 3Q,'02,5; 1Q,'01,5

[N] **C1730** Catheter, electrophysiology, diagnostic, other than 3D mapping (19 or fewer electrodes) [N1]
MED: 100-4,4,61.1; 100-4,4,61.2
AHA: 3Q,'02,5; 1Q,'01,5

[N] **C1731** Catheter, electrophysiology, diagnostic, other than 3D mapping (20 or more electrodes) [N1]
MED: 100-4,4,61.1; 100-4,4,61.2
AHA: 3Q,'02,5; 1Q,'01,5

[N] **C1732** Catheter, electrophysiology, diagnostic/ablation, 3D or vector mapping [N1]
MED: 100-4,4,61.1; 100-4,4,61.2
AHA: 1Q,'01,5

[N] **C1733** Catheter, electrophysiology, diagnostic/ablation, other than 3D or vector mapping, other than cool-tip [N1]
MED: 100-4,4,61.1; 100-4,4,61.2
AHA: 3Q,'02,5; 1Q,'01,5

[N] **C1750** Catheter, hemodialysis/peritoneal, long-term [N1]
MED: 100-4,4,61.1
AHA: 4Q,'03,8; 3Q,'02,5; 1Q,'01,5

[N] **C1751** Catheter, infusion, inserted peripherally, centrally or midline (other than hemodialysis) [N1]
MED: 100-4,4,61.1; 100-4,4,61.2
AHA: 4Q,'03,8; 3Q,'02,5; 3Q,'01,5

[N] **C1752** Catheter, hemodialysis/peritoneal, short-term [N1]
MED: 100-4,4,61.1
AHA: 4Q,'03,8; 3Q,'02,5; 1Q,'01,5

[N] **C1753** Catheter, intravascular ultrasound [N1]
MED: 100-4,4,61.1
AHA: 4Q,'03,8; 3Q,'02,5; 1Q,'01,5

[N] **C1754** Catheter, intradiscal [N1]
MED: 100-4,4,61.1
AHA: 4Q,'03,8; 3Q,'02,5; 1Q,'01,5

[N] **C1755** Catheter, intraspinal [N1]
MED: 100-4,4,61.1
AHA: 4Q,'03,8; 3Q,'02,5; 1Q,'01,5

[N] **C1756** Catheter, pacing, transesophageal [N1]
MED: 100-4,4,61.1
AHA: 4Q,'03,8; 3Q,'02,5; 1Q,'01,5

[N] **C1757** Catheter, thrombectomy/embolectomy [N1]
MED: 100-4,4,61.1; 100-4,4,61.2
AHA: 4Q,'03,8; 3Q,'02,5; 1Q,'01,5

[N] **C1758** Catheter, ureteral [N1]
MED: 100-4,4,61.1
AHA: 4Q,'03,8; 3Q,'02,5; 1Q,'01,6

[N] **C1759** Catheter, intracardiac echocardiography [N1]
MED: 100-4,4,61.1
AHA: 4Q,'03,8; 3Q,'02,5; 1Q,'01,5; 3Q,'01,4

[N] **C1760** Closure device, vascular (implantable/insertable) [N1]
MED: 100-4,4,61.1
AHA: 4Q,'03,8; 3Q,'02,5; 1Q,'01,6

[N] **C1762** Connective tissue, human (includes fascia lata) [N1]
MED: 100-4,4,61.1
AHA: 3Q,'03,12; 4Q,'03,8; 3Q,'02,5; 1Q,'01,6

---

Special Coverage Instructions Noncovered by Medicare Carrier Discretion  ☑ Quantity Alert ● New Code ○ Recycled/Reinstated ▲ Revised Code

**Outpatient PPS**

**C1763 — C1878**

[N] **C1763** Connective tissue, nonhuman (includes synthetic) [M]
MED: 100-4,4,61.1
AHA: 3Q,'03,12; 4Q,'03,8; 3Q,'02,5; 1Q,'01,6

[N] **C1764** Event recorder, cardiac (implantable) [N1]
MED: 100-4,4,61.1
AHA: 4Q,'03,8; 3Q,'02,5; 1Q,'01,6

[N] **C1765** Adhesion barrier [N1]
MED: 100-4,4,61.1

[N] **C1766** Introducer/sheath, guiding, intracardiac electrophysiological, steerable, other than peel-away [N1]
MED: 100-4,4,61.1; 100-4,4,61.2
AHA: 3Q,'02,5; 3Q,'01,5

[N] **C1767** Generator, neurostimulator (implantable), nonrechargeable [N1]
MED: 100-4,4,61.1; 100-4,4,61.2
AHA: 4Q,'03,8; 1Q,'02,9; 3Q,'02,5

[N] **C1768** Graft, vascular [N1]
MED: 100-4,4,61.1
AHA: 4Q,'03,8; 3Q,'02,5; 1Q,'01,6

[N] **C1769** Guide wire [N1]
MED: 100-4,4,61.1
AHA: 4Q,'03,8; 3Q,'02,5; 1Q,'01,6; 3Q,'01,4

[N] **C1770** Imaging coil, magnetic resonance (insertable) [N1]
MED: 100-4,4,61.1
AHA: 4Q,'03,8; 3Q,'02,5; 1Q,'01,6

[N] **C1771** Repair device, urinary, incontinence, with sling graft [N1]
MED: 100-4,4,61.1
AHA: 4Q,'03,8; 3Q,'02,5; 1Q,'01,6

[N] **C1772** Infusion pump, programmable (implantable) [N1]
MED: 100-4,4,61.1; 100-4,4,61.2
AHA: 3Q,'02,5; 1Q,'01,6

[N] **C1773** Retrieval device, insertable (used to retrieve fractured medical devices) [N1]
MED: 100-4,4,61.1
AHA: 4Q,'03,8; 3Q,'02,5; 1Q,'01,6

[N] **C1776** Joint device (implantable) [N1]
MED: 100-4,4,61.1; 100-4,4,61.2
AHA: 3Q,'02,5; 1Q,'01,6; 3Q,'01,5

[N] **C1777** Lead, cardioverter-defibrillator, endocardial single coil (implantable) [N1]
MED: 100-4,4,61.1; 100-4,4,61.2
AHA: 3Q,'02,5; 1Q,'01,6

[N] **C1778** Lead, neurostimulator (implantable) [N1]
MED: 100-4,4,61.1
AHA: 3Q,'02,5; 1Q,'02,9

[N] **C1779** Lead, pacemaker, transvenous VDD single pass [N1]
MED: 100-4,4,61.1; 100-4,4,61.2
AHA: 3Q,'02,5; 1Q,'01,6

[N] **C1780** Lens, intraocular (new technology) [N1]
MED: 100-4,4,61.1
AHA: 3Q,'02,5; 1Q,'01,6

[N] **C1781** Mesh (implantable) [N1]
MED: 100-4,4,61.1
AHA: 3Q,'02,5; 1Q,'01,6

[N] **C1782** Morcellator [N1]
MED: 100-4,4,61.1
AHA: 3Q,'02,5; 1Q,'01,6

[N] **C1783** Ocular implant, aqueous drainage assist device [N1]
MED: 100-4,4,61.1

[N] **C1784** Ocular device, intraoperative, detached retina [N1]
MED: 100-4,4,61.1
AHA: 3Q,'02,5; 1Q,'01,6

[N] **C1785** Pacemaker, dual chamber, rate-responsive (implantable) [N1]
MED: 100-4,3,10.4; 100-4,4,61.1
AHA: 4Q,'03,8; 3Q,'02,5; 1Q,'01,6

[N] **C1786** Pacemaker, single chamber, rate-responsive (implantable) [N1]
MED: 100-2,1,40; 100-4,4,61.1; 100-4,4,61.2
AHA: 4Q,'03,8; 3Q,'02,5; 1Q,'01,6

[N] **C1787** Patient programmer, neurostimulator [N1]
MED: 100-4,4,61.1
AHA: 4Q,'03,8; 3Q,'02,5; 1Q,'01,6

[N] **C1788** Port, indwelling (implantable) [N1]
MED: 100-4,4,61.1; 100-4,4,61.2
AHA: 4Q,'03,8; 3Q,'02,5; 1Q,'01,6; 3Q,'01,4

[N] **C1789** Prosthesis, breast (implantable) [N1]
MED: 100-4,4,61.1
AHA: 4Q,'03,8; 3Q,'02,5; 1Q,'01,6

[N] **C1813** Prosthesis, penile, inflatable [N1]
MED: 100-4,4,61.1
AHA: 4Q,'03,8; 3Q,'02,5; 1Q,'01,6

[N] **C1814** Retinal tamponade device, silicone oil [N1]
MED: 100-4,4,61.1

[N] **C1815** Prosthesis, urinary sphincter (implantable) [N1]
MED: 100-4,4,61.1
AHA: 4Q,'03,8; 3Q,'02,5; 1Q,'01,6

[N] **C1816** Receiver and/or transmitter, neurostimulator (implantable) [N1]
MED: 100-4,4,61.1
AHA: 4Q,'03,8; 3Q,'02,5; 1Q,'01,6

[N] **C1817** Septal defect implant system, intracardiac [N1]
MED: 100-4,4,61.1
AHA: 4Q,'03,8; 3Q,'02,5; 1Q,'01,6

[N] **C1818** Integrated keratoprosthesis [N1]
MED: 100-4,4,61.1
AHA: 4Q,'03,4

[N] **C1819** Surgical tissue localization and excision device (implantable) [N1]
MED: 100-4,4,61.1

[N] **C1820** Generator, neurostimulator (implantable), with rechargeable battery and charging system [N1]
MED: 100-4,4,10.12

[H] **C1821** Interspinous process distraction device (implantable) [J7]

[N] **C1874** Stent, coated/covered, with delivery system [N1]
MED: 100-4,4,61.1; 100-4,4,61.2
AHA: 4Q,'03,8; 1Q,'01,6

[N] **C1875** Stent, coated/covered, without delivery system [N1]
MED: 100-4,4,61.1; 100-4,4,61.2
AHA: 4Q,'03,8; 1Q,'01,6

[N] **C1876** Stent, noncoated/noncovered, with delivery system [N1]
MED: 100-4,4,61.1; 100-4,4,61.2
AHA: 4Q,'03,8; 3Q,'02,5; 1Q,'01,6; 3Q,'01,4

[N] **C1877** Stent, noncoated/noncovered, without delivery system [N1]
MED: 100-4,4,61.1; 100-4,4,61.2
AHA: 4Q,'03,8; 3Q,'02,5; 1Q,'01,6; 3Q,'01,4

[N] **C1878** Material for vocal cord medialization, synthetic (implantable) [N1]
MED: 100-4,4,61.1
AHA: 3Q,'02,5; 1Q,'01,6

Special Coverage Instructions    Noncovered by Medicare    Carrier Discretion    ☑ Quantity Alert    ● New Code    ○ Recycled/Reinstated    ▲ Revised Code

**22 — C Codes**    [A] Age Edit    [M] Maternity Edit    ♀ Female Only    ♂ Male Only    [A]-[Y] OPPS Status Indicators    **2008 HCPCS**

N | **C1879** Tissue marker (implantable) | N1
MED: 100-4,4,61.1
AHA: 4Q,'03,8; 3Q,'02,5; 1Q,'01,6

N | **C1880** Vena cava filter | N1
MED: 100-4,4,61.1
AHA: 4Q,'03,8; 3Q,'02,5; 1Q,'01,6

N | **C1881** Dialysis access system (implantable) | N1
MED: 100-4,4,61.1
AHA: 4Q,'03,8; 3Q,'02,5; 1Q,'01,6

N | **C1882** Cardioverter-defibrillator, other than single or dual chamber (implantable) | N1
MED: 100-4,4,61.1; 100-4,4,61.2
AHA: 3Q,'02,5; 1Q,'01,5

N | **C1883** Adaptor/extension, pacing lead or neurostimulator lead (implantable) | N1
MED: 100-4,4,61.1
AHA: 1Q,'02,9; 3Q,'02,5; 1Q,'01,5

N | **C1884** Embolization protective system | N1
MED: 100-4,4,61.1

N | **C1885** Catheter, transluminal angioplasty, laser | N1
MED: 100-4,4,61.1; 100-4,4,61.2
AHA: 4Q,'03,8; 3Q,'02,5; 1Q,'01,5

N | **C1887** Catheter, guiding (may include infusion/perfusion capability) | N1
MED: 100-4,4,61.1; 100-4,4,61.2
AHA: 3Q,'02,5; 1Q,'01,5

N | **C1888** Catheter, ablation, noncardiac, endovascular (implantable) | N1
MED: 100-4,4,61.1

N | **C1891** Infusion pump, nonprogrammable, permanent (implantable) | N1
MED: 100-4,4,61.1; 100-4,4,61.2
AHA: 4Q,'03,8; 3Q,'02,5; 1Q,'01,6

N | **C1892** Introducer/sheath, guiding, intracardiac electrophysiological, fixed-curve, peel-away | N1
MED: 100-4,4,61.1; 100-4,4,61.2
AHA: 3Q,'02,5; 1Q,'01,6

N | **C1893** Introducer/sheath, guiding, intracardiac electrophysiological, fixed-curve, other than peel-away | N1
MED: 100-4,4,61.1; 100-4,4,61.2
AHA: 3Q,'02,5; 1Q,'01,6; 3Q,'01,4

N | **C1894** Introducer/sheath, other than guiding, other than intracardiac electrophysiological, nonlaser | N1
MED: 100-4,4,61.1; 100-4,4,61.2
AHA: 3Q,'02,5

N | **C1895** Lead, cardioverter-defibrillator, endocardial dual coil (implantable) | N1
MED: 100-4,4,61.1; 100-4,4,61.2
AHA: 3Q,'02,5; 1Q,'01,6

N | **C1896** Lead, cardioverter-defibrillator, other than endocardial single or dual coil (implantable) | N1
MED: 100-4,4,61.1; 100-4,4,61.2
AHA: 3Q,'02,5; 1Q,'01,6

N | **C1897** Lead, neurostimulator test kit (implantable) | N1
MED: 100-4,4,61.1
AHA: 1Q,'02,9; 3Q,'02,5; 1Q,'01,6

N | **C1898** Lead, pacemaker, other than transvenous VDD single pass | N1
MED: 100-4,4,61.1
AHA: 1Q,'01,6; 3Q,'01,4

N | **C1899** Lead, pacemaker/cardioverter-defibrillator combination (implantable) | N1
MED: 100-4,4,61.1; 100-4,4,61.2
AHA: 3Q,'02,5; 1Q,'01,6

N | **C1900** Lead, left ventricular coronary venous system | N1
MED: 100-4,4,61.1; 100-4,4,61.2

N | **C2614** Probe, percutaneous lumbar discectomy | N1
MED: 100-4,4,61.1

N | **C2615** Sealant, pulmonary, liquid | N1
MED: 100-4,4,61.1
AHA: 3Q,'02,5; 1Q,'01,6

▲ K ☑ | **C2616** Brachytherapy source, nonstranded, yttrium-90, per source | H2 ⊘
MED: 100-4,4,61.1
AHA: 3Q,'03,11; 3Q,'02,5

N | **C2617** Stent, noncoronary, temporary, without delivery system | N1
MED: 100-4,4,61.1; 100-4,4,61.2
AHA: 4Q,'03,8; 3Q,'02,5; 1Q,'01,6

N | **C2618** Probe, cryoablation | N1
MED: 100-4,4,61.1; 100-4,4,61.2
AHA: 4Q,'03,8; 3Q,'02,5; 1Q,'01,6

N | **C2619** Pacemaker, dual chamber, nonrate-responsive (implantable) | N1
MED: 100-4,4,61.1
AHA: 3Q,'02,5; 1Q,'01,6; 3Q,'01,4

N | **C2620** Pacemaker, single chamber, nonrate-responsive (implantable) | N1
MED: 100-4,3,10.4; 100-4,4,61.1; 100-4,4,61.2
AHA: 4Q,'03,8; 3Q,'02,5; 1Q,'01,6

N | **C2621** Pacemaker, other than single or dual chamber (implantable) | N1
MED: 100-4,3,10.4; 100-4,4,61.1
AHA: 4Q,'03,8; 1Q,'01,6

N | **C2622** Prosthesis, penile, noninflatable | N1
MED: 100-4,4,61.1
AHA: 4Q,'03,8; 3Q,'02,5; 1Q,'01,6

N | **C2625** Stent, noncoronary, temporary, with delivery system | N1
MED: 100-4,4,61.1; 100-4,4,61.2
AHA: 4Q,'03,8; 3Q,'02,5; 1Q,'01,6

N | **C2626** Infusion pump, nonprogrammable, temporary (implantable) | N1
MED: 100-4,4,61.1; 100-4,4,61.2
AHA: 3Q,'02,5; 1Q,'01,6

N | **C2627** Catheter, suprapubic/cystoscopic | N1
MED: 100-4,4,61.1
AHA: 4Q,'03,8; 3Q,'02,5; 1Q,'01,5

N | **C2628** Catheter, occlusion | N1
MED: 100-4,4,61.1; 100-4,4,61.2
AHA: 4Q,'03,8; 3Q,'02,5; 1Q,'01,5

N | **C2629** Introducer/sheath, other than guiding, intracardiac electrophysiological, laser | N1
MED: 100-4,4,61.1
AHA: 3Q,'02,5; 1Q,'01,6

N | **C2630** Catheter, electrophysiology, diagnostic/ablation, other than 3D or vector mapping, cool-tip | N1
MED: 100-4,4,61.1
AHA: 3Q,'02,5; 1Q,'01,5

N | **C2631** Repair device, urinary, incontinence, without sling graft | N1
MED: 100-4,4,61.1
AHA: 4Q,'03,8; 3Q,'02,5; 1Q,'01,6

---

Special Coverage Instructions | Noncovered by Medicare | Carrier Discretion | ☑ Quantity Alert | ● New Code | ○ Recycled/Reinstated | ▲ Revised Code

**Outpatient PPS**

**C2633 — C9003**

C2633  ~~Brachytherapy source, cesium-131, per source~~
See code(s) C2642-C2643.

▲ K ☑ C2634  Brachytherapy source, nonstranded, high activity, iodine-125, greater than 1.01 mCi (NIST), per source H2 ⊘
MED: 100-4,4,61.1
AHA: 2Q,'05,8

▲ K ☑ C2635  Brachytherapy source, nonstranded, high activity, palladium-103, greater than 2.2 mCi (NIST), per source H2 ⊘
MED: 100-4,4,61.1
AHA: 2Q,'05,8

▲ K ☑ C2636  Brachytherapy linear source, nonstranded, palladium-103, per 1 mm H2 ⊘
MED: 100-4,4,61.1

▲ B ☑ C2637  Brachytherapy source, nonstranded, ytterbium-169, per source ⊘
AHA: 3Q,'05,7

● K ☑ C2638  Brachytherapy source, stranded, iodine-125, per source H2

● K ☑ C2639  Brachytherapy source, nonstranded, iodine-125, per source H2

● K ☑ C2640  Brachytherapy source, stranded, palladium-103, per source H2

● K ☑ C2641  Brachytherapy source, nonstranded, palladium-103, per source H2

● K ☑ C2642  Brachytherapy source, stranded, cesium-131, per source H2

● K ☑ C2643  Brachytherapy source, nonstranded, cesium-131, per source H2

● K ☑ C2698  Brachytherapy source, stranded, not otherwise specified, per source H2

● K ☑ C2699  Brachytherapy source, nonstranded, not otherwise specified, per source H2

S C8900  Magnetic resonance angiography with contrast, abdomen Z2 ⊘
MED: 100-4,13,40.1.2

S C8901  Magnetic resonance angiography without contrast, abdomen Z2 ⊘
MED: 100-4,13,40.1.2

S C8902  Magnetic resonance angiography without contrast followed by with contrast, abdomen Z2 ⊘
MED: 100-4,13,40.1.2

S C8903  Magnetic resonance imaging with contrast, breast; unilateral Z2 ⊘

S C8904  Magnetic resonance imaging without contrast, breast; unilateral Z2 ⊘

S C8905  Magnetic resonance imaging without contrast followed by with contrast, breast; unilateral Z2 ⊘

S C8906  Magnetic resonance imaging with contrast, breast; bilateral Z2 ⊘

S C8907  Magnetic resonance imaging without contrast, breast; bilateral Z2 ⊘

S C8908  Magnetic resonance imaging without contrast followed by with contrast, breast; bilateral Z2 ⊘

S C8909  Magnetic resonance angiography with contrast, chest (excluding myocardium) Z2 ⊘
MED: 100-4,13,40.1.2

S C8910  Magnetic resonance angiography without contrast, chest (excluding myocardium) Z2 ⊘
MED: 100-4,13,40.1.2

S C8911  Magnetic resonance angiography without contrast followed by with contrast, chest (excluding myocardium) Z2 ⊘
MED: 100-4,13,40.1.2

S C8912  Magnetic resonance angiography with contrast, lower extremity Z2 ⊘
MED: 100-4,13,40.1.2

S C8913  Magnetic resonance angiography without contrast, lower extremity Z2 ⊘
MED: 100-4,13,40.1.2

S C8914  Magnetic resonance angiography without contrast followed by with contrast, lower extremity Z2 ⊘
MED: 100-4,13,40.1.2

S C8918  Magnetic resonance angiography with contrast, pelvis Z2 ⊘
MED: 100-4,13,40.1.2

S C8919  Magnetic resonance angiography without contrast, pelvis Z2 ⊘
MED: 100-4,13,40.1.2
AHA: 4Q,'03,4

S C8920  Magnetic resonance angiography without contrast followed by with contrast, pelvis Z2 ⊘
MED: 100-4,13,40.1.2
AHA: 4Q,'03,4

● S C8921  Transthoracic echocardiography with contrast for congenital cardiac anomalies; complete

● S C8922  Transthoracic echocardiography with contrast for congenital cardiac anomalies; follow-up or limited study

● S C8923  Transthoracic echocardiography with contrast, real-time with image documentation (2D) with or without M-mode recording; complete

● S C8924  Transthoracic echocardiography with contrast, real-time with image documentation (2D) with or without M-mode recording; follow-up or limited study

● S C8925  Transesophageal echocardiography (TEE) with contrast, real time with image documentation (2D) (with or without M-mode recording); including probe placement, image acquisition, interpretation and report

● S C8926  Transesophageal echocardiography (TEE) with contrast for congenital cardiac anomalies; including probe placement, image acquisition, interpretation and report

● S C8927  Transesophageal echocardiography (TEE) with contrast for monitoring purposes, including probe placement, real time 2-dimensional image acquisition and interpretation leading to ongoing (continuous) assessment of (dynamically changing) cardiac pumping function and to therapeutic measures on an immediate time basis

● S C8928  Transthoracic echocardiography with contrast, real time with image documentation (2D), with or without M-mode recording, during rest and cardiovascular stress test using treadmill, bicycle exercise and/or pharmacologically induced stress, with interpretation and report

S C8957  Intravenous infusion for therapy/diagnosis; initiation of prolonged infusion (more than eight hours), requiring use of portable or implantable pump
MED: 100-4,4,230.2.1; 100-4,4,230.2.3

K ☑ C9003  Palivizumab-RSV-IgM, per 50 mg K2
Use this code for Synagis.

N     **C9113**   Injection, pantoprazole sodium, per vial    N1
Use this code for Protonix.

K ☑   **C9121**   Injection, argatroban, per 5 mg    K2

~~C9232~~   ~~Injection, idursulfase, 1 mg~~
See J1743.

~~C9233~~   ~~Injection, ranibizumab, 0.5 mg~~
See J2778.

~~C9234~~   ~~Injection, alglucosidase alfa, 10 mg~~
See J0220.

~~C9235~~   ~~Injection, panitumumab, 10 mg~~
See J9303.

~~C9236~~   ~~Injection, eculizumab, 10 mg~~
See J1300.

● ☑   C9237   Injection, lanreotide acetate, 1 mg

● K ☑☑   **C9238**   Injection, levetiracetam, 10 mg
Use this code for Keppra.

● G ☑   **C9239**   Injection, temsirolimus, 1 mg
Use this code for Torisel.

● ☑   C9240   Injection, ixabepilone, 1 mg
Use this code for Ixempra.

~~C9350~~   ~~Microporous collagen tube of nonhuman origin, per centimeter length~~
See C9352-C9353.

~~C9351~~   ~~Acellular dermal tissue matrix of nonhuman origin, per square centimeter (Do not report C9351 in conjunction with J7345)~~
J4348-J4349.

● G ☑   **C9352**   Microporous collagen implantable tube (NeuraGen Nerve Guide), per cm. length

● G ☑   **C9353**   Microporous collagen implantable slit tube (NeuraWrap Nerve Protector), per cm. length

● ☑   C9354   Acellular pericardial tissue matrix of nonhuman origin (Veritas), per square centimeter

● ☑   C9355   Collagen nerve cuff (NeuroMatrix), per 0.5 centimeter length

A    **C9399**   Unclassified drugs or biologicals    K7

T    **C9716**   Creations of thermal anal lesions by radiofrequency energy    G2

S    **C9723**   Dynamic infrared blood perfusion imaging (DIRI)

T    **C9724**   Endoscopic full-thickness plication in the gastric cardia using endoscopic plication system (EPS); includes endoscopy    G2

S    **C9725**   Placement of endorectal intracavitary applicator for high intensity brachytherapy    G2 ⊘
AHA: 3Q,'05,7

S    **C9726**   Placement and removal (if performed) of applicator into breast for radiation therapy    G2

S ☑   **C9727**   Insertion of implants into the soft palate; minimum of three implants    G2

● T    **C9728**   Placement of interstitial device(s) for radiation therapy/surgery guidance (eg, fiducial markers, dosimeter), other than prostate (any approach), single or multiple    R2

Special Coverage Instructions    Noncovered by Medicare    Carrier Discretion    ☑ Quantity Alert    ● New Code    ○ Recycled/Reinstated    ▲ Revised Code

**2008 HCPCS**    R2-Z3 ASC Payment Indicators    **MED:** Pub 100/NCD References    ⚕ DMEPOS Paid    ⊘ SNF Excluded    P0 PQRI    **C Codes — 25**

## DENTAL PROCEDURES D0000–D9999

The D, or dental, codes are a separate category of national codes. The Current Dental Terminology (CDT-2007/2008) code set is copyrighted by the American Dental Association (ADA). CDT-2007/2008 is included in HCPCS Level II. Decisions regarding the modification, deletion, or addition of CDT-2007/2008 codes are made by the ADA and not the national panel responsible for the administration of HCPCS.

The Department of Health and Human Services has an agreement with the AMA pertaining to the use of the CPT codes for physician services; it also has an agreement with the ADA to include CDT-2007/2008 as a set of HCPCS Level II codes for use in billing for dental services.

Please refer to you CPT book for possible alternate code(s).

## DIAGNOSTIC D0100–D0999

### CLINICAL ORAL EVALUATION

**E** **D0120** Periodic oral evaluation — established patient

This procedure is covered if its purpose is to identify a patient's existing infections prior to kidney transplantation.

**E** **D0140** Limited oral evaluation — problem focused

**E** **D0145** Oral evaluation for a patient under three years of age and counseling with primary caregiver

**S** **D0150** Comprehensive oral evaluation — new or established patient ⊘

This procedure is covered if its purpose is to identify a patient's existing infections prior to kidney transplantation.

MED: 100-2,15,150; 100-2,16,140; 100-3,260.6; 100-4,4,20.5

**E** **D0160** Detailed and extensive oral evaluation — problem focused, by report

Pertinent documentation to evaluate medical appropriateness should be included when this code is reported.

**E** **D0170** Re-evaluation — limited, problem focused (established patient; not postoperative visit)

**E** **D0180** Comprehensive periodontal evaluation — new or established patient

See also equivalent CPT E&M codes.

### RADIOGRAPHS

**E** **D0210** Intraoral — complete series (including bitewings)

**E** ☑ **D0220** Intraoral — periapical, first film

**E** ☑ **D0230** Intraoral — periapical, each additional film

**S** **D0240** Intraoral — occlusal film ⊘

MED: 100-2,15,150; 100-2,16,140; 100-4,4,20.5

**S** ☑ **D0250** Extraoral — first film ⊘

MED: 100-2,15,150; 100-2,16,140; 100-4,4,20.5

**S** ☑ **D0260** Extraoral — each additional film ⊘

MED: 100-2,15,150; 100-2,16,140; 100-4,4,20.5

**S** ☑ **D0270** Bitewing — single film ⊘

MED: 100-2,15,150; 100-2,16,140; 100-4,4,20.5

**S** ☑ **D0272** Bitewings — two films ⊘

MED: 100-2,15,150; 100-2,16,140; 100-4,4,20.5

**E** **D0273** Bitewings — three films

**S** ☑ **D0274** Bitewings — four films ⊘

MED: 100-2,15,150; 100-2,16,140; 100-4,4,20.5

**S** ☑ **D0277** Vertical bitewings - 7 to 8 films

MED: 100-2,15,150; 100-2,16,140; 100-4,4,20.5

**E** **D0290** Posterior-anterior or lateral skull and facial bone survey film

**E** **D0310** Sialography

**E** **D0320** Temporomandibular joint arthrogram, including injection

**E** **D0321** Other temporomandibular joint films, by report

**E** **D0322** Tomographic survey

MED: 100-3,260.6

**E** **D0330** Panoramic film

**E** **D0340** Cephalometric film

**E** **D0350** Oral/facial photographic images

This code excludes conventional radiographs.

**E** **D0360** Cone beam CT — craniofacial data capture

**E** **D0362** Cone beam — two-dimensional image reconstruction using existing data, includes multiple images

**E** **D0363** Cone beam — three-dimensional image reconstruction using existing data, includes multiple images

### TEST AND LABORATORY EXAMINATIONS

**E** **D0415** Collection of microorganisms for culture and sensitivity

This procedure is covered if its purpose is to identify a patient's existing infections prior to kidney transplantation.

See code(s): D0410

**B** **D0416** Viral culture

**B** **D0421** Genetic test for susceptibility to oral diseases

**E** **D0425** Caries susceptibility tests

This procedure is covered by Medicare if its purpose is to identify a patient's existing infections prior to kidney transplantation.

**B** **D0431** Adjunctive pre-diagnostic test that aids In detection of mucosal abnormalities including premalignant and malignant lesions, not to include cytology or biopsy procedures

**S** **D0460** Pulp vitality tests ⊘

This procedure is covered by Medicare if its purpose is to identify a patient's existing infections prior to kidney transplantation.

MED: 100-2,15,150; 100-2,16,140; 100-3,260.6; 100-4,4,20.5

**E** **D0470** Diagnostic casts

**B** **D0472** Accession of tissue, gross examination, preparation, and transmission of written report

MED: 100-2,15,150; 100-2,16,140; 100-3,260.6; 100-4,4,20.5

**B** **D0473** Accession of tissue, gross and microscopic examination, preparation and transmission of written report

MED: 100-2,15,150; 100-2,16,140; 100-3,260.6; 100-4,4,20.5

**B** **D0474** Accession of tissue, gross and microscopic examination, including assessment of surgical margins for presence of disease, preparation and transmission of written report

MED: 100-2,15,150; 100-2,16,140; 100-3,260.6; 100-4,4,20.5

**B** **D0475** Decalcification procedure

MED: 100-4,4,20.5

**B** **D0476** Special stains for microorganisms

MED: 100-4,4,20.5

**B** **D0477** Special stains, not for microorganisms

MED: 100-4,4,20.5

**B** **D0478** Immunohistochemical stains

MED: 100-4,4,20.5

---

Special Coverage Instructions    Noncovered by Medicare    Carrier Discretion    ☑ Quantity Alert    ● New Code    ○ Recycled/Reinstated    ▲ Revised Code

**2008 HCPCS**    N2–N1 ASC Payment Indicators    **MED:** Pub 100/NCD References    ☒ DMEPOS Paid    ⊘ SNF Excluded    PQRI PQRI    **D Codes — 27**

**D0120 — D0478**

**Dental Procedures**

**D0479 — D2662**

B **D0479** Tissue in-situ hybridization, including interpretation

MED: 100-4,4,20.5

B **D0480** Accession of exfoliative cytologic smears, microscopic examination, preparation and transmission of written report

MED: 100-2,15,150; 100-2,16,140; 100-3,260.6; 100-4,4,20.5

B **D0481** Electron microscopy - diagnostic

MED: 100-4,4,20.5

B **D0482** Direct immunofluorescence

MED: 100-4,4,20.5

B **D0483** Indirect immunofluorescence

MED: 100-4,4,20.5

B **D0484** Consultation on slides prepared elsewhere

MED: 100-4,4,20.5

B **D0485** Consultation, including preparation of slides from biopsy material supplied by referring source

MED: 100-4,4,20.5

E **D0486** Accession of brush biopsy sample, microscopic examination, preparation and transmission of written report

B **D0502** Other oral pathology procedures, by report  ⊘

Pertinent documentation to evaluate medical appropriateness should be included when this code is reported. This procedure is covered by Medicare if its purpose is to identify a patient's existing infections prior to kidney transplantation.

MED: 100-2,15,150; 100-2,16,140; 100-3,260.6; 100-4,4,20.5

B **D0999** Unspecified diagnostic procedure, by report  ⊘

Determine if an alternative HCPCS Level II or a CPT code better describes the service being reported. This code should be used only if a more specific code is unavailable.

MED: 100-2,15,150; 100-2,16,140; 100-3,260.6; 100-4,4,20.5

## PREVENTIVE D1000-D1999

### DENTAL PROPHYLAXIS

E **D1110** Prophylaxis — adult  A

E **D1120** Prophylaxis — child  A

### TOPICAL FLUORIDE TREATMENT (OFFICE PROCEDURE)

E **D1203** Topical application of fluoride (prophylaxis not included) — child  A

E **D1204** Topical application of fluoride (prophylaxis not included) — adult  A

E **D1206** Topical fluoride varnish; therapeutic application for moderate to high caries risk patients

### OTHER PREVENTIVE SERVICES

E **D1310** Nutritional counseling for the control of dental disease

MED: 100-2,16,10

E **D1320** Tobacco counseling for the control and prevention of oral disease

MED: 100-2,16,10

E **D1330** Oral hygiene instruction

MED: 100-2,16,10

E ☑ **D1351** Sealant — per tooth

## SPACE MAINTENANCE (PASSIVE APPLIANCES)

S **D1510** Space maintainer — fixed-unilateral  ⊘

MED: 100-2,16,140; 100-4,4,20.5

S **D1515** Space maintainer — fixed-bilateral  ⊘

MED: 100-2,15,150; 100-2,16,140; 100-4,4,20.5

S **D1520** Space maintainer — removable-unilateral  ⊘

MED: 100-2,15,150; 100-2,16,140; 100-4,4,20.5

S **D1525** Space maintainer — removable-bilateral  ⊘

MED: 100-2,15,150; 100-2,16,140; 100-4,4,20.5

S **D1550** Recementation of space maintainer  ⊘

MED: 100-2,15,150; 100-2,16,140; 100-4,4,20.5

E **D1555** Removal of fixed space maintainer

E ☑ **D2140** Amalgam—one surface, primary or permanent

E ☑ **D2150** Amalgam—two surfaces, primary or permanent

E ☑ **D2160** Amalgam—three surfaces, primary or permanent

E ☑ **D2161** Amalgam—four or more surfaces, primary or permanent

### RESIN RESTORATIONS

E ☑ **D2330** Resin — one surface, anterior

E ☑ **D2331** Resin — two surfaces, anterior

E ☑ **D2332** Resin — three surfaces, anterior

E ☑ **D2335** Resin — four or more surfaces or involving incisal angle (anterior)

E ☑ **D2390** Resin-based composite crown, anterior

E ☑ **D2391** Resin-based composite — one surface, posterior

E ☑ **D2392** Resin-based composite — two surfaces, posterior

E ☑ **D2393** Resin-based composite — three surfaces, posterior

E ☑ **D2394** Resin-based composite — four or more surfaces, posterior

### GOLD FOIL RESTORATIONS

E ☑ **D2410** Gold foil — one surface

E ☑ **D2420** Gold foil — two surfaces

E ☑ **D2430** Gold foil — three surfaces

### INLAY/ONLAY RESTORATIONS

E ☑ **D2510** Inlay — metallic — one surface

E ☑ **D2520** Inlay — metallic — two surfaces

E ☑ **D2530** Inlay — metallic — three or more surfaces

E ☑ **D2542** Onlay — metallic — two surfaces

E ☑ **D2543** Onlay — metallic — three surfaces

E ☑ **D2544** Onlay — metallic — four or more surfaces

E ☑ **D2610** Inlay — porcelain/ceramic — one surface

E ☑ **D2620** Inlay — porcelain/ceramic — two surfaces

E ☑ **D2630** Inlay — porcelain/ceramic — three or more surfaces

E ☑ **D2642** Onlay — porcelain/ceramic — two surfaces

E ☑ **D2643** Onlay — porcelain/ceramic — three surfaces

E ☑ **D2644** Onlay — porcelain/ceramic — four or more surfaces

E ☑ **D2650** Inlay — resin-based composite — one surface

E ☑ **D2651** Inlay — resin-based composite — two surfaces

E ☑ **D2652** Inlay — resin-based composite — three or more surfaces

E ☑ **D2662** Onlay — resin-based composite — two surfaces

Special Coverage Instructions   Noncovered by Medicare   Carrier Discretion   ☑ Quantity Alert   ● New Code   ○ Recycled/Reinstated   ▲ Revised Code

**28 — D Codes**   A Age Edit   M Maternity Edit   ♀ Female Only   ♂ Male Only   A-Y OPPS Status Indicators   **2008 HCPCS**

E ☑ **D2663** Onlay — resin-based composite — three surfaces

E ☑ **D2664** Onlay — resin-based composite — four or more surfaces

## CROWNS - SINGLE RESTORATION ONLY

E **D2710** Crown — resin-based composite (indirect)

E **D2712** Crown — 3/4 resin-based composite (indirect)

E **D2720** Crown — resin with high noble metal

E **D2721** Crown — resin with predominantly base metal

E **D2722** Crown — resin with noble metal

E **D2740** Crown — porcelain/ceramic substrate

E **D2750** Crown — porcelain fused to high noble metal

E **D2751** Crown — porcelain fused to predominantly base metal

E **D2752** Crown — porcelain fused to noble metal

E **D2780** Crown — 3/4 cast high noble metal

E **D2781** Crown — 3/4 cast predominately base metal

E **D2782** Crown — 3/4 cast noble metal

E **D2783** Crown - 3/4 porcelain/ceramic

E **D2790** Crown — full cast high noble metal

E **D2791** Crown — full cast predominantly base metal

E **D2792** Crown — full cast noble metal

E **D2794** Crown — titanium

E **D2799** Provisional crown
**Do not use this code to report a temporary crown for routine prosthetic restoration.**

## OTHER RESTORATIVE SERVICES

E **D2910** Recement inlay, onlay or partial coverage restoration

E **D2915** Recement cast or prefabricated post and core

E **D2920** Recement crown

E **D2930** Prefabricated stainless steel crown — primary tooth

E **D2931** Prefabricated stainless steel crown — permanent tooth

E **D2932** Prefabricated resin crown

E **D2933** Prefabricated stainless steel crown with resin window

E **D2934** Prefabricated esthetic coated stainless steel crown - primary tooth

E **D2940** Sedative filling

E **D2950** Core buildup, including any pins

E **D2951** Pin retention — per tooth, in addition to restoration

E **D2952** Post and core in addition to crown, indirectly fabricated

E **D2953** Each additional indirectly fabricated post — same tooth
**Report in addition to code D2952.**

E **D2954** Prefabricated post and core in addition to crown

E **D2955** Post removal (not in conjunction with endodontic therapy)

E **D2957** Each additional prefabricated post — same tooth
**Report in addition to code D2954.**

E **D2960** Labial veneer (resin laminate) — chairside

E **D2961** Labial veneer (resin laminate) — laboratory

E **D2962** Labial veneer (porcelain laminate) — laboratory

○ E **D2970** Temporary crown (fractured tooth)

E **D2971** Additional procedures to construct new crown under existing partial denture framework

E **D2975** Coping

E **D2980** Crown repair, by report
**Pertinent documentation to evaluate medical appropriateness should be included when this code is reported.**

S **D2999** Unspecified restorative procedure, by report ⊘
**Determine if an alternative HCPCS Level II or a CPT code better describes the service being reported. This code should be used only if a more specific code is unavailable.**
MED: 100-2,15,150; 100-2,16,140; 100-4,4,20.5

## ENDODONTICS D3000-D3999

### PULP CAPPING

E **D3110** Pulp cap — direct (excluding final restoration)

E **D3120** Pulp cap — indirect (excluding final restoration)

### PULPOTOMY

E **D3220** Therapeutic pulpotomy (excluding final restoration) — removal of pulp coronal to the dentinocemental junction and application of medicament
**Do not use this code to report the first stage of root canal therapy.**

E **D3221** Pulpal debridement, primary and permanent teeth

### PULPAL THERAPY ON PRIMARY TEETH (INCLUDES PRIMARY TEETH WITH SUCCEDANEOUS TEETH AND PLACEMENT OF RESORBABLE FILLING)

E **D3230** Pulpal therapy (resorbable filling) — anterior, primary tooth (excluding final restoration)

E **D3240** Pulpal therapy (resorbable filling) — posterior, primary tooth (excluding final restoration)

### ROOT CANAL THERAPY (INCLUDING TREATMENT PLAN, CLINICAL PROCEDURES, AND FOLLOW-UP CARE, INCLUDES PRIMARY TEETH WITHOUT SUCCEDANEOUS TEETH AND PERMANENT TEETH)

E **D3310** Anterior (excluding final restoration)

E **D3320** Bicuspid (excluding final restoration)

E **D3330** Molar (excluding final restoration)

E **D3331** Treatment of root canal obstruction; nonsurgical access

E **D3332** Incomplete endodontic therapy; inoperable, unrestorable or fractured tooth

E **D3333** Internal root repair of perforation defects

E **D3346** Retreatment of previous root canal therapy — anterior

E **D3347** Retreatment of previous root canal therapy — bicuspid

E **D3348** Retreatment of previous root canal therapy — molar

E **D3351** Apexification/recalcification — initial visit (apical closure/calcific repair of perforations, root resorption, etc.)

E **D3352** Apexification/recalcification — interim medication replacement (apical closure/calcific repair of perforations, root resorption, etc.)

Special Coverage Instructions | Noncovered by Medicare | Carrier Discretion | ☑ Quantity Alert | ● New Code | ○ Recycled/Reinstated | ▲ Revised Code

**2008 HCPCS** | ASC Payment Indicators | **MED:** Pub 100/NCD References | DMEPOS Paid | ⊘ SNF Excluded | PQRI | **D Codes — 29**

**Dental Procedures**

**D3353 — D4999**

E D3353 Apexification/recalcification — final visit (includes completed root canal therapy — apical closure/calcific repair of perforations, root resorption, etc.)

## APICOECTOMY/PERIRADICULAR SERVICES

E D3410 Apicoectomy/periradicular surgery — anterior

E D3421 Apicoectomy/periradicular surgery — bicuspid (first root)

E D3425 Apicoectomy/periradicular surgery — molar (first root)

E ☑ D3426 Apicoectomy/periradicular surgery (each additional root)

E ☑ D3430 Retrograde filling — per root

E ☑ D3450 Root amputation — per root

S D3460 Endodontic endosseous implant ⊘
MED: 100-2,15,150; 100-2,16,140; 100-4,4,20.5

E D3470 Intentional replantation (including necessary splinting)

## OTHER ENDODONTIC PROCEDURES

E D3910 Surgical procedure for isolation of tooth with rubber dam

E D3920 Hemisection (including any root removal), not including root canal therapy

E D3950 Canal preparation and fitting of preformed dowel or post

S D3999 Unspecified endodontic procedure, by report ⊘
**Determine if an alternative HCPCS Level II a CPT code better describes the service being reported. This code should be used only if a more specific code is unavailable.**
MED: 100-2,15,150; 100-2,16,140; 100-4,4,20.5

## PERIODONTICS D4000-D4999

## SURGICAL SERVICES (INCLUDING USUAL POSTOPERATIVE SERVICES)

E ☑ D4210 Gingivectomy or gingivoplasty - Four or more contiguous teeth or bounded teeth spaces per quadrant

E ☑ D4211 Gingivectomy or gingivoplasty - one to three contiguous teeth or bounded teeth spaces per quadrant

E D4230 Anatomical crown exposure - Four or more contiguous teeth per quadrant

E D4231 Anatomical crown exposure — one to three teeth per quadrant

E ☑ D4240 Gingival flap procedure, including root planing — four or more contiguous teeth or bounded teeth spaces per quadrant

E D4241 Gingival flap procedure, including root planing — one to three contiguous teeth or bounded teeth spaces per quadrant

E D4245 Apically positioned flap

E D4249 Clinical crown lengthening — hard tissue

S ☑ D4260 Osseous surgery (including flap entry and closure) — four or more contiguous teeth or bounded teeth spaces per quadrant ⊘
MED: 100-2,15,150; 100-2,16,140; 100-4,4,20.5

E D4261 Osseous surgery (including flap entry and closure) — one to three contiguous teeth or bounded teeth spaces per quadrant

S ☑ D4263 Bone replacement graft — first site in quadrant ⊘
MED: 100-2,15,150; 100-2,16,140; 100-3,260.6; 100-4,4,20.5

S ☑ D4264 Bone replacement graft — each additional site in quadrant ⊘
MED: 100-2,15,150; 100-2,16,140; 100-3,260.6; 100-4,4,20.5

E D4265 Biologic materials to aid in soft and osseous tissue regeneration

E ☑ D4266 Guided tissue regeneration — resorbable barrier, per site

E ☑ D4267 Guided tissue regeneration — nonresorbable barrier, per site (includes membrane removal)

S ☑ D4268 Surgical revision procedure, per tooth
MED: 100-2,15,150; 100-2,16,140

S D4270 Pedicle soft tissue graft procedure ⊘
MED: 100-2,15,150; 100-2,16,140; 100-4,4,20.5

S D4271 Free soft tissue graft procedure (including donor site surgery) ⊘
MED: 100-2,15,150; 100-2,16,140; 100-4,4,20.5

S D4273 Subepithelial connective tissue graft procedures, per tooth ⊘
MED: 100-2,15,150; 100-2,16,140; 100-3,260.6; 100-4,4,20.5

E D4274 Distal or proximal wedge procedure (when not performed in conjunction with surgical procedures in the same anatomical area)

E D4275 Soft tissue allograft

E D4276 Combined connective tissue and double pedicle graft, per tooth

## ADJUNCTIVE PERIODONTAL SERVICES

E D4320 Provisional splinting — intracoronal

E D4321 Provisional splinting — extracoronal

E ☑ D4341 Periodontal scaling and root planing — four or more teeth per quadrant

E ☑ D4342 Periodontal scaling and root planing — one to three teeth, per quadrant

S D4355 Full mouth debridement to enable comprehensive evaluation and diagnosis ⊘
**This procedure is covered by Medicare if its purpose is to identify a patient's existing infections prior to kidney transplantation.**
MED: 100-2,15,150; 100-2,16,140; 100-3,260.6; 100-4,4,20.5

S D4381 Localized delivery of antimicrobial agents via a controlled release vehicle into diseased crevicular tissue, per tooth, by report ⊘
**Pertinent documentation to evaluate medical appropriateness should be included when this code is reported.**
MED: 100-2,15,150; 100-2,16,140; 100-3,260.6; 100-4,4,20.5

## OTHER PERIODONTAL SERVICES

E D4910 Periodontal maintenance

E D4920 Unscheduled dressing change (by someone other than treating dentist)

E D4999 Unspecified periodontal procedure, by report
**Determine if an alternative HCPCS Level II or a CPT code better describes the service being reported. This code should be used only if a more specific code is unavailable.**

---

Special Coverage Instructions    Noncovered by Medicare    Carrier Discretion    ☑ Quantity Alert    ● New Code    ○ Recycled/Reinstated    ▲ Revised Code

## PROSTHODONTICS (REMOVABLE) D5000-D5899

### COMPLETE DENTURES (INCLUDING ROUTINE POST DELIVERY CARE)

- [E] **D5110** Complete denture — maxillary
- [E] **D5120** Complete denture — mandibular
- [E] **D5130** Immediate denture — maxillary
- [E] **D5140** Immediate denture — mandibular

### PARTIAL DENTURES (INCLUDING ROUTINE POST DELIVERY CARE)

- [E] **D5211** Maxillary partial denture — resin base (including any conventional clasps, rests and teeth)
- [E] **D5212** Mandibular partial denture — resin base (including any conventional clasps, rests and teeth)
- [E] **D5213** Maxillary partial denture — cast metal framework with resin denture bases (including any conventional clasps, rests and teeth)
- [E] **D5214** Mandibular partial denture — cast metal framework with resin denture bases (including any conventional clasps, rests and teeth)
- [E] **D5225** Maxillary partial denture - flexible base (including any clasps, rests and teeth)
- [E] **D5226** Mandibular partial denture — flexible base (including any clasps, rests and teeth)
- [E] **D5281** Removable unilateral partial denture — one piece cast metal (including clasps and teeth)

### ADJUSTMENTS TO REMOVABLE PROSTHESES

- [E] **D5410** Adjust complete denture — maxillary
- [E] **D5411** Adjust complete denture — mandibular
- [E] **D5421** Adjust partial denture — maxillary
- [E] **D5422** Adjust partial denture — mandibular

### REPAIRS TO COMPLETE DENTURES

- [E] **D5510** Repair broken complete denture base
- [E] **D5520** Replace missing or broken teeth — complete denture (each tooth)

### REPAIRS TO PARTIAL DENTURES

- [E] **D5610** Repair resin denture base
- [E] **D5620** Repair cast framework
- [E] **D5630** Repair or replace broken clasp
- [E] ☑ **D5640** Replace broken teeth — per tooth
- [E] **D5650** Add tooth to existing partial denture
- [E] **D5660** Add clasp to existing partial denture
- [E] **D5670** Replace all teeth and acrylic on cast metal framework (maxillary)
- [E] **D5671** Replace all teeth and acrylic on cast metal framework (mandibular)

### DENTURE REBASE PROCEDURES

- [E] **D5710** Rebase complete maxillary denture
- [E] **D5711** Rebase complete mandibular denture
- [E] **D5720** Rebase maxillary partial denture
- [E] **D5721** Rebase mandibular partial denture

### DENTURE RELINE PROCEDURES

- [E] **D5730** Reline complete maxillary denture (chairside)
- [E] **D5731** Reline lower complete mandibular denture (chairside)
- [E] **D5740** Reline maxillary partial denture (chairside)
- [E] **D5741** Reline mandibular partial denture (chairside)
- [E] **D5750** Reline complete maxillary denture (laboratory)
- [E] **D5751** Reline complete mandibular denture (laboratory)
- [E] **D5760** Reline maxillary partial denture (laboratory)
- [E] **D5761** Reline mandibular partial denture (laboratory)

### OTHER REMOVABLE PROSTHETIC SERVICES

- [E] **D5810** Interim complete denture (maxillary)
- [E] **D5811** Interim complete denture (mandibular)
- [E] **D5820** Interim partial denture (maxillary)
- [E] **D5821** Interim partial denture (mandibular)
- [E] **D5850** Tissue conditioning, maxillary
- [E] **D5851** Tissue conditioning, mandibular
- [E] **D5860** Overdenture — complete, by report
  Pertinent documentation to evaluate medical appropriateness should be included when this code is reported.
- [E] **D5861** Overdenture — partial, by report
  Pertinent documentation to evaluate medical appropriateness should be included when this code is reported.
- [E] **D5862** Precision attachment, by report
  Pertinent documentation to evaluate medical appropriateness should be included when this code is reported.
- [E] **D5867** Replacement of replaceable part of semi-precision or precision attachment (male or female component)
- [E] **D5875** Modification of removable prosthesis following implant surgery
- [E] **D5899** Unspecified removable prosthodontic procedure, by report
  Determine if an alternative HCPCS Level II or a CPT code better describes the service being reported. This code should be used only if a more specific code is unavailable.

## MAXILLOFACIAL PROSTHETICS D5900-D5999

- [S] **D5911** Facial moulage (sectional) ⊘
  MED: 100-2,15,120; 100-2,15,150; 100-4,4,20.5
- [S] **D5912** Facial moulage (complete) ⊘
  MED: 100-2,15,120; 100-4,4,20.5
- [E] **D5913** Nasal prosthesis
- [E] **D5914** Auricular prosthesis
- [E] **D5915** Orbital prosthesis
  See code(s): L8611
- [E] **D5916** Ocular prosthesis
  See code(s): V2623, V2629
- [E] **D5919** Facial prosthesis
- [E] **D5922** Nasal septal prosthesis
- [E] **D5923** Ocular prosthesis, interim
- [E] **D5924** Cranial prosthesis
- [E] **D5925** Facial augmentation implant prosthesis
- [E] **D5926** Nasal prosthesis, replacement
- [E] **D5927** Auricular prosthesis, replacement

| Special Coverage Instructions | Noncovered by Medicare | Carrier Discretion | ☑ Quantity Alert | ● New Code | ○ Recycled/Reinstated | ▲ Revised Code |

**2008 HCPCS**  A2-Z3 ASC Payment Indicators  **MED:** Pub 100/NCD References  & DMEPOS Paid  ⊘ SNF Excluded  PQ PQRI  **D Codes — 31**

**Dental Procedures**

**D5928 — D6078**

| | | |
|---|---|---|
| E | D5928 | Orbital prosthesis, replacement |
| E | D5929 | Facial prosthesis, replacement |
| E | D5931 | Obturator prosthesis, surgical |
| E | D5932 | Obturator prosthesis, definitive |
| E | D5933 | Obturator prosthesis, modification |
| E | D5934 | Mandibular resection prosthesis with guide flange |
| E | D5935 | Mandibular resection prosthesis without guide flange |
| E | D5936 | Obturator/prosthesis, interim |
| E | D5937 | Trismus appliance (not for TM treatment) |

MED: 100-2,15,120

| | | | |
|---|---|---|---|
| E | D5951 | Feeding aid | ⊘ |

MED: 100-2,15,120; 100-2,16,140

| | | |
|---|---|---|
| E | D5952 | Speech aid prosthesis, pediatric |
| E | D5953 | Speech aid prosthesis, adult |
| E | D5954 | Palatal augmentation prosthesis |
| E | D5955 | Palatal lift prosthesis, definitive |
| E | D5958 | Palatal lift prosthesis, interim |
| E | D5959 | Palatal lift prosthesis, modification |
| E | D5960 | Speech aid prosthesis, modification |
| E | D5982 | Surgical stent |

| | | | |
|---|---|---|---|
| S | D5983 | Radiation carrier | ⊘ |

MED: 100-2,15,150; 100-2,16,140; 100-4,4,20.5

| | | | |
|---|---|---|---|
| S | D5984 | Radiation shield | ⊘ |

MED: 100-2,15,150; 100-2,16,140; 100-4,4,20.5

| | | | |
|---|---|---|---|
| S | D5985 | Radiation cone locator | ⊘ |

MED: 100-2,15,150; 100-2,16,140; 100-4,4,20.5

| | | |
|---|---|---|
| E | D5986 | Fluoride gel carrier |

| | | | |
|---|---|---|---|
| S | D5987 | Commissure splint | ⊘ |

MED: 100-2,15,150; 100-2,16,140; 100-4,4,20.5; 100-4,4,240

| | | |
|---|---|---|
| E | D5988 | Surgical splint |

MED: 100-4,4,240

| | | |
|---|---|---|
| E | D5999 | Unspecified maxillofacial prosthesis, by report **Determine if an alternative HCPCS Level II or a CPT code better describes the service being reported. This code should be used only if a more specific code is unavailable.** |

## IMPLANT SERVICES D6000-D6199

| | | |
|---|---|---|
| E | D6010 | Surgical placement of implant body: endosteal implant |
| E | D6012 | Surgical placement of interim implant body for transitional prosthesis: endosteal implant |
| E | D6040 | Surgical placement: eposteal implant |
| E | D6050 | Surgical placement: transosteal implant |
| E | D6053 | Implant/abutment supported removable denture for completely edentulous arch |

MED: 100-2,15,150

| | | |
|---|---|---|
| E | D6054 | Implant/abutment supported removable denture for partially edentulous arch |

MED: 100-2,15,150

| | | |
|---|---|---|
| E | D6055 | Dental implant supported connecting bar |

MED: 100-2,15,150

| | | |
|---|---|---|
| E | D6056 | Prefabricated abutment - includes placement |

MED: 100-2,15,150

| | | |
|---|---|---|
| E | D6057 | Custom abutment — includes placement |

MED: 100-2,15,150

| | | |
|---|---|---|
| E | D6058 | Abutment supported porcelain/ceramic crown |

MED: 100-2,15,150

| | | |
|---|---|---|
| E | D6059 | Abutment supported porcelain fused to metal crown (high noble metal) |

MED: 100-2,15,150

| | | |
|---|---|---|
| E | D6060 | Abutment supported porcelain fused to metal crown (predominantly base metal) |

MED: 100-2,15,150

| | | |
|---|---|---|
| E | D6061 | Abutment supported porcelain fused to metal crown (noble metal) |

MED: 100-2,15,150

| | | |
|---|---|---|
| E | D6062 | Abutment supported cast metal crown (high noble metal) |

MED: 100-2,15,150

| | | |
|---|---|---|
| E | D6063 | Abutment supported cast metal crown (predominantly base metal) |

MED: 100-2,15,150

| | | |
|---|---|---|
| E | D6064 | Abutment supported cast metal crown (noble metal) |

MED: 100-2,15,150

| | | |
|---|---|---|
| E | D6065 | Implant supported porcelain/ceramic crown |

MED: 100-2,15,150

| | | |
|---|---|---|
| E | D6066 | Implant supported porcelain fused to metal crown (titanium, titanium alloy, high noble metal) |

MED: 100-2,15,150

| | | |
|---|---|---|
| E | D6067 | Implant supported metal crown (titanium, titanium alloy, high noble metal) |

MED: 100-2,15,150

| | | |
|---|---|---|
| E | D6068 | Abutment supported retainer for porcelain/ceramic FPD |

MED: 100-2,15,150

| | | |
|---|---|---|
| E | D6069 | Abutment supported retainer for porcelain fused to metal FPD (high noble metal) |

MED: 100-2,15,150

| | | |
|---|---|---|
| E | D6070 | Abutment supported retainer for porcelain fused to metal FPD (predominantly base metal) |

MED: 100-2,15,150

| | | |
|---|---|---|
| E | D6071 | Abutment supported retainer for porcelain fused to metal FPD (noble metal) |

MED: 100-2,15,150

| | | |
|---|---|---|
| E | D6072 | Abutment supported retainer for cast metal FPD (high noble metal) |

MED: 100-2,15,150

| | | |
|---|---|---|
| E | D6073 | Abutment supported retainer for cast metal FPD (predominantly base metal) |

MED: 100-2,15,150

| | | |
|---|---|---|
| E | D6074 | Abutment supported retainer for cast metal FPD (noble metal) |

MED: 100-2,15,150

| | | |
|---|---|---|
| E | D6075 | Implant supported retainer for ceramic FPD |

MED: 100-2,15,150

| | | |
|---|---|---|
| E | D6076 | Implant supported retainer for porcelain fused to metal FPD (titanium, titanium alloy, or high noble metal) |

MED: 100-2,15,150

| | | |
|---|---|---|
| E | D6077 | Implant supported retainer for cast metal FPD (titanium, titanium alloy, or high noble metal) |

MED: 100-2,15,150

| | | |
|---|---|---|
| E | D6078 | Implant/abutment supported fixed denture for completely edentulous arch |

MED: 100-2,15,150

---

| | | |
|---|---|---|
| ▨ Special Coverage Instructions | ▨ Noncovered by Medicare | ▨ Carrier Discretion | ☑ Quantity Alert | ● New Code | ○ Recycled/Reinstated | ▲ Revised Code |

E **D6079** Implant/abutment supported fixed denture for partially edentulous arch
MED: 100-2,15,150

E **D6080** Implant maintenance procedures, including removal of prosthesis, cleansing of prosthesis and abutments, reinsertion of prosthesis
MED: 100-2,15,150

E **D6090** Repair implant supported prosthesis, by report
Pertinent documentation to evaluate medical appropriateness should be included when this code is reported.

E **D6091** Replacement of semi-precision or precision attachment (male or female component) of implant/abutment supported prosthesis, per attachment

E **D6092** Recement implant/abutment supported crown

E **D6093** Recement implant/abutment supported fixed partial denture

E **D6094** Abutment supported crown - (titanium)

E **D6095** Repair implant abutment, by report
Pertinent documentation to evaluate medical appropriateness should be included when this code is reported.

E **D6100** Implant removal, by report
Pertinent documentation to evaluate medical appropriateness should be included when this code is reported.

E **D6190** Radiographic/surgical implant index, by report

E **D6194** Abutment supported retainer crown for FPD - (titanium)

E **D6199** Unspecified implant procedure, by report

E **D6205** Pontic — indirect resin based composite

## PROSTHODONTICS (FIXED) D6200-D6999

### FIXED PARTIAL DENTURE PONTICS

E **D6210** Pontic — cast high noble metal
Each abutment and each pontic constitute a unit in a prosthesis. An alloy of at least 60 percent gold (Au), palladium (Pd), or platinum (Pt) is considered a high noble metal.

E **D6211** Pontic — cast predominantly base metal
Each abutment and each pontic constitute a unit in a prosthesis. An alloy of less than 25 percent gold (Au), palladium (Pd), or platinum (Pt) is considered a high noble metal.

E **D6212** Pontic — cast noble metal
Each abutment and each pontic constitute a unit in a prosthesis. An alloy of at least 25 percent gold (Au), palladium (Pd), or platinum (Pt) is considered a high noble metal.

E **D6214** Pontic — titanium

E **D6240** Pontic — porcelain fused to high noble metal
Each abutment and each pontic constitute a unit in a prosthesis. An alloy of at least 60 percent gold (Au), palladium (Pd), or platinum (Pt) is considered a high noble metal.

E **D6241** Pontic — porcelain fused to predominantly base metal
Each abutment and each pontic constitute a unit in a prosthesis. An alloy of less than 25 percent gold (Au), palladium (Pd), or platinum (Pt) is considered a high noble metal.

E **D6242** Pontic — porcelain fused to noble metal
Each abutment and each pontic constitute a unit in a prosthesis. An alloy of at least 60 percent gold (Au), palladium (Pd), or platinum (Pt) is considered a high noble metal.

E **D6245** Pontic — porcelain/ceramic
MED: 100-2,15,150

E **D6250** Pontic — resin with high noble metal
Each abutment and each pontic constitute a unit in a prosthesis. An alloy of at least 60 percent gold (Au), palladium (Pd), or platinum (Pt) is considered a high noble metal.

E **D6251** Pontic — resin with predominantly base metal
Each abutment and each pontic constitute a unit in a prosthesis. An alloy of less than 25 percent gold (Au), palladium (Pd), or platinum (Pt) is considered a high noble metal.

E **D6252** Pontic — resin with noble metal
Each abutment and each pontic constitute a unit in a prosthesis. An alloy of at least 25 percent gold (Au), palladium (Pd), or platinum (Pt) is considered a high noble metal.

E **D6253** Provisional pontic

E **D6545** Retainer — cast metal for resin bonded fixed prosthesis

E **D6548** Retainer — porcelain/ceramic for resin bonded fixed prosthesis
MED: 100-2,15,150

E **D6600** Inlay — porcelain/ceramic, two surfaces
MED: 100-2,15,150

E **D6601** Inlay — porcelain/ceramic, three or more surfaces
MED: 100-2,15,150

E **D6602** Inlay — cast high noble metal, two surfaces
MED: 100-2,15,150

E **D6603** Inlay — cast high noble metal, three or more surfaces
MED: 100-2,15,150

E **D6604** Inlay — cast predominantly base metal, two surfaces
MED: 100-2,15,150

E **D6605** Inlay — cast predominantly base metal, three or more surfaces
MED: 100-2,15,150

E **D6606** Inlay — cast noble metal, two surfaces
MED: 100-2,15,150

E **D6607** Inlay — cast noble metal, three or more surfaces
MED: 100-2,15,150

E **D6608** Onlay — porcelain/ceramic, two surfaces
MED: 100-2,15,150

E **D6609** Onlay — porcelain/ceramic, three or more surfaces
MED: 100-2,15,150

E **D6610** Onlay — cast high noble metal, two surfaces
MED: 100-2,15,150

E **D6611** Onlay — cast high noble metal, three or more surfaces
MED: 100-2,15,150

E **D6612** Onlay — cast predominantly base metal, two surfaces
MED: 100-2,15,150

E **D6613** Onlay — cast predominantly base metal, three or more surfaces
MED: 100-2,15,150

---

Special Coverage Instructions    Noncovered by Medicare    Carrier Discretion    ☑ Quantity Alert    ● New Code    ○ Recycled/Reinstated    ▲ Revised Code

**2008 HCPCS**    N2-Z3 ASC Payment Indicators    **MED:** Pub 100/NCD References    ⅙ DMEPOS Paid    ⊘ SNF Excluded    PQRI PQRI    **D Codes — 33**

**Dental Procedures**

**D6614 — D7270**

E | **D6614** Onlay — cast noble metal, two surfaces
MED: 100-2,15,150

E | **D6615** Onlay — cast noble metal, three or more surfaces
MED: 100-2,15,150

E | **D6624** Inlay — titanium

E | **D6634** Onlay — titanium

E | **D6710** Crown — indirect resin based composite

## FIXED PARTIAL DENTURE RETAINERS - CROWNS

E | **D6720** Crown — resin with high noble metal
An alloy of at least 60 percent gold (Au), palladium (Pd), or platinum (Pt) is considered a high noble metal.

E | **D6721** Crown — resin with predominantly base metal
An alloy of less than 25 percent gold (Au), palladium (Pd), or platinum (Pt) is considered a base metal.

E | **D6722** Crown — resin with noble metal
An alloy of at least 25 percent gold (Au), palladium (Pd), or platinum (Pt) is considered a noble metal.

E | **D6740** Crown — porcelain/ceramic
MED: 100-2,15,150

E | **D6750** Crown — porcelain fused to high noble metal
An alloy of at least 60 percent gold (Au), palladium (Pd), or platinum (Pt) is considered a high noble metal.

E | **D6751** Crown — porcelain fused to predominantly base metal
An alloy of less than 25 percent gold (Au), palladium (Pd), or platinum (Pt) is considered a base metal.

E | **D6752** Crown — porcelain fused to noble metal
An alloy of at least 25 percent gold (Au), palladium (Pd), or platinum (Pt) is considered a noble metal.

E | **D6780** Crown — 3/4 cast high noble metal
An alloy of at least 60 percent gold (Au), palladium (Pd), or platinum (Pt) is considered a high noble metal.

E | **D6781** Crown — 3/4 cast predominately base metal
An alloy of less than 25 percent gold (Au), palladium (Pd), or platinum (Pt) is considered a base metal.
MED: 100-2,15,150

E | **D6782** Crown — 3/4 cast noble metal
An alloy of at least 25 percent gold (Au), palladium (Pd), or platinum (Pt) is considered a noble metal.
MED: 100-2,15,150

E | **D6783** Crown — 3/4 porcelain/ceramic
MED: 100-2,15,150

E | **D6790** Crown — full cast high noble metal
An alloy of at least 60 percent gold (Au), palladium (Pd), or platinum (Pt) is considered a high noble metal.

E | **D6791** Crown — full cast predominantly base metal
An alloy of less than 25 percent gold (Au), palladium (Pd), or platinum (Pt) is considered a base metal.

E | **D6792** Crown — full cast noble metal
An alloy of at least 25 percent gold (Au), palladium (Pd), or platinum (Pt) is considered a noble metal.

E | **D6793** Provisional retainer crown

E | **D6794** Crown — titanium

## OTHER FIXED PARTIAL DENTURE SERVICES

S | **D6920** Connector bar ⊘
MED: 100-2,15,150; 100-2,16,140; 100-3,260.6; 100-4,4,20.5

E | **D6930** Recement bridge

E | **D6940** Stress breaker

E | **D6950** Precision attachment

E | **D6970** Post and core in addition to fixed partial denture retainer, indirectly fabricated

E | **D6972** Prefabricated post and core in addition to bridge retainer

E | **D6973** Core build up for retainer, including any pins

E | **D6975** Coping — metal

E | **D6976** Each additional indirectly fabricated post — same tooth
Report this code in addition to codes D6970 or D6971.
MED: 100-2,15,150

E | **D6977** Each additional prefabricated post — same tooth
Report this code in addition to code D6972.
MED: 100-2,15,150

E | **D6980** Bridge repair, by report
Pertinent documentation to evaluate medical appropriateness should be included when this code is reported.

E | **D6985** Pediatric partial denture, fixed ▢A

E | **D6999** Unspecified fixed prosthodontic procedure, by report
Determine if an alternative HCPCS Level II or a CPT code better describes the service being reported. This code should be used only if a more specific code is unavailable.

S | **D7111** Extraction, coronal remnants — deciduous tooth
MED: 100-2,16,140; 100-4,4,20.5

S | **D7140** Extraction, erupted tooth or exposed root (elevation and/or forceps removal)
MED: 100-2,16,140; 100-4,4,20.5

## SURGICAL EXTRACTIONS (INCLUDES LOCAL ANESTHESIA AND ROUTINE POSTOPERATIVE CARE)

S | **D7210** Surgical removal of erupted tooth requiring elevation of mucoperiosteal flap and removal of bone and/or section of tooth ⊘
MED: 100-2,15,150; 100-2,16,140; 100-4,4,20.5

S | **D7220** Removal of impacted tooth — soft tissue ⊘
MED: 100-2,15,150; 100-2,16,140; 100-4,4,20.5

S | **D7230** Removal of impacted tooth — partially bony ⊘
MED: 100-2,15,150; 100-2,16,140; 100-4,4,20.5

S | **D7240** Removal of impacted tooth — completely bony ⊘
MED: 100-2,15,150; 100-2,16,140; 100-4,4,20.5

S | **D7241** Removal of impacted tooth — completely bony, with unusual surgical complications ⊘
MED: 100-2,15,150; 100-2,16,140; 100-4,4,20.5

S | **D7250** Surgical removal of residual tooth roots (cutting procedure) ⊘
MED: 100-2,15,150; 100-2,16,140; 100-4,4,20.5

## OTHER SURGICAL PROCEDURES

S | **D7260** Oral antral fistula closure ⊘
MED: 100-2,15,150; 100-2,16,140; 100-4,4,20.5

S | **D7261** Primary closure of a sinus perforation
See equivalent CPT code for repair of mucous membranes.
MED: 100-2,16,140

E | **D7270** Tooth reimplantation and/or stabilization of accidentally evulsed or displaced tooth

---

Special Coverage Instructions | Noncovered by Medicare | Carrier Discretion | ☑ Quantity Alert ● New Code ○ Recycled/Reinstated ▲ Revised Code

E  **D7272** Tooth transplantation (includes reimplantation from one site to another and splinting and/or stabilization)

E  **D7280** Surgical access of an unerupted tooth

E  **D7282** Mobilization of erupted or malpositioned tooth to aid eruption

B  **D7283** Placement of device to facilitate eruption of impacted tooth

E  **D7285** Biopsy of oral tissue — hard (bone, tooth)

E  **D7286** Biopsy of oral tissue — soft

E  **D7287** Exfoliative cytological sample collection

B  **D7288** Brush biopsy — transepithelial sample collection

E  **D7290** Surgical repositioning of teeth

S  **D7291** Transseptal fiberotomy/supra crestal fiberotomy, by report  ⊘

Pertinent documentation to evaluate medical appropriateness should be included when this code is reported.

MED: 100-2,15,150; 100-2,16,140; 100-4,4,20.5

E  **D7292** Surgical placement: temporary anchorage device (screw retained plate) requiring surgical flap

E  **D7293** Surgical placement: temporary anchorage device requiring surgical flap

E  **D7294** Surgical placement: temporary anchorage device without surgical flap

## ALVEOLOPLASTY - SURGICAL PREPARATION OF RIDGE FOR DENTURES

E ☑  **D7310** Alveoloplasty in conjunction with extractions—four or more teeth or tooth spaces, per quadrant

E ☑  **D7311** Alveoloplasty in conjunction with extractions — one to three teeth or tooth spaces, per quadrant

E ☑  **D7320** Alveoloplasty not in conjunction with extractions—four or more teeth or tooth spaces, per quadrant

B ☑  **D7321** Alveoloplasty not in conjunction with extractions — one to three teeth or tooth spaces, per quadrant

## VESTIBULOPLASTY

E  **D7340** Vestibuloplasty — ridge extension (second epithelialization)

E  **D7350** Vestibuloplasty — ridge extension (including soft tissue grafts, muscle reattachments, revision of soft tissue attachment and management of hypertrophied and hyperplastic tissue)

## SURGICAL EXCISION OF REACTIVE INFLAMMATORY LESIONS (SCAR TISSUE OR LOCALIZED CONGENITAL LESIONS)

E  **D7410** Excision of benign lesion up to 1.25 cm

E  **D7411** Excision of benign lesion greater than 1.25 cm

E  **D7412** Excision of benign lesion, complicated

E  **D7413** Excision of malignant lesion up to 1.25 cm

E  **D7414** Excision of malignant lesion greater than 1.25 cm

E  **D7415** Excision of malignant lesion, complicated

E ☑  **D7440** Excision of malignant tumor — lesion diameter up to 1.25 cm

E ☑  **D7441** Excision of malignant tumor — lesion diameter greater than 1.25 cm

E ☑  **D7450** Removal of benign odontogenic cyst or tumor — lesion diameter up to 1.25 cm

E ☑  **D7451** Removal of benign odontogenic cyst or tumor — lesion diameter greater than 1.25 cm

E ☑  **D7460** Removal of benign nonodontogenic cyst or tumor — lesion diameter up to 1.25 cm

E ☑  **D7461** Removal of benign nonodontogenic cyst or tumor — lesion diameter greater than 1.25 cm

E  **D7465** Destruction of lesion(s) by physical or chemical method, by report

Pertinent documentation to evaluate medical appropriateness should be included when this code is reported.

E ☑  **D7471** Removal of lateral exostosis (maxilla or mandible)

E  **D7472** Removal of torus palatinus

E  **D7473** Removal of torus mandibularis

E  **D7485** Surgical reduction of osseous tuberosity

E  **D7490** Radical resection of maxilla or mandible

## SURGICAL INCISION

E  **D7510** Incision and drainage of abscess — intraoral soft tissue

B  **D7511** Incision and drainage of abscess — intraoral soft tissue — complicated (includes drainage of multiple fascial spaces)

E  **D7520** Incision and drainage of abscess — extraoral soft tissue

B  **D7521** Incision and drainage of abscess — extraoral soft tissue — complicated (includes drainage of multiple fascial spaces)

E  **D7530** Removal of foreign body from mucosa, skin, or subcutaneous alveolar tissue

E  **D7540** Removal of reaction-producing foreign bodies, musculoskeletal system

E  **D7550** Partial ostectomy/sequestrectomy for removal of nonvital bone

E  **D7560** Maxillary sinusotomy for removal of tooth fragment or foreign body

## TREATMENT OF FRACTURES - SIMPLE

E  **D7610** Maxilla — open reduction (teeth immobilized, if present)

E  **D7620** Maxilla — closed reduction (teeth immobilized, if present)

E  **D7630** Mandible — open reduction (teeth immobilized, if present)

E  **D7640** Mandible — closed reduction (teeth immobilized, if present)

E  **D7650** Malar and/or zygomatic arch — open reduction

E  **D7660** Malar and/or zygomatic arch — closed reduction

E  **D7670** Alveolus - closed reduction, may include stabilization of teeth

E  **D7671** Alveolus - open reduction, may include stabilization of teeth

E  **D7680** Facial bones — complicated reduction with fixation and multiple surgical approaches

## TREATMENT OF FRACTURES - COMPOUND

E  **D7710** Maxilla — open reduction

E  **D7720** Maxilla — closed reduction

E  **D7730** Mandible — open reduction

E  **D7740** Mandible — closed reduction

E  **D7750** Malar and/or zygomatic arch — open reduction

Special Coverage Instructions | Noncovered by Medicare | Carrier Discretion | ☑ Quantity Alert | ● New Code | ○ Recycled/Reinstated | ▲ Revised Code

**2008 HCPCS**   A2–Z3 ASC Payment Indicators   **MED:** Pub 100/NCD References   ♿ DMEPOS Paid   ⊘ SNF Excluded   PQ PQRI   **D Codes — 35**

D7272 — D7750

**Dental Procedures**

**D7760 — D8020**

E   D7760   Malar and/or zygomatic arch — closed reduction

E   D7770   Alveolus — open reduction stabilization of teeth

E   D7771   Alveolus, closed reduction stabilization of teeth

E   D7780   Facial bones — complicated reduction with fixation and multiple surgical approaches

## REDUCTION OF DISLOCATION AND MANAGEMENT OF OTHER TEMPOROMANDIBULAR JOINT DYSFUNCTIONS

Procedures which are an integral part of a primary procedure should not be reported separately.

E   D7810   Open reduction of dislocation

E   D7820   Closed reduction of dislocation

E   D7830   Manipulation under anesthesia

E   D7840   Condylectomy

E   D7850   Surgical discectomy; with/without implant

E   D7852   Disc repair

E   D7854   Synovectomy

E   D7856   Myotomy

E   D7858   Joint reconstruction

E   D7860   Arthrotomy
     MED: 100-2,15,150; 100-2,16,140

E   D7865   Arthroplasty

E   D7870   Arthrocentesis

E   D7871   Nonarthroscopic lysis and lavage

E   D7872   Arthroscopy — diagnosis, with or without biopsy

E   D7873   Arthroscopy — surgical: lavage and lysis of adhesions

E   D7874   Arthroscopy — surgical: disc repositioning and stabilization

E   D7875   Arthroscopy — surgical: synovectomy

E   D7876   Arthroscopy — surgical: discectomy

E   D7877   Arthroscopy — surgical: debridement

E   D7880   Occlusal orthotic appliance

E   D7899   Unspecified TMD therapy, by report
     Determine if an alternative HCPCS Level II or a CPT code better describes the service being reported. This code should be used only if a more specific code is unavailable.

## REPAIR OF TRAUMATIC WOUNDS

E ☑   D7910   Suture of recent small wounds up to 5 cm

## COMPLICATED SUTURING (RECONSTRUCTION REQUIRING DELICATE HANDLING OF TISSUES AND WIDE UNDERMINING FOR METICULOUS CLOSURE)

E   D7911   Complicated suture — up to 5 cm

E   D7912   Complicated suture — greater than 5 cm

## OTHER REPAIR PROCEDURES

E   D7920   Skin graft (identify defect covered, location and type of graft)

S   D7940   Osteoplasty — for orthognathic deformities   ⊘
     MED: 100-2,15,150; 100-2,16,140; 100-4,4,20.5

E   D7941   Osteotomy — mandibular rami

E   D7943   Osteotomy — mandibular rami with bone graft; includes obtaining the graft

E ☑   D7944   Osteotomy-segmented or subapical

E   D7945   Osteotomy — body of mandible

E   D7946   LeFort I (maxilla — total)

E   D7947   LeFort I (maxilla — segmented)

E   D7948   LeFort II or LeFort III (osteoplasty of facial bones for midface hypoplasia or retrusion) — without bone graft

E   D7949   LeFort II or LeFort III — with bone graft

E   D7950   Osseous, osteoperiosteal, or cartilage graft of the mandible or maxilla—autogenous or nonautogenous, by report
     Pertinent documentation to evaluate medical appropriateness should be included when this code is reported.

E   D7951   Sinus augmentation with bone or bone substitutes

E ☑   D7953   Bone replacement graft for ridge preservation - per site

E   D7955   Repair of maxillofacial soft and/or hard tissue defect

E   D7960   Frenulectomy (frenectomy or frenotomy) — separate procedure

E   D7963   Frenuloplasty

E ☑   D7970   Excision of hyperplastic tissue — per arch

E   D7971   Excision of pericoronal gingiva

E   D7972   Surgical reduction of fibrous tuberosity

E   D7980   Sialolithotomy

E   D7981   Excision of salivary gland, by report
     Pertinent documentation to evaluate medical appropriateness should be included when this code is reported.

E   D7982   Sialodochoplasty

E   D7983   Closure of salivary fistula

E   D7990   Emergency tracheotomy

E   D7991   Coronoidectomy

E   D7995   Synthetic graft — mandible or facial bones, by report
     Pertinent documentation to evaluate medical appropriateness should be included when this code is reported.

E   D7996   Implant — mandible for augmentation purposes (excluding alveolar ridge), by report
     Pertinent documentation to evaluate medical appropriateness should be included when this code is reported.

E   D7997   Appliance removal (not by dentist who placed appliance), includes removal of archbar

E   D7998   Intraoral placement of a fixation device not in conjunction with a fracture

E   D7999   Unspecified oral surgery procedure, by report
     Determine if an alternative HCPCS Level II or a CPT code better describes the service being reported. This code should be used only if a more specific code is unavailable.

## ORTHODONTICS D8000-D8999

E   D8010   Limited orthodontic treatment of the primary dentition

E   D8020   Limited orthodontic treatment of the transitional dentition

---

| Special Coverage Instructions | Noncovered by Medicare | Carrier Discretion | ☑ Quantity Alert | ● New Code | ○ Recycled/Reinstated | ▲ Revised Code |

| | | | |
|---|---|---|---|
| E | D8030 | Limited orthodontic treatment of the adolescent dentition | A |
| E | D8040 | Limited orthodontic treatment of the adult dentition | A |
| E | D8050 | Interceptive orthodontic treatment of the primary dentition | A |
| E | D8060 | Interceptive orthodontic treatment of the transitional dentition | |
| E | D8070 | Comprehensive orthodontic treatment of the transitional dentition | |
| E | D8080 | Comprehensive orthodontic treatment of the adolescent dentition | A |
| E | D8090 | Comprehensive orthodontic treatment of the adult dentition | A |

## MINOR TREATMENT TO CONTROL HARMFUL HABITS

| | | |
|---|---|---|
| E | D8210 | Removable appliance therapy |
| E | D8220 | Fixed appliance therapy |

## OTHER ORTHODONTIC SERVICES

| | | |
|---|---|---|
| E | D8660 | Preorthodontic treatment visit |
| E | D8670 | Periodic orthodontic treatment visit (as part of contract) |
| E | D8680 | Orthodontic retention (removal of appliances, construction and placement of retainer(s)) |
| E | D8690 | Orthodontic treatment (alternative billing to a contract fee) |
| E | D8691 | Repair of orthodontic appliance |
| E | D8692 | Replacement of lost or broken retainer |
| E | D8693 | Rebonding or recementing; and/or repair, as required, of fixed retainers |
| E | D8999 | Unspecified orthodontic procedure, by report |

Determine if an alternative HCPCS Level II or a CPT code better describes the service being reported. This code should be used only if a more specific code is unavailable.

## ADJUNCTIVE GENERAL SERVICES D9110-D9999

## UNCLASSIFIED TREATMENT

| | | | |
|---|---|---|---|
| N | D9110 | Palliative (emergency) treatment of dental pain — minor procedure | ⊘ |

MED: 100-2,15,150; 100-2,16,140

| | | |
|---|---|---|
| E | D9120 | Fixed partial denture sectioning |

## ANESTHESIA

| | | | |
|---|---|---|---|
| E | D9210 | Local anesthesia not in conjunction with operative or surgical procedures | |
| E | D9211 | Regional block anesthesia | |
| E | D9212 | Trigeminal division block anesthesia | |
| E | D9215 | Local anesthesia | |
| E ☑ | D9220 | Deep sedation/general anesthesia — first 30 minutes | |
| E ☑ | D9221 | Deep sedation/general anesthesia — each additional 15 minutes | |

MED: 100-2,15,150; 100-2,16,140

| | | | |
|---|---|---|---|
| N | D9230 | Analgesia, anxiolysis, inhalation of nitrous oxide | ⊘ |

MED: 100-2,15,150; 100-2,16,140

| | | | |
|---|---|---|---|
| E ☑ | D9241 | Intravenous conscious sedation/analgesia — first 30 minutes | |
| E ☑ | D9242 | Intravenous conscious sedation/analgesia — each additional 15 minutes | |
| N | D9248 | Nonintravenous conscious sedation | |

## PROFESSIONAL CONSULTATION

| | | |
|---|---|---|
| E | D9310 | Consultation—diagnostic service provided by dentist or physician other than requesting dentist or physician |

## PROFESSIONAL VISITS

| | | |
|---|---|---|
| E | D9410 | House/extended care facility call |
| E | D9420 | Hospital call |
| E | D9430 | Office visit for observation (during regularly scheduled hours) — no other services performed |
| E | D9440 | Office visit — after regularly scheduled hours |
| E | D9450 | Case presentation, detailed and extensive treatment planning |

## DRUGS

| | | |
|---|---|---|
| E | D9610 | Therapeutic parenteral drug, single administration |

Pertinent documentation to evaluate medical appropriateness should be included when this code is reported.

| | | |
|---|---|---|
| E | D9612 | Therapeutic parenteral drugs, two or more administrations, different medications |
| S | D9630 | Other drugs and/or medicaments, by report ⊘ |

Determine if an alternative HCPCS Level II or a CPT code better describes the service being reported. This code should be used only if a more specific code is unavailable.

MED: 100-2,15,150; 100-2,16,140; 100-4,4,20.5

## MISCELLANEOUS SERVICES

| | | | |
|---|---|---|---|
| E | D9910 | Application of desensitizing medicament | |
| E ☑ | D9911 | Application of desensitizing resin for cervical and/or root surface, per tooth | |
| E | D9920 | Behavior management, by report | |

Pertinent documentation to evaluate medical appropriateness should be included when this code is reported.

| | | | |
|---|---|---|---|
| S | D9930 | Treatment of complications (postsurgical) — unusual circumstances, by report | ⊘ |

MED: 100-2,15,150; 100-2,16,140; 100-4,4,20.5

| | | | |
|---|---|---|---|
| S | D9940 | Occlusal guards, by report | ⊘ |

Pertinent documentation to evaluate medical appropriateness should be included when this code is reported.

MED: 100-2,15,150; 100-2,16,140; 100-4,4,20.5

| | | | |
|---|---|---|---|
| E | D9941 | Fabrication of athletic mouthguard | |
| E | D9942 | Repair and/or reline of occlusal guard | |
| S | D9950 | Occlusion analysis — mounted case | ⊘ |

MED: 100-2,15,150; 100-2,16,140; 100-4,4,20.5

| | | | |
|---|---|---|---|
| S | D9951 | Occlusal adjustment — limited | ⊘ |

MED: 100-2,15,150; 100-2,16,140; 100-4,4,20.5

| | | | |
|---|---|---|---|
| S | D9952 | Occlusal adjustment — complete | ⊘ |

MED: 100-2,15,150; 100-2,16,140; 100-4,4,20.5

| | | | |
|---|---|---|---|
| E | D9970 | Enamel microabrasion | |
| E ☑ | D9971 | Odontoplasty 1-2 teeth; includes removal of enamel projections | |
| E ☑ | D9972 | External bleaching — per arch | |
| E ☑ | D9973 | External bleaching — per tooth | |

▨ Special Coverage Instructions    ▨ Noncovered by Medicare    ▨ Carrier Discretion    ☑ Quantity Alert    ● New Code    ○ Recycled/Reinstated    ▲ Revised Code

**2008 HCPCS**    A2-Z3 ASC Payment Indicators    **MED:** Pub 100/NCD References    ⅋ DMEPOS Paid    ⊘ SNF Excluded    P0 PQRI    **D Codes — 37**

Ⓔ ☑ **D9974** Internal bleaching — per tooth

Ⓔ **D9999** Unspecified adjunctive procedure, by report
Determine if an alternative HCPCS Level II or a CPT code better describes the service being reported. This code should be used only if a more specific code is unavailable.

Special Coverage Instructions    Noncovered by Medicare    Carrier Discretion    ☑ Quantity Alert  ● New Code   ○ Recycled/Reinstated   ▲ Revised Code

**38 — D Codes**    Ⓐ Age Edit    Ⓜ Maternity Edit  ♀ Female Only  ♂ Male Only   Ⓐ-Ⓨ OPPS Status Indicators    **2008 HCPCS**

## DURABLE MEDICAL EQUIPMENT E0100-E9999

E codes include durable medical equipment such as canes, crutches, walkers, commodes, decubitus care, bath and toilet aids, hospital beds, oxygen and related respiratory equipment, monitoring equipment, pacemakers, patient lifts, safety equipment, restraints, traction equipment, fracture frames, wheelchairs, and artificial kidney machines.

## CANES

Ⓨ **E0100** Cane, includes canes of all materials, adjustable or fixed, with tip &
White canes for the blind are not covered under Medicare.
MED: 100-2,15,110.1; 100-3,280.1; 100-3,280.2

Ⓨ **E0105** Cane, quad or three-prong, includes canes of all materials, adjustable or fixed, with tips &
MED: 100-2,15,110.1; 100-3,280.1; 100-3,280.5

## CRUTCHES

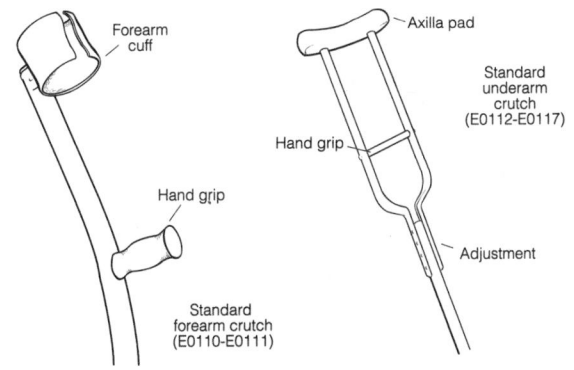

Forearm cuff

Axilla pad

Standard underarm crutch (E0112-E0117)

Hand grip

Hand grip

Adjustment

Standard forearm crutch (E0110-E0111)

Ⓨ ☑ **E0110** Crutches, forearm, includes crutches of various materials, adjustable or fixed, pair, complete with tips and handgrips &
MED: 100-2,15,110.1; 100-3,280.1

Ⓨ ☑ **E0111** Crutch, forearm, includes crutches of various materials, adjustable or fixed, each, with tip and handgrip &
MED: 100-2,15,110.1; 100-3,280.1

Ⓨ ☑ **E0112** Crutches, underarm, wood, adjustable or fixed, pair, with pads, tips and handgrips &
MED: 100-2,15,110.1; 100-3,280.1

Ⓨ ☑ **E0113** Crutch, underarm, wood, adjustable or fixed, each, with pad, tip and handgrip &
MED: 100-2,15,110.1; 100-3,280.1

Ⓨ ☑ **E0114** Crutches, underarm, other than wood, adjustable or fixed, pair, with pads, tips and handgrips &
MED: 100-2,15,110.1; 100-3,280.1

Ⓨ ☑ **E0116** Crutch, underarm, other than wood, adjustable or fixed, with pad, tip, handgrip, with or without shock absorber, each &
MED: 100-2,15,110.1; 100-3,280.1

Ⓨ ☑ **E0117** Crutch, underarm, articulating, spring assisted, each &
MED: 100-2,15,110.1

Ⓔ ☑ **E0118** Crutch substitute, lower leg platform, with or without wheels, each
Medicare covers walkers if patient's ambulation is impaired.

Ⓨ **E0130** Walker, rigid (pickup), adjustable or fixed height
MED: 100-2,15,110.1; 100-3,280.1

Ⓨ **E0135** Walker, folding (pickup), adjustable or fixed height &
Medicare covers walkers if patient's ambulation is impaired.
MED: 100-2,15,110.1; 100-3,280.1

Ⓨ **E0140** Walker, with trunk support, adjustable or fixed height, any type &
MED: 100-2,15,110.1; 100-3,280.1

Ⓨ **E0141** Walker, rigid, wheeled, adjustable or fixed height &
Medicare covers walkers if patient's ambulation is impaired.
MED: 100-2,15,110.1; 100-3,280.1

Ⓨ **E0143** Walker, folding, wheeled, adjustable or fixed height &
Medicare covers walkers if patient's ambulation is impaired.
MED: 100-2,15,110.1; 100-3,280.1

Ⓨ **E0144** Walker, enclosed, four sided framed, rigid or folding, wheeled with posterior seat &
MED: 100-2,15,110.1; 100-3,280.1

Ⓨ **E0147** Walker, heavy duty, multiple braking system, variable wheel resistance &
Medicare covers safety roller walkers only in patients with severe neurological disorders or restricted use of one hand. In some cases, coverage will be extended to patients with a weight exceeding the limits of a standard wheeled walker.
MED: 100-2,15,110.1; 100-3,280.5

Ⓨ **E0148** Walker, heavy duty, without wheels, rigid or folding, any type, each &

Ⓨ **E0149** Walker, heavy duty, wheeled, rigid or folding, any type &

Ⓨ ☑ **E0153** Platform attachment, forearm crutch, each &

Ⓨ ☑ **E0154** Platform attachment, walker, each &

Ⓨ **E0155** Wheel attachment, rigid pick-up walker, per pair &

## ATTACHMENTS

Ⓨ **E0156** Seat attachment, walker &

Ⓨ ☑ **E0157** Crutch attachment, walker, each &

Ⓨ ☑ **E0158** Leg extensions for walker, per set of four (4) &

Ⓨ ☑ **E0159** Brake attachment for wheeled walker, replacement, each &

## COMMODES

Ⓨ **E0160** Sitz type bath or equipment, portable, used with or without commode &
Medicare covers sitz baths if medical record indicates that the patient has an infection or injury of the perineal area and the sitz bath is prescribed by the physician.
MED: 100-3,280.1

Ⓨ **E0161** Sitz type bath or equipment, portable, used with or without commode, with faucet attachment(s) &
Medicare covers sitz baths if medical record indicates that the patient has an infection or injury of the perineal area and the sitz bath is prescribed by the physician.
MED: 100-3,280.1

Ⓨ **E0162** Sitz bath chair &
Medicare covers sitz baths if medical record indicates that the patient has an infection or injury of the perineal area and the sitz bath is prescribed by the physician.
MED: 100-3,280.1

■ Special Coverage Instructions   ■ Noncovered by Medicare   ■ Carrier Discretion   ☑ Quantity Alert   ● New Code   ○ Recycled/Reinstated   ▲ Revised Code

**2008 HCPCS**   **N2-Z3** ASC Payment Indicators   **MED:** Pub 100/NCD References   & DMEPOS Paid   ⊘ SNF Excluded   🅟 PQRI   **E Codes — 39**

**Durable Medical Equipment**

**E0163 — E0202**

Y **E0163** Commode chair, mobile or stationary, with fixed arms
Medicare covers commodes for patients confined to their beds or rooms, for patients without indoor bathroom facilities, and to patients who cannot climb or descend the stairs necessary to reach the bathrooms in their homes.
MED: 100-2,15,110.1; 100-3,280.1

Y **E0165** Commode chair, mobile or stationary, with detachable arms
Medicare covers commodes for patients confined to their beds or rooms, for patients without indoor bathroom facilities, and to patients who cannot climb or descend the stairs necessary to reach the bathrooms in their homes.
MED: 100-2,15,110.1; 100-3,280.1

Y **E0167** Pail or pan for use with commode chair, replacement only
Medicare covers commodes for patients confined to their beds or rooms, for patients without indoor bathroom facilities, and to patients who cannot climb or descend the stairs necessary to reach the bathrooms in their homes.
MED: 100-3,280.1

Y **E0168** Commode chair, extra wide and/or heavy duty, stationary or mobile, with or without arms, any type, each

Y **E0170** Commode chair with integrated seat lift mechanism, electric, any type

Y **E0171** Commode chair with integrated seat lift mechanism, non-electric, any type

E **E0172** Seat lift mechanism placed over or on top of toilet, any type

Y ☑ **E0175** Foot rest, for use with commode chair, each

## DECUBITUS CARE EQUIPMENT

Y **E0181** Powered pressure reducing mattress overlay/pad, alternating, with pump, includes heavy duty
Medicare covers pads if physicians supervise their use in patients who have decubitus ulcers or susceptibility to them. Prior authorization is required by Medicare for this item.
MED: 100-3,280.1; 100-8,5,5.2.3

Y **E0182** Pump for alternating pressure pad, for replacement only
Medicare covers pads if physicians supervise their use in patients who have decubitus ulcers or susceptibility to them. Prior authorization is required by Medicare for this item.
MED: 100-3,280.1; 100-8,5,5.2.3

Y **E0184** Dry pressure mattress
Medicare covers pads if physicians supervise their use in patients who have decubitus ulcers or susceptibility to them. Prior authorization is required by Medicare for this item.
MED: 100-3,280.1; 100-8,5,5.2.3

Y **E0185** Gel or gel-like pressure pad for mattress, standard mattress length and width
Medicare covers pads if physicians supervise their use in patients who have decubitus ulcers or susceptibility to them. Prior authorization is required by Medicare for this item.
MED: 100-3,280.1; 100-8,5,5.2.3

Y **E0186** Air pressure mattress
Medicare covers pads if physicians supervise their use in patients who have decubitus ulcers or susceptibility to them.
MED: 100-3,280.1

Y **E0187** Water pressure mattress
Medicare covers pads if physicians supervise their use in patients who have decubitus ulcers or susceptibility to them.
MED: 100-3,280.1

Y **E0188** Synthetic sheepskin pad
Medicare covers pads if physicians supervise their use in patients who have decubitus ulcers or susceptibility to them. Prior authorization is required by Medicare for this item.
MED: 100-3,280.1; 100-8,5,5.2.3

Y **E0189** Lambswool sheepskin pad, any size
Medicare covers pads if physicians supervise their use in patients who have decubitus ulcers or susceptibility to them. Prior authorization is required by Medicare for this item.
MED: 100-3,280.1; 100-8,5,5.2.3

E **E0190** Positioning cushion/pillow/wedge, any shape or size, includes all components and accessories
MED: 100-2,15,110.1

Y ☑ **E0191** Heel or elbow protector, each

Y **E0193** Powered air flotation bed (low air loss therapy)

Y **E0194** Air fluidized bed
An air fluidized bed is covered by Medicare if the patient has a stage 3 or stage 4 pressure sore and, without the bed, would require institutionalization. A physician's prescription is required.
MED: 100-3,280.8

Y **E0196** Gel pressure mattress
Medicare covers pads if physicians supervise their use in patients who have decubitus ulcers or susceptibility to them.
MED: 100-3,280.1

Y **E0197** Air pressure pad for mattress, standard mattress length and width
Medicare covers pads if physicians supervise their use in patients who have decubitus ulcers or susceptibility to them.
MED: 100-3,280.1

Y **E0198** Water pressure pad for mattress, standard mattress length and width
Medicare covers pads if physicians supervise their use in patients who have decubitus ulcers or susceptibility to them.
MED: 100-3,280.1

Y **E0199** Dry pressure pad for mattress, standard mattress length and width
Medicare covers pads if physicians supervise their use in patients who have decubitus ulcers or susceptibility to them.
MED: 100-3,280.1

## HEAT/COLD APPLICATION

Y **E0200** Heat lamp, without stand (table model), includes bulb, or infrared element
MED: 100-2,15,110.1; 100-3,280.1

Y **E0202** Phototherapy (bilirubin) light with photometer

---

Special Coverage Instructions    Noncovered by Medicare    Carrier Discretion     ☑ Quantity Alert    ● New Code    ○ Recycled/Reinstated    ▲ Revised Code

| E | E0203 | Therapeutic lightbox, minimum 10,000 lux, table top model |

| Y | E0205 | Heat lamp, with stand, includes bulb, or infrared element |

MED: 100-2,15,110.1; 100-3,280.1

| Y | E0210 | Electric heat pad, standard |

MED: 100-3,280.1

| Y | E0215 | Electric heat pad, moist |

MED: 100-3,280.1

| Y | E0217 | Water circulating heat pad with pump |

MED: 100-3,280.1

| Y | E0218 | Water circulating cold pad with pump |

MED: 100-3,280.1

| Y | E0220 | Hot water bottle |

| Y | E0221 | Infrared heating pad system |

MED: 100-3,270.2

| Y | E0225 | Hydrocollator unit, includes pads |

MED: 100-2,15,230; 100-3,280.1

| Y | E0230 | Ice cap or collar |

| E | E0231 | Noncontact wound warming device (temperature control unit, AC adapter and power cord) for use with warming card and wound cover |

MED: 100-2,16,20

| E | E0232 | Warming card for use with the noncontact wound warming device and noncontact wound warming wound cover |

| Y | E0235 | Paraffin bath unit, portable (see medical supply code A4265 for paraffin) |

MED: 100-2,15,230; 100-3,280.1

| Y | E0236 | Pump for water circulating pad |

MED: 100-3,280.1

| Y | E0238 | Nonelectric heat pad, moist |

MED: 100-3,280.1

| Y | E0239 | Hydrocollator unit, portable |

MED: 100-2,15,230; 100-3,280.1

## BATH AND TOILET AIDS

| E | E0240 | Bath/shower chair, with or without wheels, any size |

MED: 100-3,280.1

| E ☑ | E0241 | Bathtub wall rail, each |

MED: 100-2,15,110.1; 100-3,280.1

| E | E0242 | Bathtub rail, floor base |

MED: 100-2,15,110.1; 100-3,280.1

| E ☑ | E0243 | Toilet rail, each |

MED: 100-2,15,110.1; 100-3,280.1

| E | E0244 | Raised toilet seat |

MED: 100-3,280.1

| E | E0245 | Tub stool or bench |

MED: 100-3,280.1

| E | E0246 | Transfer tub rail attachment |

| E | E0247 | Transfer bench for tub or toilet with or without commode opening |

MED: 100-3,280.1

| E | E0248 | Transfer bench, heavy duty, for tub or toilet with or without commode opening |

MED: 100-3,280.1

| Y | E0249 | Pad for water circulating heat unit |

MED: 100-3,280.1

## HOSPITAL BEDS AND ACCESSORIES

| E | E0250 | Hospital bed, fixed height, with any type side rails, with mattress |

MED: 100-2,15,110.1; 100-3,280.7

| E | E0251 | Hospital bed, fixed height, with any type side rails, without mattress |

MED: 100-2,15,110.1; 100-3,280.7

| E | E0255 | Hospital bed, variable height, hi-lo, with any type side rails, with mattress |

MED: 100-2,15,110.1; 100-3,280.7

| E | E0256 | Hospital bed, variable height, hi-lo, with any type side rails, without mattress |

MED: 100-2,15,110.1; 100-3,280.7

| E | E0260 | Hospital bed, semi-electric (head and foot adjustment), with any type side rails, with mattress |

MED: 100-2,15,110.1; 100-3,280.7

| E | E0261 | Hospital bed, semi-electric (head and foot adjustment), with any type side rails, without mattress |

MED: 100-2,15,110.1; 100-3,280.7

| E | E0265 | Hospital bed, total electric (head, foot, and height adjustments), with any type side rails, with mattress |

MED: 100-2,15,110.1; 100-3,280.7

| E | E0266 | Hospital bed, total electric (head, foot, and height adjustments), with any type side rails, without mattress |

MED: 100-2,15,110.1; 100-3,280.7

| E | E0270 | Hospital bed, institutional type includes: oscillating, circulating and Stryker frame, with mattress |

MED: 100-3,280.1

| E | E0271 | Mattress, innerspring |

MED: 100-3,280.1; 100-3,280.7

| E | E0272 | Mattress, foam rubber |

MED: 100-3,280.1; 100-3,280.7

| E | E0273 | Bed board |

MED: 100-3,280.1

| E | E0274 | Over-bed table |

MED: 100-3,280.1

| Y | E0275 | Bed pan, standard, metal or plastic |

Reusable, autoclavable bedpans are covered by Medicare for bed-confined patients.

MED: 100-3,280.1

| Y | E0276 | Bed pan, fracture, metal or plastic |

Reusable, autoclavable bedpans are covered by Medicare for bed-confined patients.

MED: 100-3,280.1

| Y | E0277 | Powered pressure-reducing air mattress |

MED: 100-3,280.1

| Y | E0280 | Bed cradle, any type |

| E | E0290 | Hospital bed, fixed height, without side rails, with mattress |

MED: 100-2,15,110.1; 100-3,280.7

| Y | E0291 | Hospital bed, fixed height, without side rails, without mattress |

MED: 100-2,15,110.1; 100-3,280.7

| E | E0292 | Hospital bed, variable height, hi-lo, without side rails, with mattress |

MED: 100-2,15,110.1; 100-3,280.7

---

Special Coverage Instructions    Noncovered by Medicare    Carrier Discretion    ☑ Quantity Alert    ● New Code    ○ Recycled/Reinstated    ▲ Revised Code

Y **E0293** Hospital bed, variable height, hi-lo, without side rails, without mattress ♿
MED: 100-2,15,110.1; 100-3,280.7

E **E0294** Hospital bed, semi-electric (head and foot adjustment), without side rails, with mattress ♿
MED: 100-2,15,110.1; 100-3,280.7

Y **E0295** Hospital bed, semi-electric (head and foot adjustment), without side rails, without mattress ♿
MED: 100-2,15,110.1; 100-3,280.7

E **E0296** Hospital bed, total electric (head, foot, and height adjustments), without side rails, with mattress ♿
MED: 100-2,15,110.1; 100-3,280.7

Y **E0297** Hospital bed, total electric (head, foot, and height adjustments), without side rails, without mattress ♿
MED: 100-2,15,110.1; 100-3,280.7

Y **E0300** Pediatric crib, hospital grade, fully enclosed ♿

Y **E0301** Hospital bed, heavy duty, extra wide, with weight capacity greater than 350 pounds, but less than or equal to 600 pounds, with any type side rails, without mattress ♿
MED: 100-3,280.7

Y **E0302** Hospital bed, extra heavy duty, extra wide, with weight capacity greater than 600 pounds, with any type side rails, without mattress ♿
MED: 100-3,280.7

E **E0303** Hospital bed, heavy duty, extra wide, with weight capacity greater than 350 pounds, but less than or equal to 600 pounds, with any type side rails, with mattress ♿
MED: 100-3,280.7

E **E0304** Hospital bed, extra heavy duty, extra wide, with weight capacity greater than 600 pounds, with any type side rails, with mattress ♿
MED: 100-3,280.7

E **E0305** Bedside rails, half-length ♿
MED: 100-3,280.7

E **E0310** Bedside rails, full-length ♿
MED: 100-3,280.7

E **E0315** Bed accessory: board, table, or support device, any type
MED: 100-3,280.1

Y **E0316** Safety enclosure frame/canopy for use with hospital bed, any type ♿

Y **E0325** Urinal; male, jug-type, any material ♂♿
MED: 100-3,280.1

Y **E0326** Urinal; female, jug-type, any material ♀♿
MED: 100-3,280.1

● Y **E0328** Hospital bed, pediatric, manual, 360 degree side enclosures, top of headboard, footboard, and side rails up to 24 in. above the spring, includes mattress

● Y **E0329** Hospital bed, pediatric, electric or semi-electric, 360 degree side enclosures, top of headboard, footboard, and side rails up to 24 in. above the spring, includes mattress

E **E0350** Control unit for electronic bowel irrigation/evacuation system

E **E0352** Disposable pack (water reservoir bag, speculum, valving mechanism, and collection bag/box) for use with the electronic bowel irrigation/evacuation system

E **E0370** Air pressure elevator for heel

Y **E0371** Nonpowered advanced pressure reducing overlay for mattress, standard mattress length and width ♿

Y **E0372** Powered air overlay for mattress, standard mattress length and width ♿

Y **E0373** Nonpowered advanced pressure reducing mattress ♿

## OXYGEN AND RELATED RESPIRATORY EQUIPMENT

Y **E0424** Stationary compressed gaseous oxygen system, rental; includes container, contents, regulator, flowmeter, humidifier, nebulizer, cannula or mask, and tubing ♿
For the first claim filed for home oxygen equipment or therapy, submit a certificate of medical necessity that includes the oxygen flow rate, anticipated frequency and duration of oxygen therapy, and physician signature. Medicare accepts oxygen therapy as medically necessary in cases documenting any of the following: erythocythemia with a hematocrit greater than 56 percent; a P pulmonale on EKG; or dependent edema consistent with congestive heart failure.
MED: 100-3,240.2

E **E0425** Stationary compressed gas system, purchase; includes regulator, flowmeter, humidifier, nebulizer, cannula or mask, and tubing
MED: 100-3,240.2

E **E0430** Portable gaseous oxygen system, purchase; includes regulator, flowmeter, humidifier, cannula or mask, and tubing
MED: 100-3,240.2

Y **E0431** Portable gaseous oxygen system, rental; includes portable container, regulator, flowmeter, humidifier, cannula or mask, and tubing ♿
MED: 100-3,240.2

Y **E0434** Portable liquid oxygen system, rental; includes portable container, supply reservoir, humidifier, flowmeter, refill adaptor, contents gauge, cannula or mask, and tubing ♿
MED: 100-3,240.2

E **E0435** Portable liquid oxygen system, purchase; includes portable container, supply reservoir, flowmeter, humidifier, contents gauge, cannula, or mask, tubing and refill adaptor
MED: 100-3,240.2

Y **E0439** Stationary liquid oxygen system, rental; includes container, contents, regulator, flowmeter, humidifier, nebulizer, cannula or mask, & tubing ♿
MED: 100-3,240.2

E **E0440** Stationary liquid oxygen system, purchase; includes use of reservoir, contents indicator, regulator, flowmeter, humidifier, nebulizer, cannula or mask, and tubing
MED: 100-3,240.2

Y ☑ **E0441** Oxygen contents, gaseous (for use with owned gaseous stationary systems or when both a stationary and portable gaseous system are owned), one month's supply = 1 unit ♿
MED: 100-3,240.2

Y ☑ **E0442** Oxygen contents, liquid (for use with owned liquid stationary systems or when both a stationary and portable liquid system are owned), one month's supply = 1 unit ♿
MED: 100-3,240.2

---

Special Coverage Instructions    Noncovered by Medicare    Carrier Discretion    ☑ Quantity Alert    ● New Code    ○ Recycled/Reinstated    ▲ Revised Code

**42 — E Codes**    Ⓐ Age Edit    Ⓜ Maternity Edit    ♀ Female Only    ♂ Male Only    Ⓐ-Ⓨ OPPS Status Indicators    **2008 HCPCS**

Y ☑ **E0443** Portable oxygen contents, gaseous (for use only with portable gaseous systems when no stationary gas or liquid system is used), one month's supply = 1 unit         ♿

MED: 100-3,240.2

Y ☑ **E0444** Portable oxygen contents, liquid (for use only with portable liquid systems when no stationary gas or liquid system is used), one month's supply = 1 unit    ♿

MED: 100-3,240.2

A **E0445** Oximeter device for measuring blood oxygen levels non-invasively

Y **E0450** Volume control ventilator, without pressure support mode, may include pressure control mode, used with invasive interface (e.g., tracheostomy tube)    ♿

MED: 100-3,280.1

Y **E0455** Oxygen tent, excluding croup or pediatric tents

MED: 100-3,240.2

Y **E0457** Chest shell (cuirass)    ♿

Y **E0459** Chest wrap    ♿

Y **E0460** Negative pressure ventilator; portable or stationary    ♿

MED: 100-3,280.1

Y **E0461** Volume control ventilator, without pressure support mode, may include pressure control mode, used with noninvasive interface (e.g., mask)    ♿

MED: 100-3,280.1

Y **E0462** Rocking bed, with or without side rails    ♿

Y **E0463** Pressure support ventilator with volume control mode, may include pressure control mode, used with invasive interface (e.g., tracheostomy tube)

Y **E0464** Pressure support ventilator with volume control mode, may include pressure control mode, used with noninvasive interface (e.g., mask)

Y **E0470** Respiratory assist device, bi-level pressure capability, without backup rate feature, used with noninvasive interface, e.g., nasal or facial mask (intermittent assist device with continuous positive airway pressure device)    ♿

MED: 100-3,280.1

Y **E0471** Respiratory assist device, bi-level pressure capability, with back-up rate feature, used with noninvasive interface, e.g., nasal or facial mask (intermittent assist device with continuous positive airway pressure device)    ♿

MED: 100-3,280.1

Y **E0472** Respiratory assist device, bi-level pressure capability, with backup rate feature, used with invasive interface, e.g., tracheostomy tube (intermittent assist device with continuous positive airway pressure device)    ♿

MED: 100-3,280.1

Y **E0480** Percussor, electric or pneumatic, home model    ♿

MED: 100-3,280.1

E **E0481** Intrapulmonary percussive ventilation system and related accessories

MED: 100-3,240.5

Y **E0482** Cough stimulating device, alternating positive and negative airway pressure    ♿

Y ☑ **E0483** High frequency chest wall oscillation air-pulse generator system, (includes hoses and vest), each    ♿

Y ☑ **E0484** Oscillatory positive expiratory pressure device, nonelectric, any type, each    ♿

Y **E0485** Oral device/appliance used to reduce upper airway collapsibility, adjustable or non-adjustable, prefabricated, includes fitting and adjustment

Y **E0486** Oral device/appliance used to reduce upper airway collapsibility, adjustable or non-adjustable, custom fabricated, includes fitting and adjustment

## IPPB MACHINES

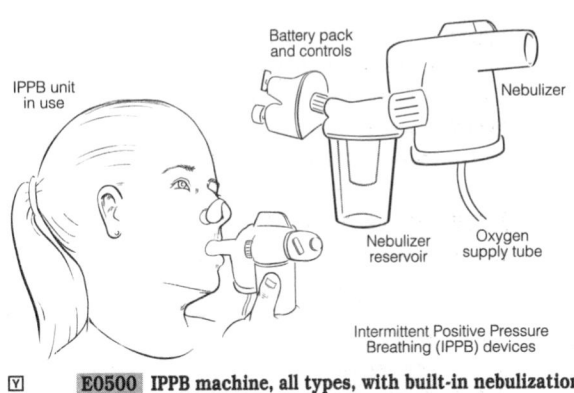

Battery pack and controls

Nebulizer

IPPB unit in use

Nebulizer reservoir

Oxygen supply tube

Intermittent Positive Pressure Breathing (IPPB) devices

Y **E0500** IPPB machine, all types, with built-in nebulization; manual or automatic valves; internal or external power source    ♿

MED: 100-3,280.1

## HUMIDIFIERS/COMPRESSORS/NEBULIZERS FOR USE WITH OXYGEN IPPB EQUIPMENT

Y **E0550** Humidifier, durable for extensive supplemental humidification during IPPB treatments or oxygen delivery    ♿

MED: 100-3,280.1

Y **E0555** Humidifier, durable, glass or autoclavable plastic bottle type, for use with regulator or flowmeter    ♿

MED: 100-3,280.1

Y **E0560** Humidifier, durable for supplemental humidification during IPPB treatment or oxygen delivery    ♿

MED: 100-3,280.1

Y **E0561** Humidifier, nonheated, used with positive airway pressure device    ♿

Y **E0562** Humidifier, heated, used with positive airway pressure device    ♿

Y **E0565** Compressor, air power source for equipment which is not self-contained or cylinder driven    ♿

Y **E0570** Nebulizer, with compressor    ♿

MED: 100-3,280.1

Y **E0571** Aerosol compressor, battery powered, for use with small volume nebulizer    ♿

MED: 100-3,280.1

Y **E0572** Aerosol compressor, adjustable pressure, light duty for intermittent use    ♿

Y **E0574** Ultrasonic/electronic aerosol generator with small volume nebulizer    ♿

Y **E0575** Nebulizer, ultrasonic, large volume    ♿

MED: 100-3,280.1

Y **E0580** Nebulizer, durable, glass or autoclavable plastic, bottle type, for use with regulator or flowmeter    ♿

MED: 100-3,280.1

Y **E0585** Nebulizer, with compressor and heater    ♿

MED: 100-3,280.1

Special Coverage Instructions    Noncovered by Medicare    Carrier Discretion    ☑ Quantity Alert    ● New Code    ○ Recycled/Reinstated    ▲ Revised Code

**2008 HCPCS**    A2– A3 ASC Payment Indicators    **MED:** Pub 100/NCD References    ♿ DMEPOS Paid    Ⓢ SNF Excluded    PQ PQRI    **E Codes — 43**

**Durable Medical Equipment**

**E0600 — E0671**

## SUCTION PUMP/ROOM VAPORIZERS

**E0600** Respiratory suction pump, home model, portable or stationary, electric ♿
MED: 100-3,280.1

**E0601** Continuous airway pressure (CPAP) device ♿
MED: 100-3,240.4

**E0602** Breast pump, manual, any type ♀♿

**E0603** Breast pump, electric (AC and/or DC), any type ♀

▲ **E0604** Breast pump, hospital grade, electric (AC and/or DC), any type ♀

**E0605** Vaporizer, room type ♿
MED: 100-3,280.1

**E0606** Postural drainage board ♿
MED: 100-3,280.1

## MONITORING EQUIPMENT

**E0607** Home blood glucose monitor ♿
Medicare covers home blood testing devices for diabetic patients when the devices are prescribed by the patients' physicians. Many commercial payers provide this coverage to non-insulin dependent diabetics as well.
MED: 100.3,230.16

## PACEMAKER MONITOR

**E0610** Pacemaker monitor, self-contained, (checks battery depletion, includes audible and visible check systems) ♿
MED: 100-3,20.8; 100-3,20.8.1; 100-3,20.8.2

**E0615** Pacemaker monitor, self-contained, checks battery depletion and other pacemaker components, includes digital/visible check systems ♿
MED: 100-3,20.8; 100-3,20.8.1; 100-3,20.8.2

**E0616** Implantable cardiac event recorder with memory, activator, and programmer NI

**E0617** External defibrillator with integrated electrocardiogram analysis ♿

**E0618** Apnea monitor, without recording feature

**E0619** Apnea monitor, with recording feature

**E0620** Skin piercing device for collection of capillary blood, laser, each ♿

## PATIENT LIFTS

**E0621** Sling or seat, patient lift, canvas or nylon ♿
MED: 100-3,280.1

**E0625** Patient lift, bathroom or toilet, not otherwise classified
MED: 100-3,280.1

**E0627** Seat lift mechanism incorporated into a combination lift-chair mechanism ♿
MED: 100-3,280.4; 100-4,20,100; 100-4,20,130.2; 100-4,20,130.3; 100-4,20,130.4; 100-4,20,130.5

**E0628** Separate seat lift mechanism for use with patient owned furniture — electric ♿
MED: 100-3,280.4; 100-4,20,100; 100-4,20,130.2; 100-4,20,130.3; 100-4,20,130.4; 100-4,20,130.5

**E0629** Separate seat lift mechanism for use with patient owned furniture — nonelectric ♿
MED: 100-4,20,100; 100-4,20,130.2; 100-4,20,130.3; 100-4,20,130.4; 100-4,20,130.5

▲ **E0630** Patient lift, hydraulic or mechanical, includes any seat, sling, strap(s), or pad(s) ♿
MED: 100-3,280.1

**E0635** Patient lift, electric, with seat or sling ♿
MED: 100-3,280.1

**E0636** Multipositional patient support system, with integrated lift, patient accessible controls ♿

**E0637** Combination sit to stand system, any size including pediatric, with seatlift feature, with or without wheels
MED: 100-3,280.1

**E0638** Standing frame system, one position (e.g., upright, supine, or prone stander), any size including pediatric, with or without wheels ♿
MED: 100-3,280.1

**E0639** Patient lift, moveable from room to room with disassembly and reassembly, includes all components/accessories

**E0640** Patient lift, fixed system, includes all components/accessories

**E0641** Standing frame System, multi-position (e.g. three-way stander), any size including pediatric, with or without wheels

**E0642** Standing frame system, mobile (dynamic stander), any size including pediatric

## PNEUMATIC COMPRESSOR AND APPLIANCES

**E0650** Pneumatic compressor, nonsegmental home model ♿
MED: 100-3,280.6

**E0651** Pneumatic compressor, segmental home model without calibrated gradient pressure ♿
MED: 100-3,280.6

**E0652** Pneumatic compressor, segmental home model with calibrated gradient pressure ♿
MED: 100-3,280.6

**E0655** Nonsegmental pneumatic appliance for use with pneumatic compressor, half arm ♿
MED: 100-3,280.6

**E0660** Nonsegmental pneumatic appliance for use with pneumatic compressor, full leg ♿
MED: 100-3,280.6

**E0665** Nonsegmental pneumatic appliance for use with pneumatic compressor, full arm ♿
MED: 100-3,280.6

**E0666** Nonsegmental pneumatic appliance for use with pneumatic compressor, half leg ♿
MED: 100-3,280.6

**E0667** Segmental pneumatic appliance for use with pneumatic compressor, full leg ♿
MED: 100-3,280.6

**E0668** Segmental pneumatic appliance for use with pneumatic compressor, full arm ♿
MED: 100-3,280.6

**E0669** Segmental pneumatic appliance for use with pneumatic compressor, half leg ♿
MED: 100-3,280.6

**E0671** Segmental gradient pressure pneumatic appliance, full leg ♿
MED: 100-3,280.6

---

Special Coverage Instructions    Noncovered by Medicare    Carrier Discretion    ☑ Quantity Alert    ● New Code    ○ Recycled/Reinstated    ▲ Revised Code

**44 — E Codes**    Ⓐ Age Edit    Ⓜ Maternity Edit    ♀ Female Only    ♂ Male Only    Ⓐ-Ⓨ OPPS Status Indicators    **2008 HCPCS**

[Y] **E0672** Segmental gradient pressure pneumatic appliance, full arm &

MED: 100-3,280.6

[Y] **E0673** Segmental gradient pressure pneumatic appliance, half leg &

MED: 100-3,280.6

[Y] **E0675** Pneumatic compression device, high pressure, rapid inflation/deflation cycle, for arterial insufficiency (unilateral or bilateral system) &

[Y] **E0676** Intermittent limb compression device (includes all accessories), not otherwise specified &

[Y] **E0691** Ultraviolet light therapy system panel, includes bulbs/lamps, timer, and eye protection; treatment area 2 sq. ft. or less &

[Y] **E0692** Ultraviolet light therapy system panel, includes bulbs/lamps, timer, and eye protection, 4 ft. panel &

[Y] **E0693** Ultraviolet light therapy system panel, includes bulbs/lamps, timer, and eye protection, 6 ft. panel &

[Y] **E0694** Ultraviolet multidirectional light therapy system in 6 ft. cabinet, includes bulbs/lamps, timer, and eye protection &

## SAFETY EQUIPMENT

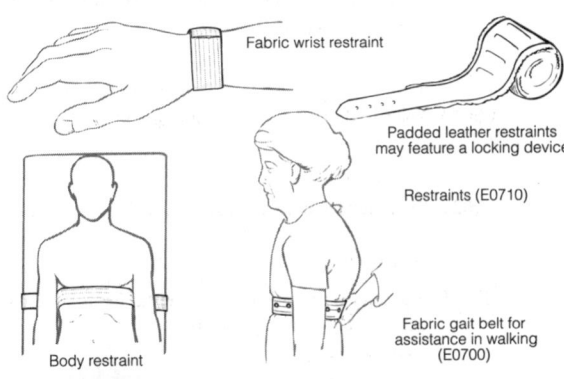

Fabric wrist restraint

Padded leather restraints may feature a locking device

Restraints (E0710)

Fabric gait belt for assistance in walking (E0700)

Body restraint

[E] **E0700** Safety equipment (e.g., belt, harness, or vest)

▲ [B] [☑] **E0705** Transfer device, any type, each

## RESTRAINTS

[E] **E0710** Restraints, any type (body, chest, wrist, or ankle)

## TRANSCUTANEOUS AND/OR NEUROMUSCULAR ELECTRICAL NERVE STIMULATORS - TENS

[Y] **E0720** Transcutaneous electrical nerve stimulation (TENS) device, two lead, localized stimulation &

While TENS is covered when employed to control chronic pain, it is not covered for experimental treatment, as in motor function disorders like MS. Prior authorization is required by Medicare for this item.

MED: 100-3,40.5; 100-3,130.5; 100-3,130.6; 100-3,160.2; 100-3,160.7.1; 100-3,230.1; 100-8,5,5.2.3

[Y] **E0730** Transcutaneous electrical nerve stimulation (TENS) device, four or more leads, for multiple nerve stimulation &

While TENS is covered when employed to control chronic pain, it is not covered for experimental treatment, as in motor function disorders like MS. Prior authorization is required by Medicare for this item.

MED: 100-3,40.5; 100-3,130.5; 100-3,130.6; 100-3,160.2; 100-3,160.7.1; 100-3,230.1; 100-8,5,5.2.3

[Y] **E0731** Form-fitting conductive garment for delivery of TENS or NMES (with conductive fibers separated from the patient's skin by layers of fabric) &

MED: 100-3,160.13

[Y] **E0740** Incontinence treatment system, pelvic floor stimulator, monitor, sensor, and/or trainer &

MED: 100-3,230.8

[Y] **E0744** Neuromuscular stimulator for scoliosis &

[Y] **E0745** Neuromuscular stimulator, electronic shock unit &

MED: 100-3,160.12

[A] **E0746** Electromyography (EMG), biofeedback device

Biofeedback therapy is covered by Medicare only for re-education of specific muscles or for treatment of incapacitating muscle spasm or weakness. Medicare jurisdiction: local contractor.

MED: 100-3,30.1; 100-3,30.1.1

[Y] **E0747** Osteogenesis stimulator, electrical, noninvasive, other than spinal applications &

Medicare covers noninvasive osteogenic stimulation for nonunion of long bone fractures, failed fusion, or congenital pseudoarthroses.

MED: 100-3,150.2

[Y] **E0748** Osteogenesis stimulator, electrical, noninvasive, spinal applications &

Medicare covers noninvasive osteogenic stimulation as an adjunct to spinal fusion surgery for patients at high risk of pseudoarthroses due to previously failed spinal fusion, or for those undergoing fusion of three or more vertebrae.

MED: 100-3,150.2

[N] **E0749** Osteogenesis stimulator, electrical, surgically implanted [N1] &

Medicare covers invasive osteogenic stimulation for nonunion of long bone fractures or as an adjunct to spinal fusion surgery for patients at high risk of pseudoarthroses due to previously failed spinal fusion, or for those undergoing fusion of three or more vertebrae.

MED: 100-3,150.2; 100-4,4,20.5; 100-4,4,190

[E] **E0755** Electronic salivary reflex stimulator (intraoral/noninvasive)

[Y] **E0760** Osteogenesis stimulator, low intensity ultrasound, noninvasive &

MED: 100-3,150.2

[E] **E0761** Nonthermal pulsed high frequency radiowaves, high peak power electromagnetic energy treatment device

[B] **E0762** Transcutaneous electrical joint stimulation device system, includes all accessories &

[Y] **E0764** Functional neuromuscular stimulator, transcutaneous stimulation of muscles of ambulation with computer control, used for walking by spinal cord injured, entire system, after completion of training program

[Y] **E0765** FDA approved nerve stimulator, with replaceable batteries, for treatment of nausea and vomiting &

[B] **E0769** Electrical stimulation or electromagnetic wound treatment device, not otherwise classified

MED: 100-4,32,11.1

## INFUSION SUPPLIES

[Y] **E0776** IV pole &

[Y] **E0779** Ambulatory infusion pump, mechanical, reusable, for infusion 8 hours or greater

Special Coverage Instructions | Noncovered by Medicare | Carrier Discretion | ☑ Quantity Alert ● New Code ○ Recycled/Reinstated ▲ Revised Code

**2008 HCPCS** [A2]-[Z3] ASC Payment Indicators  **MED:** Pub 100/NCD References  & DMEPOS Paid  ⊘ SNF Excluded  [PQ] PQRI  **E Codes — 45**

**Durable Medical Equipment**

**E0780 — E0952**

[Y] **E0780** Ambulatory infusion pump, mechanical, reusable, for infusion less than 8 hours

[Y] **E0781** Ambulatory infusion pump, single or multiple channels, electric or battery operated, with administrative equipment, worn by patient
**Medicare jurisdiction: DME local or regional contractor. Bill Medicare claims for regional contractor when the infusion is initiated in the physician's office but the patient does not return during the same day of business.**

MED: 100-3,280.14

[N] **E0782** Infusion pump, implantable, non-programmable (includes all components, e.g., pump, catheter, connectors, etc.)
**Medicare jurisdiction: local contractor.**

MED: 100-3,280.14; 100-4,4,20.5; 100-4,4,190

[N] **E0783** Infusion pump system, implantable, programmable (includes all components, e.g., pump, catheter, connectors, etc.)
**Medicare jurisdiction: local contractor.**

MED: 100-3,280.14; 100-4,4,20.5; 100-4,4,190

[Y] **E0784** External ambulatory infusion pump, insulin
**Covered by some commercial payers with preauthorization.**

MED: 100-3,280.14

[N] **E0785** Implantable intraspinal (epidural/intrathecal) catheter used with implantable infusion pump, replacement
**Medicare jurisdiction: local contractor.**

MED: 100-3,280.14; 100-4,4,20.5; 100-4,4,190

[N] **E0786** Implantable programmable infusion pump, replacement (excludes implantable intraspinal catheter)
**Medicare jurisdiction: local contractor.**

MED: 100-3,280.14

[Y] ▲ **E0791** Parenteral infusion pump, stationary, single, or multi-channel

MED: 100-2,15,120; 100-3,180.2; 100-4,20,100.2.2

## TRACTION - ALL TYPES

[N] **E0830** Ambulatory traction device, all types, each

MED: 100-3,280.1

## TRACTION - CERVICAL

[Y] **E0840** Traction frame, attached to headboard, cervical traction

MED: 100-3,280.1

[Y] **E0849** Traction equipment, cervical, free-standing stand/frame, pneumatic, applying traction force to other than mandible

[Y] **E0850** Traction stand, freestanding, cervical traction

MED: 100-3,280.1

[Y] **E0855** Cervical traction equipment not requiring additional stand or frame

● [Y] **E0856** Cervical traction device, cervical collar with inflatable air bladder

## TRACTION - OVERDOOR

[Y] **E0860** Traction equipment, overdoor, cervical

MED: 100-3,280.1

## TRACTION - EXTREMITY

[Y] **E0870** Traction frame, attached to footboard, extremity traction (e.g., Buck's)

MED: 100-3,280.1

[Y] **E0880** Traction stand, freestanding, extremity traction (e.g., Buck's)

MED: 100-3,280.1

## TRACTION - PELVIC

[Y] **E0890** Traction frame, attached to footboard, pelvic traction

MED: 100-3,280.1

[Y] **E0900** Traction stand, freestanding, pelvic traction (e.g., Buck's)

MED: 100-3,280.1

## TRAPEZE EQUIPMENT, FRACTURE FRAME, AND OTHER ORTHOPEDIC DEVICES

[Y] **E0910** Trapeze bars, also known as Patient Helper, attached to bed, with grab bar

MED: 100-3,280.1

[Y] **E0911** Trapeze bar, heavy duty, for patient weight capacity greater than 250 pounds, attached to bed, with grab bar

[Y] **E0912** Trapeze bar, heavy duty, for patient weight capacity greater than 250 pounds, free standing, complete with grab bar

[Y] **E0920** Fracture frame, attached to bed, includes weights

MED: 100-3,280.1

[Y] **E0930** Fracture frame, freestanding, includes weights

MED: 100-3,280.1

[Y] **E0935** Continuous passive motion exercise device for use on knee only

MED: 100-3,280.1

[E] **E0936** Continuous passive motion exercise device for use other than knee

[Y] **E0940** Trapeze bar, freestanding, complete with grab bar

MED: 100-3,280.1

[Y] **E0941** Gravity assisted traction device, any type

MED: 100-3,280.1

[Y] **E0942** Cervical head harness/halter

[Y] **E0944** Pelvic belt/harness/boot

[Y] **E0945** Extremity belt/harness

[Y] **E0946** Fracture frame, dual with cross bars, attached to bed (e.g., Balken, Four Poster)

MED: 100-3,280.1

[Y] **E0947** Fracture frame, attachments for complex pelvic traction

MED: 100-3,280.1

[Y] **E0948** Fracture frame, attachments for complex cervical traction

MED: 100-3,280.1

[A] **E0950** Wheelchair accessory, tray, each

MED: 100-3,280.1

[A] ☑ **E0951** Heel loop/holder, any type, with or without ankle strap, each

[A] ☑ **E0952** Toe loop/holder, any type, each

MED: 100-3,280.1

Special Coverage Instructions     Noncovered by Medicare     Carrier Discretion     ☑ Quantity Alert   ● New Code   ○ Recycled/Reinstated   ▲ Revised Code

**46 — E Codes**        [A] Age Edit     [M] Maternity Edit    ♀ Female Only   ♂ Male Only   [A]-[Y] OPPS Status Indicators        **2008 HCPCS**

Y ☑ **E0955** Wheelchair accessory, headrest, cushioned, any type, including fixed mounting hardware, each ♿

Y ☑ **E0956** Wheelchair accessory, lateral trunk or hip support, any type, including fixed mounting hardware, each ♿

Y ☑ **E0957** Wheelchair accessory, medial thigh support, any type, including fixed mounting hardware, each ♿

A ☑ **E0958** Manual wheelchair accessory, one-arm drive attachment, each ♿
MED: 100-3,280.1

B ☑ **E0959** Manual wheelchair accessory, adapter for amputee, each ♿
MED: 100-3,280.1

Y **E0960** Wheelchair accessory, shoulder harness/straps or chest strap, including any type mounting hardware ♿

B ☑ **E0961** Manual wheelchair accessory, wheel lock brake extension (handle), each ♿
MED: 100-3,280.1

B ☑ **E0966** Manual wheelchair accessory, headrest extension, each ♿
MED: 100-3,280.1

Y ☑ **E0967** Manual wheelchair accessory, hand rim with projections, any type, each ♿
MED: 100-3,280.1

Y **E0968** Commode seat, wheelchair ♿
MED: 100-3,280.1

Y **E0969** Narrowing device, wheelchair ♿
MED: 100-3,280.1

E **E0970** No. 2 footplates, except for elevating leg rest ♿
See code(s): K0037, K0042
MED: 100-3,280.1

B ☑ **E0971** Manual wheelchair accessory, anti-tipping device, each ♿
DME fee schedule reflects a base billing unit of each.
MED: 100-3,280.1

B ☑ **E0973** Wheelchair accessory, adjustable height, detachable armrest, complete assembly, each ♿
MED: 100-3,280.1

B ☑ **E0974** Manual wheelchair accessory, anti-rollback device, each ♿
MED: 100-3,280.1

B ☑ **E0978** Wheelchair accessory, positioning belt/safety belt/pelvic strap, each ♿

Y **E0980** Safety vest, wheelchair ♿

Y ☑ **E0981** Wheelchair accessory, seat upholstery, replacement only, each ♿

Y ☑ **E0982** Wheelchair accessory, back upholstery, replacement only, each ♿

Y **E0983** Manual wheelchair accessory, power add-on to convert manual wheelchair to motorized wheelchair, joystick control ♿

Y **E0984** Manual wheelchair accessory, power add-on to convert manual wheelchair to motorized wheelchair, tiller control ♿

Y **E0985** Wheelchair accessory, seat lift mechanism ♿

Y ☑ **E0986** Manual wheelchair accessory, push activated power assist, each ♿

B ☑ **E0990** Wheelchair accessory, elevating leg rest, complete assembly, each ♿
MED: 100-3,280.1

B **E0992** Manual wheelchair accessory, solid seat insert ♿

Y ☑ **E0994** Armrest, each ♿
MED: 100-3,280.1

B ☑ **E0995** Wheelchair accessory, calf rest/pad, each ♿
MED: 100-3,280.1

Y **E1002** Wheelchair accessory, power seating system, tilt only ♿

Y **E1003** Wheelchair accessory, power seating system, recline only, without shear reduction ♿

Y **E1004** Wheelchair accessory, power seating system, recline only, with mechanical shear reduction ♿

Y **E1005** Wheelchair accessory, power seatng System, recline only, with power shear reduction ♿

Y **E1006** Wheelchair accessory, power seating system, combination tilt and recline, without shear reduction ♿

Y **E1007** Wheelchair accessory, power seating system, combination tilt and recline, with mechanical shear reduction ♿

Y **E1008** Wheelchair accessory, power seating system, combination tilt and recline, with power shear reduction ♿

Y ☑ **E1009** Wheelchair accessory, addition to power seating system, mechanically linked leg elevation system, including pushrod and leg rest, each ♿

Y ☑ **E1010** Wheelchair accessory, addition to power seating system, power leg elevation system, including leg rest, pair ♿

Y **E1011** Modification to pediatric size wheelchair, width adjustment package (not to be dispensed with initial chair) ♿
MED: 100-3,280.1

Y **E1014** Reclining back, addition to pediatric size wheelchair ♿
MED: 100-3,280.1

Y **E1015** Shock absorber for manual wheelchair, each ♿
MED: 100-3,280.1

Y **E1016** Shock absorber for power wheelchair, each ♿
MED: 100-3,280.1

Y ☑ **E1017** Heavy duty shock absorber for heavy duty or extra heavy duty manual wheelchair, each ♿
MED: 100-3,280.1

Y ☑ **E1018** Heavy duty shock absorber for heavy duty or extra heavy duty power wheelchair, each ♿
MED: 100-3,280.1

Y **E1020** Residual limb support system for wheelchair ♿
MED: 100-3,280.3

Y **E1028** Wheelchair accessory, manual swingaway, retractable or removable mounting hardware for joystick, other control interface or positioning accessory ♿

Y **E1029** Wheelchair accessory, ventilator tray, fixed ♿

Y **E1030** Wheelchair accessory, ventilator tray, gimbaled ♿

## ROLLABOUT CHAIR

Y **E1031** Rollabout chair, any and all types with castors 5 in. or greater ♿
MED: 100-3,280.1

Y **E1035** Multi-positional patient transfer system, with integrated seat, operated by care giver ♿
MED: 100-2,15,110

---

Special Coverage Instructions    Noncovered by Medicare    Carrier Discretion    ☑ Quantity Alert    ● New Code    ○ Recycled/Reinstated    ▲ Revised Code

**2008 HCPCS**    A2-Z3 ASC Payment Indicators    **MED:** Pub 100/NCD References    ♿ DMEPOS Paid    ⊘ SNF Excluded    PQRI PQRI    **E Codes — 47**

**Durable Medical Equipment**

**E1037 — E1225**

| Y | E1037 | Transport chair, pediatric size |
MED: 100-3,280.1

| Y | E1038 | Transport chair, adult size, patient weight capacity up to and including 300 pounds |
MED: 100-3,280.1

| Y | E1039 | Transport chair, adult size, heavy duty, patient weight capacity greater than 300 pounds |

## WHEELCHAIRS - FULLY RECLINING

| A | E1050 | Fully reclining wheelchair; fixed full-length arms, swing-away, detachable, elevating legrests |
MED: 100-3,280.1

| A | E1060 | Fully reclining wheelchair; detachable arms, desk, or full-length, swing-away, detachable, elevating leg rests |
MED: 100-3,280.1

| A | E1070 | Fully reclining wheelchair; detachable arms, desk or full-length, swing-away, detachable footrests |
MED: 100-3,280.1

| A | E1083 | Hemi-wheelchair; fixed full-length arms, swing-away, detachable, elevating legrests |
MED: 100-3,280.1

| A | E1084 | Hemi-wheelchair; detachable arms, desk, or full-length, swing-away, detachable, elevating leg rests |
MED: 100-3,280.1

| E | E1085 | Hemi-wheelchair; fixed full-length arms, swing-away, detachable footrests
See code(s): K0002 |
MED: 100-3,280.1

| E | E1086 | Hemi-wheelchair; detachable arms, desk or full-length, swing-away, detachable footrests
See code(s): K0002 |
MED: 100-3,280.1

| A | E1087 | High-strength lightweight wheelchair; fixed full-length arms, swing-away, detachable, elevating legrests |
MED: 100-3,280.1

| A | E1088 | High strength lightweight wheelchair, detachable arms desk or full length, swing away detachable elevating leg rests |
MED: 100-3,280.1

| E | E1089 | High-strength lightweight wheelchair; fixed-length arms, swing-away, detachable footrests
See code(s): K0004 |
MED: 100-3,280.1

| E | E1090 | High-strength lightweight wheelchair; detachable arms, desk or full-length, swing-away, detachable footrests
See code(s): K0004 |
MED: 100-3,280.1

| A | E1092 | Wide heavy duty wheel chair, detachable arms (desk or full length), swing away detachable elevating leg rests |
MED: 100-3,280.1

| A | E1093 | Wide, heavy-duty wheelchair; detachable arms, desk or full-length arms, swing-away, detachable footrests |
MED: 100-3,280.1

## WHEELCHAIR - SEMI-RECLINING

| A | E1100 | Semi-reclining wheelchair, fixed full-length arms, swing away detachable elevating leg rests |
MED: 100-3,280.1

| A | E1110 | Semi-reclining wheelchair; detachable arms, desk or full-length, elevating legrest |
MED: 100-3,280.1

## WHEELCHAIR - STANDARD

| E | E1130 | Standard wheelchair; fixed full-length arms, fixed or swing-away, detachable footrests
See code(s): K0001 |
MED: 100-3,280.1

| E | E1140 | Wheelchair; detachable arms, desk or full-length, swing-away, detachable footrests
See code(s): K0001 |
MED: 100-3,280.1

| Y | E1150 | Wheelchair, detachable arms, desk or full-length swing away detachable elevating leg rests |
MED: 100-3,280.1

| A | E1160 | Wheelchair, fixed full-length arms, swing away detachable elevating leg rests |
MED: 100-3,280.1

| A | E1161 | Manual adult size wheelchair, includes tilt in space |

## WHEELCHAIR - AMPUTEE

| A | E1170 | Amputee wheelchair, fixed full-length arms, swing away detachable elevating leg rests |
MED: 100-3,280.1

| A | E1171 | Amputee wheelchair, fixed full-length arms, without footrests or leg rest |
MED: 100-3,280.1

| A | E1172 | Amputee wheelchair, detachable arms (desk or full-length) without footrests or leg rest |
MED: 100-3,280.1

| A | E1180 | Amputee wheelchair, detachable arms (desk or full-length) swing away detachable foot rests |
MED: 100-3,280.1

| A | E1190 | Amputee wheelchair, detachable arms (desk or full-length) swing away detachable elevating leg rests |
MED: 100-3,280.1

| A | E1195 | Heavy duty wheelchair, fixed full-length arms, swing away detachable elevating leg rests |
MED: 100-3,280.1

| A | E1200 | Amputee wheelchair, fixed full-length arms, swing away detachable footrest |
MED: 100-3,280.1

## WHEELCHAIR - SPECIAL SIZE

| A | E1220 | Wheelchair; specially sized or constructed (indicate brand name, model number, if any, and justification) |
MED: 100-3,280.3

| A | E1221 | Wheelchair with fixed arm, footrests |
MED: 100-3,280.3

| A | E1222 | Wheelchair with fixed arm, elevating leg rests |
MED: 100-3,280.3

| A | E1223 | Wheelchair with detachable arms, footrests |
MED: 100-3,280.3

| A | E1224 | Wheelchair with detachable arms, elevating leg rests |
MED: 100-3,280.3

| Y | E1225 | Wheelchair accessory, manual semi-reclining back, (recline greater than 15 degrees, but less than 80 degrees), each |
MED: 100-3,280.3

Special Coverage Instructions  Noncovered by Medicare  Carrier Discretion  ☑ Quantity Alert  ● New Code  ○ Recycled/Reinstated  ▲ Revised Code

48 — E Codes   A Age Edit  M Maternity Edit  ♀ Female Only  ♂ Male Only  A-Y OPPS Status Indicators   2008 HCPCS

**Durable Medical Equipment**

B  **E1226**  Wheelchair accessory, manual fully reclining back, (recline greater than 80 degrees), each ♿
See also K0028
MED: 100-3,280.1

Y  **E1227**  Special height arms for wheelchair ♿
MED: 100-3,280.3

Y  **E1228**  Special back height for wheelchair ♿
MED: 100-3,280.3

Y  **E1229**  Wheelchair, pediatric size, not otherwise specified

Y  **E1230**  Power operated vehicle (three- or four-wheel nonhighway), specify brand name and model number ♿
Prior authorization is required by Medicare for this item.
MED: 100-8,5,5.2.3

Y  **E1231**  Wheelchair, pediatric size, tilt-in-space, rigid, adjustable, with seating system ♿
MED: 100-3,280.1

Y  **E1232**  Wheelchair, pediatric size, tilt-in-space, folding, adjustable, with seating system ♿
MED: 100-3,280.1

Y  **E1233**  Wheelchair, pediatric size, tilt-in-space, rigid, adjustable, without seating system ♿
MED: 100-3,280.1

Y  **E1234**  Wheelchair, pediatric size, tilt-in-space, folding, adjustable, without seating system ♿
MED: 100-3,280.1

Y  **E1235**  Wheelchair, pediatric size, rigid, adjustable, with seating system ♿
MED: 100-3,280.1

Y  **E1236**  Wheelchair, pediatric size, folding, adjustable, with seating system ♿
MED: 100-3,280.1

Y  **E1237**  Wheelchair, pediatric size, rigid, adjustable, without seating system ♿
MED: 100-3,280.1

Y  **E1238**  Wheelchair, pediatric size, folding, adjustable, without seating system ♿
MED: 100-3,280.1

Y  **E1239**  Power wheelchair, pediatric size, not otherwise specified

## WHEELCHAIR - LIGHTWEIGHT

A  **E1240**  Lightweight wheelchair, detachable arms, (desk or full length) swing away detachable, elevating leg rest
MED: 100-3,280.1

E  **E1250**  Lightweight wheelchair; fixed full-length arms, swing-away, detachable footrests
See code(s): K0003
MED: 100-3,280.1

E  **E1260**  Lightweight wheelchair; detachable arms, desk or full-length, swing-away, detachable footrests
See code(s): K0003
MED: 100-3,280.1

A  **E1270**  Lightweight wheelchair, fixed full length arms, swing away detachable elevating leg rests
MED: 100-3,280.1

## WHEELCHAIR - HEAVY-DUTY

A  **E1280**  Heavy duty wheelchair, detachable arms (desk or full length) elevating leg rests
MED: 100-3,280.1

E  **E1285**  Heavy-duty wheelchair; fixed full-length arms, swing-away, detachable footrests
See code(s): K0006
MED: 100-3,280.1

E  **E1290**  Heavy-duty wheelchair; detachable arms, desk or full-length, swing-away, detachable footrests
See code(s): K0006
MED: 100-3,280.1

A  **E1295**  Heavy duty wheelchair, fixed full length arms, elevating leg rest
MED: 100-3,280.1

Y  **E1296**  Special wheelchair seat height from floor ♿
MED: 100-3,280.3

Y  **E1297**  Special wheelchair seat depth, by upholstery ♿
MED: 100-3,280.3

Y  **E1298**  Special wheelchair seat depth and/or width, by construction ♿
MED: 100-3,280.3

## WHIRLPOOL - EQUIPMENT

E  **E1300**  Whirlpool, portable (overtub type)
MED: 100-3,280.1

Y  **E1310**  Whirlpool, nonportable (built-in type) ♿
MED: 100-3,280.1

## REPAIRS AND REPLACEMENT SUPPLIES

Y ☑  **E1340**  Repair or nonroutine service for durable medical equipment requiring the skill of a technician, labor component, per 15 minutes
Medicare jurisdiction: local contractor if repair or implanted DME.
MED: 100-2,15,110.2

## ADDITIONAL OXYGEN RELATED EQUIPMENT

Y  **E1353**  Regulator ♿
MED: 100-3,240.2

Y  **E1355**  Stand/rack ♿
MED: 100-3,240.2

Y  **E1372**  Immersion external heater for nebulizer ♿
MED: 100-3,240.2

Y  **E1390**  Oxygen concentrator, single delivery port, capable of delivering 85 percent or greater oxygen concentration at the prescribed flow rate ♿
MED: 100-3,240.2

Y ☑  **E1391**  Oxygen concentrator, dual delivery port, capable of delivering 85 percent or greater oxygen concentration at the prescribed flow rate, each ♿
MED: 100-3,240.2

Y  **E1392**  Portable oxygen concentrator, rental ♿

Y  **E1399**  Durable medical equipment, miscellaneous ♿
Determine if an alternative HCPCS Level II or a CPT code better describes the service being reported. This code should be used only if a more specific code is unavailable. Medicare jurisdiction: local contractor if repair or implanted DME.

Y  **E1405**  Oxygen and water vapor enriching system with heated delivery ♿
MED: 100-3,240.2; 100-4,20,20; 100-4,20,20.4

Y  **E1406**  Oxygen and water vapor enriching system without heated delivery ♿
MED: 100-3,240.2; 100-4,20,20; 100-4,20,20.4

Special Coverage Instructions   Noncovered by Medicare   Carrier Discretion   ☑ Quantity Alert   ● New Code   ○ Recycled/Reinstated   ▲ Revised Code

**2008 HCPCS**   N2-N3 ASC Payment Indicators   **MED:** Pub 100/NCD References   ♿ DMEPOS Paid   ⊘ SNF Excluded   PQ PQRI   **E Codes — 49**

**E1226 — E1406**

**Durable Medical Equipment**

**E1500 — E2201**

## ARTIFICIAL KIDNEY MACHINES AND ACCESSORIES

[A] **E1500** Centrifuge, for dialysis ⊘

[A] **E1510** Kidney, dialysate delivery system kidney machine, pump recirculating, air removal system, flowrate meter, power off, heater and temp control with alarm, IV poles, pressure gauge, concentrate container ⊘

[A] **E1520** Heparin infusion pump for hemodialysis ⊘

[A] ☑ **E1530** Air bubble detector for hemodialysis, each, replacement ⊘

[A] ☑ **E1540** Pressure alarm for hemodialysis, each, replacement ⊘

[A] ☑ **E1550** Bath conductivity meter for hemodialysis, each ⊘

[A] ☑ **E1560** Blood leak detector for hemodialysis, each, replacement ⊘

[A] **E1570** Adjustable chair, for ESRD patients ⊘

[A] ☑ **E1575** Transducer protectors/fluid barriers, for hemodialysis, any size, per 10 ⊘

[A] **E1580** Unipuncture control system for hemodialysis ⊘

[A] **E1590** Hemodialysis machine ⊘

[A] **E1592** Automatic intermittent peritoneal dialysis system ⊘

[A] **E1594** Cycler dialysis machine for peritoneal dialysis ⊘

[A] **E1600** Delivery and/or installation charges for hemodialysis equipment ⊘

[A] **E1610** Reverse osmosis water purification system, for hemodialysis ⊘
MED: 100-3,230.7

[A] **E1615** Deionizer water purification system, for hemodialysis ⊘
MED: 100-3,230.7

[A] **E1620** Blood pump for hemodialysis, replacement ⊘

[A] **E1625** Water softening system, for hemodialysis ⊘
MED: 100-3,230.7

[A] **E1630** Reciprocating peritoneal dialysis system ⊘

[A] ☑ **E1632** Wearable artificial kidney, each ⊘

[B] ☑ **E1634** Peritoneal dialysis clamps, each ⊘

[A] **E1635** Compact (portable) travel hemodialyzer system ⊘

[A] ☑ **E1636** Sorbent cartridges, for hemodialysis, per 10 ⊘

[A] ☑ **E1637** Hemostats, each ⊘

[A] ☑ **E1639** Scale, each ⊘

[A] **E1699** Dialysis equipment, not otherwise specified ⊘
Determine if an alternative HCPCS Level II or a CPT code better describes the service being reported. This code should be used only if a more specific code is unavailable. Pertinent documentation to evaluate medical appropriateness should be included when this code is reported.

## JAW MOTION REHABILITATION SYSTEM AND ACCESSORIES

[Y] **E1700** Jaw motion rehabilitation system ᕂ
Medicare jurisdiction: local contractor.

[Y] ☑ **E1701** Replacement cushions for jaw motion rehabilitation system, package of six ᕂ
Medicare jurisdiction: local contractor.

[Y] ☑ **E1702** Replacement measuring scales for jaw motion rehabilitation system, package of 200 ᕂ
Medicare jurisdiction: local contractor.

## OTHER ORTHOPEDIC DEVICES

[Y] **E1800** Dynamic adjustable elbow extension/flexion device, includes soft interface material ᕂ

▲ [Y] **E1801** Static progressive stretch elbow device, extension and/or flexion, with or without range of motion adjustment, includes all components and accessories ᕂ

[Y] **E1802** Dynamic adjustable forearm pronation/supination device, includes soft interface material ᕂ

[Y] **E1805** Dynamic adjustable wrist extension/flexion device, includes soft interface material ᕂ

▲ [Y] **E1806** Static progressive stretch wrist device, flexion and/or extension, with or without range of motion adjustment, includes all components and accessories ᕂ

[Y] **E1810** Dynamic adjustable knee extension/flexion device, includes soft interface material ᕂ

▲ [Y] **E1811** Static progressive stretch knee device, extension and/or flexion, with or without range of motion adjustment, includes all components and accessories ᕂ

[Y] **E1812** Dynamic knee, extension/flexion device with active resistance control

[Y] **E1815** Dynamic adjustable ankle extension/flexion device, includes soft interface material ᕂ

▲ [Y] **E1816** Static progressive stretch ankle device, flexion and/or extension, with or without range of motion adjustment, includes all components and accessories ᕂ

▲ [Y] **E1818** Static progressive stretch forearm pronation/supination device, with or without range of motion adjustment, includes all components and accessories ᕂ

[Y] **E1820** Replacement soft interface material, dynamic adjustable extension/flexion device ᕂ

[Y] **E1821** Replacement soft interface material/cuffs for bi-directional static progressive stretch device ᕂ

[Y] **E1825** Dynamic adjustable finger extension/flexion device, includes soft interface material ᕂ

[Y] **E1830** Dynamic adjustable toe extension/flexion device, includes soft interface material ᕂ

[Y] **E1840** Dynamic adjustable shoulder flexion/abduction/rotation device, includes soft interface material ᕂ

▲ [Y] **E1841** Static progressive stretch shoulder device, with or without range of motion adjustment, includes all components and accessories

[A] **E1902** Communication board, non-electronic augmentative or alternative communication device

[Y] **E2000** Gastric suction pump, home model, portable or stationary, electric ᕂ

[Y] **E2100** Blood glucose monitor with integrated voice synthesizer ᕂ
MED: 100.3,230.16

[Y] **E2101** Blood glucose monitor with integrated lancing/blood sample ᕂ
MED: 100.3,230.16

[Y] **E2120** Pulse generator system for tympanic treatment of inner ear endolymphatic fluid

[Y] ☑ **E2201** Manual wheelchair accessory, nonstandard seat frame, width greater than or equal to 20 inches and less than 24 inches ᕂ

---

| Special Coverage Instructions | Noncovered by Medicare | Carrier Discretion | ☑ Quantity Alert | ● New Code | ○ Recycled/Reinstated | ▲ Revised Code |

Y ☑ **E2202** Manual wheelchair accessory, nonstandard seat frame width, 24–27 in. ⓖ

Y ☑ **E2203** Manual wheelchair accessory, nonstandard seat frame depth, 20 to less than 22 inches ⓖ

Y ☑ **E2204** Manual wheelchair accessory, nonstandard seat frame depth, 22 to 25 inches ⓖ

▲ Y ☑ **E2205** Manual wheelchair accessory, handrim without projections (includes ergonomic or contoured), any type, replacement only, each

Y ☑ **E2206** Manual wheelchair accessory, wheel Lock assembly, complete, each

Y ☑ **E2207** Wheelchair accessory, crutch and cane holder, each

Y ☑ **E2208** Wheelchair accessory, cylinder tank carrier, each

Y ☑ **E2209** Accessory, arm trough, with or without hand support, each

Y ☑ **E2210** Wheelchair accessory, bearings, any type, replacement only, each

Y ☑ **E2211** Manual wheelchair accessory, pneumatic propulsion tire, any size, each

Y ☑ **E2212** Manual wheelchair accessory, tube for pneumatic propulsion tire, any size, each

Y ☑ **E2213** Manual wheelchair accessory, insert for pneumatic propulsion tire (removable), any type, any size, each

Y ☑ **E2214** Manual wheelchair accessory, pneumatic caster tire, any size, each

Y ☑ **E2215** Manual wheelchair accessory, tube for pneumatic caster tire, any size, each

Y ☑ **E2216** Manual wheelchair accessory, foam filled propulsion tire, any size, each

Y ☑ **E2217** Manual wheelchair accessory, foam filled caster tire, any size, each

Y ☑ **E2218** Manual wheelchair accessory, foam propulsion tire, any size, each

Y ☑ **E2219** Manual wheelchair accessory, foam caster tire, any size, each

Y ☑ **E2220** Manual wheelchair accessory, solid (rubber/plastic) propulsion tire, any size, each

Y ☑ **E2221** Manual wheelchair accessory, solid (rubber/plastic) caster tire (removable), any size, each

Y ☑ **E2222** Manual wheelchair accessory, solid (rubber/plastic) caster tire with integrated wheel, any size, each

Y ☑ **E2223** Manual wheelchair accessory, valve, any type, replacement only, each

Y ☑ **E2224** Manual wheelchair accessory, propulsion wheel excludes tire, any size, each

Y ☑ **E2225** Manual wheelchair accessory, caster wheel excludes tire, any size, replacement only, each

Y ☑ **E2226** Manual wheelchair accessory, caster fork, any size, replacement only, each

● Y ☑ **E2227** Manual wheelchair accessory, gear reduction drive wheel, each

● Y ☑ **E2228** Manual wheelchair accessory, wheel braking system and lock, complete, each

Y **E2291** Back, planar, for pediatric size wheelchair including fixed attaching hardware

Y **E2292** Seat, planar, for pediatric size wheelchair including fixed attaching hardware

Y **E2293** Back, contoured, for pediatric size wheelchair including fixed attaching hardware

Y **E2294** Seat, contoured, for pediatric size wheelchair including fixed attaching hardware

Y **E2300** Power wheelchair accessory, power seat elevation system

Y **E2301** Power wheelchair accessory, power standing system

Y **E2310** Power wheelchair accessory, electronic connection between wheelchair controller and one power seating system motor, including all related electronics, indicator feature, mechanical function selection switch, and fixed mounting hardware ⓖ

Y **E2311** Power wheelchair accessory, electronic connection between wheelchair controller and two or more power seating system motors, including all related electronics, indicator feature, mechanical function selection switch, and fixed mounting hardware ⓖ

● Y **E2312** Power wheelchair accessory, hand or chin control interface, mini-proportional remote joystick, proportional, including fixed mounting hardware

● Y **E2313** Power wheelchair accessory, harness for upgrade to expandable controller, including all fasteners, connectors and mounting hardware, each

Y **E2321** Power wheelchair accessory, hand control interface, remote joystick, nonproportional, including all related electronics, mechanical stop switch, and fixed mounting hardware ⓖ

Y **E2322** Power wheelchair accessory, hand control interface, multiple mechanical switches, nonproportional, including all related electronics, mechanical stop switch, and fixed mounting hardware ⓖ

Y **E2323** Power wheelchair accessory, specialty joystick handle for hand control interface, prefabricated ⓖ

Y **E2324** Power wheelchair accessory, chin cup for chin control interface ⓖ

Y **E2325** Power wheelchair accessory, sip and puff interface, nonproportional, including all related electronics, mechanical stop switch, and manual swingaway mounting hardware ⓖ

Y **E2326** Power wheelchair accessory, breath tube kit for sip and puff interface ⓖ

Y **E2327** Power wheelchair accessory, head control interface, mechanical, proportional, including all related electronics, mechanical direction change switch, and fixed mounting hardware ⓖ

Y **E2328** Power wheelchair accessory, head control or extremity control interface, electronic, proportional, including all related electronics and fixed mounting hardware ⓖ

Y **E2329** Power wheelchair accessory, head control interface, contact switch mechanism, nonproportional, including all related electronics, mechanical stop switch, mechanical direction change switch, head array, and fixed mounting hardware ⓖ

Y **E2330** Power wheelchair accessory, head control interface, proximity switch mechanism, nonproportional, including all related electronics, mechanical stop switch, mechanical direction change switch, head array, and fixed mounting hardware ⓖ

Y **E2331** Power wheelchair accessory, attendant control, proportional, including all related electronics and fixed mounting hardware

Y ☑ **E2340** Power wheelchair accessory, nonstandard seat frame width, 20–23 in. ⓖ

☑ Special Coverage Instructions    ☐ Noncovered by Medicare    ☐ Carrier Discretion    ☑ Quantity Alert    ● New Code    ○ Recycled/Reinstated    ▲ Revised Code

**2008 HCPCS**    A2-Z3 ASC Payment Indicators    **MED:** Pub 100/NCD References    ⓖ DMEPOS Paid    ⊘ SNF Excluded    PQ PQRI    **E Codes — 51**

Ⓨ ☑ **E2341** Power wheelchair accessory, nonstandard seat frame width, 24–27 in. &

Ⓨ ☑ **E2342** Power wheelchair accessory, nonstandard seat frame depth, 20 or 21 in. &

Ⓨ ☑ **E2343** Power wheelchair accessory, nonstandard seat frame depth, 22–25 in. &

Ⓨ **E2351** Power wheelchair accessory, electronic interface to operate speech generating device using power wheelchair control interface

Ⓨ ☑ **E2360** Power wheelchair accessory, 22 NF nonsealed lead acid battery, each &

Ⓨ ☑ **E2361** Power wheelchair accessory, 22 NF sealed lead acid battery, each, (e.g., gel cell, absorbed glassmat) &

Ⓨ ☑ **E2362** Power wheelchair accessory, group 24 nonsealed lead acid battery, each &

Ⓨ ☑ **E2363** Power wheelchair accessory, group 24 sealed lead acid battery, each (e.g., gel cell, absorbed glassmat) &

Ⓨ ☑ **E2364** Power wheelchair accessory, U-1 nonsealed lead acid battery, each &

Ⓨ ☑ **E2365** Power wheelchair accessory, U-1 sealed lead acid battery, each (e.g., gel cell, absorbed glassmat) &

Ⓨ ☑ **E2366** Power wheelchair accessory, battery charger, single mode, for use with only one battery type, sealed or non-sealed, each &

Ⓨ ☑ **E2367** Power wheelchair accessory, battery charger, dual mode, for use with either battery type, sealed or nonsealed, each

Ⓨ **E2368** Power wheelchair component, motor, replacement only

Ⓨ **E2369** Power wheelchair component, gear box, replacement only

Ⓨ **E2370** Power wheelchair component, motor and gear box combination, replacement only

Ⓨ ☑ **E2371** Power wheelchair accessory, group 27 sealed lead acid battery, (e.g., gel cell, absorbed glassmat), each &

Ⓨ ☑ **E2372** Power wheelchair accessory, group 27 nonsealed lead acid battery, each

▲ Ⓨ **E2373** Power wheelchair accessory, hand or chin control interface, compact remote joystick, proportional, including fixed mounting hardware &

Ⓨ **E2374** Power wheelchair accessory, hand or chin control interface, standard remote joystick (not including controller), proportional, including all related electronics and fixed mounting hardware, replacement only &

Ⓨ **E2375** Power wheelchair accessory, nonexpandable controller, including all related electronics and mounting hardware, replacement only &

Ⓨ **E2376** Power wheelchair accessory, expandable controller, including all related electronics and mounting hardware, replacement only &

Ⓨ **E2377** Power wheelchair accessory, expandable controller, including all related electronics and mounting hardware, upgrade provided at initial issue &

Ⓨ ☑ **E2381** Power wheelchair accessory, pneumatic drive wheel tire, any size, replacement only, each &

Ⓨ ☑ **E2382** Power wheelchair accessory, tube for pneumatic drive wheel tire, any size, replacement only, each &

Ⓨ ☑ **E2383** Power wheelchair accessory, insert for pneumatic drive wheel tire (removable), any type, any size, replacement only, each &

Ⓨ ☑ **E2384** Power wheelchair accessory, pneumatic caster tire, any size, replacement only, each &

Ⓨ ☑ **E2385** Power wheelchair accessory, tube for pneumatic caster tire, any size, replacement only, each &

Ⓨ ☑ **E2386** Power wheelchair accessory, foam filled drive wheel tire, any size, replacement only, each &

Ⓨ ☑ **E2387** Power wheelchair accessory, foam filled caster tire, any size, replacement only, each &

Ⓨ ☑ **E2388** Power wheelchair accessory, foam drive wheel tire, any size, replacement only, each &

Ⓨ ☑ **E2389** Power wheelchair accessory, foam caster tire, any size, replacement only, each &

Ⓨ ☑ **E2390** Power wheelchair accessory, solid (rubber/plastic) drive wheel tire, any size, replacement only, each &

Ⓨ ☑ **E2391** Power wheelchair accessory, solid (rubber/plastic) caster tire (removable), any size, replacement only, each &

Ⓨ ☑ **E2392** Power wheelchair accessory, solid (rubber/plastic) caster tire with integrated wheel, any size, replacement only, each &

Ⓨ ☑ **E2393** Power wheelchair accessory, valve for pneumatic tire tube, any type, replacement only, each &

Ⓨ ☑ **E2394** Power wheelchair accessory, drive wheel excludes tire, any size, replacement only, each &

Ⓨ ☑ **E2395** Power wheelchair accessory, caster wheel excludes tire, any size, replacement only, each &

Ⓨ ☑ **E2396** Power wheelchair accessory, caster fork, any size, replacement only, each &

● Ⓨ ☑ **E2397** Power wheelchair accessory, lithium-based battery, each

Ⓨ **E2399** Power wheelchair accessory, not otherwise classified interface, including all related electronics and any type mounting hardware &

Ⓨ **E2402** Negative pressure wound therapy electrical pump, stationary or portable &

Ⓨ ☑ **E2500** Speech generating device, digitized speech, using pre-recorded messages, less than or equal to eight minutes recording time &

　　MED: 100-3,50.1

Ⓨ ☑ **E2502** Speech generating device, digitized speech, using prerecorded messages, greater than eight minutes but less than or equal to 20 minutes recording time &

　　MED: 100-3,50.1

Ⓨ ☑ **E2504** Speech generating device, digitized speech, using prerecorded messages, greater than 20 minutes but less than or equal to 40 minutes recording time &

　　MED: 100-3,50.1

Ⓨ ☑ **E2506** Speech generating device, digitized speech, using prerecorded messages, greater than 40 minutes recording time &

　　MED: 100-3,50.1

Ⓨ **E2508** Speech generating device, synthesized speech, requiring message formulation by spelling and access by physical contact with the device &

　　MED: 100-3,50.1

Ⓨ **E2510** Speech generating device, synthesized speech, permitting multiple methods of message formulation and multiple methods of device access &

　　MED: 100-3,50.1

　Special Coverage Instructions　　　Noncovered by Medicare　　　Carrier Discretion　　☑ Quantity Alert　　● New Code　　○ Recycled/Reinstated　　▲ Revised Code

**52 — E Codes**　　Ⓐ Age Edit　　Ⓜ Maternity Edit　　♀ Female Only　　♂ Male Only　　Ⓐ-Ⓨ OPPS Status Indicators　　**2008 HCPCS**

Y **E2511** Speech generating software program, for personal computer or personal digital assistant &
MED: 100-3,50.1

Y **E2512** Accessory for speech generating device, mounting system &
MED: 100-3,50.1

Y **E2599** Accessory for speech generating device, not otherwise classified
MED: 100-3,50.1

Y **E2601** General use wheelchair seat cushion, width less than 22 in., any depth

Y **E2602** General use wheelchair seat cushion, width 22 in. or greater, any depth

Y **E2603** Skin protection wheelchair seat cushion, width less than 22 in., any depth

Y **E2604** Skin protection wheelchair seat cushion, width 22 in. or greater, any depth

Y **E2605** Positioning wheelchair seat cushion, width less than 22 in., any depth

Y **E2606** Positioning wheelchair seat cushion, width 22 in. or greater, any depth

Y **E2607** Skin protection and positioning wheelchair seat cushion, width less than 22 in., any depth

Y **E2608** Skin protection and positioning wheelchair seat cushion, width 22 in. or greater, any depth

Y **E2609** Custom fabricated wheelchair seat cushion, any size

B **E2610** Wheelchair seat cushion, powered

Y **E2611** General use wheelchair back cushion, width less than 22 in., any height, including any type mounting hardware

Y **E2612** General use wheelchair back cushion, width 22 in. or greater, any height, including any type mounting hardware

Y **E2613** Positioning wheelchair back cushion, posterior, width less than 22 in., any height, including any type mounting hardware

Y **E2614** Positioning wheelchair back cushion, posterior, width 22 in. or greater, any height, including any type mounting hardware

Y **E2615** Positioning wheelchair back cushion, posterior-lateral, width less than 22 in., any height, including any type mounting hardware

Y **E2616** Positioning wheelchair back cushion, posterior-lateral, width 22 in. or greater, any height, including any type mounting hardware

Y **E2617** Custom fabricated wheelchair back cushion, any size, including any type mounting hardware

~~E2618 Wheelchair accessory, solid seat support base (replaces sling seat), for use with manual wheelchair or lightweight power wheelchair, includes any type mounting hardware~~

Y **E2619** Replacement cover for wheelchair seat cushion or back cushion, each

Y **E2620** Positioning wheelchair back cushion, planar back with lateral supports, width less than 22 in., any height, including any type mounting hardware

Y **E2621** Positioning wheelchair back cushion, planar back with lateral supports, width 22 in. or greater, any height, including any type mounting hardware

E **E8000** Gait trainer, pediatric size, posterior support, includes all accessories and components

E **E8001** Gait trainer, pediatric size, upright support, includes all accessories and components

E **E8002** Gait trainer, pediatric size, anterior support, includes all accessories and components

Special Coverage Instructions    Noncovered by Medicare    Carrier Discretion    ☑ Quantity Alert    ● New Code    ○ Recycled/Reinstated    ▲ Revised Code

**2008 HCPCS**    A2-Z3 ASC Payment Indicators    **MED:** Pub 100/NCD References    & DMEPOS Paid    ⊘ SNF Excluded    PQ PQRI    **E Codes — 53**

## PROCEDURES/PROFESSIONAL SERVICES (TEMPORARY)
## G0000-G9999

The G codes are used to identify professional health care procedures and services that would otherwise be coded in CPT but for which there are no CPT codes.

Please refer to you CPT book for possible alternate code(s).

[S] **G0008** Administration of influenza virus vaccine ⊘
MED: 100-2,6,10; 100-4,4,240

[S] **G0009** Administration of pneumococcal vaccine ⊘
MED: 100-2,6,10; 100-4,4,240

[B] **G0010** Administration of hepatitis B vaccine ⊘
MED: 100-2,6,10; 100-4,4,240

[A] **G0027** Semen analysis; presence and/or motility of sperm excluding huhner

[V] **G0101** Cervical or vaginal cancer screening; pelvic and clinical breast examination ♀⊘
G0101 can be reported with an E/M code when a separately identifiable E/M service was provided.
MED: 100-2,6,10; 100-4,4,240
AHA: 4Q,'02,8; 3Q,'01,6

[N] **G0102** Prostate cancer screening; digital rectal examination ♂⊘
MED: 100-2,6,10; 100-3,210.1; 100-4,4,240

[A] **G0103** Prostate cancer screening; prostate specific antigen test (PSA) ♂⊘
MED: 100-2,6,10; 100-3,210.1; 100-4,4,240

[S] **G0104** Colorectal cancer screening; flexible sigmoidoscopy [P3]⊘
Medicare covers colorectal screening for cancer via flexible sigmoidoscopy once every four years for patients 50 years or older.
MED: 100-2,6,10; 100-4,4,240; 100-4,18,60.1; 100-4,18,60.2; 100-4,18,60.2.1; 100-4,18,60.6

[T] **G0105** Colorectal cancer screening; colonoscopy on individual at high risk [A2]⊘
An individual with ulcerative enteritis or a history of a malignant neoplasm of the lower gastrointestinal tract is considered at high-risk for colorectal cancer, as defined by CMS.
MED: 100-2,6,10; 100-4,4,240; 100-4,18,60.1; 100-4,18,60.2; 100-4,18,60.2.1; 100-4,18,60.6
AHA: 3Q,'01,6

[S] **G0106** Colorectal cancer screening; alternative to G0104, screening sigmoidoscopy, barium enema ⊘
MED: 100-2,6,10; 100-4,4,240; 100-4,18,60.1; 100-4,18,60.2; 100-4,18,60.2.1; 100-4,18,60.6

[A] ☑ **G0108** Diabetes outpatient self-management training services, individual, per 30 minutes ⊘
MED: 100-2,6,10; 100-4,4,240

[A] ☑ **G0109** Diabetes outpatient self-management training services, group session (2 or more), per 30 minutes ⊘
MED: 100-2,6,10; 100-4,4,240

[S] **G0117** Glaucoma screening for high risk patients furnished by an optometrist or ophthalmologist ⊘
MED: 100-2,15,280.1
AHA: 1Q,'02,4; 3Q,'01,12

[S] **G0118** Glaucoma screening for high risk patient furnished under the direct supervision of an optometrist or ophthalmologist ⊘
MED: 100-2,15,280.1
AHA: 1Q,'02,4; 3Q,'01,12

[S] **G0120** Colorectal cancer screening; alternative to G0105, screening colonoscopy, barium enema ⊘
MED: 100-2,6,10; 100-4,18,60.1; 100-4,18,60.2; 100-4,18,60.2.1; 100-4,18,60.6

[T] **G0121** Colorectal cancer screening; colonoscopy on individual not meeting criteria for high risk [A2]⊘
MED: 100-2,6,10; 100-4,4,240; 100-4,18,60.1; 100-4,18,60.2; 100-4,18,60.2.1; 100-4,18,60.6
AHA: 1Q,'02,4; 3Q,'01,12

[E] **G0122** Colorectal cancer screening; barium enema
MED: 100-4,18,60.2; 100-4,18,60.2.1; 100-4,18,60.6

[A] **G0123** Screening cytopathology, cervical or vaginal (any reporting system), collected in preservative fluid, automated thin layer preparation, screening by cytotechnologist under physician supervision ♀⊘
See also P3000-P3001.
MED: 100-2,6,10; 100-3,190.2; 100-4,4,240

[B] **G0124** Screening cytopathology, cervical or vaginal (any reporting system), collected in preservative fluid, automated thin layer preparation, requiring interpretation by physician ♀⊘
See also P3000-P3001.
MED: 100-2,6,10; 100-3,190.2; 100-4,4,240

[T] ☑ **G0127** Trimming of dystrophic nails, any number [P3]⊘
MED: 100-2,15,290

[B] ☑ **G0128** Direct (face-to-face with patient) skilled nursing services of a registered nurse provided in a comprehensive outpatient rehabilitation facility, each 10 minutes beyond the first 5 minutes ⊘

[P] **G0129** Occupational therapy requiring the skills of a qualified occupational therapist, furnished as a component of a partial hospitalization treatment program, per day

[X] **G0130** Single energy x-ray absorptiometry (SEXA) bone density study, one or more sites; appendicular skeleton (peripheral) (e.g., radius, wrist, heel) [Z3]
MED: 100-2,6,10; 100-3,150.3; 100-4,4,240; 100-4,13,140

[B] **G0141** Screening cytopathology smears, cervical or vaginal, performed by automated system, with manual rescreening, requiring interpretation by physician ♀⊘
MED: 100-2,6,10

[A] **G0143** Screening cytopathology, cervical or vaginal (any reporting system), collected in preservative fluid, automated thin layer preparation, with manual screening and rescreening by cytotechnologist under physician supervision ♀⊘
MED: 100-2,6,10

[A] **G0144** Screening cytopathology, cervical or vaginal (any reporting system), collected in preservative fluid, automated thin layer preparation, with screening by automated system, under physician supervision ♀⊘
MED: 100-2,6,10

[A] **G0145** Screening cytopathology, cervical or vaginal (any reporting system), collected in preservative fluid, automated thin layer preparation, with screening by automated system and manual rescreening under physician supervision ♀⊘
MED: 100-2,6,10

[A] **G0147** Screening cytopathology smears, cervical or vaginal, performed by automated system under physician supervision ♀⊘
MED: 100-2,6,10

---

Special Coverage Instructions   Noncovered by Medicare   Carrier Discretion   ☑ Quantity Alert   ● New Code   ○ Recycled/Reinstated   ▲ Revised Code

**2008 HCPCS**   [A2]-[Z3] ASC Payment Indicators   **MED:** Pub 100/NCD References   ᓚ DMEPOS Paid   ⊘ SNF Excluded   [P3] PQRI   **G Codes — 55**

**Procedures/Professional Services (Temporary)**

**G0148 — G0245**

Ⓐ **G0148** Screening cytopathology smears, cervical or vaginal, performed by automated system with manual rescreening ♀ ⊘
MED: 100-2,6,10

Ⓑ ☑ **G0151** Services of physical therapist in home health setting, each 15 minutes

Ⓑ ☑ **G0152** Services of occupational therapist in home health setting, each 15 minutes

Ⓑ ☑ **G0153** Services of speech and language pathologist in home health setting, each 15 minutes

Ⓑ ☑ **G0154** Services of skilled nurse in home health setting, each 15 minutes

Ⓑ ☑ **G0155** Services of clinical social worker in home health setting, each 15 minutes

Ⓑ ☑ **G0156** Services of home health aide in home health setting, each 15 minutes

Ⓣ ☑ **G0166** External counterpulsation, per treatment session ⊘
MED: 100-3,20.20; 100-4,4,20.5

Ⓑ **G0168** Wound closure utilizing tissue adhesive(s) only ⊘
AHA: 3Q,'01,13; 4Q,'01,12

Ⓢ **G0173** Linear accelerator based stereotactic radiosurgery, complete course of therapy in one session ⊘
MED: 100-4,4,220.3

Ⓥ **G0175** Scheduled interdisciplinary team conference (minimum of three exclusive of patient care nursing staff) with patient present

Ⓟ **G0176** Activity therapy, such as music, dance, art or play therapies not for recreation, related to the care and treatment of patient's disabling mental health problems, per session (45 minutes or more)

Ⓝ **G0177** Training and educational services related to the care and treatment of patient's disabling mental health problems per session (45 minutes or more)

Ⓜ **G0179** Physician re-certification for Medicare-covered home health services under a home health plan of care (patient not present), including contacts with home health agency and review of reports of patient status required by physicians to affirm the initial implementation of the plan of care that meets patient's needs, per re-certification period ⊘
MED: 100-4,11,40.1.3.1; 100-4,12,180; 100-4,12,180.1

Ⓜ **G0180** Physician certification for Medicare-covered home health services under a home health plan of care (patient not present), including contacts with home health agency and review of reports of patient status required by physicians to affirm the initial implementation of the plan of care that meets patient's needs, per certification period ⊘
MED: 100-4,11,40.1.3.1; 100-4,12,180; 100-4,12,180.1

Ⓜ **G0181** Physician supervision of a patient receiving Medicare-covered services provided by a participating home health agency (patient not present) requiring complex and multidisciplinary care modalities involving regular physician development and/or revision of care plans, review of subsequent reports of patient status, review of laboratory and other studies, communication (including telephone calls) with other health care professionals involved in the patient's care, integration of new information into the medical treatment plan and/or adjustment of medical therapy, within a calendar month, 30 minutes or more ⊘
MED: 100-4,11,40.1.3.1; 100-4,12,180; 100-4,12,180.1

Ⓜ **G0182** Physician supervision of a patient under a Medicare-approved hospice (patient not present) requiring complex and multidisciplinary care modalities involving regular physician development and/or revision of care plans, review of subsequent reports of patient status, review of laboratory and other studies, communication (including telephone calls) with other health care professionals involved in the patient's care, integration of new information into the medical treatment plan and/or adjustment of medical therapy, within a calendar month, 30 minutes or more ⊘
MED: 100-4,11,40.1.3.1; 100-4,12,180; 100-4,12,180.1

Ⓣ **G0186** Destruction of localized lesion of choroid (for example, choroidal neovascularization); photocoagulation, feeder vessel technique (one or more sessions) ⊘

Ⓐ **G0202** Screening mammography, producing direct digital image, bilateral, all views ⊘
MED: 100-2,6,10; 100-4,4,240
AHA: 1Q,'02,3

Ⓐ **G0204** Diagnostic mammography, producing direct digital image, bilateral, all views
AHA: 1Q,'03,7

Ⓐ **G0206** Diagnostic mammography, producing direct digital image, unilateral, all views
AHA: 1Q,'03,7

Ⓔ **G0219** PET imaging whole body; melanoma for noncovered indications
MED: 100-3,220.6
AHA: 1Q,'02,10

Ⓔ **G0235** PET imaging, any site, not otherwise specified
MED: 100-4,13,60.14

Ⓢ ☑ **G0237** Therapeutic procedures to increase strength or endurance of respiratory muscles, face-to-face, one-on-one, each 15 minutes (includes monitoring)

Ⓢ ☑ **G0238** Therapeutic procedures to improve respiratory function, other than described by G0237, one-on-one, face-to-face, per 15 minutes (includes monitoring)

Ⓢ **G0239** Therapeutic procedures to improve respiratory function or increase strength or endurance of respiratory muscles, two or more individuals (includes monitoring)

Ⓥ **G0245** Initial physician evaluation and management of a diabetic patient with diabetic sensory neuropathy resulting in a loss of protective sensation (LOPS) which must include: (1) the diagnosis of LOPS, (2) a patient history, (3) a physical examination that consists of at least the following elements: (a) visual inspection of the forefoot, hindfoot, and toe web spaces, (b) evaluation of a protective sensation, (c) evaluation of foot structure and biomechanics, (d) evaluation of vascular status and skin integrity, and (e) evaluation and recommendation of footwear, and (4) patient education ⊘
MED: 100-3,70.2.1
AHA: 4Q,'02,9

Special Coverage Instructions　Noncovered by Medicare　Carrier Discretion　☑ Quantity Alert　● New Code　○ Recycled/Reinstated　▲ Revised Code

**56 — G Codes**　Ⓐ Age Edit　Ⓜ Maternity Edit　♀ Female Only　♂ Male Only　Ⓐ-Ⓨ OPPS Status Indicators　**2008 HCPCS**

[V] **G0246** Follow-up physician evaluation and management of a diabetic patient with diabetic sensory neuropathy resulting in a loss of protective sensation (LOPS) to include at least the following: (1) a patient history, (2) a physical examination that includes: (a) visual inspection of the forefoot, hindfoot, and toe web spaces, (b) evaluation of protective sensation, (c) evaluation of foot structure and biomechanics, (d) evaluation of vascular status and skin integrity, and (e) evaluation and recommendation of footwear, and (3) patient education ⊘

MED: 100-3,70.2.1

AHA: 4Q,'02,9

[T] **G0247** Routine foot care by a physician of a diabetic patient with diabetic sensory neuropathy resulting in a loss of protective sensation (LOPS) to include, the local care of superficial wounds (i.e., superficial to muscle and fascia) and at least the following if present: (1) local care of superficial wounds, (2) debridement of corns and calluses, and (3) trimming and debridement of nails [P3]⊘

MED: 100-3,70.2.1

AHA: 4Q,'02,9

[V] **G0248** Demonstration, at initial use, of home INR monitoring for patient with mechanical heart valve(s) who meets Medicare coverage criteria, under the direction of a physician; includes: demonstrating use and care of the INR monitor, obtaining at least one blood sample, provision of instructions for reporting home INR test results, and documentation of patient ability to perform testing

MED: 100-3,210.1

AHA: 4Q,'02,9

[V] **G0249** Provision of test materials and equipment for home INR monitoring to patient with mechanical heart valve(s) who meets Medicare coverage criteria; includes provision of materials for use in the home and reporting of test results to physician; per four tests

MED: 100-3,210.1

AHA: 4Q,'02,9

[M] **G0250** Physician review, interpretation and patient management of home INR testing for a patient with mechanical heart valve(s) who meets other coverage criteria; per four tests (does not require face-to-face service) ⊘

MED: 100-3,210.1

AHA: 4Q,'02,9

[S] ☑ **G0251** Linear accelerator based stereotactic radiosurgery, delivery including collimator changes and custom plugging, fractionated treatment, all lesions, per session, maximum five sessions per course of treatment [P2]⊘

MED: 100-4,4,220.3

[E] **G0252** PET imaging, full and partial-ring PET scanners only, for initial diagnosis of breast cancer and/or surgical planning for breast cancer (e.g., initial staging of axillary lymph nodes)

MED: 100-3,220.6

[E] **G0255** Current perception threshold/sensory nerve conduction test, (SNCT) per limb, any nerve

MED: 100-3,160.23

AHA: 4Q,'02,9

[S] **G0257** Unscheduled or emergency dialysis treatment for an ESRD patient in a hospital outpatient department that is not certified as an ESRD facility

AHA: 1Q,'03,9; 4Q,'02,9

[N] **G0259** Injection procedure for sacroiliac joint; arthrography [N1]

AHA: 4Q,'02,9

[T] **G0260** Injection procedure for sacroiliac joint; provision of anesthetic, steroid and/or other therapeutic agent, with or without arthrography [A2]

AHA: 4Q,'02,9

~~G0265~~ ~~Cryopreservation, freezing and storage of cells for therapeutic use, each cell line~~
See CPT code 38207.

~~G0266~~ ~~Thawing and expansion of frozen cells for therapeutic use, each aliquot~~
See CPT code 38208-38209.

~~G0267~~ ~~Bone marrow or peripheral stem cell harvest, modification or treatment to eliminate cell type(s) (e.g., T-cells, metastatic carcinoma)~~
See CPT code 38210-38215.

[N] **G0268** Removal of impacted cerumen (one or both ears) by physician on same date of service as audiologic function testing [N1]⊘

AHA: 1Q,'03,12

[N] **G0269** Placement of occlusive device into either a venous or arterial access site, post surgical or interventional procedure (e.g., angioseal plug, vascular plug) [N1]⊘

[A] ☑ **G0270** Medical nutrition therapy; reassessment and subsequent intervention(s) following second referral in same year for change in diagnosis, medical condition or treatment regimen (including additional hours needed for renal disease), individual, face-to-face with the patient, each 15 minutes ⊘ [P0]

[A] ☑ **G0271** Medical nutrition therapy, reassessment and subsequent intervention(s) following second referral in same year for change in diagnosis, medical condition, or treatment regimen (including additional hours needed for renal disease), group (2 or more individuals), each 30 minutes ⊘ [P0]

[N] **G0275** Renal artery angiography (unilateral or bilateral) performed at the time of cardiac catheterization, includes catheter placement, injection of dye, flush aortogram and radiologic supervision and interpretation and production of images (list separately in addition to primary procedure) ⊘

[N] **G0278** Iliac artery angiography performed at the same time of cardiac catheterization, includes catheter placement, injection of dye, radiologic supervision and interpretation and production of images (list separately in addition to primary procedure) ⊘

[A] **G0281** Electrical stimulation, (unattended), to one or more areas, for chronic Stage III and Stage IV pressure ulcers, arterial ulcers, diabetic ulcers, and venous stasis ulcers not demonstrating measurable signs of healing after 30 days of conventional care, as part of a therapy plan of care

MED: 100-4,32,11.1

AHA: 1Q,'03,7; 2Q,'03,7

[E] **G0282** Electrical stimulation, (unattended), to one or more areas, for wound care other than described in G0281 ⊘

MED: 100-3,270.1

AHA: 1Q,'03,7; 2Q,'03,7

[A] **G0283** Electrical stimulation (unattended), to one or more areas for indication(s) other than wound care, as part of a therapy plan of care

AHA: 1Q,'03,7; 2Q,'03,7

[N] **G0288** Reconstruction, computed tomographic angiography of aorta for surgical planning for vascular surgery [N1]

---

| Special Coverage Instructions | Noncovered by Medicare | Carrier Discretion | ☑ Quantity Alert | ● New Code | ○ Recycled/Reinstated | ▲ Revised Code |

**2008 HCPCS**  [A2]-[P2] ASC Payment Indicators  **MED:** Pub 100/NCD References  ⓓ DMEPOS Paid  ⊘ SNF Excluded  [P0] PQRI  **G Codes — 57**

Ⓝ **G0289** Arthroscopy, knee, surgical, for removal of loose body, foreign body, debridement/shaving of articular cartilage (chondroplasty) at the time of other surgical knee arthroscopy in a different compartment of the same knee  Ⓜ⊘

Ⓣ **G0290** Transcatheter placement of a drug eluting intracoronary stent(s), percutaneous, with or without other therapeutic intervention, any method; single vessel  ⊘

AHA: 3Q,'03,11; 4Q,'03,7; 4Q,'02,9

Ⓣ **G0291** Transcatheter placement of a drug eluting intracoronary stent(s), percutaneous, with or without other therapeutic intervention, any method; each additional vessel  ⊘

AHA: 3Q,'03,11; 4Q,'03,7; 4Q,'02,9

Ⓧ ☑ **G0293** Noncovered surgical procedure(s) using conscious sedation, regional, general, or spinal anesthesia in a Medicare qualifying clinical trial, per day  ⊘

AHA: 4Q,'02,9

Ⓧ ☑ **G0294** Noncovered procedure(s) using either no anesthesia or local anesthesia only, in a Medicare qualifying clinical trial, per day  ⊘

AHA: 4Q,'02,9

Ⓔ **G0295** Electromagnetic therapy, to one or more areas, for wound care other than described in G0329 or for other uses

MED: 100-3,270.1

AHA: 1Q,'03,7

Ⓓ **G0297** Insertion of single chamber pacing cardioverter defibrillator pulse generator  ⊘

MED: 100-4,4,61.2

~~G0298~~ ~~Insertion of dual chamber pacing cardioverter~~ ~~defibrillator pulse generator~~
See CPT code 33240.

MED: 100-4,4,61.2

~~G0299~~ ~~Insertion or repositioning of electrode lead for single~~ ~~chamber pacing cardioverter defibrillator and insertion~~ ~~of pulse generator~~
See CPT code 33240.

MED: 100-4,4,61.2

Ⓓ **G0300** Insertion or repositioning of electrode lead(s) for dual chamber pacing cardioverter defibrillator and insertion of pulse generator  ⊘

MED: 100-4,4,61.2

Ⓢ ☑ **G0302** Preoperative pulmonary surgery services for preparation for LVRS, complete course of services, to include a minimum of 16 days of services

Ⓢ ☑ **G0303** Preoperative pulmonary surgery services for preparation for LVRS, 10 to 15 days of services

Ⓢ ☑ **G0304** Preoperative pulmonary surgery services for preparation for LVRS, 1 to 9 days of services

Ⓢ ☑ **G0305** Postdischarge pulmonary surgery services after LVRS, minimum of 6 days of services

Ⓐ **G0306** Complete CBC, automated (HgB, HCT, RBC, WBC, without platelet count) and automated WBC differential count

Ⓐ **G0307** Complete CBC, automated (HgB, HCT, RBC, WBC; without platelet count)

Ⓑ **G0308** ESRD related services during the course of treatment, for patients under 2 years of age to include monitoring for the adequacy of nutrition, assessment of growth and development, and counseling of parents; with 4 or more face-to-face physician visits per month.  Ⓐ⊘

MED: 100-2,11,130; 100-2,11,130.1; 100-4,12,190

Ⓑ **G0309** ESRD related services during the course of treatment, for patients under 2 years of age to include monitoring for the adequacy of nutrition, assessment of growth and development, and counseling of parents; with 2 or 3 face-to-face physician visits per month.  Ⓐ⊘

MED: 100-2,11,130; 100-2,11,130.1; 100-4,12,190

Ⓑ **G0310** ESRD related services during the course of treatment, for patients under 2 years of age to include monitoring for the adequacy of nutrition, assessment of growth and development, and counseling of parents; with 1 face-to-face physician visit per month  Ⓐ⊘

MED: 100-2,11,130; 100-2,11,130.1

Ⓑ **G0311** ESRD related services during the course of treatment, for patients between 2 and 11 years of age to include monitoring for the adequacy of nutrition, assessment of growth and development, and counseling of parents; with 4 or more face-to-face physician visits per month  Ⓐ⊘

MED: 100-2,11,130; 100-2,11,130.1; 100-4,12,190

Ⓑ **G0312** ESRD related services during the course of treatment, for patients between 2 and 11 years of age to include monitoring for the adequacy of nutrition, assessment of growth and development, and counseling of parents; with 2 or 3 face-to-face physician visits per month  Ⓐ⊘

MED: 100-2,11,130; 100-2,11,130.1; 100-4,12,190

Ⓑ **G0313** ESRD related services during the course of treatment, for patients between 2 and 11 years of age to include monitoring for the adequacy of nutrition, assessment of growth and development, and counseling of parents; with 1 face-to-face physician visit per month  Ⓐ⊘

MED: 100-2,11,130; 100-2,11,130.1

Ⓑ **G0314** ESRD related services during the course of treatment, for patients between 12 and 19 years of age to include monitoring for the adequacy of nutrition, assessment of growth and development, and counseling of parents; with 4 or more face-to-face physician visits per month  Ⓐ⊘ ⑰

MED: 100-2,11,130; 100-2,11,130.1; 100-4,12,190

Ⓑ **G0315** End Stage Renal disease (ESRD) related services during the course of treatment, for patients between 12 and 19 years of age to include monitoring for the adequacy of nutrition, assessment of growth and development, and counseling of parents; with two or three face-to-face physician visits per month  Ⓐ⊘ ⑰

MED: 100-2,11,130; 100-2,11,130.1; 100-4,12,190

Ⓑ **G0316** End Stage Renal disease (ESRD) related services during the course of treatment, for patients between 12 and 19 years of age to include monitoring for the adequacy of nutrition, assessment of growth and development, and counseling of parents; with one face-to-face physician visit per month  Ⓐ⊘ ⑰

MED: 100-2,11,130; 100-2,11,130.1

Ⓑ **G0317** End Stage Renal disease (ESRD) related services during the course of treatment, for patients 20 years of age and over; with four or more face-to-face physician visits per month  Ⓐ⊘ ⑰

MED: 100-2,11,130; 100-2,11,130.1; 100-4,12,190

Ⓑ **G0318** ESRD related services during the course of treatment, for patients 20 years of age and over; with 2 or 3 face-to-face physician visits per month  Ⓐ⊘ ⑰

MED: 100-2,11,130; 100-2,11,130.1; 100-4,12,190

---

▮ Special Coverage Instructions   ▮ Noncovered by Medicare   ▮ Carrier Discretion     ☑ Quantity Alert   ● New Code   ○ Recycled/Reinstated   ▲ Revised Code

58 — G Codes     Ⓐ Age Edit   Ⓜ Maternity Edit   ♀ Female Only   ♂ Male Only     Ⓐ-Ⓨ OPPS Status Indicators     2008 HCPCS

B **G0319** End Stage Renal disease (ESRD) related services during the course of treatment, for patients 20 years of age and over; with one face-to-face physician visit per month ⊘ PQ
MED: 100-2,11,130; 100-2,11,130.1

B **G0320** ESRD related services for home dialysis patients per full month; for patients under 2 years of age to include monitoring for adequacy of nutrition, assessment of growth and development, and counseling of parents A⊘
MED: 100-2,11,130; 100-2,11,130.1

B **G0321** ESRD related services for home dialysis patients per full month; for patients 2 to 11 years of age to include monitoring for adequacy of nutrition, assessment of growth and development, and counseling of parents A⊘
MED: 100-2,11,130; 100-2,11,130.1

B **G0322** End Stage Renal disease (ESRD) related services for home dialysis patients per full month; for patients 12 to 19 years of age to include monitoring for adequacy of nutrition, assessment of growth and development, and counseling of parents A⊘ PQ
MED: 100-2,11,130; 100-2,11,130.1

B **G0323** End Stage Renal disease (ESRD) related services for home dialysis patients per full month; for patients 20 years of age and older A⊘ PQ
MED: 100-2,11,130; 100-2,11,130.1

B **G0324** ESRD related services for home dialysis (less than full month), per day; for patients under 2 years of age A⊘
MED: 100-2,11,130; 100-2,11,130.1

B **G0325** ESRD related services for home dialysis (less than full month), per day; for patients between 2 and 11 years of age A⊘
MED: 100-2,11,130; 100-2,11,130.1

B **G0326** ESRD related services for home dialysis (less than full month), per day; for patients between twelve and nineteen years of age A⊘ PQ
MED: 100-2,11,130; 100-2,11,130.1

B **G0327** ESRD related services for home dialysis (less than full month), per day; for patients twenty years of age and over A⊘ PQ
MED: 100-2,11,130; 100-2,11,130.1

A **G0328** Colorectalcancer screening; fecal-occult blood test, immunoassay, 1–3 simultaneous determinations. ⊘
MED: 100-4,18,60.1; 100-4,18,60.2; 100-4,18,60.2.1; 100-4,18,60.6

A **G0329** Electromagnetic therapy, to one or more areas for chronic Stage III and Stage IV pressure ulcers, arterial ulcers, diabetic ulcers and venous stasis ulcers not demonstrating measurable signs of healing after 30 days of conventional care as part of a therapay plan of care ⊘
MED: 100-4,32,11.2

S **G0332** Services for intravenous infusion of immunoglobulin prior to administration (this service is to be billed in conjunction with administration of immunoglobulin)

M **G0333** Pharmacy dispensing fee for inhalation drug(s); initial 30-day supply as a beneficiary

B **G0337** Hospice evaluation and counseling services, pre-election

S **G0339** Image guided robotic linear accelerator-based stereotactic radiosurgery, complete course of therapy in one session, or first session of fractionated treatment Z2⊘

S **G0340** Image guided robotic linear accelerator-based stereotactic radiosurgery, delivery including collimator changes and custom plugging, fractionated treatment, all lesions, per session, second through fifth sessions, maximum five sessions per course of treatment Z2⊘

C **G0341** Percutaneous islet cell transplant, includes portal vein catheterization and infusion ⊘
MED: 100-3,260.3; 100-4,32,70

C **G0342** Laparoscopy for islet cell transplant, includes portal vein catheterization and infusion ⊘
MED: 100-3,260.3; 100-4,32,70

C **G0343** Laparotomy for islet cell transplant, includes portal vein catheterization and infusion ⊘
MED: 100-3,260.3; 100-4,32,70

V **G0344** Initial preventive physical examination; face-to-face visit, services limited to new beneficiary during the first six months of Medicare enrollment ⊘
MED: 100-4,12,30.6.1.1

T **G0364** Bone marrow aspiration performed with bone marrow biopsy through the same incision on the same date of service P3⊘

S **G0365** Vessel mapping of vessels for hemodialysis access (services for preoperative vessel mapping prior to creation of hemodialysis access using an autogenous hemodialysis conduit, including arterial inflow and venous outflow)

B **G0366** Electrocardiogram, routine ECG with 12 leads; performed as a component of the initial preventive examination with interpretation and report
MED: 100-4,12,30.6.1.1

S **G0367** Tracing only, without interpretation and report, performed as a component of the initial preventive examination ⊘
MED: 100-4,12,30.6.1.1

M **G0368** Interpretation and report only, performed as a component of the initial preventive examination ⊘
MED: 100-4,12,30.6.1.1

M **G0372** Physician service required to establish and document the need for a power mobility device ⊘

~~**G0375** Smoking and tobacco use cessation counseling visit; intermediate, greater than 3 minutes up to 10 minutes~~
MED: 100-4,32,12
AHA: 3Q,'05,9

~~**G0376** Smoking and tobacco use cessation counseling visit; intensive, greater than 10 minutes~~
MED: 100-4,32,12
AHA: 3Q,'05,9

S **G0377** Administration of vaccine for Part D drug

N **G0378** Hospital observation service, per hour
MED: 100-2,6,20.5; 100-4,4,290.4.1

Q **G0379** Direct admission of patient for hospital observation care
MED: 100-2,6,20.5; 100-4,4,290.4.1

Special Coverage Instructions    Noncovered by Medicare    Carrier Discretion    ☑ Quantity Alert    ● New Code    ○ Recycled/Reinstated    ▲ Revised Code

2008 HCPCS    A2- Z3 ASC Payment Indicators    MED: Pub 100/NCD References    ⅋ DMEPOS Paid    ⊘ SNF Excluded    PQ PQRI    G Codes — 59

**Procedures/Professional Services (Temporary)**

**G0380 — G3001**

▲ Ⓥ **G0380** Level 1 hospital emergency department visit provided in a type B emergency department; (the ED must meet at least one of the following requirements: (1) it is licensed by the state in which it is located under applicable state law as an emergency room or emergency department; (2) it is held out to the public (by name, posted signs, advertising, or other means) as a place that provides care for emergency medical conditions on an urgent basis without requiring a previously scheduled appointment; or (3) during the calendar year immediately preceding the calendar year in which a determination under 42 CFR §489.24 is being made, based on a representative sample of patient visits that occurred during that calendar year, it provides at least one-third of all of its outpatient visits for the treatment of emergency medical conditions on an urgent basis without requiring a previously scheduled appointment
MED: 100-4,4,160

▲ Ⓥ **G0381** Level 2 hospital emergency department visit provided in a type B emergency department; (the ED must meet at least one of the following requirements: (1) it is licensed by the state in which it is located under applicable state law as an emergency room or emergency department; (2) it is held out to the public (by name, posted signs, advertising, or other means) as a place that provides care for emergency medical conditions on an urgent basis without requiring a previously scheduled appointment; or (3) during the calendar year immediately preceding the calendar year in which a determination under 42 CFR §489.24 is being made, based on a representative sample of patient visits that occurred during that calendar year, it provides at least one-third of all of its outpatient visits for the treatment of emergency medical conditions on an urgent basis without requiring a previously scheduled appointment
MED: 100-4,4,160

▲ Ⓥ **G0382** Level 3 hospital emergency department visit provided in a type B emergency department; (the ED must meet at least one of the following requirements: (1) it is licensed by the state in which it is located under applicable state law as an emergency room or emergency department; (2) it is held out to the public (by name, posted signs, advertising, or other means) as a place that provides care for emergency medical conditions on an urgent basis without requiring a previously scheduled appointment; or (3) during the calendar year immediately preceding the calendar year in which a determination under 42 CFR §489.24 is being made, based on a representative sample of patient visits that occurred during that calendar year, it provides at least one-third of all of its outpatient visits for the treatment of emergency medical conditions on an urgent basis without requiring a previously scheduled appointment
MED: 100-4,4,160

▲ Ⓥ **G0383** Level 4 hospital emergency department visit provided in a type B emergency department; (the ED must meet at least one of the following requirements: (1) it is licensed by the state in which it is located under applicable state law as an emergency room or emergency department; (2) it is held out to the public (by name, posted signs, advertising, or other means) as a place that provides care for emergency medical conditions on an urgent basis without requiring a previously scheduled appointment; or (3) during the calendar year immediately preceding the calendar year in which a determination under 42 CFR §489.24 is being made, based on a representative sample of patient visits that occurred during that calendar year, it provides at least one-third of all of its outpatient visits for the treatment of emergency medical conditions on an urgent basis without requiring a previously scheduled appointment
MED: 100-4,4,160

▲ Ⓥ **G0384** Level 5 hospital emergency department visit provided in a type B emergency department; (the ED must meet at least one of the following requirements: (1) it is licensed by the state in which it is located under applicable state law as an emergency room or emergency department; (2) it is held out to the public (by name, posted signs, advertising, or other means) as a place that provides care for emergency medical conditions on an urgent basis without requiring a previously scheduled appointment; or (3) during the calendar year immediately preceding the calendar year in which a determination under 42 CFR §489.24 is being made, based on a representative sample of patient visits that occurred during that calendar year, it provides at least one-third of all of its outpatient visits for the treatment of emergency medical conditions on an urgent basis without requiring a previously scheduled appointment
MED: 100-4,4,160

Ⓢ **G0389** Ultrasound B-scan and/or real time with image documentation; for abdominal aortic aneurysm (AAA) screening ⊘

Ⓢ **G0390** Trauma response team associated with hospital critical care service

Ⓣ **G0392** Transluminal balloon angioplasty, percutaneous; for maintenance of hemodialysis access, arteriovenous fistula or graft; arterial 🅐🆉

Ⓣ **G0393** Transluminal balloon angioplasty, percutaneous; for maintenance of hemodialysis access, arteriovenous fistula or graft; venous 🅐🆉

Ⓐ **G0394** Blood occult test (e.g., guaiac), feces, for single determination for colorectal neoplasm (e.g., patient was provided three cards or single triple card for consecutive collection)

● Ⓢ **G0396** Alcohol and/or substance (other than tobacco) abuse structured assessment (e.g., audit, dast), and brief intervention 15 to 30 minutes

● Ⓢ **G0397** Alcohol and/or substance (other than tobacco) abuse structured assessment (e.g., audit, dast), and intervention, greater than 30 minutes

Ⓢ ☑ **G3001** Administration and supply of tositumomab, 450 mg ⊘

## PHYSICIAN QUALITY REPORTING INDICATOR CODE (PQRI)

Physician Quality Reporting Indicator Codes (PQRI) are to be used for the physician Quality Reporting Indicator Code (PQRI) program in which CMS seeks to analyze the quality of care provided to Medicare beneficiaries. Reporting of these codes is voluntary. Physicians should not charge for these codes. Unless otherwise indicated, report these codes in addition to office visit, home visit, nursing facility,

Special Coverage Instructions    Noncovered by Medicare    Carrier Discretion    ☑ Quantity Alert   ● New Code   ○ Recycled/Reinstated   ▲ Revised Code

60 — G Codes    🅐 Age Edit   Ⓜ Maternity Edit   ♀ Female Only   ♂ Male Only   🅐–Ⓥ OPPS Status Indicators    **2008 HCPCS**

and domiciliary evaluation and management codes. For additional information, please visit the following website: http://www.cms.hhs.gov/providers/pqri

[M] **G8006** Acute myocardial infarction: patient documented to have received aspirin at arrival

[M] **G8007** Acute myocardial infarction: patient not documented to have received aspirin at arrival

[M] **G8008** Clinician documented that acute myocardial infarction patient was not an eligible candidate to receive aspirin at arrival measure

[M] **G8009** Acute myocardial infarction: patient documented to have received beta-blocker at arrival　[PQ]

[M] **G8010** Acute myocardial infarction: patient not documented to have received beta-blocker at arrival　[PQ]

[M] **G8011** Clinician documented that acute myocardial infarction patient was not an eligible candidate for beta-blocker at arrival measure　[PQ]

[M] **G8012** Pneumonia: patient documented to have received antibiotic within 4 hours of presentation

[M] **G8013** Pneumonia: patient not documented to have received antibiotic within 4 hours of presentation

[M] **G8014** Clinician documented that pneumonia patient was not an eligible candidate for antibiotic within 4 hours of presentation measure

[M] **G8015** Diabetic patient with most recent hemoglobin A1c level (within the last 6 months) documented as greater than 9%

[M] **G8016** Diabetic patient with most recent hemoglobin A1c level (within the last 6 months) documented as less than or equal to 9%

[M] **G8017** Clinician documented that diabetic patient was not eligible candidate for hemoglobin A1c measure

[M] **G8018** Clinician has not provided care for the diabetic patient for the required time for hemoglobin A1c measure (6 months)

[M] **G8019** Diabetic patient with most recent low-density lipoprotein (within the last 12 months) documented as greater than or equal to 100 mg/dl

[M] **G8020** Diabetic patient with most recent low-density lipoprotein (within the last 12 months) documented as less than 100 mg/dl

[M] **G8021** Clinician documented that diabetic patient was not eligible candidate for low-density lipoprotein measure

[M] **G8022** Clinician has not provided care for the diabetic patient for the required time for low-density lipoprotein measure (12 months)

[M] **G8023** Diabetic patient with most recent blood pressure (within the last 6 months) documented as equal to or greater than 140 systolic or equal to or greater than 80 mm Hg diastolic

[M] **G8024** Diabetic patient with most recent blood pressure (within the last 6 months) documented less than 140 systolic and less than 80 diastolic

[M] **G8025** Clinician documented that the diabetic patient was not eligible candidate for blood pressure measure

[M] **G8026** Clinician has not provided care for the diabetic patient for the required time for blood measure (within the last 6 months)

[M] **G8027** Heart failure patient with left ventricular systolic dysfunction (LVSD) documented to be on either angiotensin-converting enzyme-inhibitor or angiotensin-receptor blocker (ACE-1 or ARB) therapy

[M] **G8028** Heart failure patient with left ventricular systolic dysfunction (LVSD) not documented to be on either angiotensin-converting enzyme-inhibitor or angiotensin-receptor blocker (ACE-1 or ARB) therapy

[M] **G8029** Clinician documented that heart failure patient was not an eligible candidate for either angiotensin-converting enzyme-inhibitor or angiotensin-receptor blocker (ACE-I or ARB) therapy measure

[M] **G8030** Heart failure patient with left ventricular systolic dysfunction (LVSD) documented to be on beta-blocker therapy

[M] **G8031** Heart failure patient with left ventricular systolic dysfunction (LVSD) not documented to be on beta-blocker therapy

[M] **G8032** Clinician documented that heart failure patient was not eligible candidate for beta-blocker therapy measure

[M] **G8033** Prior myocardial infarction—coronary artery disease patient documented to be on beta-blocker therapy

[M] **G8034** Prior myocardial infarction—coronary artery disease patient not documented to be on beta-blocker therapy

[M] **G8035** Clinician documented that prior myocardial infarction—coronary artery disease patient was not eligible candidate for beta-blocker therapy measure

[M] **G8036** Coronary artery disease patient documented to be on antiplatelet therapy

[M] **G8037** Coronary artery disease patient not documented to be on antiplatelet therapy

[M] **G8038** Clinician documented that coronary artery disease patient was not eligible candidate for antiplatelet therapy measure

[M] **G8039** Coronary artery disease—patient with low-density lipoprotein documented to be greater than 100 mg/dl

[M] **G8040** Coronary artery disease—patient with low-density lipoprotein documented to be less than or equal to 100 mg/dl

[M] **G8041** Clinician documented that coronary artery disease patient was not eligible candidate for low-density lipoprotein measure　♀

[M] **G8051** Patient (female) documented to have been assessed for osteoporosis　♀

[M] **G8052** Patient (female) not documented to have been assessed for osteoporosis　♀

[M] **G8053** Clinician documented that (female) patient was not an eligible candidate for osteoporosis assessment measure　♀

[M] **G8054** Patient not documented for the assessment of falls within last 12 months

[M] **G8055** Patient documented for the assessment of falls within last 12 months

[M] **G8056** Clinician documented that patient was not an eligible candidate for the falls assessment measure within the last 12 months

[M] **G8057** Patient documented to have received hearing assessment

[M] **G8058** Patient not documented to have received hearing assessment

[M] **G8059** Clinician documented that patient was not an eligible candidate for hearing assessment measure

Special Coverage Instructions　　Noncovered by Medicare　　Carrier Discretion　　☑ Quantity Alert　● New Code　○ Recycled/Reinstated　▲ Revised Code

**2008 HCPCS**　[A2]-[A3] ASC Payment Indicators　**MED:** Pub 100/NCD References　⚥ DMEPOS Paid　⊘ SNF Excluded　[PQ] PQRI　**G Codes — 61**

Ⓜ **G8060** Patient documented for the assessment of urinary incontinence

Ⓜ **G8061** Patient not documented for the assessment of urinary incontinence

Ⓜ **G8062** Clinician documented that patient was not an eligible candidate for urinary incontinence assessment measure

Ⓜ **G8075** ESRD patient with documented dialysis dose of URR greater than or equal to 65% (or Kt/ V greater than or equal to 1.2) Ⓐ 🄿🄾

Ⓜ **G8076** ESRD patient with documented dialysis dose of URR less than 65% (or Kt/V less than 1.2) Ⓐ 🄿🄾

Ⓜ **G8077** Clinician documented that ESRD patient was not eligible candidate for URR or Kt/V measure Ⓐ 🄿🄾

Ⓜ **G8078** ESRD patient with documented hematocrit greater than or equal to 33 (or hemoglobin greater than or equal to 11) Ⓐ 🄿🄾

Ⓜ **G8079** ESRD patient with documented hematocrit less than 33 (or hemoglobin less than 11) Ⓐ 🄿🄾

Ⓜ **G8080** Clinician documented that ESRD patient was not an eligible candidate for hematocrit (hemoglobin) measure Ⓐ 🄿🄾

Ⓜ **G8081** ESRD patient requiring hemodialysis vascular access documented to have received autogenous AV fistula

Ⓜ **G8082** ESRD patient requiring hemodialysis documented to have received vascular access other than autogenous AV fistula

Ⓜ **G8085** ESRD patient requiring hemodialysis vascular access was not an eligible candidate for autogenous AV fistula

Ⓜ **G8093** Newly diagnosed chronic obstructive pulmonary disease (COPD) patient documented to have received smoking cessation intervention, within 3 months of diagnosis

Ⓜ **G8094** Newly diagnosed chronic obstructive pulmonary disease (COPD) patient not documented to have received smoking cessation intervention, within 3 months of diagnosis

Ⓜ **G8099** Osteoporosis patient documented to have been prescribed calcium and vitamin D supplements

Ⓜ **G8100** Clinician documented that osteoporosis patient was not an eligible candidate for calcium and vitamin D supplement measure

Ⓜ **G8103** Newly diagnosed osteoporosis patients documented to have been treated with antiresorptive therapy and/or PTH within three months of diagnosis

Ⓜ **G8104** Clinician documented that newly diagnosed osteoporosis patient was not an eligible candidate for antiresorptive therapy and/or PTH treatment measure within three months of diagnosis

Ⓜ **G8106** Within 6 months of suffering a nontraumatic fracture, female patient 65 years of age or older documented to have undergone bone mineral density testing or to have been prescribed a drug to treat or prevent osteoporosis

Ⓜ **G8107** Clinician documented that female patient 65 years of age or older who suffered a nontraumatic fracture within the last 6 months was not an eligible candidate for measure to test bone mineral density or drug to treat or prevent osteoporosis

Ⓜ **G8108** Patient documented to have received influenza vaccination during influenza season Ⓐ

Ⓜ **G8109** Patient not documented to have received influenza vaccination during influenza season Ⓐ

Ⓜ **G8110** Clinician documented that patient was not an eligible candidate for influenza vaccination measure Ⓐ

Ⓜ **G8111** Patient (female) documented to have received a mammogram during the measurement year or prior year to the measurement year Ⓐ ♀

Ⓜ **G8112** Patient (female) not documented to have received a mammogram during the measurement year or prior year to the measurement year Ⓐ ♀

Ⓜ **G8113** Clinician documented that female patient was not an eligible candidate for mammography measure Ⓐ

Ⓜ **G8114** Clinician did not provide care to patient for the required time of mammography measure (i.e., measurement year or prior year) Ⓐ

Ⓜ **G8115** Patient documented to have received pneumococcal vaccination Ⓐ

Ⓜ **G8116** Patient not documented to have received pneumococcal vaccination Ⓐ

Ⓜ **G8117** Clinician documented that patient was not an eligible candidate for pneumococcal vaccination measure Ⓐ

▲ Ⓜ **G8126** Patient documented as being treated with antidepressant medication during the entire 12 week acute treatment phase Ⓐ 🄿🄾

▲ Ⓜ **G8127** Patient not documented as being treated with antidepressant medication during the entire 12 weeks acute treatment phase Ⓐ 🄿🄾

▲ Ⓜ **G8128** Clinician documented that patient was not an eligible candidate for antidepressant medication during the entire 12 week acute treatment phase measure Ⓐ 🄿🄾

Ⓜ **G8129** Patient documented as being treated with antidepressant medication for at least 6 months continuous treatment phase Ⓐ

Ⓜ **G8130** Patient not documented as being treated with antidepressant medication for at least 6 months continuous treatment phase Ⓐ

Ⓜ **G8131** Clinician documented that patient was not an eligible candidate for antidepressant medication for continuous treatment phase Ⓐ

Ⓜ **G8152** Patient documented to have received antibiotic prophylaxis one hour prior to incision time (two hours for vancomycin)

Ⓜ **G8153** Patient not documented to have received antibiotic prophylaxis one hour prior to incision time (two hours for vancomycin)

Ⓜ **G8154** Clinician documented that patient was not an eligible candidate for antibiotic prophylaxis one hour prior to incision time (two hours for vancomycin) measure

Ⓜ **G8155** Patient with documented receipt of thromboembolism prophylaxis

Ⓜ **G8156** Patient without documented receipt of thromboembolism prophylaxis

Ⓜ **G8157** Clinician documented that patient was not an eligible candidate for thromboembolism prophylaxis measure

~~**G8158** Patient documented to have received coronary artery bypass graft with use of internal mammary artery~~

Ⓜ **G8159** Patient documented to have received coronary artery bypass graft without use of internal mammary artery

---

Ⓢ Special Coverage Instructions    Ⓝ Noncovered by Medicare    Ⓒ Carrier Discretion    ☑ Quantity Alert    ● New Code    ○ Recycled/Reinstated    ▲ Revised Code

**62 — G Codes**    Ⓐ Age Edit    Ⓜ Maternity Edit    ♀ Female Only    ♂ Male Only    Ⓐ-Ⓨ OPPS Status Indicators    **2008 HCPCS**

G8160 ~~Clinician documented that patient was not an eligible candidate for coronary artery bypass graft with use of internal mammary artery measure~~

G8161 ~~Patient with isolated coronary artery bypass graft documented to have received pre-operative beta-blockade~~

Ⓜ G8162 Patient with isolated coronary artery bypass graft not documented to have received pre-operative beta-blockade

G8163 ~~Clinician documented that patient with isolated coronary artery bypass graft was not an eligible candidate for pre-operative beta-blockade measure~~

Ⓜ G8164 Patient with isolated coronary artery bypass graft documented to have prolonged intubation

Ⓜ G8165 Patient with isolated coronary artery bypass graft not documented to have prolonged intubation

Ⓜ G8166 Patient with isolated coronary artery bypass graft documented to have required surgical re-exploration

Ⓜ G8167 Patient with isolated coronary artery bypass graft did not require surgical re-exploration

Ⓜ G8170 Patient with isolated coronary artery bypass graft documented to have been discharged on aspirin or clopidogrel

Ⓜ G8171 Patient with isolated coronary artery bypass graft not documented to have been discharged on aspirin or clopidogrel

Ⓜ G8172 Clinician documented that patient with isolated coronary artery bypass graft was not an eligible candidate for antiplatelet therapy at discharge measure

Ⓜ G8182 Clinician has not provided care for the cardiac patient for the required time for low-density lipoprotein measure (6 months)

Ⓜ G8183 Patient with heart failure and atrial fibrillation documented to be on warfarin therapy

Ⓜ G8184 Clinician documented that patient with heart failure and atrial fibrillation was not an eligible candidate for warfarin therapy measure

Ⓜ G8185 Patients diagnosed with symptomatic osteoarthritis with documented annual assessment of function and pain

Ⓜ G8186 Clinician documented that symptomatic osteoarthritis patient was not an eligible candidate for annual assessment of function and pain measure

G8191 ~~Clinician documented to have given order for prophylactic antibiotic to be given within one hour (if vancomycin, two hours) prior to surgical incision (or start of procedure when no incision is required)~~

G8192 ~~Clinician documented to have given the prophylactic antibiotic within one hour (if vancomycin, two hours) prior to the surgical incision (or start of procedure when no incision is required)~~

Ⓜ G8193 Clinician did not document that an order for prophylactic antibiotic to be given within one hour (if vancomycin, two hours) prior to surgical incision (or start of procedure when no incision is required) was given

G8194 ~~Clinician documented that patient was not an eligible candidate for prophylactic antibiotic~~

G8195 ~~Clinician documented to have given the prophylactic antibiotic within one hour (if vancomycin, two hours) prior to the surgical incision (or start of procedure when no incision is required)~~

▲ Ⓜ G8196 Clinician did not document a prophylactic antibiotic was administered within one hour (if vancomycin, two hours) prior to surgical incision (or start of procedure when no incision is required)

G8197 ~~Patient documented to have order for prophylactic antibiotic to be given within one hour (if vancomycin, two hours) prior to surgical incision (or start of procedure when no incision is required)~~

G8198 ~~Patient documented to have order for cefazolin or cefuroxime for antimicrobial prophylaxis~~

G8199 ~~Clinician documented to have given cefazolin or cefuroxime for antimicrobial prophylaxis~~

Ⓜ G8200 Order for cefazolin or cefuroxime for antimicrobial prophylaxis not documented

G8201 ~~Patient was not an eligible candidate for cefazolin or cefuroxime for antimicrobial prophylaxis~~

G8202 ~~Clinician documented an order was given to discontinue prophylactic antibiotics within 24 hours of surgical end time~~

G8203 ~~Clinician documented that prophylactic antibiotics were discontinued within 24 hours of surgical end time~~

Ⓜ G8204 Clinician did not document an order was given to discontinue prophylactic antibiotics within 24 hours of surgical end time

G8205 ~~Clinician documented that patient was not an eligible candidate for prophylactic antibiotic discontinuation within 24 hours of surgical end time~~

G8206 ~~Clinician documented that prophylactic antibiotic was given~~

G8207 ~~Clinician documented an order was given to discontinue prophylactic antibiotics within 48 hours of surgical end time~~

G8208 ~~Clinician documented that prophylactic antibiotics were discontinued within 48 hours of surgical end time~~

Ⓜ G8209 Clinician did not document an order was given to discontinue prophylactic antibiotics within 48 hours of surgical end time

G8210 ~~Clinician documented Patient was not an eligible candidate for discontinuation of prophylactic antibiotic discontinuation within 48 hours of surgical end time~~

G8211 ~~Clinician documented that prophylactic antibiotic was given~~

G8212 ~~Clinician documented an order was given for appropriate venous thromboembolism (VTE) prophylaxis to be given within 24 hrs prior to incision time or 24 hours after surgery end time~~

G8213 ~~Clinician documented to have given VTE prophylaxis within 24 hrs prior to incision time or 24 hours after surgery end time~~

Ⓜ G8214 Clinician did not document an order was given for appropriate venous thromboembolism (VTE) prophylaxis to be given within 24 hrs prior to incision time or 24 hours after surgery end time

G8215 ~~Clinician documented that Patient was not an eligible candidate for venous thromboembolism (VTE) prophylaxis to be given within 24 hours prior to incision time or 24 hours after surgery end time~~

G8216 ~~Patient documented to have received DVT prophylaxis by end of hospital day two~~

Ⓜ G8217 Patient not documented to have received DVT prophylaxis by end of hospital day two

---

| Special Coverage Instructions | Noncovered by Medicare | Carrier Discretion | ☑ Quantity Alert | ● New Code | ○ Recycled/Reinstated | ▲ Revised Code |

**2008 HCPCS**  N2-Z3 ASC Payment Indicators  **MED:** Pub 100/NCD References  ⅋ DMEPOS Paid  ⊘ SNF Excluded  PQ PQRI  **G Codes — 63**

~~G8218 Patient was not an eligible candidate for DVT prophylaxis by end of hospital day two, including physician documentation that patient is ambulatory~~

[M] **G8219** Patient documented to have received DVT prophylaxis by end of hospital day two

[M] **G8220** Patient not documented to have received DVT prophylaxis by end of hospital day two

[M] **G8221** Clinician documented that patient was not an eligible candidate for DVT prophylaxis by the end of hospital day two, including physician documentation that patient is ambulatory

~~G8222 Patient documented to have been prescribed antiplatelet therapy at discharge~~

[M] **G8223** Patient not documented to have received prescription for antiplatelet therapy at discharge

~~G8224 Clinician documented that patient was not an eligible candidate for antiplatelet therapy at discharge, including identification from medical record that patient is on anticoagulation therapy~~

~~G8225 Patient documented to have been prescribed an anticoagulant at discharge~~

[M] **G8226** Patient not documented to have received prescription for anticoagulant therapy at discharge

~~G8227 Patient not documented to have permanent, persistent, or paroxysmal atrial fibrillation~~

~~G8228 Clinician documented that patient was not an eligible candidate for anticoagulant therapy at discharge~~

~~G8229 Patient documented to have been administered or considered for TPA~~

~~G8230 Patient not eligible for TPA administration, ischemic stroke symptom onset of more than 3 hours~~

[M] **G8231** Patient not documented to have received TPA or not documented to have been considered a candidate for TPA administration

~~G8232 Patient documented to have received dysphagia screening prior to taking any foods, fluids or medication by mouth~~

[M] **G8234** Patient not documented to have received dysphagia screening

~~G8235 Patient not receiving or ineligible to receive food, fluids or medication by mouth, or documentation of NPO (nothing by mouth) order~~

~~G8236 Clinician documented that patient was not an eligible candidate for dysphagia screening prior to taking any foods, fluids or medication by mouth~~

~~G8237 Patient documented to have received order for rehabilitation services or documentation of consideration for rehabilitation services~~

[M] **G8238** Patient not documented to have received order for or consideration for rehabilitation services

~~G8239 Internal carotid stenosis patient below 30%, reference to measurements of distal internal carotid diameter as the denominator for stenosis measurement not necessary~~

▲ [M] **G8240** Internal carotid stenosis patient in the 30-99% range, and no documentation of reference to measurements of distal internal carotid diameter as the denominator for stenosis measurement

~~G8241 Clinician documented that patient whose final report of the carotid imaging study performed (neck MRA, neck CTA, neck duplex ultrasound, carotid angiogram), with characterization of an internal carotid stenosis in the 30-99% range, was not an eligible candidate for reference to measurements of distal internal carotid diameter as the denominator for stenosis measurement~~

~~G8242 Patient documented to have received CT or MRI with presence or absence of hemorrhage, mass lesion and acute infarction documented in the final report~~

[M] **G8243** Patient not documented to have received CT or MRI and the presence or absence of hemorrhage, mass lesion and acute infarction not documented in the final report

~~G8245 Clinician documented presence or absence alarm symptoms~~

[M] **G8246** Patient was not an eligible candidate for medical history review with assessment of new or changing moles

~~G8247 Patient with alarm symptom(s) documented to have had upper endoscopy performed or referral for upper endoscopy~~

[M] **G8248** Patient with at least one alarm symptom not documented to have had upper endoscopy or referral for upper endoscopy

~~G8249 Clinician documented that patient was not an eligible candidate for upper endoscopy~~

~~G8250 Patient with suspicion of Barrett's esophagus in endoscopy report and documented to have received an esophageal biopsy~~

[M] **G8251** Patient not documented to have received an esophageal biopsy when suspicion of Barrett's esophagus is indicated in the endoscopy report

~~G8252 Clinician documented that patient was not an eligible candidate for esophageal biopsy~~

~~G8253 Patient documented to have received an order for a barium swallow test~~

▲ [M] **G8254** Patient with no documented order for barium swallow test

~~G8255 Clinician documentation that patient was an eligible candidate for barium swallow test~~

~~G8256 Clinician documented reconciliation of discharge medications with current medication list in medical record~~

[M] **G8257** Clinician has not documented reconciliation of discharge medications with current medication list in medical record

~~G8258 Patient was not an eligible candidate for discharge medications review~~

~~G8259 Patient documented to have surrogate decision maker or advance care plan in medical record~~

[M] **G8260** Patient not documented to have surrogate decision maker or advance care plan in medical record

~~G8261 Clinician documented that patient was not an eligible candidate for surrogate decision maker or advance care plan~~

~~G8262 Patient documented to have been assessed for presence or absence of urinary incontinence~~

[M] **G8263** Patient not documented to have been assessed for presence or absence of urinary incontinence

~~G8264 Clinician documented that patient was not an eligible candidate for an assessment of the presence or absence of urinary incontinence~~

Special Coverage Instructions | Noncovered by Medicare | Carrier Discretion | ☑ Quantity Alert | ● New Code | ○ Recycled/Reinstated | ▲ Revised Code

64 — G Codes | [A] Age Edit | [M] Maternity Edit | ♀ Female Only | ♂ Male Only | [A]-[Y] OPPS Status Indicators | 2008 HCPCS

~~G8265 Patient documented to have received characterization of urinary incontinence~~

[M] **G8266** Patient not documented to have received characterization of urinary incontinence

~~G8267 Patient documented to have received a plan of care for urinary incontinence~~

[M] **G8268** Patient not documented to have received plan of care for urinary incontinence

~~G8269 Clinician has not provided care for the patient for the required time to develop plan of care for urinary incontinence~~

~~G8270 Patient documented to have received screening for fall risk (two or more falls in the past year or any fall with injury in the past year)~~

▲ [M] **G8271** Patient with no documentation of screening for fall risks (two or more falls in the past year or any fall with injury in the past year)

~~G8272 Clinician documentation that patient was not an eligible candidate for fall risk screening~~

~~G8273 Clinician has not provided care for the patient for the required time to screen for fall risk~~

[M] **G8274** Clinician has not documented presence or absence of alarm symptoms

~~G8275 Patient documented to have medical history taken which included assessment of new or changing moles~~

[M] **G8276** Patient not documented to have received medical history with assessment of new or changing moles

~~G8277 Patient was not an eligible candidate for medical history review with assessment of new or changing moles~~

~~G8278 Patient documented to have received complete physical skin exam~~

[M] **G8279** Patient not documented to have received a complete physical skin exam

~~G8280 Patient was not an eligible candidate for complete physical skin exam during the reporting year~~

~~G8281 Patient documented to have received counseling to perform a self-examination~~

[M] **G8282** Patient not documented to have received counseling to perform a self-examination

~~G8283 Patient was not an eligible candidate for counseling to perform self-examination~~

~~G8284 Patient documented to have received a prescription for pharmacologic therapy for osteoporosis~~

[M] **G8285** Patient not documented to have received pharmacologic therapy

~~G8286 Clinician documented that patient was not an eligible candidate for pharmacologic therapy~~

~~G8287 Clinician has not provided care for the patient for the required time for the pharmacologic therapy measure~~

~~G8288 Patient documented to have received calcium and vitamin D or counseling on both calcium and vitamin D use, and exercise~~

[M] **G8289** Patient with no documentation of calcium and vitamin D use or counseling regarding both calcium and vitamin D use, or exercise

~~G8290 Clinician documentation that patient was not an eligible candidate for calcium and vitamin D, and exercise during the reporting year~~

~~G8291 Clinician has not provided care for the patient for the required time for the calcium, vitamin D, and exercise measure~~

~~G8292 COPD patient with spirometry results documented~~

[M] **G8293** COPD patient without spirometry results documented

~~G8294 COPD patient was not eligible for spirometry results~~

~~G8295 COPD patient documented to have received inhaled bronchodilator therapy~~

[M] **G8296** COPD patient not documented to have inhaled bronchodilator therapy prescribed

~~G8297 COPD patient was not eligible for inhaled bronchodilator therapy~~

[M] **G8298** Patient documented to have received optic nerve head evaluation

[M] **G8299** Patient not documented to have received optic nerve head evaluation

~~G8300 Clinician documented that patient was not an eligible candidate for optic nerve head evaluation during the reporting year~~

~~G8301 Clinician has not provided care for the primary open-angle glaucoma patient for the required time for optic nerve head evaluation measure~~

[M] **G8302** Patient documented to have a specific target intraocular pressure range goal

[M] **G8303** Patient not documented to have a specific target intraocular pressure range goal

[M] **G8304** Clinician documented that patient was not an eligible candidate for a specific target intraocular pressure range goal

[M] **G8305** Clinician has not provided care for the primary open-angle glaucoma patient for the required time for treatment range goal documentation measurement

[M] **G8306** Primary open-angle glaucoma patient with intraocular pressure above the target range goal documented to have received plan of care

[M] **G8307** Primary open-angle glaucoma patient with intraocular pressure at or below goal, no plan of care necessary

[M] **G8308** Primary open-angle glaucoma patient with intraocular pressure above the target range goal, and not documented to have received plan of care during the reporting year

~~G8309 Patient documented to have been prescribed/recommended antioxidant vitamin or mineral supplement~~

▲ [M] **G8310** Patient not documented to have been prescribed/recommended at least one antioxidant vitamin or mineral supplement during the reporting year

~~G8311 Clinician documentation that patient was not an eligible candidate for antioxidant vitamin or mineral supplement during the reporting year~~

~~G8312 Clinician has not provided care for the age-related macular degeneration patient for the required time for antioxidant supplement prescription/recommended measure~~

~~G8313 Patient documented to have received macular exam, including documentation of the presence or absence of macular thickening or hemorrhage and the Level of macular degeneration severity~~

Special Coverage Instructions    Noncovered by Medicare    Carrier Discretion    ☑ Quantity Alert   ● New Code   ○ Recycled/Reinstated   ▲ Revised Code

**2008 HCPCS**   [P2-P3] ASC Payment Indicators   **MED:** Pub 100/NCD References   ⅍ DMEPOS Paid   ⊘ SNF Excluded   [PQ] PQRI   **G Codes — 65**

**Procedures/Professional Services (Temporary)**

**G8314 — G8356**

☒ **G8314** Patient not documented to have received macular exam with documentation of presence or absence of macular thickening or hemorrhage and no documentation of Level of macular degeneration severity

~~G8315 Clinician documentation that patient was not an eligible candidate for macular examination during the reporting year~~

~~G8316 Clinician has not provided care for the age-related macular degeneration patient for the required time for macular examination measurement~~

~~G8317 Patient documented to have visual functional status assessed~~

☒ **G8318** Patient documented not to have visual functional status assessed

~~G8319 Clinician documented that patient was not an eligible candidate for assessment of visual functional status~~

~~G8320 Clinician has not provided care for the cataract patient for the required time for assessment of visual functional status measurement~~

~~G8321 Patient documented to have had pre-surgical axial length, corneal power measurement and method of intraocular lens power calculation~~

☒ **G8322** Patient not documented to have had pre-surgical axial length, corneal power measurement and method of intraocular lens power calculation

~~G8323 Clinician documentation that patient was not an eligible candidate for pre-surgical axial length, corneal power measurement and method of intraocular lens power calculation~~

~~G8324 Clinician has not provided care for the cataract patient for the required time for pre-surgical measurement and intraocular lens power calculation measure~~

~~G8325 Patient documented to have received fundus evaluation within six months prior to cataract surgery~~

▲ ☒ **G8326** Patient not documented to have received fundus evaluation within six months prior to cataract surgery

~~G8327 Patient was not an eligible candidate for pre-surgical fundus evaluation~~

~~G8328 Clinician has not provided care for the cataract patient for the required time for fundus evaluation measurement~~

~~G8329 Patient documented to have received dilated macular or fundus exam with level of severity of retinopathy and the presence or absence of macular edema documented~~

☒ **G8330** Patient not documented to have received dilated macular or fundus exam with level of severity of retinopathy and the presence or absence of macular edema not documented

~~G8331 Clinician documentation that patient was not an eligible candidate for dilated macular or fundus exam during the reporting year~~

~~G8332 Clinician has not provided care for the diabetic retinopathy patient for the required time for macular edema and retinopathy measurement~~

~~G8333 Patient documented to have had findings of macular or fundus exam communicated to the physician managing the diabetes care~~

☒ **G8334** Documentation of findings of macular or fundus exam not communicated to the physician managing the patient's ongoing diabetes care

~~G8335 Clinician documentation that patient was not an eligible candidate for the findings of their macular or fundus exam being communicated to the physician managing their diabetes care during the reporting year~~

~~G8336 Clinician has not provided care for the diabetic retinopathy patient for the required time for physician communication measurement~~

~~G8337 Clinician documented that communication was sent to the physician managing ongoing care of patient that a fracture occurred and that the patient was or should be tested or treated for osteoporosis~~

☒ **G8338** Clinician has not documented that communication was sent to the physician managing ongoing care of patient that a fracture occurred and that the patient was or should be tested or treated for osteoporosis

~~G8339 Patient was not an eligible candidate for communication with the physician managing the patient's ongoing care that a fracture occurred and that the patient was or should be tested or treated for osteoporosis~~

~~G8340 Patient documented to have had central DEXA performed and results documented or central DEXA ordered or pharmacologic therapy prescribed~~

▲ ☒ **G8341** Patient not documented to have had central DEXA measurement or pharmacologic therapy

~~G8342 Clinician documented that patient was not an eligible candidate for central DEXA measurement or prescribing pharmacologic~~

~~G8343 Clinician has not provided care for the patient for the required time for central DEXA measurement or pharmacological therapy measure~~

~~G8344 Patient documented to have had central DEXA ordered or performed and results documented or pharmacological therapy prescribed~~

▲ ☒ **G8345** Patient not documented to have had central DEXA measurement ordered or performed or pharmacologic therapy

~~G8346 Clinician documented that patient was not an eligible candidate for central DEXA measurement or pharmacologic therapy~~

~~G8347 Clinician has not provided care for the patient for the required time for central DEXA measurement or pharmacological therapy measure~~

~~G8348 Internal carotid stenosis patient in the 30-99% range documented to have reference to measurements of distal internal carotid diameter as the denominator for stenosis measurement~~

~~G8349 Patient was not an eligible candidate for documentation of presence or absence of alarm symptoms~~

~~G8350 Patient documented to have had 12-lead ECG performed~~

☒ **G8351** Patient not documented to have had ECG

~~G8352 Clinician documented that patient was not an eligible candidate for ECG~~

~~G8353 Patient documented to have received or taken aspirin 24 hours before emergency department arrival or during emergency department stay~~

▲ ☒ **G8354** Patient not documented to have received or taken aspirin 24 hours before emergency department arrival or during emergency department stay

~~G8355 Clinician documented that patient was not an eligible candidate to receive aspirin~~

~~G8356 Patient documented to have had ECG performed~~

▮ Special Coverage Instructions   ▮ Noncovered by Medicare   ▮ Carrier Discretion    ☑ Quantity Alert   ● New Code   ○ Recycled/Reinstated   ▲ Revised Code

**66 — G Codes**    Ⓐ Age Edit    Ⓜ Maternity Edit   ♀ Female Only   ♂ Male Only   Ⓐ-Ⓨ OPPS Status Indicators    **2008 HCPCS**

▲ Ⓜ G8357 Patient not documented to have had ECG

~~G8358 Clinician documented that patient was not an eligible candidate for ECG~~

~~G8359 Patient documented to have had vital signs recorded and reviewed~~

Ⓜ G8360 Patient not documented to have vital signs recorded and reviewed

~~G8361 Patient documented to have oxygen saturation assessed~~

Ⓜ G8362 Patient not documented to have oxygen saturation assessed

~~G8363 Clinician documented that patient was not an eligible candidate for oxygen saturation assessment~~

~~G8364 Patient documented to have mental status assessed~~

Ⓜ G8365 Patient not documented to have mental status assessed

~~G8366 Patient documented to have appropriate empiric antibiotic prescribed~~

Ⓜ G8367 Patient not documented to have appropriate empiric antibiotic prescribed

~~G8368 Clinician documented that patient was not an eligible candidate for appropriate empiric antibiotic~~

● Ⓜ G8370 Asthma patients with numeric frequency of symptoms or patient completion of an asthma assessment tool/survey/questionnaire not documented

● Ⓜ G8371 Chemotherapy documented as not received or prescribed for Stage III colon cancer patients Ⓐ ᴾᵠ

● Ⓜ G8372 Chemotherapy documented as received or prescribed for Stage III colon cancer patients Ⓐ ᴾᵠ

● Ⓜ G8373 Chemotherapy plan documented prior to chemotherapy administration ᴾᵠ

● Ⓜ G8374 Chemotherapy plan not documented prior to chemotherapy administration ᴾᵠ

● Ⓜ G8375 Chronic lymphocytic leukemia (CLL) patient with no documentation of baseline flow cytometry performed

● Ⓜ G8376 Clinician documentation that breast cancer patient was not eligible for tamoxifen or aromatase inhibitor therapy measure Ⓐ ♀ ᴾᵠ

● Ⓜ G8377 Clinician documentation that colon cancer patient is not eligible for the chemotherapy measure Ⓐ ᴾᵠ

● Ⓜ G8378 Clinician documentation that patient was not an eligible candidate for radiation therapy measure Ⓐ ᴾᵠ

● Ⓜ G8379 Documentation of radiation therapy recommended within 12 months of first office visit Ⓐ ᴾᵠ

● Ⓜ G8380 For patients with ER or PR positive, Stage IC-III breast cancer, clinician did not document that the patient received or was prescribed tamoxifen or aromatase inhibitor Ⓐ ♀ ᴾᵠ

● Ⓜ G8381 For patients with ER or PR positive, Stage IC-III breast cancer, clinician documented or prescribed that the patient is receiving tamoxifen or aromatase inhibitor Ⓐ ♀ ᴾᵠ

● Ⓜ G8382 Multiple myeloma patients with no documentation of prescribed or received intravenous bisphosphonate therapy

● Ⓜ G8383 No documentation of radiation therapy recommended within 12 months of first office visit Ⓐ ᴾᵠ

● Ⓜ G8384 Baseline cytogenetic testing not performed in patients with myelodysplastic syndrome (MDS) or acute leukemias

● Ⓜ G8385 Diabetic patients with no documentation of hemoglobin A1c level (within the last 12 months)

● Ⓜ G8386 Diabetic patients with no documentation of low-density lipoprotein (within the last 12 months)

● Ⓜ G8387 ESRD patient with a hematocrit or hemoglobin not documented Ⓐ ᴾᵠ

● Ⓜ G8388 ESRD patient with URR or Kt/V value not documented, but otherwise eligible for measure Ⓐ ᴾᵠ

● Ⓜ G8389 Myelodysplastic syndrome (MDS) patients with no documentation of iron stores prior to receiving erythropoietin therapy

● Ⓜ G8390 Diabetic patients with no documentation of blood pressure measurement (within the last 12 months)

● Ⓜ G8391 Patients with persistent asthma, no documentation of preferred long term control medication or acceptable alternative treatment prescribed

● Ⓜ G8395 Left ventricular ejection fraction (LVEF) >= 40% or documentation as normal or mildly depressed left ventricular systolic function

● Ⓜ G8396 Left ventricular ejection fraction (LVEF) not performed or documented

● Ⓜ G8397 Dilated macular or fundus exam performed, including documentation of the presence or absence of macular edema and level of severity of retinopathy

● Ⓜ G8398 Dilated macular or fundus exam not performed

● Ⓜ G8399 Patient with central dual-energy x-ray absorptiometry (DXA) results documented or ordered or pharmacologic therapy (other than minerals/vitamins) for osteoporosis prescribed

● Ⓜ G8400 Patient with central dual-energy x-ray absorptiometry (DEXA) results not documented or not ordered or pharmacologic therapy (other than minerals/vitamins) for osteoporosis not prescribed

● Ⓜ G8401 Clinician documented that patient was not an eligible candidate for screening or therapy for osteoporosis for women measure ♀

● Ⓜ G8402 Tobacco (smoke) use cessation intervention, counseling

● Ⓜ G8403 Tobacco (smoke) use cessation intervention not counseled

● Ⓜ G8404 Lower extremity neurological exam performed and documented

● Ⓜ G8405 Lower extremity neurological exam not performed

● Ⓜ G8406 Clinician documented that patient was not an eligible candidate for lower extremity neurological exam measure

● Ⓜ G8407 ABI measured and documented

● Ⓜ G8408 ABI measurement was not obtained

● Ⓜ G8409 Clinician documented that patient was not an eligible candidate for ABI measurement measure

● Ⓜ G8410 Footwear evaluation performed and documented

● Ⓜ G8415 Footwear evaluation was not performed

● Ⓜ G8416 Clinician documented that patient was not an eligible candidate for footwear evaluation measure

● Ⓜ G8417 BMI >= 30 was calculated and a follow-up plan was documented in the medical record

● Ⓜ G8418 BMI < 22 was calculated and a follow-up plan was documented in the medical record

● Ⓜ G8419 BMI >= 30 or < 22 was calculated, but no follow-up plan was documented in the medical record

---

Special Coverage Instructions    Noncovered by Medicare    Carrier Discretion    ☑ Quantity Alert    ● New Code    ○ Recycled/Reinstated    ▲ Revised Code

*(left margin)* Procedures/Professional Services (Temporary)    G8420 — G8463

● Ⓜ **G8420** BMI < 30 and >= 22 was calculated and documented

● Ⓜ **G8421** BMI not calculated

● Ⓜ **G8422** Patient not eligible for BMI calculation

● Ⓜ **G8423** Documented that patient was screened and either influenza vaccination status is current or patient was counseled

● Ⓜ **G8424** Influenza vaccine status was not screened

● Ⓜ **G8425** Influenza vaccine status screened, patient not current and counseling was not provided

● Ⓜ **G8426** Documented that patient was not appropriate for screening and/or counseling about the influenza vaccine (e.g., allergy to eggs)

● Ⓜ **G8427** Written provider documentation was obtained confirming that current medications with dosages (includes prescription, over-the-counter, herbals, vitamin/mineral/dietary (nutritional) supplements) were verified with the patient or authorized representative or patient assessed and is not currently on any medications

● Ⓜ **G8428** Current medications with dosages (includes prescription, over-the-counter, herbals, vitamin/mineral/dietary (nutritional) supplements) were documented without documented patient verification

● Ⓜ **G8429** Incomplete or no documentation that patient's current medications with dosages (includes prescription, over-the-counter, herbals, vitamin/mineral/dietary (nutritional) supplements) were assessed

● Ⓜ **G8430** Documentation that patient is not eligible for medication assessment

● Ⓜ **G8431** Documentation of clinical depression screening using a standardized tool

● Ⓜ **G8432** No documentation of clinical depression screening using a standardized tool

● Ⓜ **G8433** Patient not eligible/not appropriate for clinical depression screening

● Ⓜ **G8434** Documentation of cognitive impairment screening using a standardized tool

● Ⓜ **G8435** No documentation of cognitive impairment screening using a standardized tool

● Ⓜ **G8436** Patient not eligible/not appropriate for cognitive impairment screening

● Ⓜ **G8437** Documentation of clinician and patient involvement with the development of a treament plan/plan of care including signature by the practitioner and either a co-signature by the patient or documented verbal agreement obtained from the patient or, when necessary, an authorized representative

● Ⓜ **G8438** No documentation of clinician and patient involvement with the development of a treatment plan/plan of care including signature by the practitioner and either a co-signature by the patient or documented verbal agreement obtained from the patient or, when necessary, an authorized representative

● Ⓜ **G8439** Documentation that patient is not eligible for co-developing a treatment plan/plan of care including signature by the practitioner and either a co-signature by the patient or documented verbal agreement obtained from the patient or, when necessary, an authorized representative

● Ⓜ **G8440** Documentation of pain assessment (including location, intensity and description) prior to initiation of treatment or documentation of the absence of pain as a result of assessment

● Ⓜ **G8441** No documentation of pain assessment (including location, intensity and description) prior to initiation of treatment

● Ⓜ **G8442** Documentation that patient is not eligible for pain assessment

● Ⓜ **G8443** All prescriptions created during the encounter were generated using a qualified e-prescribing system

● Ⓜ **G8445** No prescriptions were generated during the encounter, provider does have access to a qualified e-prescribing system

● Ⓜ **G8446** Some or all prescriptions generated during the encounter were handwritten or phoned in due to one of the following: required by state law, patient request, or qualified e-prescribing system being temporarily inoperable

● Ⓜ **G8447** Patient encounter was documented using a CCHIT certified EMR

● Ⓜ **G8448** Patient encounter was documented using a non-CCHIT certified EMR; to qualify, the system must be capable of all of the following: generating a medication list, generating a problem list, entering laboratory tests as discrete searchable data elements

● Ⓜ **G8449** Patient encounter was not documented using an EMR due to system reasons such as, the system being inoperable at the time of the visit; use of this code implies that an EMR is in place and generally available

● Ⓜ **G8450** Beta-blocker therapy prescribed for patients with left ventricular ejection fraction (LVEF) <40% or documentation as moderately or severely depressed left ventricular systolic function

● Ⓜ **G8451** Clinician documented patient with left ventricular ejection fraction (LVEF) <40% or documentation as moderately or severely depressed left ventricular systolic function was not eligible candidate for beta-blocker therapy

● Ⓜ **G8452** Beta-blocker therapy not prescribed for patients with left ventricular ejection fraction (LVEF) <40% or documentation as moderately or severely depressed left ventricular systolic function

● Ⓜ **G8453** Tobacco use cessation intervention, counseling

● Ⓜ **G8454** Tobacco use cessation intervention not counseled, reason not specified

● Ⓜ **G8455** Current tobacco smoker

● Ⓜ **G8456** Current smokeless tobacco user

● Ⓜ **G8457** Tobacco nonuser

● Ⓜ **G8458** Clinician documented that patient is not an eligible candidate for genotype testing; patient not receiving antiviral treatment for hepatitis C

● Ⓜ **G8459** Clinician documented that patient is receiving antiviral treatment for hepatitis C

● Ⓜ **G8460** Clinician documented that patient is not an eligible candidate for quantitative RNA testing at week 12; patient not receiving antiviral treatment for hepatitis C

● Ⓜ **G8461** Patient receiving antiviral treatment for hepatitis C

● Ⓜ **G8462** Clinician documented that patient is not an eligible candidate for counseling regarding contraception prior to antiviral treatment; patient not receiving antiviral treatment for hepatitis C

● Ⓜ **G8463** Patient receiving antiviral treatment for hepatitis C documented

---

▒ Special Coverage Instructions    ▒ Noncovered by Medicare    ▒ Carrier Discretion    ☑ Quantity Alert    ● New Code    ○ Recycled/Reinstated    ▲ Revised Code

**68 — G Codes**    Ⓐ Age Edit    Ⓜ Maternity Edit    ♀ Female Only    ♂ Male Only    Ⓐ-Ⓨ OPPS Status Indicators    **2008 HCPCS**

● Ⓜ **G8464** Clinician documented that prostate cancer patient is not an eligible candidate for adjuvant hormonal therapy; low or intermediate risk of recurrence or risk of recurrence not determined

● Ⓜ **G8465** High risk of recurrence of prostate cancer

● Ⓜ **G8466** Clinician documented that patient is not an eligible candidate for suicide risk assessment; major depressive disorder, in remission

● Ⓜ **G8467** Documentation of new diagnosis of initial or recurrent episode of major depressive disorder

● Ⓜ **G8468** Angiotensin converting enzyme (ACE) inhibitor or angiotensin receptor blocker (ARB) therapy prescribed for patients with a left ventricular ejection fraction (LVEF) <40% or documentation of moderately or severely depressed left ventricular systolic function

● Ⓜ **G8469** Clinician documented that patient with a left ventricular ejection fraction (LVEF) <40% or documentation of moderately or severely depressed left ventricular systolic function was not an eligible candidate for angiotensin converting enzyme (ACE) inhibitor or angiotensin receptor blocker (ARB) therapy

● Ⓜ **G8470** Patient with left ventricular ejection fraction (LVEF) >=40% or documentation as normal or mildly depressed left ventricular systolic function

● Ⓜ **G8471** Left ventricular ejection fraction (LVEF) was not performed or documented

● Ⓜ **G8472** Angiotensin converting enzyme (ACE) inhibitor or angiotensin receptor blocker (ARB) therapy not prescribed for patients with a left ventricular ejection fraction (LVEF) <40% or documentation of moderately or severely depressed left ventricular systolic function, reason not specified

● Ⓜ **G8473** Angiotensin converting enzyme (ACE) inhibitor or angiotensin receptor blocker (ARB) therapy prescribed

● Ⓜ **G8474** Angiotensin converting enzyme (ACE) inhibitor or angiotensin receptor blocker (ARB) therapy not prescribed for reasons documented by the clinician

● Ⓜ **G8475** Angiotensin converting enzyme (ACE) inhibitor or angiotensin receptor blocker (ARB) therapy not prescribed, reason not specified

● Ⓜ **G8476** Most recent blood pressure has a systolic measurement of <130 mm/Hg and a diastolic measurement of <80 mm/Hg

● Ⓜ **G8477** Most recent blood pressure has a systolic measurement of >=130 mm/Hg and/or a diastolic measurement of >=80 mm/Hg

● Ⓜ **G8478** Blood pressure measurement not performed or documented, reason not specified

● Ⓜ **G8479** Clinician prescribed angiotensin converting enzyme (ACE) inhibitor or angiotensin receptor blocker (ARB) therapy

● Ⓜ **G8480** Clinician documented that patient was not an eligible candidate for angiotensin converting enzyme (ACE) inhibitor or angiotensin receptor blocker (ARB) therapy

● Ⓜ **G8481** Clinician did not prescribe angiotensin converting enzyme (ACE) inhibitor or angiotensin receptor blocker (ARB) therapy, reason not specified

● Ⓜ **G8482** Influenza immunization was ordered or administered

● Ⓜ **G8483** Influenza immunization was not ordered or administered for reasons documented by clinician

● Ⓜ **G8484** Influenza immunization was not ordered or administered, reason not specified

Ⓑ **G9001** Coordinated care fee, initial rate ⊘

Ⓑ **G9002** Coordinated care fee, maintenance rate ⊘

Ⓑ **G9003** Coordinated care fee, risk adjusted high, initial ⊘

Ⓑ **G9004** Coordinated care fee, risk adjusted low, initial ⊘

Ⓑ **G9005** Coordinated care fee, risk adjusted maintenance ⊘

Ⓑ **G9006** Coordinated care fee, home monitoring ⊘

Ⓑ **G9007** Coordinated care fee, scheduled team conference ⊘

Ⓑ **G9008** Coordinated care fee, physician coordinated care oversight services ⊘

Ⓑ **G9009** Coordinated care fee, risk adjusted maintenance, Level 3 ⊘

Ⓑ **G9010** Coordinated care fee, risk adjusted maintenance, Level 4 ⊘

Ⓑ **G9011** Coordinated care fee, risk adjusted maintenance, Level 5 ⊘

▲ Ⓑ **G9012** Other specified case management service not elsewhere classified ⊘

Ⓔ **G9013** ESRD demo basic bundle Level I

Ⓔ **G9014** ESRD demo expanded bundle including venous access and related services

Ⓔ **G9016** Smoking cessation counseling, individual, in the absence of or in addition to any other evaluation and management service, per session (6–10 minutes) [demonstration project code only] ⊘

▲ Ⓐ **G9017** Amantadine HCl, oral, per 100 mg (for use in a Medicare-approved demonstration project)

Ⓐ **G9018** Zanamivir, inhalation powder, administered through inhaler, generic, 10 mg (for use in a Medicare-approved demonstration project)

Ⓐ **G9019** Oseltamivir phosphate, oral, generic, 75 mg (for use in a Medicare-approved demonstration project)

▲ Ⓐ **G9020** Rimantadine HCl, oral, per 100 mg (for use in a Medicare-approved demonstration project)

Ⓐ **G9033** Amantadine HCl, oral brand, per 100 mg (for use in a Medicare-approved demonstration project)

Ⓐ **G9034** Zanamivir, inhalation powder, administered through inhaler, brand name, 10 mg (for use in a Medicare-approved demonstration project)

Ⓐ **G9035** Oseltamivir phosphate, oral, brand name, 75 mg (for use in a Medicare-approved demonstration project)

Ⓐ **G9036** Rimantadine HCl, oral, brand name, 100 mg (for use in a Medicare-approved demonstration project)

Ⓐ **G9041** Rehabilitation services for low vision by qualified occupational therapist, direct one-on-one contact, each 15 minutes

Ⓐ **G9042** Rehabilitation services for low vision by certified orientation and mobility specialists, direct one-on-one contact, each 15 minutes

Ⓐ **G9043** Rehabilitation services for low vision by certified low vision rehabilitation therapist, direct one-on-one contact, each 15 minutes

Ⓐ **G9044** Rehabilitation services for low vision by certified low vision rehabilitation teacher, direct one-on-one contact, each 15 minutes

Ⓔ **G9050** Oncology; primary focus of visit; work-up, evaluation, or staging at the time of cancer diagnosis or recurrence (for use in a Medicare-approved demonstration project)

Special Coverage Instructions    Noncovered by Medicare    Carrier Discretion    ☑ Quantity Alert    ● New Code    ○ Recycled/Reinstated    ▲ Revised Code

**2008 HCPCS**    Ⓐ²–Ⓩ³ ASC Payment Indicators    **MED:** Pub 100/NCD References    🖎 DMEPOS Paid    ⊘ SNF Excluded    🄟 PQRI    **G Codes — 69**

**Procedures/Professional Services (Temporary)**

**G9051 — G9074**

E **G9051** Oncology; primary focus of visit; treatment decision-making after disease is staged or restaged, discussion of treatment options, supervising/coordinating active cancer-directed therapy or managing consequences of cancer-directed therapy (for use in a Medicare-approved demonstration project)

E **G9052** Oncology; primary focus of visit; surveillance for disease recurrence for patient who has completed definitive cancer-directed therapy and currently lacks evidence of recurrent disease; cancer-directed therapy might be considered in the future (for use in a Medicare-approved demonstration project)

E **G9053** Oncology; primary focus of visit; expectant management of patient with evidence of cancer for whom no cancer-directed therapy is being administered or arranged at present; cancer-directed therapy might be considered in the future (for use in a Medicare-approved demonstration project)

E **G9054** Oncology; primary focus of visit; supervising, coordinating or managing care of patient with terminal cancer or for whom other medical illness prevents further cancer treatment; includes symptom management, end-of-life care planning, management of palliative therapies (for use in a Medicare-approved demonstration project)

E **G9055** Oncology; primary focus of visit; other, unspecified service not otherwise listed (for use in a Medicare-approved demonstration project)

E **G9056** Oncology; practice guidelines; management adheres to guidelines (for use in a Medicare-approved demonstration project)

E **G9057** Oncology; practice guidelines; management differs from guidelines as a result of patient enrollment in an institutional review board-approved clinical trial (for use in a Medicare-approved demonstration project)

E **G9058** Oncology; practice guidelines; management differs from guidelines because the treating physician disagrees with guideline recommendations (for use in a Medicare-approved demonstration project)

E **G9059** Oncology; practice guidelines; management differs from guidelines because the patient, after being offered treatment consistent with guidelines, has opted for alternative treatment or management, including no treatment (for use in a Medicare-approved demonstration project)

E **G9060** Oncology; practice guidelines; management differs from guidelines for reason(s) associated with patient comorbid illness or performance status not factored into guidelines (for use in a Medicare-approved demonstration project)

E **G9061** Oncology; practice guidelines; patient's condition not addressed by available guidelines (for use in a Medicare-approved demonstration project)

E **G9062** Oncology; practice guidelines; management differs from guidelines for other reason(s) not listed (for use in a Medicare-approved demonstration project)

M **G9063** Oncology; disease status; limited to nonsmall cell lung cancer; extent of disease initially established as Stage I (prior to neo-adjuvant therapy, if any) with no evidence of disease progression, recurrence, or metastases (for use in a Medicare-approved demonstration project)

M **G9064** Oncology; disease status; limited to nonsmall cell lung cancer; extent of disease initially established as Stage II (prior to neo-adjuvant therapy, if any) with no evidence of disease progression, recurrence, or metastases (for use in a Medicare-approved demonstration project)

M **G9065** Oncology; disease status; limited to nonsmall cell lung cancer; extent of disease initially established as Stage III a (prior to neo-adjuvant therapy, if any) with no evidence of disease progression, recurrence, or metastases (for use in a Medicare-approved demonstration project)

M **G9066** Oncology; disease status; limited to nonsmall cell lung cancer; Stage III B-IV at diagnosis, metastatic, locally recurrent, or progressive (for use in a Medicare-approved demonstration project)

M **G9067** Oncology; disease status; limited to nonsmall cell lung cancer; extent of disease unknown, staging in progress, or not listed (for use in a Medicare-approved demonstration project)

M **G9068** Oncology; disease status; limited to small cell and combined small cell/nonsmall cell; extent of disease initially established as limited with no evidence of disease progression, recurrence, or metastases (for use in a Medicare-approved demonstration project)

M **G9069** Oncology; disease status; small cell lung cancer, limited to small cell and combined small cell/nonsmall cell; extensive Stage at diagnosis, metastatic, locally recurrent, or progressive (for use in a Medicare-approved demonstration project)

M **G9070** Oncology; disease status; small cell lung cancer, limited to small cell and combined small cell/nonsmall; extent of disease unknown, staging in progress, or not listed (for use in a Medicare-approved demonstration project)

M **G9071** Oncology; disease status; invasive female breast cancer (does not include ductal carcinoma in situ); adenocarcinoma as predominant cell type; stage I or stage IIA-IIB; or T3, N1, M0; and ER and/or PR positive; with no evidence of disease progression, recurrence, or metastases (for use in a Medicare-approved demonstration project) ♀

M **G9072** Oncology; disease status; invasive female breast cancer (does not include ductal carcinoma in situ); adenocarcinoma as predominant cell type; stage I, or stage IIA-IIB; or T3, N1, M0; and ER and PR negative; with no evidence of disease progression, recurrence, or metastases (for use in a Medicare-approved demonstration project) ♀

M **G9073** Oncology; disease status; invasive female breast cancer (does not include ductal carcinoma in situ); adenocarcinoma as predominant cell type; stage IIIA-IIIB; and not T3, N1, M0; and ER and/or PR positive; with no evidence of disease progression, recurrence, or metastases (for use in a Medicare-approved demonstration project) ♀

M **G9074** Oncology; disease status; invasive female breast cancer (does not include ductal carcinoma in situ); adenocarcinoma as predominant cell type; stage IIIA-IIIB; and not T3, N1, M0; and ER and PR negative; with no evidence of disease progression, recurrence, or metastases (for use in a Medicare-approved demonstration project) ♀

---

Special Coverage Instructions    Noncovered by Medicare    Carrier Discretion    ☑ Quantity Alert    ● New Code    ○ Recycled/Reinstated    ▲ Revised Code

Ⓜ **G9075** Oncology; disease status; invasive female breast cancer (does not include ductal carcinoma in situ); adenocarcinoma as predominant cell type; M1 at diagnosis, metastatic locally recurrent, or progressive (for use in a Medicare-approved demonstration project) ♀

Ⓜ **G9077** Oncology; disease status; prostate cancer, limited to adenocarcinoma as predominant cell type; T1-T2C and Gleason 2-7 and PSA < or equal to 20 at diagnosis with no evidence of disease progression, recurrence, or metastases (for use in a Medicare-approved demonstration project) ♂

Ⓜ **G9078** Oncology; disease status; prostate cancer, limited to adenocarcinoma as predominant cell type; T2 or T3a Gleason 8-10 or PSA >20 at diagnosis with no evidence of disease progression, recurrence, or metastases (for use in a Medicare-approved demonstration project) ♂

Ⓜ **G9079** Oncology; disease status; prostate cancer, limited to adenocarcinoma as predominant cell type; T3B-T4, any N; any T, N1 at diagnosis with no evidence of disease progression, recurrence, or metastases (for use in a Medicare-approved demonstration project) ♂

Ⓜ **G9080** Oncology; disease status; prostate cancer, limited to adenocarcinoma; after initial treatment with rising PSA or failure of PSA decline (for use in a Medicare-approved demonstration project) ♂

Ⓜ **G9083** Oncology; disease status; prostate cancer, limited to adenocarcinoma; extent of disease unknown, staging in progress, or not listed (for use in a Medicare-approved demonstration project) ♂

Ⓜ **G9084** Oncology; disease status; colon cancer, limited to invasive cancer, adenocarcinoma as predominant cell type; extent of disease initially established as T1-3, N0, M0 with no evidence of disease progression, recurrence or metastases (for use in a Medicare-approved demonstration project)

Ⓜ **G9085** Oncology; disease status; colon cancer, limited to invasive cancer, adenocarcinoma as predominant cell type; extent of disease initially established as T4, N0, M0 with no evidence of disease progression, recurrence, or metastases (for use in a Medicare-approved demonstration project)

Ⓜ **G9086** Oncology; disease status; colon cancer, limited to invasive cancer, adenocarcinoma as predominant cell type; extent of disease initially established as T1-4, N1-2, M0 with no evidence of disease progression, recurrence, or metastases (for use in a Medicare-approved demonstration project)

Ⓜ **G9087** Oncology; disease status; colon cancer, limited to invasive cancer, adenocarcinoma as predominant cell type; M1 at diagnosis, metastatic locally recurrent, or progressive with current clinical, radiologic, or biochemical evidence of disease (for use in a Medicare-approved demonstration project)

Ⓜ **G9088** Oncology; disease status; colon cancer, limited to invasive cancer, adenocarcinoma as predominant cell type; M1 at diagnosis, metastatic, locally recurrent, or progressive without current clinical, radiologic, or biochemical evidence of disease (for use in a Medicare-approved demonstration project)

Ⓜ **G9089** Oncology; disease status; colon cancer, limited to invasive cancer; adenocarcinoma as predominant cell type; extent of disease unknown, staging in progress, or not listed (for use in a Medicare-approved demonstration project)

Ⓜ **G9090** Oncology; disease status; rectal cancer, limited to invasive cancer, adenocarcinoma as predominant cell type; extent of disease initially established as T1-2, N0, M0 (prior to neoadjuvant therapy, if any) with no evidence of disease progression, recurrence, or metastases (for use in a Medicare-approved demonstration project)

Ⓜ **G9091** Oncology; disease status; rectal cancer, limited to invasive cancer, adenocarcinoma as predominant cell type; extent of disease initially established as T3, N0, M0 (prior to neoadjuvant therapy, if any) with no evidence of disease progression, recurrence, or metastases (for use in a Medicare-approved demonstration project)

Ⓜ **G9092** Oncology; disease status; rectal cancer, limited to invasive cancer, adenocarcinoma as predominant cell type; extent of disease initially established as T1-3, N1-2, M0 (prior to neoadjuvant therapy, if any) with no evidence of disease progression, recurrence or metastases (for use in a Medicare-approved demonstration project)

Ⓜ **G9093** Oncology; disease status; rectal cancer, limited to invasive cancer, adenocarcinoma as predominant cell type; extent of disease initially established as T4, any N, M0 (prior to neoadjuvant therapy, if any) with no evidence of disease progression, recurrence, or metastases (for use in a Medicare-approved demonstration project)

Ⓜ **G9094** Oncology; disease status; rectal cancer, limited to invasive cancer, adenocarcinoma as predominant cell type; M1 at diagnosis, metastatic, locally recurrent, or progressive (for use in a Medicare-approved demonstration project)

Ⓜ **G9095** Oncology; disease status; rectal cancer, limited to invasive cancer; adenocarcinoma as predominant cell type; extent of disease unknown, staging in progress, or not listed (for use in a Medicare-approved demonstration project)

Ⓜ **G9096** Oncology; disease status; esophageal cancer, limited to adenocarcinoma or squamous cell carcinoma as predominant cell type; extent of disease initially established as T1-T3, N0-N1 or NX (prior to neoadjuvant therapy, if any) with no evidence of disease progression, recurrence, or metastases (for use in a Medicare-approved demonstration project)

Ⓜ **G9097** Oncology; disease status; esophageal cancer, limited to adenocarcinoma or squamous cell carcinoma as predominant cell type; extent of disease initially established as T4, any N, M0 (prior to neoadjuvant therapy, if any) with no evidence of disease progression, recurrence, or metastases (for use in a Medicare-approved demonstration project)

Ⓜ **G9098** Oncology; disease status; esophageal cancer, limited to adenocarcinoma or squamous cell carcinoma as predominant cell type; M1 at diagnosis, metastatic, locally recurrent, or progressive (for use in a Medicare-approved demonstration project)

Ⓜ **G9099** Oncology; disease status; esophageal cancer, limited to adenocarcinoma or squamous cell carcinoma as predominant cell type; extent of disease unknown, staging in progress, or not listed (for use in a Medicare-approved demonstration project)

Ⓜ **G9100** Oncology; disease status; gastric cancer, limited to adenocarcinoma as predominant cell type; post R0 resection (with or without neoadjuvant therapy) with no evidence of disease recurrence, progression, or metastases (for use in a Medicare-approved demonstration project)

Special Coverage Instructions    Noncovered by Medicare    Carrier Discretion    ☑ Quantity Alert    ● New Code    ○ Recycled/Reinstated    ▲ Revised Code

**2008 HCPCS**    A2-Z3 ASC Payment Indicators    **MED:** Pub 100/NCD References    ⅋ DMEPOS Paid    ⊘ SNF Excluded    PQRI    **G Codes — 71**

**Procedures/Professional Services (Temporary)**

**G9101 — G9132**

Ⓜ **G9101** Oncology; disease status; gastric cancer, limited to adenocarcinoma as predominant cell type; post R1 or R2 resection (with or without neoadjuvant therapy) with no evidence of disease progression, or metastases (for use in a Medicare-approved demonstration project)

Ⓜ **G9102** Oncology; disease status; gastric cancer, limited to adenocarcinoma as predominant cell type; clinical or pathologic M0, unresectable with no evidence of disease progression, or metastases (for use in a Medicare-approved demonstration project)

Ⓜ **G9103** Oncology; disease status; gastric cancer, limited to adenocarcinoma as predominant cell type; clinical or pathologic M1 at diagnosis, metastatic, locally recurrent, or progressive (for use in a Medicare-approved demonstration project)

Ⓜ **G9104** Oncology; disease status; gastric cancer, limited to adenocarcinoma as predominant cell type; extent of disease unknown, staging in progress, or not listed (for use in a Medicare-approved demonstration project)

Ⓜ **G9105** Oncology; disease status; pancreatic cancer, limited to adenocarcinoma as predominant cell type; post R0 resection without evidence of disease progression, recurrence, or metastases (for use in a Medicare-approved demonstration project)

Ⓜ **G9106** Oncology; disease status; pancreatic cancer, limited to adenocarcinoma; post R1 or R2 resection with no evidence of disease progression, or metastases (for use in a Medicare-approved demonstration project)

Ⓜ **G9107** Oncology; disease status; pancreatic cancer, limited to adenocarcinoma; unresectable at diagnosis, M1 at diagnosis, metastatic, locally recurrent, or progressive (for use in a Medicare-approved demonstration project)

Ⓜ **G9108** Oncology; disease status; pancreatic cancer, limited to adenocarcinoma; extent of disease unknown, staging in progress, or not listed (for use in a Medicare-approved demonstration project)

Ⓜ **G9109** Oncology; disease status; head and neck cancer, limited to cancers of oral cavity, pharynx and larynx with squamous cell as predominant cell type; extent of disease initially established as T1-T2 and N0, M0 (prior to neoadjuvant therapy, if any) with no evidence of disease progression, recurrence, or metastases (for use in a Medicare-approved demonstration project)

Ⓜ **G9110** Oncology; disease status; head and neck cancer, limited to cancers of oral cavity, pharynx and larynx with squamous cell as predominant cell type; extent of disease initially established as T3-4 and/or N1-3, M0 (prior to neoadjuvant therapy, if any) with no evidence of disease progression, recurrence, or metastases (for use in a Medicare-approved demonstration project)

Ⓜ **G9111** Oncology; disease status; head and neck cancer, limited to cancers of oral cavity, pharynx and larynx with squamous cell as predominant cell type; M1 at diagnosis, metastatic, locally recurrent, or progressive (for use in a Medicare-approved demonstration project)

Ⓜ **G9112** Oncology; disease status; head and neck cancer, limited to cancers of oral cavity, pharynx and larynx with squamous cell as predominant cell type; extent of disease unknown, staging in progress, or not listed (for use in a Medicare-approved demonstration project)

Ⓜ **G9113** Oncology; disease status; ovarian cancer, limited to epithelial cancer; pathologic state 1A-B (Grade 1) without evidence of disease progression, recurrence, or metastases (for use in a Medicare-approved demonstration project) ♀

Ⓜ **G9114** Oncology; disease status; ovarian cancer, limited to epithelial cancer; pathologic stage IA-B (grade 2-3); or stage IC (all grades); or stage II; without evidence of disease progression, recurrence, or metastases (for use in a Medicare-approved demonstration project) ♀

Ⓜ **G9115** Oncology; disease status; ovarian cancer, limited to epithelial cancer; pathologic stage III-IV; without evidence of progression, recurrence, or metastases (for use in a Medicare-approved demonstration project) ♀

Ⓜ **G9116** Oncology; disease status; ovarian cancer, limited to epithelial cancer; evidence of disease progression, or recurrence, and/or platinum resistance (for use in a Medicare-approved demonstration project) ♀

Ⓜ **G9117** Oncology; disease status; ovarian cancer, limited to epithelial cancer; extent of disease unknown, staging in progress, or not listed (for use in a Medicare-approved demonstration project) ♀

Ⓜ **G9123** Oncology; disease status; chronic myelogenous leukemia, limited to Philadelphia chromosome positive and/or BCR-ABL positive; chronic phase not in hematologic, cytogenetic, or molecular remission (for use in a Medicare-approved demonstration project)

Ⓜ **G9124** Oncology; disease status; chronic myelogenous leukemia, limited to Philadelphia chromosome positive and /or BCR-ABL positive; accelerated phase not in hematologic cytogenetic, or molecular remission (for use in a Medicare-approved demonstration project)

Ⓜ **G9125** Oncology; disease status; chronic myelogenous leukemia, limited to Philadelphia chromosome positive and /or BCR-ABL positive; blast phase not in hematologic, cytogenetic, or molecular remission (for use in a Medicare-approved demonstration project)

Ⓜ **G9126** Oncology; disease status; chronic myelogenous leukemia, limited to Philadelphia chromosome positive and /or BCR-ABL positive; in hematologic, cytogenetic, or molecular remission (for use in a Medicare-approved demonstration project)

Ⓜ **G9128** Oncology; disease status; limited to multiple myeloma, systemic disease; smoldering, stage I (for use in a Medicare-approved demonstration project)

Ⓜ **G9129** Oncology; disease status; limited to multiple myeloma, systemic disease; stage II or higher (for use in a Medicare-approved demonstration project)

Ⓜ **G9130** Oncology; disease status; limited to multiple myeloma, systemic disease; extent of disease unknown, staging in progress, or not listed (for use in a Medicare-approved demonstration project)

Ⓜ **G9131** Oncology; disease status; invasive female breast cancer (does not include ductal carcinoma in situ); adenocarcinoma as predominant cell type; extent of disease unknown, staging in progress, or not listed (for use in a Medicare-approved demonstration project) ♀

Ⓜ **G9132** Oncology; disease status; prostate cancer, limited to adenocarcinoma; hormone-refractory/androgen-independent (e.g., rising PSA on anti-androgen therapy or post-orchiectomy); clinical metastases (for use in a Medicare-approved demonstration project) ♂

⬛ Special Coverage Instructions   ⬛ Noncovered by Medicare   Carrier Discretion   ☑ Quantity Alert   ● New Code   ○ Recycled/Reinstated   ▲ Revised Code

**72 — G Codes**   Ⓐ Age Edit   Ⓜ Maternity Edit   ♀ Female Only   ♂ Male Only   Ⓐ-Ⓨ OPPS Status Indicators   **2008 HCPCS**

Ⓜ **G9133** Oncology; disease status; prostate cancer, limited to adenocarcinoma; hormone-responsive; clinical metastases or M1 at diagnosis (for use in a Medicare-approved demonstration project) ♂

Ⓜ **G9134** Oncology; disease status; non-Hodgkin's lymphoma, any cellular classification; Stage I, II at diagnosis, not relapsed, not refractory (for use in a Medicare-approved demonstration project)

Ⓜ **G9135** Oncology; disease status; non-Hodgkin's lymphoma, any cellular classification; Stage III, IV, not relapsed, not refractory (for use in a Medicare-approved demonstration project)

Ⓜ **G9136** Oncology; disease status; non-Hodgkin's lymphoma, transformed from original cellular diagnosis to a second cellular classification (for use in a medicare-approved demonstration project)

Ⓜ **G9137** Oncology; disease status; non-Hodgkin's lymphoma, any cellular classification; relapsed/refractory (for use in a medicare-approved demonstration project)

Ⓜ **G9138** Oncology; disease status; non-Hodgkin's lymphoma, any cellular classification; diagnostic evaluation, stage not determined, evaluation of possible relapse or nonresponse to therapy, or not listed (for use in a Medicare-approved demonstration project)

Ⓜ **G9139** Oncology; disease status; chronic myelogenous leukemia, limited to Philadelphia chromosome positive and/or BCR-ABL positive; extent of disease unknown, staging in progress, not listed (for use in a Medicare-approved demonstration project)

● Ⓜ ☑ **G9140** Frontier extended stay clinic demonstration; for a patient stay in a clinic approved for the CMS demonstration project; the following measures should be present: the stay must be equal to or greater than 4 hours; weather or other conditions must prevent transfer or the case falls into a category of monitoring and observation cases that are permitted by the rules of the demonstration; there is a maximum frontier extended stay clinic (FESC) visit of 48 hours, except in the case when weather or other conditions prevent transfer; payment is made on each period up to 4 hrs., after the first 4 hrs.

Special Coverage Instructions    Noncovered by Medicare    Carrier Discretion    ☑ Quantity Alert    ● New Code    ○ Recycled/Reinstated    ▲ Revised Code

**2008 HCPCS**    A2-Z3 ASC Payment Indicators    **MED:** Pub 100/NCD References    ⅋ DMEPOS Paid    ⊘ SNF Excluded    P8 PQRI    **G Codes — 73**

## ALCOHOL AND DRUG ABUSE TREATMENT SERVICES
### H0001–H2037

The H codes are used by those state Medicaid agencies that are mandated by state law to establish separate codes for identifying mental health services that include alcohol and drug treatment services.

**H0001** Alcohol and/or drug assessment

**H0002** Behavioral health screening to determine eligibility for admission to treatment program

**H0003** Alcohol and/or drug screening; laboratory analysis of specimens for presence of alcohol and/or drugs

☑ **H0004** Behavioral health counseling and therapy, per 15 minutes

**H0005** Alcohol and/or drug services; group counseling by a clinician

**H0006** Alcohol and/or drug services; case management

**H0007** Alcohol and/or drug services; crisis intervention (outpatient)

**H0008** Alcohol and/or drug services; subacute detoxification (hospital inpatient)

**H0009** Alcohol and/or drug services; acute detoxification (hospital inpatient)

**H0010** Alcohol and/or drug services; subacute detoxification (residential addiction program inpatient)

**H0011** Alcohol and/or drug services; acute detoxification (residential addiction program inpatient)

**H0012** Alcohol and/or drug services; subacute detoxification (residential addiction program outpatient)

**H0013** Alcohol and/or drug services; acute detoxification (residential addiction program outpatient)

**H0014** Alcohol and/or drug services; ambulatory detoxification

**H0015** Alcohol and/or drug services; intensive outpatient (treatment program that operates at least 3 hours/day and at least 3 days/week and is based on an individualized treatment plan), including assessment, counseling; crisis intervention, and activity therapies or education

**H0016** Alcohol and/or drug services; medical/somatic (medical intervention in ambulatory setting)

☑ **H0017** Behavioral health; residential (hospital residential treatment program), without room and board, per diem

☑ **H0018** Behavioral health; short-term residential (nonhospital residential treatment program), without room and board, per diem

☑ **H0019** Behavioral health; long-term residential (nonmedical, nonacute care in a residential treatment program where stay is typically longer than 30 days), without room and board, per diem

**H0020** Alcohol and/or drug services; methadone administration and/or service (provision of the drug by a licensed program)

**H0021** Alcohol and/or drug training service (for staff and personnel not employed by providers)

**H0022** Alcohol and/or drug intervention service (planned facilitation)

**H0023** Behavioral health outreach service (planned approach to reach a targeted population)

**H0024** Behavioral health prevention information dissemination service (one-way direct or nondirect contact with service audiences to affect knowledge and attitude)

**H0025** Behavioral health prevention education service (delivery of services with target population to affect knowledge, attitude and/or behavior)

**H0026** Alcohol and/or drug prevention process service, community-based (delivery of services to develop skills of impactors)

**H0027** Alcohol and/or drug prevention environmental service (broad range of external activities geared toward modifying systems in order to mainstream prevention through policy and law)

**H0028** Alcohol and/or drug prevention problem identification and referral service (e.g., student assistance and employee assistance programs), does not include assessment

**H0029** Alcohol and/or drug prevention alternatives service (services for populations that exclude alcohol and other drug use e.g., alcohol free social events)

**H0030** Behavioral health hotline service

**H0031** Mental health assessment, by nonphysician

**H0032** Mental health service plan development by nonphysician

**H0033** Oral medication administration, direct observation

☑ **H0034** Medication training and support, per 15 minutes

☑ **H0035** Mental health partial hospitalization, treatment, less than 24 hours

☑ **H0036** Community psychiatric supportive treatment, face-to-face, per 15 minutes

☑ **H0037** Community psychiatric supportive treatment program, per diem

☑ **H0038** Self-help/peer services, per 15 minutes

☑ **H0039** Assertive community treatment, face-to-face, per 15 minutes

☑ **H0040** Assertive community treatment program, per diem

☑ **H0041** Foster care, child, non-therapeutic, per diem   A

☑ **H0042** Foster care, child, non-therapeutic, per month   A

☑ **H0043** Supported housing, per diem

☑ **H0044** Supported housing, per month

☑ **H0045** Respite care services, not in the home, per diem

**H0046** Mental health services, not otherwise specified

**H0047** Alcohol and/or other drug abuse services, not otherwise specified

**H0048** Alcohol and/or other drug testing: collection and handling only, specimens other than blood

**H0049** Alcohol and/or drug screening

☑ **H0050** Alcohol and/or drug services, brief intervention, per 15 minutes

**H1000** Prenatal care, at-risk assessment   M♀

**H1001** Prenatal care, at-risk enhanced service; antepartum management   M♀

**H1002** Prenatal care, at risk enhanced service; care coordination   M♀

**H1003** Prenatal care, at-risk enhanced service; education   M♀

**H1004** Prenatal care, at-risk enhanced service; follow-up home visit   M♀

Special Coverage Instructions    Noncovered by Medicare    Carrier Discretion    ☑ Quantity Alert    ● New Code    ○ Recycled/Reinstated    ▲ Revised Code

**2008 HCPCS**    A2 Z3 ASC Payment Indicators    **MED:** Pub 100/NCD References    ⚖ DMEPOS Paid    ⊘ SNF Excluded    PQ PQRI    **H Codes — 75**

**H1005** Prenatal care, at-risk enhanced service package (includes H1001–H1004) Ⓜ ♀

☑ **H1010** Nonmedical family planning education, per session

**H1011** Family assessment by licensed behavioral health professional for state defined purposes

**H2000** Comprehensive multidisciplinary evaluation

☑ **H2001** Rehabilitation program, per 1/2 day

☑ **H2010** Comprehensive medication services, per 15 minutes

☑ **H2011** Crisis intervention service, per 15 minutes

☑ **H2012** Behavioral health day treatment, per hour

☑ **H2013** Psychiatric health facility service, per diem

☑ **H2014** Skills training and development, per 15 minutes

☑ **H2015** Comprehensive community support services, per 15 minutes

☑ **H2016** Comprehensive community support services, per diem

☑ **H2017** Psychosocial rehabilitation services, per 15 minutes

☑ **H2018** Psychosocial rehabilitation services, per diem

☑ **H2019** Therapeutic behavioral services, per 15 minutes

☑ **H2020** Therapeutic behavioral services, per diem

☑ **H2021** Community-based wrap-around services, per 15 minutes

☑ **H2022** Community-based wrap-around services, per diem

☑ **H2023** Supported employment, per 15 minutes

☑ **H2024** Supported employment, per diem

☑ **H2025** Ongoing support to maintain employment, per 15 minutes

☑ **H2026** Ongoing support to maintain employment, per diem

☑ **H2027** Psychoeducational service, per 15 minutes

☑ **H2028** Sexual offender treatment service, per 15 minutes

☑ **H2029** Sexual offender treatment service, per diem

☑ **H2030** Mental health clubhouse services, per 15 minutes

☑ **H2031** Mental health clubhouse services, per diem

☑ **H2032** Activity therapy, per 15 minutes

☑ **H2033** Multisystemic therapy for juveniles, per 15 minutes

☑ **H2034** Alcohol and/or drug abuse halfway house services, per diem

☑ **H2035** Alcohol and/or other drug treatment program, per hour

☑ **H2036** Alcohol and/or other drug treatment program, per diem

☑ **H2037** Developmental delay prevention activities, dependent child of client, per 15 minutes Ⓐ

Special Coverage Instructions  Noncovered by Medicare  Carrier Discretion  ☑ Quantity Alert  ● New Code  ○ Recycled/Reinstated  ▲ Revised Code

**76 — H Codes**  Ⓐ Age Edit  Ⓜ Maternity Edit  ♀ Female Only  ♂ Male Only  Ⓐ-Ⓨ OPPS Status Indicators  **2008 HCPCS**

## DRUGS ADMINISTERED OTHER THAN ORAL METHOD
## J0000-J9999

J codes include drugs that ordinarily cannot be self-administered, chemotherapy drugs, immunosuppressive drugs, inhalation solutions, and other miscellaneous drugs and solutions.

**N** ☑ **J0120** Injection, tetracycline, up to 250 mg **N1**
MED: 100-2,15,50

**K** ☑ **J0128** Injection, abarelix, 10 mg **K2**
Use this code for Planaxis.

**G** ☑ **J0129** Injection, abatacept, 10 mg **K2**
Use this code for Orencia

**K** ☑ **J0130** Injection abciximab, 10 mg **K2**
Use this code for ReoPro.
MED: 100-2,15,50

**N** ☑ **J0132** Injection, acetylcysteine, 100 mg **N1**
Use this code for Acetadote.

**N** ☑ **J0133** Injection, acyclovir, 5 mg **N1**
Use this code for Zovirax.
MED: 100-4,4,230.1

**K** ☑ **J0135** Injection, adalimumab, 20 mg **K2**
Use this code for Humira.

**K** ☑ **J0150** Injection, adenosine for therapeutic use, 6 mg (not to be used to report any adenosine phosphate compounds, instead use A9270) **K2**
Use this code for Adenocard, Adenoscan
MED: 100-2,15,50; 100-4,4,230.1
AHA: 2Q,'02,10

**K** ☑ **J0152** Injection, adenosine for diagnostic use, 30 mg (not to be used to report any adenosine phosphate compounds; instead use A9270) **K2**
Use this code for Adenoscan, Adenoscan
MED: 100-4,4,230.1

**N** ☑ **J0170** Injection, adrenalin, epinephrine, up to 1 ml ampule **N1**
Use this code for Adrenalin Chloride, Epipen, Sus-Phrine.
MED: 100-2,15,50

**K** ☑ **J0180** Injection, agalsidase beta, 1 mg **K2**
Use this code for Fabrazyme.

**K** ☑ **J0190** Injection, biperiden lactate, per 5 mg **K2**
MED: 100-2,15,50

**N** ☑ **J0200** Injection, alatrofloxacin mesylate, 100 mg **N1**
MED: 100-2,15,50.5

**K** ☑ **J0205** Injection, alglucerase, per 10 units **K2**
Use this code for Ceredase.
MED: 100-2,15,50

**K** ☑ **J0207** Injection, amifostine, 500 mg **K2**
Use this code for Ethyol.
MED: 100-2,15,50

**K** ☑ **J0210** Injection, methyldopa HCl, up to 250 mg **K2**
Use this code for Aldomet.
MED: 100-2,15,50

**K** ☑ **J0215** Injection, alefacept, 0.5 mg **K2**
Use this for Amevive.
MED: 100-4,4,230.1

● **K** ☑ **J0220** Injection, alglucosidase alfa, 10 mg **K2**
Use this code for Myozime

**K** ☑ **J0256** Injection, alpha 1-proteinase inhibitor — human, 10 mg **K2**
Use this code for Prolastin, Zemira.
MED: 100-2,15,50

**B** ☑ **J0270** Injection, alprostadil, 1.25 mcg (code may be used for Medicare when drug administered under direct supervision of a physician, not for use when drug is self-administered)
Use this code for Alprostadil, Caverject, Edex, Prostin VR Pediatric.
MED: 100-2,15,50

**B** **J0275** Alprostadil urethral suppository (code may be used for Medicare when drug administered under direct supervision of a physician, not for use when drug is self-administered)
Use this code for Muse.
MED: 100-2,15,50

**N** ☑ **J0278** Injection, amikacin sulfate, 100 mg **N1**
Use this code for Amikin.

**N** ☑ **J0280** Injection, aminophyllin, up to 250 mg **N1**
MED: 100-2,15,50

**N** ☑ **J0282** Injection, amiodarone HCl, 30 mg **N1**
Use this code for Cordarone IV.
MED: 100-2,15,50

**N** ☑ **J0285** Injection, amphotericin B, 50 mg **N1**
Use this for Abelcet, Amphocin, Fungizone
MED: 100-2,15,50

**K** ☑ **J0287** Injection, amphotericin B lipid complex, 10 mg **K2**
MED: 100-2,15,50

**K** ☑ **J0288** Injection, amphotericin B cholesteryl sulfate complex, 10 mg **K2**
Use this code for Amphotec.
MED: 100-2,15,50

**K** ☑ **J0289** Injection, amphotericin B liposome, 10 mg **K2**
Use this code for Ambisome.
MED: 100-2,15,50

**N** ☑ **J0290** Injection, ampicillin sodium, 500 mg **N1**
MED: 100-2,15,50

**N** ☑ **J0295** Injection, ampicillin sodium/sulbactam sodium, per 1.5 g **N1**
Use this code for Unasyn.
MED: 100-2,15,50

**N** ☑ **J0300** Injection, amobarbital, up to 125 mg **N1**
Use this code for Amytal.
MED: 100-2,15,50

**N** ☑ **J0330** Injection, succinylcholine chloride, up to 20 mg **N1**
Use this code for Anectine, Quelicin.
MED: 100-2,15,50

**G** ☑ **J0348** Injection, anadulafungin, 1 mg **K2**
Use this code for Eraxis.

**K** ☑ **J0350** Injection, anistreplase, per 30 units **K2**
Use this code for Eminase.
MED: 100-2,15,50

**N** ☑ **J0360** Injection, hydralazine HCl, up to 20 mg **N1**
MED: 100-2,15,50

**N** ☑ **J0364** Injection, apomorphine hydrochloride, 1 mg **N1**
Use this code for Apokyn.

| Special Coverage Instructions | Noncovered by Medicare | Carrier Discretion | ☑ Quantity Alert | ● New Code | ○ Recycled/Reinstated | ▲ Revised Code |

**2008 HCPCS**　**K2-Z3** ASC Payment Indicators　**MED:** Pub 100/NCD References　& DMEPOS Paid　⊘ SNF Excluded　**PQ** PQRI　**J Codes — 77**

K ☑ **J0365** Injection, aprotonin, 10,000 kiu  K2
Use this code for Trasylol.
MED: 100-2,15,50; 100-4,4,230.1

N ☑ **J0380** Injection, metaraminol bitartrate, per 10 mg  N1
Use this code for Aramine.
MED: 100-2,15,50

N ☑ **J0390** Injection, chloroquine HCl, up to 250 mg  N1
Use this code for Aralen.
MED: 100-2,15,50

N ☑ **J0395** Injection, arbutamine HCl, 1 mg  N1
MED: 100-2,15,50

● K ☑ **J0400** Injection, aripiprazole, intramuscular, 0.25 mg  K2
Use this code for Abilify.

N ☑ **J0456** Injection, azithromycin, 500 mg  N1
Use this code for Zithromax.
MED: 100-2,15,50.5

N ☑ **J0460** Injection, atropine sulfate, up to 0.3 mg  N1
Use this code for Atropen.
MED: 100-2,15,50

N ☑ **J0470** Injection, dimercaprol, per 100 mg  N1
Use this code for BAL
MED: 100-2,15,50

K ☑ **J0475** Injection, baclofen, 10 mg  K2
Use this code for Lioresal.
MED: 100-2,15,50; 100-4,4,230.1

K ☑ **J0476** Injection, baclofen, 50 mcg for intrathecal trial  K2
Use this code for Lioresal for intrathecal trial.
MED: 100-2,15,50; 100-4,4,230.1

K **J0480** Injection, basiliximab, 20 mg  K2
Use this code for Simulect.
MED: 100-2,15,50; 100-4,4,230.1; 100-4,4,240

N ☑ **J0500** Injection, dicyclomine HCl, up to 20 mg  N1
Use this code for Bentyl.
MED: 100-2,15,50

N ☑ **J0515** Injection, benztropine mesylate, per 1 mg  N1
Use this code for Cogentin.
MED: 100-2,15,50

N ☑ **J0520** Injection, bethanechol chloride, Mytonachol or Urecholine, up to 5 mg  N1
MED: 100-2,15,50

N ☑ **J0530** Injection, penicillin G benzathine and penicillin G procaine, up to 600,000 units  N1
Use this code for Bicillin C-R.
MED: 100-2,15,50

N ☑ **J0540** Injection, penicillin G benzathine and penicillin G procaine, up to 1,200,000 units  N1
Use this code for Bicillin C-R, Bicillin C-R 900/300.
MED: 100-2,15,50

N ☑ **J0550** Injection, penicillin G benzathine and penicillin G procaine, up to 2,400,000 units  N1
Use this code for Bicillin C-R.
MED: 100-2,15,50

N ☑ **J0560** Injection, penicillin G benzathine, up to 600,000 units  N1
Use this code for Bicillin L-A, Permapen.
MED: 100-2,15,50

N ☑ **J0570** Injection, penicillin G benzathine, up to 1,200,000 units  N1
Use this code for Bicillin L-A, Permapen.
MED: 100-2,15,50

N ☑ **J0580** Injection, penicillin G benzathine, up to 2,400,000 units  N1
Use this code for Bicillin L-A, Permapen.
MED: 100-2,15,50

K ☑ **J0583** Injection, bivalirudin, 1 mg  K2
Use this code for Angiomax.

K ☑ **J0585** Botulinum toxin type A, per unit  K2
Use this code for Botox.
MED: 100-2,15,50

K ☑ **J0587** Botulinum toxin type B, per 100 units  K2
Use this code for Myobloc.
MED: 100-2,15,50
AHA: 2Q,'02,8

N ☑ **J0592** Injection, buprenorphine HCl, 0.1 mg  N1
Use this code for Buprenex.
MED: 100-2,15,50

K ☑ **J0594** Injection, busulfan, 1 mg  K2
Use this code for Busulfex.

N ☑ **J0595** Injection, butorphanol tartrate, 1 mg  N1
Use this code for Stadol.

K ☑ **J0600** Injection, edetate calcium disodium, up to 1000 mg  K2
Use this code for Calcium Disodium Versenate, Calcium EDTA.
MED: 100-2,15,50

N ☑ **J0610** Injection, calcium gluconate, per 10 ml  N1
MED: 100-2,15,50

N ☑ **J0620** Injection, calcium glycerophosphate and calcium lactate, per 10 ml  N1
MED: 100-2,15,50

N ☑ **J0630** Injection, calcitonin salmon, up to 400 units  N1
Use this code for Calcimar, Miacalcin.
MED: 100-2,15,50

N ☑ **J0636** Injection, calcitriol, 0.1 mcg  N1
Use this code for Calcijex.
MED: 100-2,15,50

K **J0637** Injection, caspofungin acetate, 5 mg  K2
Use this code for Cancidas.

N ☑ **J0640** Injection, leucovorin calcium, per 50 mg  N1
MED: 100-2,15,50

N ☑ **J0670** Injection, mepivacaine HCl, per 10 ml  N1
Use this code for Carbocaine, Polocaine, Isocaine HCl, Scandonest
MED: 100-2,15,50

N ☑ **J0690** Injection, cefazolin sodium, 500 mg  N1
Use this code for Ancef, Kefzol
MED: 100-2,15,50

N ☑ **J0692** Injection, cefepime HCl, 500 mg  N1
Use this code for Maxipime.

N ☑ **J0694** Injection, cefoxitin sodium, 1 g  N1
MED: 100-2,15,50

N ☑ **J0696** Injection, ceftriaxone sodium, per 250 mg  N1
Use this code for Rocephin.
MED: 100-2,15,50

---

Special Coverage Instructions    Noncovered by Medicare    Carrier Discretion    ☑ Quantity Alert   ● New Code   ○ Recycled/Reinstated   ▲ Revised Code

N ☑ **J0697** Injection, sterile cefuroxime sodium, per 750 mg   N1
Use this code for Zinacef.

MED: 100-2,15,50

N ☑ **J0698** Cefotaxime sodium, per g   N1
Use this code for Claforan.

MED: 100-2,15,50

▲ N ☑ **J0702** Injection, betamethasone acetate 3 mg and betamethasone sodium phosphate 3 mg   N1
Use this code for Celestone Soluspan.

MED: 100-2,15,50

N ☑ **J0704** Injection, betamethasone sodium phosphate, per 4 mg   N1

MED: 100-2,15,50

N ☑ **J0706** Injection, caffeine citrate, 5 mg   N1
Use this code for Cafcit.

AHA: 2Q,'02,8

N ☑ **J0710** Injection, cephapirin sodium, up to 1 g   N1

MED: 100-2,15,50

N ☑ **J0713** Injection, ceftazidime, per 500 mg   N1
Use this code for Ceptax, Fortaz, Tazicef

MED: 100-2,15,50

N ☑ **J0715** Injection, ceftizoxime sodium, per 500 mg   N1
Use this code for Cefizox.

MED: 100-2,15,50

N ☑ **J0720** Injection, chloramphenicol sodium succinate, up to 1 g   N1
Use this code for Chlormycetin.

MED: 100-2,15,50

N ☑ **J0725** Injection, chorionic gonadotropin, per 1,000 USP units   N1

MED: 100-2,15,50

K ☑ **J0735** Injection, clonidine HCl, 1 mg   K2
Use this code for Clorpres, Duraclon, Iopidine

MED: 100-2,15,50

K ☑ **J0740** Injection, cidofovir, 375 mg   K2
Use this code for Vistide.

MED: 100-2,15,50

N ☑ **J0743** Injection, cilastatin sodium; imipenem, per 250 mg   N1
Use this code for Primaxin I.M., Primaxin I.V.

MED: 100-2,15,50

N ☑ **J0744** Injection, ciprofloxacin for intravenous infusion, 200 mg   N1
Use this code for Cipro.

N ☑ **J0745** Injection, codeine phosphate, per 30 mg   N1

MED: 100-2,15,50

N ☑ **J0760** Injection, colchicine, per 1 mg   N1

MED: 100-2,15,50

N ☑ **J0770** Injection, colistimethate sodium, up to 150 mg   N1
Use this code for Coly-Mycin M.

MED: 100-2,15,50

N ☑ **J0780** Injection, prochlorperazine, up to 10 mg   N1
Use this code for Compazine, Cotranzine, Compa-Z, Ultrazine-10.

MED: 100-2,15,50

K ☑ **J0795** Injection, corticorelin ovine triflutate, 1 microgram   K2
Use this code for Acthrel.

MED: 100-2,15,50; 100-4,4,230.1

K ☑ **J0800** Injection, corticotropin, up to 40 units   K2
Use this code for H.P. Acthar gel

MED: 100-2,15,50

K ☑ **J0835** Injection, cosyntropin, per 0.25 mg   K2
Use this code for Cortrosyn.

MED: 100-2,15,50

K ☑ **J0850** Injection, cytomegalovirus immune globulin intravenous (human), per vial   K2
Use this code for Cytogam.

MED: 100-2,15,50; 100-4,4,240

K ☑ **J0878** Injection, daptomycin, 1 mg   K2
Use this code for Cubicin.

K ☑ **J0881** Injection, darbepoetin alfa, 1 mcg (non-ESRD use)   K2
Use this code for Aranesp.

MED: 100-2,6,10; 100-4,4,230.1; 100-4,4,240

A ☑ **J0882** Injection, darbepoetin alfa, 1 microgram (for ESRD on dialysis)   ⊘
Use this code for Aranesp.

MED: 100-2,6,10; 100-4,4,240

K ☑ **J0885** Injection, epoetin alfa, (for non-ESRD use), 1000 units   K2
Use this code for Epogen/Procrit.

MED: 100-2,6,10; 100-2,15,50; 100-4,4,230.1; 100-4,4,240

A ☑ **J0886** Injection, epoetin alfa, 1000 units (for ESRD on dialysis)   ⊘
Use this code for Epogen/Procrit.

MED: 100-2,6,10; 100-4,4,240

G ☑ **J0894** Injection, decitabine, 1 mg   K2
Use this code for Dacogen.

N ☑ **J0895** Injection, deferoxamine mesylate, 500 mg   N1
Use this code for Desferal.

MED: 100-2,15,50

N ☑ **J0900** Injection, testosterone enanthate and estradiol valerate, up to 1 cc   N1

MED: 100-2,15,50

N ☑ **J0945** Injection, brompheniramine maleate, per 10 mg   N1

MED: 100-2,15,50

N ☑ **J0970** Injection, estradiol valerate, up to 40 mg   N1
Use this code for Clinagen LA, Clinagen, LA-10, Clinagen LA-20, Clinagen LA-40, Delestrogen

MED: 100-2,15,50

N ☑ **J1000** Injection, depo-estradiol cypionate, up to 5 mg   N1
Use this code for depGynogen, Depogen, Estradiol Cypionate

MED: 100-2,15,50

N ☑ **J1020** Injection, methylprednisolone acetate, 20 mg   N1
Use this code for Depo-Medrol.

MED: 100-2,15,50; 100-4,4,240

N ☑ **J1030** Injection, methylprednisolone acetate, 40 mg   N1
Use this code for DepoMedalone40, Depo-Medrol, Sano-Drol

MED: 100-2,15,50; 100-4,4,240

N ☑ **J1040** Injection, methylprednisolone acetate, 80 mg   N1
Use this code for Cortimed, DepMedalone, DepoMedalone 80, Depo-Medrol, Duro Cort, Methylcotolone, Pri-Methylate, Sano-Drol

MED: 100-2,15,50; 100-4,4,240

---

Special Coverage Instructions    Noncovered by Medicare    Carrier Discretion    ☑ Quantity Alert    ● New Code    ○ Recycled/Reinstated    ▲ Revised Code

**2008 HCPCS**    A2-Z3 ASC Payment Indicators    **MED:** Pub 100/NCD References    ⅄ DMEPOS Paid    ⊘ SNF Excluded    PQ PQRI    **J Codes — 79**

**Drugs Administered Other Than Oral Method**

**J1051 — J1380**

**J1051** Injection, medroxyprogesterone acetate, 50 mg
Use this code for Depo-Provera.
MED: 100-2,15,50

**J1055** Injection, medroxyprogesterone acetate for contraceptive use, 150 mg ♀
Use this code for Depo-Provera.

**J1056** Injection, medroxyprogesterone acetate/estradiol cypionate, 5 mg/25 mg ♀
Use this code for Lunelle monthly contraceptive.

**J1060** Injection, testosterone cypionate and estradiol cypionate, up to 1 ml
Use this code for Depo-Testadiol, Duo-Span, Duo-Span II.
MED: 100-2,15,50

**J1070** Injection, testosterone cypionate, up to 100 mg
Use this code for Depo Testosterone Cypionate
MED: 100-2,15,50

**J1080** Injection, testosterone cypionate, 1 cc, 200 mg
Use this code for Depandrante, Depo-Testosterone, Virilon
MED: 100-2,15,50

**J1094** Injection, dexamethasone acetate, 1 mg
Use this code for Cortastat LA, Dalalone L.A., Dexamethasone Acetate Anhydrous, Dexone LA.
MED: 100-2,15,50

**J1100** Injection, dexamethasone sodium phosphate, 1 mg
Use this code for Cortastat, Dalalone, Decaject, Dexone, Solurex, Adrenocort, Primethasone, Dexasone, Dexim, Medidex, Spectro-Dex.
MED: 100-2,15,50

**J1110** Injection, dihydroergotamine mesylate, per 1 mg
Use this code for D.H.E. 45.
MED: 100-2,15,50

**J1120** Injection, acetazolamide sodium, up to 500 mg
Use this code for Diamox.
MED: 100-2,15,50

**J1160** Injection, digoxin, up to 0.5 mg
Use this code for Lanoxin.
MED: 100-2,15,50

**J1162** Injection, digoxin immune fab (ovine), per vial
Use this code for Digibind, Digifab.
MED: 100-2,15,50; 100-4,4,230.1

**J1165** Injection, phenytoin sodium, per 50 mg
Use this code for Dilantin.
MED: 100-2,15,50

**J1170** Injection, hydromorphone, up to 4 mg
Use this code for Dilaudid, Dilaudid-HP.
MED: 100-2,15,50

**J1180** Injection, dyphylline, up to 500 mg
MED: 100-2,15,50

**J1190** Injection, dexrazoxane HCl, per 250 mg
Use this code for Toltect, Zinecard.
MED: 100-2,15,50; 100-4,4,230.1

**J1200** Injection, diphenhydramine HCl, up to 50 mg
Use this code for Benadryl, Benahist 10, Benahist 50, Benoject-10, Benoject-50, Bena-D 10, Bena-D 50, Nordryl, Dihydrex, Dimine, Diphenacen-50, Hyrexin-50, Truxadryl, Wehdryl.
MED: 100-2,15,50
AHA: 1Q,'02,2

**J1205** Injection, chlorothiazide sodium, per 500 mg
Use this code for Diuril Sodium.
MED: 100-2,15,50

**J1212** Injection, DMSO, dimethyl sulfoxide, 50%, 50 ml
Use this code for Rimso 50. DMSO is covered only as a treatment of interstitial cystitis.
MED: 100-2,15,50; 100-3,230.12

**J1230** Injection, methadone HCl, up to 10 mg
Use this code for Dolophine HCl.
MED: 100-2,15,50

**J1240** Injection, dimenhydrinate, up to 50 mg
Use this code for Dramamine, Dinate, Dommanate, Dramanate, Dramilin, Dramocen, Dramoject, Dymenate, Hydrate, Marmine, Wehamine.
MED: 100-2,15,50

**J1245** Injection, dipyridamole, per 10 mg
Use this code for Persantine IV.
MED: 100-2,15,50

**J1250** Injection, dobutamine HCl, per 250 mg
MED: 100-2,15,50

**J1260** Injection, dolasetron mesylate, 10 mg
Use this code for Anzemet.
MED: 100-2,15,50

**J1265** Injection, dopamine HCl, 40 mg
MED: 100-4,4,230.1

**J1270** Injection, doxercalciferol, 1 mcg
Use this code for Hectorol.

● **J1300** Injection, eculizumab, 10 mg
Use this code for Soliris.

**J1320** Injection, amitriptyline HCl, up to 20 mg
Use this code for Elavil
MED: 100-2,15,50

**J1324** Injection, enfuvirtide, 1 mg
Use this code for Fuzeon.

**J1325** Injection, epoprostenol, 0.5 mg
Use this code for Flolan. See K0455 for infusion pump for epoprosterol.
MED: 100-2,15,50

**J1327** Injection, eptifibatide, 5 mg
Use this code for Integrilin.
MED: 100-2,15,50

**J1330** Injection, ergonovine maleate, up to 0.2 mg
Medicare jurisdiction: local contractor. Use this code for Ergotrate Maleate.
MED: 100-2,15,50

**J1335** Injection, ertapenem sodium, 500 mg
Use this code for Invanz.

**J1364** Injection, erythromycin lactobionate, per 500 mg
MED: 100-2,15,50

**J1380** Injection, estradiol valerate, up to 10 mg
Use this code for Delestrogen, Dioval, Dioval XX, Dioval 40, Duragen-10, Duragen-20, Duragen-40, Estradiol L.A., Estradiol L.A. 20, Estradiol L.A. 40, Gynogen L.A. 10, Gynogen L.A. 20, Gynogen L.A. 40, Valergen 10, Valergen 20, Valergen 40, Estra-L 20, Estra-L 40, L.A.E. 20.
MED: 100-2,15,50

---

▨ Special Coverage Instructions    ▨ Noncovered by Medicare    ▨ Carrier Discretion     ☑ Quantity Alert    ● New Code    ○ Recycled/Reinstated    ▲ Revised Code

N ☑ **J1390** Injection, estradiol valerate, up to 20 mg   N1
Use this code for Delestrogen, Dioval, Dioval XX, Dioval 40, Duragen-10, Duragen-20, Duragen-40, Estradiol L.A., Estradiol L.A. 20, Estradiol L.A. 40, Gynogen L.A. 10, Gynogen L.A. 20, Gynogen L.A. 40, Valergen 10, Valergen 20, Valergen 40, Estra-L 20, Estra-L 40, L.A.E. 20.
MED: 100-2,15,50

K ☑ **J1410** Injection, estrogen conjugated, per 25 mg   K2
Use this code for Natural Estrogenic Substance, Premarin Intravenous, Primestrin Aqueous.
MED: 100-2,15,50

K **J1430** Injection, ethanolamine oleate, 100 mg   K2
Use this code for Ethamiolin.
MED: 100-2,15,50; 100-4,4,230.1

N ☑ **J1435** Injection, estrone, per 1 mg   N1
Use this code for Estone Aqueous, Estragyn, Estro-A, Estrone, Estronol, Theelin Aqueous, Estone 5, Kestrone 5.
MED: 100-2,15,50

K ☑ **J1436** Injection, etidronate disodium, per 300 mg   K2
Use this code for Didronel.
MED: 100-2,15,50

K ☑ **J1438** Injection, etanercept, 25 mg (code may be used for Medicare when drug administered under the direct supervision of a physician, not for use when drug is self-administered)   K2
Use this code for Enbrel.
MED: 100-2,15,50

K ☑ **J1440** Injection, filgrastim (G-CSF), 300 mcg   K2
Use this code for Neupogen.
MED: 100-2,15,50

K ☑ **J1441** Injection, filgrastim (G-CSF), 480 mcg   K2
Use this code for Neupogen.
MED: 100-2,15,50

N ☑ **J1450** Injection, fluconazole, 200 mg   N1
Use this code for Diflucan.
MED: 100-2,15,50.5

K ☑ **J1451** Injection, fomepizole, 15 mg   K2
Use this code for Antizol.
MED: 100-2,15,50; 100-4,4,230.1

N ☑ **J1452** Injection, fomivirsen sodium, intraocular, 1.65 mg   N1
Use this code for Vitavene.
MED: 100-2,15,50.4.2

N ☑ **J1455** Injection, foscarnet sodium, per 1,000 mg   N1
Use this code for Foscavir.

K ☑ **J1457** Injection, gallium nitrate, 1 mg   K2
Use this code for Ganite.

K ☑ **J1458** Injection, galsulfase, 1 mg   K2
Use this code for Naglazyme.

K ☑ **J1460** Injection, gamma globulin, intramuscular, 1 cc   K2
Use this code for Baygam, Gammar, Gamastan, Flebogamma.
MED: 100-2,15,50

K ☑ **J1470** Injection, gamma globulin, intramuscular, 2 cc   K2
Use this code for Gammar, Gamastan.
MED: 100-2,15,50

K ☑ **J1480** Injection, gamma globulin, intramuscular, 3 cc   K2
Use this code for Gammar, Gamastan.
MED: 100-2,15,50

K ☑ **J1490** Injection, gamma globulin, intramuscular, 4 cc   K2
Use this code for Gammar, Gamastan.
MED: 100-2,15,50

K ☑ **J1500** Injection, gamma globulin, intramuscular, 5 cc   K2
Use this code for Gammar, Gamastan.
MED: 100-2,15,50

K ☑ **J1510** Injection, gamma globulin, intramuscular, 6 cc   K2
Use this code for Gammar, Gamastan.
MED: 100-2,15,50

K ☑ **J1520** Injection, gamma globulin, intramuscular, 7 cc   K2
Use this code for Gammar, Gamastan.
MED: 100-2,15,50

K ☑ **J1530** Injection, gamma globulin, intramuscular, 8 cc   K2
Use this code for Gammar, Gamastan.
MED: 100-2,15,50

K ☑ **J1540** Injection, gamma globulin, intramuscular, 9 cc   K2
Use this code for Gammar, Gamastan.
MED: 100-2,15,50

K ☑ **J1550** Injection, gamma globulin, intramuscular, 10 cc   K2
Use this code for Gammar, Gamastan.
MED: 100-2,15,50

K ☑ **J1560** Injection, gamma globulin, intramuscular, over 10 cc   K2
Use this code for Gammar, Gamastan.
MED: 100-2,15,50

● K ☑ **J1561** Injection, immune globulin, (Gamunex), intravenous, nonlyophilized (e.g., liquid), 500 mg   K2

▲ K ☑ **J1562** Injection, immune globulin (Vivaglobin), 100 mg   K2
Use this code for Vivaglobin.

K ☑ **J1565** Injection, respiratory syncytial virus immune globulin, intravenous, 50 mg   K2
Use this code for Respigam.
MED: 100-2,15,50

▲ K ☑ **J1566** Injection, immune globulin, intravenous, lyophilized (e.g., powder), not otherwise specified, 500 mg   K2
Use this code for Carimune.
MED: 100-2,15,50; 100-4,4,230.1

~~J1567~~ ~~Injection, immune globulin, intravenous, nonlyophilized (e.g., liquid), 500 mg~~
See J1561, J1568-J1569.
MED: 100-2,15,50; 100-4,4,230.1

● K ☑ **J1568** Injection, immune globulin, (Octagam), intravenous, nonlyophilized (e.g., liquid), 500 mg

● K ☑ **J1569** Injection, immune globulin, (Gammagard liquid), intravenous, nonlyophilized, (e.g., liquid), 500 mg

N ☑ **J1570** Injection, ganciclovir sodium, 500 mg   N1
Use this code for Cytovene.
MED: 100-2,15,50

● K ☑ **J1571** Injection, hepatitis B immune globulin (Hepagam B), intramuscular, 0.5 ml

● K ☑ **J1572** Injection, immune globulin, (Flebogamma), intravenous, nonlyophilized (e.g., liquid), 500 mg

● K ☑ **J1573** Injection, hepatitis B immune globulin (Hepagam B), intravenous, 0.5 ml

N ☑ **J1580** Injection, garamycin, gentamicin, up to 80 mg   N1
Use this code for Gentamicin Sulfate, Jenamicin.
MED: 100-2,15,50

N ☑ **J1590** Injection, gatifloxacin, 10 mg   N1

---

Special Coverage Instructions    Noncovered by Medicare    Carrier Discretion    ☑ Quantity Alert    ● New Code    ○ Recycled/Reinstated    ▲ Revised Code

**2008 HCPCS**    A2-Z3 ASC Payment Indicators    **MED:** Pub 100/NCD References    ⓖ DMEPOS Paid    ⊘ SNF Excluded    PQ PQRI    **J Codes — 81**

K ☑ | **J1595** | Injection, glatiramer acetate, 20 mg   K2
Use this code for Copaxone.
MED: 100-2,15,50

N ☑ | **J1600** | Injection, gold sodium thiomalate, up to 50 mg   N1
Use this code for Myochrysine.
MED: 100-2,15,50

K ☑ | **J1610** | Injection, glucagon HCl, per 1 mg   K2
Use this code for Glucagen.
MED: 100-2,15,50

K ☑ | **J1620** | Injection, gonadorelin HCl, per 100 mcg   K2
Use this code for Factrel, Lutrepulse.
MED: 100-2,15,50; 100-4,4,230.1

K ☑ | **J1626** | Injection, granisetron HCl, 100 mcg   K2
Use this code for Kytril.
MED: 100-2,15,50

N ☑ | **J1630** | Injection, haloperidol, up to 5 mg   N1
Use this code for Haldol.
MED: 100-2,15,50

N ☑ | **J1631** | Injection, haloperidol decanoate, per 50 mg   N1
Use this code for Haldol Decanoate-50.
MED: 100-2,15,50

K ☑ | **J1640** | Injection, hemin, 1 mg   K2
Use this code for Panhematin.
MED: 100-2,15,50; 100-4,4,230.1

N ☑ | **J1642** | Injection, heparin sodium, (heparin lock flush), per 10 units   N1
Use this code for Hep-Lock, Hep-Lock U/P, Hep-Pak, Lok-Pak.
MED: 100-2,15,50

N ☑ | **J1644** | Injection, Heparin sodium, per 1000 units   N1
Use this code for Heparin Sodium, Liquaemin Sodium.
MED: 100-2,15,50

N ☑ | **J1645** | Injection, dalteparin sodium, per 2500 IU   N1
Use this code for Fragmin.
MED: 100-2,15,50

N ☑ | **J1650** | Injection, enoxaparin sodium, 10 mg   N1
Use this code for Lovenox.

K ☑ | **J1652** | Injection, fondaparinux sodium, 0.5 mg   K2
Use this code for Atrixtra.
MED: 100-2,15,50

N ☑ | **J1655** | Injection, tinzaparin sodium, 1000 IU   N1
Use this code for Innohep.

K ☑ | **J1670** | Injection, tetanus immune globulin, human, up to 250 units   K2
Use this code for Baytet.
MED: 100-2,15,50

B | **J1675** | Injection, histrelin acetate, 10 micrograms
Use this code for Supprelin LA.
MED: 100-2,15,50

N ☑ | **J1700** | Injection, hydrocortisone acetate, up to 25 mg   N1
Use this code for Hydrocortone Acetate.
MED: 100-2,15,50

N ☑ | **J1710** | Injection, hydrocortisone sodium phosphate, up to 50 mg   N1
Use this code for Hydrocortone Phosphate.
MED: 100-2,15,50

N ☑ | **J1720** | Injection, hydrocortisone sodium succinate, up to 100 mg   N1
Use this code for Solu-Cortef, A-Hydrocort.
MED: 100-2,15,50

K ☑ | **J1730** | Injection, diazoxide, up to 300 mg   K2
MED: 100-2,15,50

G ☑ | **J1740** | Injection, ibandronate sodium, 1 mg   K2
Use this code for Boniva.

K ☑ | **J1742** | Injection, ibutilide fumarate, 1 mg   K2
Use this code for Corvert.
MED: 100-2,15,50

● G | **J1743** | Injection, idursulfase, 1 mg

K ☑ | **J1745** | Injection, infliximab, 10 mg   K2
Use this code for Remicade.
MED: 100-2,15,50

K ☑ | **J1751** | Injection, iron dextran 165, 50 mg   K2
MED: 100-4,4,230.1

K ☑ | **J1752** | Injection, iron dextran 267, 50 mg   K2
MED: 100-4,4,230.1

K ☑ | **J1756** | Injection, iron sucrose, 1 mg   K2
Use this code for Venofer.

K ☑ | **J1785** | Injection, imiglucerase, per unit   K2
Use this code for Cerezyme.
MED: 100-2,15,50

N ☑ | **J1790** | Injection, droperidol, up to 5 mg   N1
Use this code for Inapsine.
MED: 100-2,15,50

N ☑ | **J1800** | Injection, propranolol HCl, up to 1 mg   N1
Use this code for Inderal.
MED: 100-2,15,50

E ☑ | **J1810** | Injection, droperidol and fentanyl citrate, up to 2 ml ampule
MED: 100-2,15,50
AHA: 2Q,'02,8

N ☑ | **J1815** | Injection, insulin, per 5 units   N1
Use this code for Humalog, Humulin, Iletin, Insulin Lispo, Novo Nordisk, NPH, Pork insulin, Regular insulin, Ultralente, Velosulin, Humulin R, Iletin II Regular Port, Insulin Purified Pork, Relion, Lente Iletin I, Novolin R, Humulin R U-500.
MED: 100-2,15,50; 100-3,280.14

N ☑ | **J1817** | Insulin for administration through DME (i.e., insulin pump) per 50 units   N1
Use this code for Humalog, Humulin, Vesolin BR, Iletin II NPH Pork, Lantus, Lispro-PFC, Novolin, Novolog, Novolog Flexpen, Novolog Mix, Relion Novolin.

E ☑ | **J1825** | Injection, interferon beta-1a, 33 mcg
Use this code for Avonex, Rebif.

K ☑ | **J1830** | Injection interferon beta-1b, 0.25 mg (code may be used for Medicare when drug administered under direct supervision of a physician, not for use when drug is self-administered)   K2
Use this code for Actimmune and Betaseron.
MED: 100-2,15,50

K ☑ | **J1835** | Injection, itraconazole, 50 mg   K2
Use this code for Sporonox IV.

N ☑ | **J1840** | Injection, kanamycin sulfate, up to 500 mg   N1
Use this code for Kantrex.
MED: 100-2,15,50

---

Special Coverage Instructions    Noncovered by Medicare    Carrier Discretion      ☑ Quantity Alert   ● New Code   ○ Recycled/Reinstated   ▲ Revised Code

82 — J Codes      A Age Edit    M Maternity Edit   ♀ Female Only   ♂ Male Only   A-Y OPPS Status Indicators      **2008 HCPCS**

N ☑ **J1850** Injection, kanamycin sulfate, up to 75 mg　　N1
Use this code for Kantrex
MED: 100-2,15,50

N ☑ **J1885** Injection, ketorolac tromethamine, per 15 mg　　N1
MED: 100-2,15,50

N ☑ **J1890** Injection, cephalothin sodium, up to 1 g　　N1
MED: 100-2,15,50

K ☑ **J1931** Injection, laronidase, 0.1 mg　　K2
Use this code for Aldurazyme.

N ☑ **J1940** Injection, furosemide, up to 20 mg　　N1
Use this code for Lasix
MED: 100-2,15,50

K ☑ **J1945** Injection, lepirudin, 50 mg　　K2
Use this code for Refludan.
This drug is used for patients with heparin induced thrombocytopenia.
MED: 100-2,15,50; 100-4,4,230.1

K ☑ **J1950** Injection, leuprolide acetate (for depot suspension), per 3.75 mg　　K2
Use this code for Eliguard, Lupron, Lupron-3, Lupron-4, Lupron Depot.
MED: 100-2,15,50

B ☑ **J1955** Injection, levocarnitine, per 1 g
Use this code for Carnitor
MED: 100-2,15,50

N ☑ **J1956** Injection, levofloxacin, 250 mg　　N1
Use this code for Levaquin.
MED: 100-2,15,50

N ☑ **J1960** Injection, levorphanol tartrate, up to 2 mg　　N1
Use this code for Levo-Dromoran.
MED: 100-2,15,50

N ☑ **J1980** Injection, hyoscyamine sulfate, up to 0.25 mg　　N1
Use this code for Levsin.
MED: 100-2,15,50

N ☑ **J1990** Injection, chlordiazepoxide HCl, up to 100 mg　　N1
Use this code for Librium.
MED: 100-2,15,50

N ☑ **J2001** Injection, lidocaine HCl for intravenous infusion, 10 mg　　N1
Use this code for Xylocaine.
MED: 100-2,15,50

N ☑ **J2010** Injection, lincomycin HCl, up to 300 mg　　N1
Use this code for Lincocin
MED: 100-2,15,50

K ☑ **J2020** Injection, linezolid, 200 mg　　K2
Use this code for Zyvok.
AHA: 2Q,'02,8

N ☑ **J2060** Injection, lorazepam, 2 mg　　N1
Use this code for Ativan.
MED: 100-2,15,50

N ☑ **J2150** Injection, mannitol, 25% in 50 ml　　N1
Use this code for Osmitrol.
MED: 100-2,15,50

K ☑ **J2170** Injection, mecasermin, 1 mg　　K2
Use this code for Iplex, Increlex.

N ☑ **J2175** Injection, meperidine HCl, per 100 mg　　N1
Use this code for Demerol.
MED: 100-2,15,50

N ☑ **J2180** Injection, meperidine and promethazine HCl, up to 50 mg　　N1
Use this code for Mepergan Injection.
MED: 100-2,15,50

N ☑ **J2185** Injection, meropenem, 100 mg　　N1
Use this code for Merrem

N ☑ **J2210** Injection, methylergonovine maleate, up to 0.2 mg　　N1
Use this code for Methergine.
MED: 100-2,15,50

G ☑ **J2248** Injection, micafungin sodium, 1 mg　　K2
Use this code for Mycamine.

N ☑ **J2250** Injection, midazolam HCl, per 1 mg　　N1
Use this code for Versed.
MED: 100-2,15,50

N ☑ **J2260** Injection, milrinone lactate, 5 mg　　N1
Use this code for Primacor.
MED: 100-2,15,50

N ☑ **J2270** Injection, morphine sulfate, up to 10 mg　　N1
Use this code for Depodur, Infumorph
MED: 100-2,15,50

N ☑ **J2271** Injection, morphine sulfate, 100 mg　　N1
Use this code for Depodur, Infumorph
MED: 100-2,15,50; 100-3,280.14

N ☑ **J2275** Injection, morphine sulfate (preservative-free sterile solution), per 10 mg　　N1
Use this code for Astramorph PF, Duramorph, Infumorph.
MED: 100-2,15,50; 100-3,280.14

K ☑ **J2278** Injection, ziconotide, 1 microgram　　K2
Use this code for Prialt
MED: 100-4,4,230.1

N ☑ **J2280** Injection, moxifloxacin, 100 mg　　N1
Use this code for Avelox.

N ☑ **J2300** Injection, nalbuphine HCl, per 10 mg　　N1
Use this code for Nubain.
MED: 100-2,15,50

N ☑ **J2310** Injection, naloxone HCl, per 1 mg　　N1
Use this code for Narcan.
MED: 100-2,15,50

K ☑ **J2315** Injection, naltrexone, depot form, 1 mg　　K2
Use this code for Vivitrol.

N ☑ **J2320** Injection, nandrolone decanoate, up to 50 mg　　N1
MED: 100-2,15,50

N ☑ **J2321** Injection, nandrolone decanoate, up to 100 mg　　N1
MED: 100-2,15,50

N ☑ **J2322** Injection, nandrolone decanoate, up to 200 mg　　N1
MED: 100-2,15,50

● G **J2323** Injection, natalizumab, 1 mg
Use this code for Tysabri.

K ☑ **J2325** Injection, nesiritide, 0.1 mg　　K2
Use this code for Natrecor.
MED: 100-2,15,50; 100-4,4,230.1

K ☑ **J2353** Injection, octreotide, depot form for intramuscular injection, 1 mg　　K2
Use this code for Sandostatin LAR.

N ☑ **J2354** Injection, octreotide, nondepot form for subcutaneous or intravenous injection, 25 mcg　　N1
Use this code for Sandostatin.

Special Coverage Instructions　　Noncovered by Medicare　　Carrier Discretion　　☑ Quantity Alert　　● New Code　　○ Recycled/Reinstated　　▲ Revised Code

**2008 HCPCS**　　K2-Z3 ASC Payment Indicators　　**MED:** Pub 100/NCD References　　& DMEPOS Paid　　⊘ SNF Excluded　　P0 PQRI　　**J Codes — 83**

K ☑ **J2355** Injection, oprelvekin, 5 mg    K2
Use this code for Neumega.
MED: 100-2,15,50

K ☑ **J2357** Injection, omalizumab, 5 mg    K2
Use this code for Xolair.

N ☑ **J2360** Injection, orphenadrine citrate, up to 60 mg    N1
Use this code for Norflex
MED: 100-2,15,50

N ☑ **J2370** Injection, phenylephrine HCl, up to 1 ml    N1
MED: 100-2,15,50

N ☑ **J2400** Injection, chloroprocaine HCl, per 30 ml    N1
Use this code for Nesacaine, Nesacaine-MPF.
MED: 100-2,15,50

K ☑ **J2405** Injection, ondansetron HCl, per 1 mg    K2
Use this code for Zofran.
MED: 100-2,15,50

N ☑ **J2410** Injection, oxymorphone HCl, up to 1 mg    N1
Use this code for Numorphan, Oxymorphone HCl.
MED: 100-2,15,50

K ☑ **J2425** Injection, palifermin, 50 mcg    K2
Use this code for Kepivance.

K ☑ **J2430** Injection, pamidronate disodium, per 30 mg    K2
Use this code for Aredia
MED: 100-2,15,50; 100-4,4,230.1

N ☑ **J2440** Injection, papaverine HCl, up to 60 mg    N1
MED: 100-2,15,50

N ☑ **J2460** Injection, oxytetracycline HCl, up to 50 mg    N1
Use this code for Terramycin IM.
MED: 100-2,15,50

K ☑ **J2469** Injection, palonosetron HCl, 25 mcg    K2
Use this code for Aloxi.

N ☑ **J2501** Injection, paricalcitol, 1 mcg    N1
Use this code For Zemplar.
MED: 100-2,15,50

K **J2503** Injection, pegaptanib sodium, 0.3 mg    K2
Use this code for Mucagen.
MED: 100-4,4,230.1

K ☑ **J2504** Injection, pegademase bovine, 25 IU    K2
Use this code for Adagen.
MED: 100-2,15,50; 100-4,4,230.1

K ☑ **J2505** Injection, pegfilgrastim, 6 mg    K2
Use this code for Neulasta.

N ☑ **J2510** Injection, penicillin G procaine, aqueous, up to 600,000 units
Use this code for Wycillin, Duracillin A.S., Pfizerpen A.S., Crysticillin 300 A.S., Crysticillin 600 A.S.
MED: 100-2,15,50

K **J2513** Injection, pentastarch, 10% solution, 100 ml    K2
MED: 100-2,15,50; 100-4,4,230.1

N ☑ **J2515** Injection, pentobarbital sodium, per 50 mg    N1
Use this code for Nembutal Sodium Solution.
MED: 100-2,15,50

N ☑ **J2540** Injection, penicillin G potassium, up to 600,000 units    N1
Use this code for Pfizerpen.
MED: 100-2,15,50

N ☑ **J2543** Injection, piperacillin sodium/tazobactam sodium, 1 g/0.125 g (1.125 g)    N1
Use this code for Zosyn.
MED: 100-2,15,50

▲ B ☑ **J2545** Pentamidine isethionate, inhalation solution, FDA-approved final product, noncompounded, administered through DME, unit dose form, per 300 mg
Use this code for Nebupent, Pentam 300

N ☑ **J2550** Injection, promethazine HCl, up to 50 mg    N1
Use this code for Phenergan
MED: 100-2,15,50

N ☑ **J2560** Injection, phenobarbital sodium, up to 120 mg    N1
MED: 100-2,15,50

N ☑ **J2590** Injection, oxytocin, up to 10 units    N1
Use this code for Pitocin, Syntocinon.
MED: 100-2,15,50

N ☑ **J2597** Injection, desmopressin acetate, per 1 mcg    N1
Use this code for DDAVP.
MED: 100-2,15,50

N ☑ **J2650** Injection, prednisolone acetate, up to 1 ml    N1
MED: 100-2,15,50; 100-4,4,240

N ☑ **J2670** Injection, tolazoline HCl, up to 25 mg    N1
MED: 100-2,15,50

N **J2675** Injection, progesterone, per 50 mg    N1
Use this code for Gesterone, Gestrin.
MED: 100-2,15,50

N ☑ **J2680** Injection, fluphenazine decanoate, up to 25 mg    N1
MED: 100-2,15,50

N ☑ **J2690** Injection, procainamide HCl, up to 1 g    N1
Use this code for Pronestyl.
MED: 100-2,15,50

N ☑ **J2700** Injection, oxacillin sodium, up to 250 mg    N1
Use this code for Bactocill
MED: 100-2,15,50

N ☑ **J2710** Injection, neostigmine methylsulfate, up to 0.5 mg    N1
Use this code for Prostigmin.
MED: 100-2,15,50

N ☑ **J2720** Injection, protamine sulfate, per 10 mg    N1
MED: 100-2,15,50

● K **J2724** Injection, protein C concentrate, intravenous, human, 10 IU

N ☑ **J2725** Injection, protirelin, per 250 mcg    N1
Use this code for Thyrel TRH
MED: 100-2,15,50

K ☑ **J2730** Injection, pralidoxime chloride, up to 1 g    K2
Use this code for Protopam Chloride.
MED: 100-2,15,50

N ☑ **J2760** Injection, phentolamine mesylate, up to 5 mg    N1
Use this code for Regitine.
MED: 100-2,15,50

N ☑ **J2765** Injection, metoclopramide HCl, up to 10 mg    N1
Use this code for Reglan
MED: 100-2,15,50

K ☑ **J2770** Injection, quinupristin/dalfopristin, 500 mg (150/350)    K2
Use this code for Synercid.
MED: 100-2,15,50

---

Special Coverage Instructions    Noncovered by Medicare    Carrier Discretion    ☑ Quantity Alert    ● New Code    ○ Recycled/Reinstated    ▲ Revised Code

● G ☑ **J2778** Injection, ranibizumab, 0.1 mg
Use this code for Lucentis.

N ☑ **J2780** Injection, ranitidine HCl, 25 mg N1
Use this code for Zantac.
MED: 100-2,15,50

K ☑ **J2783** Injection, rasburicase, 0.5 mg K2
Use this code for Elitek.

K ☑ **J2788** Injection, Rho D immune globulin, human, minidose, 50 mcg K2
Use this code for RhoGam HYPRho-D, MICRhoGam, Ultra-Filtered
MED: 100-2,15,50

K ☑ **J2790** Injection, Rho D immune globulin, human, full dose, 300 mcg K2
Use this code for Gamulin RH, HypRho-D, BayRho-D, RhoGam.
MED: 100-2,15,50

● K ☑ **J2791** Injection, Rho( D) immune globulin (human), (Rhophylac), intramuscular or intravenouss, 10 IU

K ☑ **J2792** Injection, Rho D immune globulin, intravenous, human, solvent detergent, 100 IU K2
Use this code for WINRho SDF.
MED: 100-2,15,50

K ☑ **J2794** Injection, risperidone, long acting, 0.5 mg K2
Use this code for Risperidal Costa Long Acting.

N ☑ **J2795** Injection, ropivacaine HCl, 1 mg N1
Use this code for Naropin.

N ☑ **J2800** Injection, methocarbamol, up to 10 ml N1
Use this code for Robaxin
MED: 100-2,15,50

N ☑ **J2805** Injection, sincalide, 5 mcg N1
Use this code for Kinevac.

N ☑ **J2810** Injection, theophylline, per 40 mg N1
MED: 100-2,15,50

K ☑ **J2820** Injection, sargramostim (GM-CSF), 50 mcg K2
Use this code for Leukine
MED: 100-2,15,50

K ☑ **J2850** Injection, secretin, synthetic, human, 1 mcg K2
MED: 100-2,15,50

N ☑ **J2910** Injection, aurothioglucose, up to 50 mg N1
Use this code for Solganal.
MED: 100-2,15,50

N ☑ **J2916** Injection, sodium ferric gluconate complex in sucrose injection, 12.5 mg N1
MED: 100-2,15,50.2

N ☑ **J2920** Injection, methylprednisolone sodium succinate, up to 40 mg N1
Use this code for Solu-Medrol, A-methaPred.
MED: 100-2,15,50; 100-4,4,240

N ☑ **J2930** Injection, methylprednisolone sodium succinate, up to 125 mg N1
Use this code for Solu-Medrol, A-methaPred.
MED: 100-2,15,50; 100-4,4,240

K ☑ **J2940** Injection, somatrem, 1 mg K2
Use this code for Protropin.
MED: 100-2,15,50
AHA: 2Q,'02,8

K ☑ **J2941** Injection, somatropin, 1 mg K2
Use this code for Humatrope, Genotropin Nutropin, Biotropin, Genotropin, Genotropin Miniquick, Norditropin, Nutropin, Nutropin AQ, Saizen, Saizen Somatropin RDNA Origin, Serostim, Serostim RDNA Origin, Zorbtive.
MED: 100-2,15,50
AHA: 2Q,'02,8

N ☑ **J2950** Injection, promazine HCl, up to 25 mg N1
Use this code for Sparine, Prozine-50.
MED: 100-2,15,50

K ☑ **J2993** Injection, reteplase, 18.1 mg K2
Use this code for Retavase
MED: 100-2,15,50

K ☑ **J2995** Injection, streptokinase, per 250,000 IU K2
Use this code for Streptase
MED: 100-2,15,50

K ☑ **J2997** Injection, alteplase recombinant, 1 mg K2
Use this code for Activase, Cathflo.
MED: 100-2,15,50

N ☑ **J3000** Injection, streptomycin, up to 1 g N1
Use this code for Streptomycin Sulfate.
MED: 100-2,15,50

N ☑ **J3010** Injection, fentanyl citrate, 0.1 mg N1
Use this code for Sublimaze.
MED: 100-2,15,50

K ☑ **J3030** Injection, sumatriptan succinate, 6 mg (code may be used for Medicare when drug administered under the direct supervision of a physician, not for use when drug is self-administered) K2
Use this code for Imitrex.
MED: 100-2,15,50

N ☑ **J3070** Injection, pentazocine, 30 mg N1
Use this code for Talwin.
MED: 100-2,15,50

K ☑ **J3100** Injection, tenecteplase, 50 mg K2
Use this code for TNKase.
AHA: 2Q,'02,8

N ☑ **J3105** Injection, terbutaline sulfate, up to 1 mg N1
For terbutaline in inhalation solution, see K0525 and K0526.
MED: 100-2,15,50

B ☑ **J3110** Injection, teriparatide, 10 mcg
Use this code for Forteo.

N ☑ **J3120** Injection, testosterone enanthate, up to 100 mg N1
Use this code for Delatestryl.
MED: 100-2,15,50

N ☑ **J3130** Injection, testosterone enanthate, up to 200 mg N1
Use this code for Delatestryl.
MED: 100-2,15,50

N ☑ **J3140** Injection, testosterone suspension, up to 50 mg N1
MED: 100-2,15,50

N ☑ **J3150** Injection, testosterone propionate, up to 100 mg N1
MED: 100-2,15,50

N ☑ **J3230** Injection, chlorpromazine HCl, up to 50 mg N1
Use this code for Thorazine.
MED: 100-2,15,50

K ☑ **J3240** Injection, thyrotropin alpha, 0.9 mg, provided in 1.1 mg vial K2
Use this code for Thyrogen.
MED: 100-2,15,50

---

Special Coverage Instructions     Noncovered by Medicare     Carrier Discretion     ☑ Quantity Alert     ● New Code     ○ Recycled/Reinstated     ▲ Revised Code

**Drugs Administered Other Than Oral Method**

**J3243 — J3535**

G ☑ **J3243** Injection, tigecycline, 1 mg    K2
Use this code for Tygacil.

K ☑ **J3246** Injection, tirofiban HCl, 0.25mg    K2
Use this code for Aggrastat.

N ☑ **J3250** Injection, trimethobenzamide HCl, up to 200 mg    N1
Use this code for Tigan, Tiject-20, Arrestin.
MED: 100-2,15,50

N ☑ **J3260** Injection, tobramycin sulfate, up to 80 mg    N1
Use this code for Nebcin.
MED: 100-2,15,50

N ☑ **J3265** Injection, torsemide, 10 mg/ml    N1
Use this code for Demadex, Torsemide.
MED: 100-2,15,50

N ☑ **J3280** Injection, thiethylperazine maleate, up to 10 mg    N1
MED: 100-2,15,50

K ☑ **J3285** Injection, treprostinil, 1 mg    K2
Use this code for Remodulin.
MED: 100-4,4,230.1

N ☑ **J3301** Injection, triamcinolone acetonide, per 10 mg    N1
Use this code for Kenalog-10, Kenalog-40, Tri-Kort, Kenaject-40, Cenacort A-40, Triam-A, Trilog. For triamcinolone in inhalation solution, see K0527 and K0528.
MED: 100-2,15,50

N ☑ **J3302** Injection, triamcinolone diacetate, per 5 mg    N1
Use this code for Aristocort, Aristocort Intralesional, Aristocort Forte, Amcort, Trilone, Cenacort Forte.
MED: 100-2,15,50

N ☑ **J3303** Injection, triamcinolone hexacetonide, per 5 mg    N1
Use this code for Aristospan Intralesional, Aristospan Intra-articular.
MED: 100-2,15,50

K ☑ **J3305** Injection, trimetrexate glucuronate, per 25 mg    K2
Use this code for Neutrexin.
MED: 100-2,15,50

N ☑ **J3310** Injection, perphenazine, up to 5 mg    N1
Use this code for Trilafon.
MED: 100-2,15,50

K ☑ **J3315** Injection, triptorelin pamoate, 3.75 mg    K2
Use this code for Trelstar Depot, Trelstar Depot Plus Debioclip Kit, Trelstar LA.
MED: 100-2,15,50

N ☑ **J3320** Injection, spectinomycin dihydrochloride, up to 2 g    N1
Use this code for Trobicin.
MED: 100-2,15,50

K ☑ **J3350** Injection, urea, up to 40 g    K2
MED: 100-2,15,50

K **J3355** Injection, urofollitropin, 75 IU    K2
Use this code for Metrodin, Bravelle, Fertinex.
MED: 100-2,15,50; 100-4,4,230.1

N ☑ **J3360** Injection, diazepam, up to 5 mg    N1
Use this code for Diastat, Dizac, Valium.
MED: 100-2,15,50

N ☑ **J3364** Injection, urokinase, 5,000 IU vial    N1
Use this code for Kinlytic
MED: 100-2,15,50

K ☑ **J3365** Injection, IV, urokinase, 250,000 IU vial    K2
Use this code for Kinlytic
MED: 100-2,15,50

N ☑ **J3370** Injection, vancomycin HCl, 500 mg    N1
Use this code for Vancocin.
MED: 100-2,15,50; 100-3,280.14

K ☑ **J3396** Injection, verteporfin, 0.1 mg    K2
Use this code for Visudyne.
MED: 100-3,80.2; 100-3,80.3

N ☑ **J3400** Injection, triflupromazine HCl, up to 20 mg    N1
MED: 100-2,15,50

N ☑ **J3410** Injection, hydroxyzine HCl, up to 25 mg    N1
Use this code for Vistaril, Vistaject-25, Hyzine, Hyzine-50.
MED: 100-2,15,50

N ☑ **J3411** Injection, thiamine HCl, 100 mg    N1

N ☑ **J3415** Injection, pyridoxine HCl, 100 mg    N1

N ☑ **J3420** Injection, vitamin B-12 cyanocobalamin, up to 1,000 mcg    N1
Use this code for Sytobex, Redisol, Rubramin PC, Betalin 12, Berubigen, Cobex, Cobal, Crystal B12, Cyano, Cyanocobalamin, Hydroxocobalamin, Hydroxycobal, Nutri-Twelve.
MED: 100-2,15,50; 100-3,150.6

N ☑ **J3430** Injection, phytonadione (vitamin K), per 1 mg    N1
Use this code for AquaMephyton, Konakion, Menadione, Phytonadione.
MED: 100-2,15,50

K ☑ **J3465** Injection, voriconazole, 10 mg    K2
MED: 100-2,15,50

N ☑ **J3470** Injection, hyaluronidase, up to 150 units    N1
MED: 100-2,15,50

N ☑ **J3471** Injection, hyaluronidase, ovine, preservative free, per 1 USP unit (up to 999 USP units)    N1

K ☑ **J3472** Injection, hyaluronidase, ovine, preservative free, per 1,000 USP units    K2

G ☑ **J3473** Injection, hyaluronidase, recombinant, 1 USP unit    K2

N ☑ **J3475** Injection, magnesium sulfate, per 500 mg    N1
Use this code for Mag Sul, Sulfa Mag.
MED: 100-2,15,50

N ☑ **J3480** Injection, potassium chloride, per 2 mEq    N1
MED: 100-2,15,50

N ☑ **J3485** Injection, zidovudine, 10 mg    N1
Use this code for Retrovir, Zidovudine.
MED: 100-2,15,50

N ☑ **J3486** Injection, ziprasidone mesylate, 10 mg    N1
Use this code for Geodon.

▲ K ☑ **J3487** Injection, zoledronic acid (Zometa), 1 mg    K2

● G ☑ **J3488** Injection, zoledronic acid (Reclast), 1 mg

N **J3490** Unclassified drugs    N1
MED: 100-2,15,50

E ☑ **J3520** Edetate disodium, per 150 mg
Use this code for Endrate, Disotate, Meritate, Chealamide, E.D.T.A. This drug is used in chelation therapy, a treatment for atherosclerosis that is not covered by Medicare.
MED: 100-3,20.21; 100-3,20.22

N **J3530** Nasal vaccine inhalation    N1
MED: 100-2,15,50

E **J3535** Drug administered through a metered dose inhaler
MED: 100-2,15,50

---

Special Coverage Instructions    Noncovered by Medicare    Carrier Discretion    ☑ Quantity Alert    ● New Code    ○ Recycled/Reinstated    ▲ Revised Code

**86 — J Codes**    A Age Edit    M Maternity Edit    ♀ Female Only    ♂ Male Only    A–Y OPPS Status Indicators    **2008 HCPCS**

[E] **J3570** Laetrile, amygdalin, vitamin B-17
The FDA has found Laetrile to have no safe or effective therapeutic purpose.
MED: 100-3,30.7

[N] **J3590** Unclassified biologics [N1]

## MISCELLANEOUS DRUGS AND SOLUTIONS

[N] ☑ **J7030** Infusion, normal saline solution, 1,000 cc [N1]
MED: 100-2,15,50

[N] ☑ **J7040** Infusion, normal saline solution, sterile (500 ml = 1 unit) [N1]
MED: 100-2,15,50

[N] ☑ **J7042** 5% dextrose/normal saline (500 ml = 1 unit) [N1]
MED: 100-2,15,50

[N] ☑ **J7050** Infusion, normal saline solution, 250 cc [N1]
MED: 100-2,15,50

[N] ☑ **J7060** 5% dextrose/water (500 ml = 1 unit) [N1]
MED: 100-2,15,50

[N] ☑ **J7070** Infusion, D-5-W, 1,000 cc [N1]
MED: 100-2,15,50

[N] ☑ **J7100** Infusion, dextran 40, 500 ml [N1]
Use this code for Gentran, 10% LMD, Rheomacrodex.
MED: 100-2,15,50

[N] ☑ **J7110** Infusion, dextran 75, 500 ml [N1]
Use this code for Gentran 75.
MED: 100-2,15,50

[N] ☑ **J7120** Ringer's lactate infusion, up to 1,000 cc [N1]
MED: 100-2,15,50

[N] ☑ **J7130** Hypertonic saline solution, 50 or 100 mEq, 20 cc vial [N1]
MED: 100-2,15,50

▲ [K] **J7187** Injection, von Willebrand Factor complex (Humate-P), per IU vWF-RCO [K2]

[K] ☑ **J7189** Factor VIIa (antihemophilic factor, recombinant), per 1 mcg [K2]
MED: 100-1,1,10.1; 100-2,6,10; 100-2,15,50; 100-4,3,20.7.3; 100-4,4,230.1

[K] ☑ **J7190** Factor VIII (antihemophilic factor, human) per IU [K2]
Use this code for Monarc-M, Koate-HP, Alphanate, Hemofil-M, Koate-DVI, Kogenate, Monoclate-P.
Medicare jurisdiction: local contractor.
MED: 100-1,1,10.1; 100-2,6,10; 100-2,15,50; 100-4,3,20.7.3; 100-4,4,240; 100-4,17,80.4

[N] ☑ **J7191** Factor VIII (antihemophilic factor (porcine)), per IU [N1]
Use this code for Hyate:C. Medicare jurisdiction: local contractor.
MED: 100-1,1,10.1; 100-2,6,10; 100-2,15,50; 100-4,3,20.7.3; 100-4,4,240; 100-4,17,80.4

[K] ☑ **J7192** Factor VIII (antihemophilic factor, recombinant) per IU [K2]
Use this code for Recombinate, Kogenate, Bioclate, Helixate, Advate rAHF-PFM, Antihemophilic Factor Human Method M Monoclonal Purified, Genarc, Refacto. Medicare jurisdiction: local contractor.
MED: 100-1,1,10.1; 100-2,6,10; 100-2,15,50; 100-4,3,20.7.3; 100-4,4,240; 100-4,17,80.4

[K] ☑ **J7193** Factor IX (antihemophilic factor, purified, nonrecombinant) per IU [K2]
Use this code for AlphaNine SD, Mononine.
MED: 100-1,1,10.1; 100-2,6,10; 100-2,15,50; 100-4,3,20.7.3; 100-4,4,240; 100-4,17,80.4
AHA: 2Q,'02,8

[K] ☑ **J7194** Factor IX complex, per IU [K2]
Use this code for Konyne-80, Profilnine Heat-Treated, Proplex T, Proplex SX-T, Alphanine SD, Bebulin VH, factor IX+ complex, Profilnine SD. Medicare jurisdiction: local contractor.
MED: 100-1,1,10.1; 100-2,6,10; 100-2,15,50; 100-4,3,20.7.3; 100-4,4,240; 100-4,17,80.4

[K] ☑ **J7195** Factor IX (antihemophilic factor, recombinant) per IU [K2]
Use this code for Benefix, Konyne 80, ProplexT.
MED: 100-1,1,10.1; 100-2,6,10; 100-2,15,50; 100-4,3,20.7.3; 100-4,4,240; 100-4,17,80.4
AHA: 2Q,'02,8

[K] ☑ **J7197** Antithrombin III (human), per IU [K2]
Medicare jurisdiction: local contractor. Use this code for Throbate III, ATnativ.
MED: 100-2,15,50

[K] ☑ **J7198** Antiinhibitor, per IU [K2]
Medicare jurisdiction: local contractor. Use this code for Autoplex T, Feiba VH AICC.

[B] **J7199** Hemophilia clotting factor, not otherwise classified
Medicare jurisdiction: local contractor.

[E] **J7300** Intrauterine copper contraceptive
Use this code for Paragard T380A.

[E] ☑ **J7302** Levonorgestrel-releasing intrauterine contraceptive system, 52 mg ♀
Use this code for Mirena.

[E] ☑ **J7303** Contraceptive supply, hormone containing vaginal ring, each ♀
Use this code for Nuvaring Vaginal Ring.

[E] ☑ **J7304** Contraceptive supply, hormone containing patch, each

[E] **J7306** Levonorgestrel (contraceptive) implant system, including implants and supplies
Use this code for Norplant II.

● [E] **J7307** Etonogestrel (contraceptive) implant system, including implant and supplies
Use this code for Implanon.

[K] ☑ **J7308** Aminolevulinic acid HCl for topical administration, 20%, single unit dosage form (354 mg) [K2]

[K] ☑ **J7310** Ganciclovir, 4.5 mg, long-acting implant [K2]
Use this code for Vitrasert.
MED: 100-2,15,50

[K] **J7311** Fluocinolone acetonide, intravitreal implant [K2]
Use this code for Retisert.

~~**J7319** Hyaluronan (sodium hyaluronate) or derivative, intra-articular injection, per injection~~
See code(s) Q4083-Q4086

● [K] ☑ **J7321** Hyaluronan or derivative, Hyalgan or Supartz, for intra-articular injection, per dose

● [K] ☑ **J7322** Hyaluronan or derivative, Synvisc, for intra-articular injection, per dose

● [K] ☑ **J7323** Hyaluronan or derivative, Euflexxa, for intra-articular injection, per dose

Special Coverage Instructions    Noncovered by Medicare    Carrier Discretion    ☑ Quantity Alert    ● New Code    ○ Recycled/Reinstated    ▲ Revised Code

**2008 HCPCS** [A2-Z3] ASC Payment Indicators    **MED:** Pub 100/NCD References    ☆ DMEPOS Paid    ⊘ SNF Excluded    [PQ] PQRI    **J Codes — 87**

● K ☑ **J7324** Hyaluronan or derivative, Orthovisc, for intra-articular injection, per dose

B ☑ **J7330** Autologous cultured chondrocytes, implant
Medicare jurisdiction: local contractor. Use this code for Carticel.

K ☑ **J7340** Dermal and epidermal, (substitute) tissue of human origin, with or without bioengineered or processed elements, with metabolically active elements, per square centimeter K2
Use this code for Apligraf, Orcel, TransCyte.
MED: 100-4,4,230.1

N ☑ **J7341** Dermal (substitute) tissue of nonhuman origin, with or without other bioengineered or processed elements, with metabolically active elements, per square centimeter N1

K ☑ **J7342** Dermal (substitute) tissue of human origin, with or without other bioengineered or processed elements, with metabolically active elements, per square centimeter K2
Use this code for Dermagraft , Dermagraft TC.
MED: 100-4,4,230.1

K ☑ **J7343** Dermal and epidermal, (substitute) tissue of nonhuman origin, with or without other bioengineered or processed elements, without metabolically active elements, per square centimeter K2
MED: 100-4,4,230.1

K ☑ **J7344** Dermal (substitute) tissue of human origin, with or without other bioengineered or processed elements, without metabolically active elements, per square centimeter K2
MED: 100-4,4,230.1

~~**J7345** Dermal (substitute) tissue of nonhuman origin, with or without other bioengineered or processed elements, without metabolically active elements, per square centimeter~~
See J7347-J7349.

K ☑ **J7346** Dermal (substitute) tissue of human origin, injectable, with or without other bioengineered or processed elements, but without metabolically active elements, 1 cc K2

● K ☑ **J7347** Dermal (substitute) tissue of nonhuman origin, with or without other bioengineered or processed elements, without metabolically active elements (Integra Matrix), per sq. cm.

● G ☑ **J7348** Dermal (substitute) tissue of nonhuman origin, with or without other bioengineered or processed elements, without metabolically active elements (TissueMend), per sq. cm.

● G ☑ **J7349** Dermal (substitute) tissue of nonhuman origin, with or without other bioengineered or processed elements, without metabolically active elements (PriMatrix), per sq. cm.

N ☑ **J7500** Azathioprine, oral, 50 mg N1
Use this code for Azasan, Imuran.
MED: 100-2,15,50.5; 100-4,4,240; 100-4,17,80.3

K ☑ **J7501** Azathioprine, parenteral, 100 mg K2
MED: 100-2,6,10; 100-2,15,50; 100-4,4,230.1; 100-4,4,240; 100-4,17,80.3

K ☑ **J7502** Cyclosporine, oral, 100 mg K2
Use this code for Neoral, Sandimmune, Gengraf, Sangcya
MED: 100-2,15,50.5; 100-4,4,230.1; 100-4,4,240; 100-4,17,80.3

K ☑ **J7504** Lymphocyte immune globulin, antithymocyte globulin, equine, parenteral, 250 mg K2
Use this code for Atgam.
MED: 100-2,6,10; 100-2,15,50; 100-3,260.7; 100-4,4,240; 100-4,17,80.3

K ☑ **J7505** Muromonab-CD3, parenteral, 5 mg K2
Use this code for Orthoclone OKT3.
MED: 100-2,6,10; 100-2,15,50; 100-4,4,240; 100-4,17,80.3

N ☑ **J7506** Prednisone, oral, per 5 mg N1
Use this code for Deltasone, Liquid Pred Syrup, Levoxyl, Predone, Prednicot, Sterapred.
MED: 100-2,15,50.5; 100-4,4,240; 100-4,17,80.3

K ☑ **J7507** Tacrolimus, oral, per 1 mg K2
Use this code for Prograf.
MED: 100-2,15,50.5; 100-4,4,240; 100-4,17,80.3

N ☑ **J7509** Methylprednisolone, oral, per 4 mg N1
Use this code for Medrol, Methylpred.
MED: 100-2,15,50.5; 100-4,4,240; 100-4,17,80.3

N ☑ **J7510** Prednisolone, oral, per 5 mg N1
Use this code for Delta-Cortef, Cotolone, Pediapred, Prednoral, Prelone.
MED: 100-2,15,50.5; 100-4,4,240; 100-4,17,80.3

K ☑ **J7511** Lymphocyte immune globulin, antithymocyte globulin, rabbit, parenteral, 25 mg K2
Use this code for Thymoglobulin.
MED: 100-2,6,10; 100-4,4,240; 100-4,17,80.3
AHA: 2Q,'02,8

K ☑ **J7513** Daclizumab, parenteral, 25 mg K2
Use this code for Zenapax.
MED: 100-2,6,10; 100-2,15,50.5; 100-4,4,240; 100-4,17,80.3

N ☑ **J7515** Cyclosporine, oral, 25 mg N1
Use this code for Neoral, Sandimmune, Gengraf, Sangcya.
MED: 100-4,4,240; 100-4,17,80.3

N ☑ **J7516** Cyclosporine, parenteral, 250 mg N1
Use this code for Neoral, Sandimmune, Gengraf, Sangcya.
MED: 100-2,6,10; 100-4,4,240; 100-4,17,80.3

K ☑ **J7517** Mycophenolate mofetil, oral, 250 mg K2
Use this code for CellCept.
MED: 100-4,4,240; 100-4,17,80.3

K ☑ **J7518** Mycophenolic acid, oral, 180 mg K2
Use this code for Myfortic Delayed Release.
MED: 100-4,4,240; 100-4,17,80.3.1

K ☑ **J7520** Sirolimus, oral, 1 mg K2
Use this code for Rapamune.
MED: 100-2,15,50.5; 100-4,4,240; 100-4,17,80.3

K ☑ **J7525** Tacrolimus, parenteral, 5 mg K2
Use this code for Prograf.
MED: 100-2,6,10; 100-2,15,50.5; 100-4,4,240; 100-4,17,80.3

N **J7599** Immunosuppressive drug, NOC N1
Determine if an alternative HCPCS Level II or a CPT code better describes the service being reported. This code should be used only if a more specific code is unavailable.
MED: 100-2,6,10; 100-2,15,50.5; 100-4,4,240; 100-4,17,80.3

## INHALATION SOLUTIONS

● M ☑ **J7602** Albuterol, all formulations including separated isomers, inhalation solution, FDA-approved final product, noncompounded, administered through DME, concentrated form, per 1 mg (Albuterol) or per 0.5 mg Levalbuterol)

---

Special Coverage Instructions    Noncovered by Medicare    Carrier Discretion    ☑ Quantity Alert    ● New Code    ○ Recycled/Reinstated    ▲ Revised Code

A Age Edit    M Maternity Edit    ♀ Female Only    ♂ Male Only    A-Y OPPS Status Indicators    **2008 HCPCS**

● Ⓜ ☑ **J7603** Albuterol, all formulations including separated isomers, inhalation solution, FDA-approved final product, noncompounded, administered through DME, unit dose, per 1 mg (Albuterol) or per 0.5 mg Levalbuterol)

● Ⓜ ☑ **J7604** Acetylcysteine, inhalation solution, compounded product, administered through DME, unit dose form, per g

● Ⓜ ☑ **J7605** Arformoterol, inhalation solution, FDA approved final product, noncompounded, administered through DME, unit dose form, 15 mcg

Ⓜ ☑ **J7607** Levalbuterol, inhalation solution, compounded product, administered through DME, concentrated form, 0.5 mg

▲ Ⓜ ☑ **J7608** Acetylcysteine, inhalation solution, FDA-approved final product, noncompounded, administered through DME, unit dose form, per g
Use this code for Acetadote, Mucomyst, Mucosil.
MED: 100-2,15,110.3

Ⓜ ☑ **J7609** Albuterol, inhalation solution, compounded product, administered through DME, unit dose, 1 mg

Ⓜ ☑ **J7610** Albuterol, inhalation solution, compounded product, administered through DME, concentrated form, 1 mg

~~J7611~~ ~~Albuterol, inhalation solution, FDA-approved final product, noncompounded, administered through DME, concentrated form, 1 mg~~
MED: 100-2,15,110.3

~~J7612~~ ~~Levalbuterol, inhalation solution, FDA-approved final product, noncompounded, administered through DME, concentrated form, 0.5 mg~~
See J7602.
MED: 100-2,15,110.3

~~J7613~~ ~~Albuterol, inhalation solution, FDA-approved final product, noncompounded, administered through DME, unit dose, 1 mg~~
See J7603.
MED: 100-2,15,110.3

~~J7614~~ ~~Levalbuterol, inhalation solution, FDA-approved final product, noncompounded, administered through DME, unit dose, 0.5 mg~~
See J7603.
MED: 100-2,15,110.3

Ⓜ ☑ **J7615** Levalbuterol, inhalation solution, compounded product, administered through DME, unit dose, 0.5 mg

Ⓜ ☑ **J7620** Albuterol, up to 2.5 mg and ipratropium bromide, up to 0.5 mg, fda-approved final product, non-compounded, administered through DME
MED: 100-2,15,110.3

Ⓜ ☑ **J7622** Beclomethasone, inhalation solution, compounded product, administered through DME, unit dose form, per milligram
Use this code for Beclovent, Beconase.

Ⓜ ☑ **J7624** Betamethasone, inhalation solution, compounded product, administered through DME, unit dose form, per milligram

Ⓜ ☑ **J7626** Budesonide, inhalation solution, FDA-approved final product, noncompounded, administered through DME, unit dose form, up to 0.5 mg
Use this code for Pulmicort, Pulmicort Flexhaler, Pulmicort Respules, Vanceril.

Ⓜ ☑ **J7627** Budesonide, inhalation solution, compounded product, administered through DME, unit dose form, up to 0.5 mg

Ⓜ ☑ **J7628** Bitolterol mesylate, inhalation solution, compounded product, administered through DME, concentrated form, per milligram
MED: 100-2,15,110.3

Ⓜ ☑ **J7629** Bitolterol mesylate, inhalation solution, compounded product, administered through DME, unit dose form, per milligram
MED: 100-2,15,110.3

▲ Ⓜ ☑ **J7631** Cromolyn sodium, inhalation solution, FDA-approved final product, noncompounded, administered through DME, unit dose form, per 10 mg
Use this code for Intal, Nasalcrom
MED: 100-2,15,110.3

● Ⓜ ☑ **J7632** Cromolyn sodium, inhalation solution, compounded product, administered through DME, unit dose form, per 10 mg

Ⓜ ☑ **J7633** Budesonide, inhalation solution, FDA-approved final product, noncompounded, administered through DME, concentrated form, per 0.25 mg
Use this code for Pulmicort, Pulmicort Flexhaler, Pulmicort Respules, Vanceril

Ⓜ ☑ **J7634** Budesonide, inhalation solution, compounded product, administered through DME, concentrated form, per 0.25 mg

Ⓜ ☑ **J7635** Atropine, inhalation solution, compounded product, administered through DME, concentrated form, per mg
MED: 100-2,15,110.3

Ⓜ ☑ **J7636** Atropine, inhalation solution, compounded product, administered through DME, unit dose form, per mg
MED: 100-2,15,110.3

Ⓜ ☑ **J7637** Dexamethasone, inhalation solution, compounded product, administered through DME, concentrated form, per mg
MED: 100-2,15,110.3

Ⓜ ☑ **J7638** Dexamethasone, inhalation solution, compounded product, administered through DME, unit dose form, per mg
MED: 100-2,15,110.3

▲ Ⓜ ☑ **J7639** Dornase alpha, inhalation solution, FDA-approved final product, noncompounded, administered through DME, unit dose form, per mg
Use this code for Pulmozyme.
MED: 100-2,15,110.3

Ⓔ ☑ **J7640** Formoterol, inhalation solution, compounded product, administered through DME, unit dose form, 12 mcg

Ⓜ ☑ **J7641** Flunisolide, inhalation solution, compounded product, administered through DME, unit dose, per mg
Use this code for Aerobid, Flunisolide.

Ⓜ ☑ **J7642** Glycopyrrolate, inhalation solution, compounded product, administered through DME, concentrated form, per mg
MED: 100-2,15,110.3

Ⓜ ☑ **J7643** Glycopyrrolate, inhalation solution, compounded product, administered through DME, unit dose form, per mg
Use this code for Robinul.
MED: 100-2,15,110.3

Ⓜ ☑ **J7644** Ipratropium bromide, inhalation solution, FDA-approved final product, noncompounded, administered through DME, unit dose form, per mg
Use this code for Atrovent.
MED: 100-2,15,110.3

---

Special Coverage Instructions    Noncovered by Medicare    Carrier Discretion    ☑ Quantity Alert    ● New Code    ○ Recycled/Reinstated    ▲ Revised Code

**2008 HCPCS**    A2-Z3 ASC Payment Indicators    **MED:** Pub 100/NCD References    ⅙ DMEPOS Paid    ⊘ SNF Excluded    PQRI PQRI    **J Codes — 89**

**Drugs Administered Other Than Oral Method**

**J7645 — J8597**

M ☑ **J7645** Ipratropium bromide, inhalation solution, compounded product, administered through DME, unit dose form, per mg

M ☑ **J7647** Isoetharine HCl, inhalation solution, compounded product, administered through DME, concentrated form, per mg

M ☑ **J7648** Isoetharine HCl, inhalation solution, FDA-approved final product, noncompounded, administered through DME, concentrated form, per mg
Use this code for Beta-2.

MED: 100-2,15,110.3

M ☑ **J7649** Isoetharine HCl, inhalation solution, FDA-approved final product, noncompounded, administered through DME, unit dose form, per mg

MED: 100-2,15,110.3

M ☑ **J7650** Isoetharine HCl, inhalation solution, compounded product, administered through DME, unit dose form, per mg

M ☑ **J7657** Isoproterenol HCl, inhalation solution, compounded product, administered through DME, concentrated form, per mg

M ☑ **J7658** Isoproterenol HCl, inhalation solution, FDA-approved final product, noncompounded, administered through DME, concentrated form, per mg
Use this code for Isuprel HCl.

MED: 100-2,15,110.3

M ☑ **J7659** Isoproterenol HCl, inhalation solution, FDA-approved final product, noncompounded, administered through DME, unit dose form, per mg
Use this code for Isuprel HCl

MED: 100-2,15,110.3

M ☑ **J7660** Isoproterenol HCl, inhalation solution, compounded product, administered through DME, unit dose form, per mg

M ☑ **J7667** Metaproterenol sulfate, inhalation solution, compounded product, concentrated form, per 10 mg

M ☑ **J7668** Metaproterenol sulfate, inhalation solution, FDA-approved final product, noncompounded, administered through DME, concentrated form, per 10 mg
Use this code for Alupent

MED: 100-2,15,110.3

M ☑ **J7669** Metaproterenol sulfate, inhalation solution, FDA-approved final product, noncompounded, administered through DME, unit dose form, per 10 mg
Use this code for Alupent.

MED: 100-2,15,110.3

M ☑ **J7670** Metaproterenol sulfate, inhalation solution, compounded product, administered through DME, unit dose form, per 10 mg

N ☑ **J7674** Methacholine chloride administered as inhalation solution through a nebulizer, per 1 mg   [N1]

● M ☑ **J7676** Pentamidine isethionate, inhalation solution, compounded product, administered through DME, unit dose form, per 300 mg

M ☑ **J7680** Terbutaline sulfate, inhalation solution, compounded product, administered through DME, concentrated form, per mg
Use this code for Brethine.

MED: 100-2,15,110.3

M ☑ **J7681** Terbutaline sulfate, inhalation solution, compounded product, administered through DME, unit dose form, per mg
Use this code for Brethine.

MED: 100-2,15,110.3

M ☑ **J7682** Tobramycin, inhalation solution, FDA-approved final product, noncompounded, unit dose form, administered through DME, per 300 mg
Use this code for Tobi.

MED: 100-2,15,110.3

M ☑ **J7683** Triamcinolone, inhalation solution, compounded product, administered through DME, concentrated form, per mg
Use this code for Azmacort.

MED: 100-2,15,110.3

M ☑ **J7684** Triamcinolone, inhalation solution, compounded product, administered through DME, unit dose form, per mg
Use this code for Azmacort.

MED: 100-2,15,110.3

M ☑ **J7685** Tobramycin, inhalation solution, compounded product, administered through DME, unit dose form, per 300 mg

M **J7699** NOC drugs, inhalation solution administered through DME

MED: 100-2,15,110.3

N **J7799** NOC drugs, other than inhalation drugs, administered through DME   [N1]

MED: 100-2,15,110.3

B **J8498** Antiemetic drug, rectal/suppository, not otherwise specified

E **J8499** Prescription drug, oral, nonchemotherapeutic, NOS

MED: 100-2,15,50

K ☑ **J8501** Aprepitant, oral, 5 mg   [K2]
Use this code for Emend.

MED: 100-4,4,240; 100-4,17,80.2; 100-4,17,80.2.1; 100-4,17,80.2.4

K ☑ **J8510** Busulfan; oral, 2 mg   [K2]
Use this code for Busulfex, Myleran.

MED: 100-2,15,50.5; 100-4,4,240; 100-4,17,80.1.1

E ☑ **J8515** Cabergoline, oral, 0.25 mg
Use this code for Dostinex.

MED: 100-2,15,50.5; 100-4,4,240

K ☑ **J8520** Capecitabine, oral, 150 mg   [K2]
Use this code for Xeloda.

MED: 100-2,15,50.5; 100-4,4,240; 100-4,17,80.1.1

K ☑ **J8521** Capecitabine, oral, 500 mg   [K2]
Use this code for Xeloda.

MED: 100-2,15,50.5; 100-4,4,240; 100-4,17,80.1.1

N ☑ **J8530** Cyclophosphamide; oral, 25 mg   [N1]
Use this code for Cytoxan.

MED: 100-2,15,50.5; 100-4,4,240; 100-4,17,80.1.1

N ☑ **J8540** Dexamethasone, oral, 0.25 mg   [N1]
Use this code for Decadron.

K ☑ **J8560** Etoposide; oral, 50 mg   [K2]
Use this code for VePesid.

MED: 100-2,15,50.5; 100-4,4,230.1; 100-4,4,240; 100-4,17,80.1.1

E ☑ **J8565** Gefitinib, oral, 250 mg
Use this code for Iressa.

MED: 100-4,4,240; 100-4,17,80.1.1

N **J8597** Antiemetic drug, oral, not otherwise specified   [N1]

---

░ Special Coverage Instructions    ░ Noncovered by Medicare    ░ Carrier Discretion     ☑ Quantity Alert    ● New Code    ○ Recycled/Reinstated    ▲ Revised Code

K ☑ **J8600** Melphalan; oral, 2 mg    K2
Use this code for Alkeran.
MED: 100-2,15,50.5; 100-4,4,240; 100-4,17,80.1.1

N ☑ **J8610** Methotrexate; oral, 2.5 mg    N1
Use this code for Trexall.

Methotrexate is an anti-metabolite used in the treatment of certain neoplastic diseases, severe psoriasis, and adult rheumatoid arthritis.
MED: 100-2,15,50.5; 100-4,4,240; 100-4,17,80.1.1

K ☑ **J8650** Nabilone, oral, 1 mg    K2
Use this code for Cesamet

K ☑ **J8700** Temozolomide, oral, 5 mg    K2
Use this code for Temodar.
MED: 100-2,15,50.5; 100-4,4,240

B    **J8999** Prescription drug, oral, chemotherapeutic, NOS
Determine if an alternative HCPCS Level II or a CPT code better describes the service being reported. This code should be used only if a more specific code is unavailable.
MED: 100-2,15,50.5; 100-4,4,240; 100-4,17,80.1.1; 100-4,17,80.1.2

## CHEMOTHERAPY DRUGS J9000-J9999

These codes cover the cost of the chemotherapy drug only, not the administration. See also J8999.

N ☑ **J9000** Doxorubicin HCl, 10 mg    N1 ⊘
Use this code for Adriamycin PFS, Adriamycin RDF, Rubex.
MED: 100-2,15,50; 100-4,4,230.1; 100-4,17,80.2

K ☑ **J9001** Doxorubicin HCl, all lipid formulations, 10 mg    K2 ⊘
Use this code for Doxil.
MED: 100-2,15,50; 100-4,17,80.2

K ☑ **J9010** Alemtuzumab, 10 mg    K2 ⊘
Use this code for Campath.

K ☑ **J9015** Aldesleukin, per single use vial    K2 ⊘
Use this code for Proleukin, IL-2, Interleukin.
MED: 100-2,15,50

K ☑ **J9017** Arsenic trioxide, 1 mg    K2 ⊘
Use this code for Trisenox.
AHA: 2Q,'02,8

K ☑ **J9020** Asparaginase, 10,000 units    K2 ⊘
Use this code for Elspar.
MED: 100-2,15,50

K ☑ **J9025** Injection, azacitidine, 1 mg    K2 ⊘
Use this code for Vidaza.
MED: 100-4,4,230.1

K ☑ **J9027** Injection, clofarabine, 1 mg    K2 ⊘
Use this code for Clolar.
MED: 100-4,4,230.1

K ☑ **J9031** BCG live (intravesical), per instillation    K2
Use this code for Tice BCG, PACIS BCG, TheraCys.
MED: 100-2,15,50

K ☑ **J9035** Injection, bevacizumab, 10 mg    K2 ⊘
Use this code for Avastin.

K ☑ **J9040** Bleomycin sulfate, 15 units    K2 ⊘
Use this code for Blenoxane.
MED: 100-2,15,50; 100-4,4,230.1

K ☑ **J9041** Injection, bortezomib, 0.1 mg    K2 ⊘
Use this code for Velcade.

K ☑ **J9045** Carboplatin, 50 mg    K2 ⊘
Use this code for Paraplatin, Platinol AQ.
MED: 100-2,15,50

K ☑ **J9050** Carmustine, 100 mg    K2 ⊘
Use this code for BiCNU.
MED: 100-2,15,50; 100-4,4,230.1; 100-4,17,80.2

K ☑ **J9055** Injection, cetuximab, 10 mg    K2 ⊘
Use this code for Erbitux.

N ☑ **J9060** Cisplatin, powder or solution, per 10 mg    N1 ⊘
Use this code for Plantinol AQ.
MED: 100-2,15,50; 100-4,4,230.1; 100-4,17,80.2

N ☑ **J9062** Cisplatin, 50 mg    N1 ⊘
Use this code for Plantinol AQ.
MED: 100-2,15,50; 100-4,17,80.2

K ☑ **J9065** Injection, cladribine, per 1 mg    K2 ⊘
Use this code for Leustatin.
MED: 100-2,15,50; 100-4,4,230.1

N ☑ **J9070** Cyclophosphamide, 100 mg    N1 ⊘
Use this code for Endoxan-Asta.
MED: 100-2,15,50; 100-4,4,230.1; 100-4,17,80.2

N ☑ **J9080** Cyclophosphamide, 200 mg    N1 ⊘
Use this code for Cytoxan, Neosar.
MED: 100-2,15,50; 100-4,17,80.2

N ☑ **J9090** Cyclophosphamide, 500 mg    N1 ⊘
Use this code for Cytoxan, Neosar.
MED: 100-2,15,50; 100-4,17,80.2

N ☑ **J9091** Cyclophosphamide, 1 g    N1 ⊘
Use this code for Cytoxan, Neosar.
MED: 100-2,15,50; 100-4,17,80.2

N ☑ **J9092** Cyclophosphamide, 2 g    N1 ⊘
Use this code for Cytoxan, Neosar.
MED: 100-2,15,50; 100-4,17,80.2

N ☑ **J9093** Cyclophosphamide, lyophilized, 100 mg    N1 ⊘
Use this code for Cytoxan Lyophilized.
MED: 100-2,15,50; 100-4,4,230.1; 100-4,17,80.2

N ☑ **J9094** Cyclophosphamide, lyophilized, 200 mg    N1 ⊘
Use this code for Cytoxan Lyophilized.
MED: 100-2,15,50; 100-4,17,80.2

N ☑ **J9095** Cyclophosphamide, lyophilized, 500 mg    N1 ⊘
Use this code for Cytoxan Lyophilized.
MED: 100-2,15,50; 100-4,17,80.2

N ☑ **J9096** Cyclophosphamide, lyophilized, 1 g    N1 ⊘
Use this code for Cytoxan Lyophilized.
MED: 100-2,15,50; 100-4,17,80.2

N ☑ **J9097** Cyclophosphamide, lyophilized, 2 g    N1 ⊘
Use this code for Cytoxan Lyophilized.
MED: 100-2,15,50; 100-4,17,80.2

K ☑ **J9098** Cytarabine liposome, 10 mg    K2 ⊘
Use this code for Depocyt.

N ☑ **J9100** Cytarabine, 100 mg    N1 ⊘
Use this code for Cytosar-U, Ara-C, Tarabin CFS.
MED: 100-2,15,50; 100-4,4,230.1

N ☑ **J9110** Cytarabine, 500 mg    N1 ⊘
Use this code for Cytosar-U.
MED: 100-2,15,50

K ☑ **J9120** Dactinomycin, 0.5 mg    K2 ⊘
Use this code for Cosmegen.
MED: 100-2,15,50

---

Special Coverage Instructions    Noncovered by Medicare    Carrier Discretion    ☑ Quantity Alert   ● New Code   ○ Recycled/Reinstated   ▲ Revised Code

**2008 HCPCS**    A2-Z3 ASC Payment Indicators    **MED:** Pub 100/NCD References   ♿ DMEPOS Paid   ⊘ SNF Excluded   PQ PQRI    **J Codes — 91**

**Chemotherapy Drugs**

**J9130 — J9265**

N ☑ **J9130** Dacarbazine, 100 mg   N1 ⊘
Use this code for DTIC-Dome.
MED: 100-2,15,50; 100-4,4,230.1; 100-4,17,80.2

N ☑ **J9140** Dacarbazine, 200 mg   N1 ⊘
Use this code for DTIC-Dome.
MED: 100-2,15,50; 100-4,17,80.2

K ☑ **J9150** Daunorubicin, 10 mg   K2 ⊘
Use this code for Cerubidine.
MED: 100-2,15,50; 100-4,4,230.1

K ☑ **J9151** Daunorubicin citrate, liposomal formulation, 10 mg   K2 ⊘
Use this code for Daunoxome.
MED: 100-2,15,50

K ☑ **J9160** Denileukin diftitox, 300 mcg   K2 ⊘
Use this code for Ontak.

N ☑ **J9165** Diethylstilbestrol diphosphate, 250 mg   N1
Use this code for Stilphostrol.
MED: 100-2,15,50; 100-4,4,230.1

K ☑ **J9170** Docetaxel, 20 mg   K2 ⊘
Use this code for Taxotere.
MED: 100-2,15,50

N ☑ **J9175** Injection, Elliotts' B solution, 1 ml   N1
MED: 100-2,15,50; 100-4,4,230.1

K ☑ **J9178** Injection, epirubicin HCl, 2 mg   K2 ⊘
Use this code for Ellence.
MED: 100-4,17,80.2

N ☑ **J9181** Etoposide, 10 mg   N1 ⊘
Use this code for VePesid, Toposar.
MED: 100-2,15,50; 100-4,4,230.1

N ☑ **J9182** Etoposide, 100 mg   N1 ⊘
Use this code for VePesid, Toposar.
MED: 100-2,15,50

K ☑ **J9185** Fludarabine phosphate, 50 mg   K2 ⊘
Use this code for Fludara.
MED: 100-2,15,50

N ☑ **J9190** Fluorouracil, 500 mg   N1
Use this code for Adrucil.
MED: 100-2,15,50

K ☑ **J9200** Floxuridine, 500 mg   K2 ⊘
Use this code for FUDR.
MED: 100-2,15,50; 100-4,4,230.1

K ☑ **J9201** Gemcitabine HCl, 200 mg   K2 ⊘
Use this code for Gemzar.
MED: 100-2,15,50

K ☑ **J9202** Goserelin acetate implant, per 3.6 mg   K2
Use this code for Zoladex.
MED: 100-2,15,50

K ☑ **J9206** Irinotecan, 20 mg   K2 ⊘
Use this code for Camptosar.
MED: 100-2,15,50

K ☑ **J9208** Ifosfamide, per 1 g   K2 ⊘
Use this code for IFEX, Mitoxana.
MED: 100-2,15,50; 100-4,4,230.1

K ☑ **J9209** Mesna, 200 mg   K2
Use this code for Mesnex.
MED: 100-2,15,50; 100-4,4,230.1

K ☑ **J9211** Idarubicin HCl, 5 mg   K2 ⊘
Use this code for Idamycin.
MED: 100-2,15,50; 100-4,4,230.1

K ☑ **J9212** Injection, interferon alfacon-1, recombinant, 1 mcg   K2
Use this code for Infergen.
MED: 100-2,15,50

K ☑ **J9213** Interferon alfa-2a, recombinant, 3 million units   K2
Use this code for Roferon-A.
MED: 100-2,15,50

K ☑ **J9214** Interferon alfa-2B, recombinant, 1 million units   K2
Use this code for Intron A, Rebetron Kit.
MED: 100-2,15,50

K ☑ **J9215** Interferon alfa-N3, (human leukocyte derived), 250,000 IU   K2
Use this code for Alferon N.
MED: 100-2,15,50

K ☑ **J9216** Interferon gamma-1B, 3 million units   K2
Use this code for Actimmune.
MED: 100-2,15,50

K ☑ **J9217** Leuprolide acetate (for depot suspension), 7.5 mg   K2
Use this code for Lupron Depot, Eligard.
MED: 100-2,15,50

K ☑ **J9218** Leuprolide acetate, per 1 mg   K2
Use this code for Lupron.
MED: 100-2,15,50; 100-4,4,230.1

K ☑ **J9219** Leuprolide acetate implant, 65 mg   K2
Use this code for Lupron Implant.
MED: 100-2,15,50
AHA: 4Q,'01,5

▲ K ☑ **J9225** Histrelin implant (Vantas), 50 mg   K2 ⊘
Use this code for Supprelin LA, Vantas.
MED: 100-2,15,50

● K ☑ **J9226** Histrelin implant (Supprelin LA), 50 mg

K ☑ **J9230** Mechlorethamine HCl, (nitrogen mustard), 10 mg   K2 ⊘
Use this code for Mustargen.
MED: 100-2,15,50; 100-4,17,80.2

K ☑ **J9245** Injection, melphalan HCl, 50 mg   K2 ⊘
Use this code for Alkeran, L-phenylalanine mustard.
MED: 100-2,15,50

N ☑ **J9250** Methotrexate sodium, 5 mg   N1
Use this code for Folex, Folex PFS, Methotrexate LPF.
MED: 100-2,15,50

N ☑ **J9260** Methotrexate sodium, 50 mg   N1
Use this code for Folex, Folex PFS, Methotrexate LPF.
MED: 100-2,15,50

G ☑ **J9261** Injection, nelarabine, 50 mg   K2 ⊘
Use this code for Arranon.

K ☑ **J9263** Injection, oxaliplatin, 0.5 mg   K2 ⊘
Use this code for Eloxatin.
MED: 100-4,4,230.1

K ☑ **J9264** Injection, paclitaxel protein-bound particles, 1 mg   K2 ⊘
Use this code for Abraxane.
MED: 100-4,4,230.1

K ☑ **J9265** Paclitaxel, 30 mg   K2 ⊘
Use this code for Taxol, Nov-Onxol.
MED: 100-2,15,50; 100-4,4,230.1

---

Special Coverage Instructions   Noncovered by Medicare   Carrier Discretion   ☑ Quantity Alert   ● New Code   ○ Recycled/Reinstated   ▲ Revised Code

K ☑ **J9266** Pegaspargase, per single dose vial  K2 ⊘
Use this code for Oncaspar.

MED: 100-2,15,50

AHA: 2Q,'02,8

K ☑ **J9268** Pentostatin, per 10 mg  K2 ⊘
Use this code for Nipent.

MED: 100-2,15,50

K ☑ **J9270** Plicamycin, 2.5 mg  K2 ⊘
Use this code for Mithacin.

MED: 100-2,15,50

K ☑ **J9280** Mitomycin, 5 mg  K2 ⊘
Use this code for Mutamycin.

MED: 100-2,15,50; 100-4,4,230.1

K ☑ **J9290** Mitomycin, 20 mg  K2 ⊘
Use this code for Mutamycin.

MED: 100-2,15,50

K ☑ **J9291** Mitomycin, 40 mg  K2 ⊘
Use this code for Mutamycin.

MED: 100-2,15,50

K ☑ **J9293** Injection, mitoxantrone HCl, per 5 mg  K2 ⊘
Use this code for Navantrone.

MED: 100-2,15,50

K ☑ **J9300** Gemtuzumab ozogamicin, 5 mg  K2 ⊘
Use this code for Mylotarg.

AHA: 2Q,'02,8

● G ☑ **J9303** Injection, panitumumab, 10 mg
Use this code for Vectibix.

K ☑ **J9305** Injection, pemetrexed, 10 mg  K2 ⊘
Use this code for Alimta.

K ☑ **J9310** Rituximab, 100 mg  K2 ⊘
Use this code for RituXan.

MED: 100-2,15,50

K ☑ **J9320** Streptozocin, 1 g  K2 ⊘
Use this code for Zanosar.

MED: 100-2,15,50; 100-4,17,80.2

K ☑ **J9340** Thiotepa, 15 mg  K2 ⊘
Use this code for Thioplex.

MED: 100-2,15,50; 100-4,4,230.1

K ☑ **J9350** Topotecan, 4 mg  K2 ⊘
Use this code for Hycamtin.

MED: 100-2,15,50

K ☑ **J9355** Trastuzumab, 10 mg  K2 ⊘
Use this code for Herceptin.

K ☑ **J9357** Valrubicin, intravesical, 200 mg  K2 ⊘
Use this code for Valstar.

MED: 100-2,15,50

N ☑ **J9360** Vinblastine sulfate, 1 mg  N1 ⊘
Use this code for Velban.

MED: 100-2,15,50

N ☑ **J9370** Vincristine sulfate, 1 mg  N1 ⊘
Use this code for Oncovin, Vincasar PFS.

MED: 100-2,15,50

N ☑ **J9375** Vincristine sulfate, 2 mg  N1 ⊘
Use this code for Oncovin, Vincasar PFS.

MED: 100-2,15,50

N ☑ **J9380** Vincristine sulfate, 5 mg  N1 ⊘
Use this code for Oncovin.

MED: 100-2,15,50

K ☑ **J9390** Vinorelbine tartrate, per 10 mg  K2 ⊘
Use this code for Navelbine.

MED: 100-2,15,50; 100-4,4,230.1

K ☑ **J9395** Injection, fulvestrant, 25 mg  K2 ⊘
Use this code for Fastodex.

K ☑ **J9600** Porfimer sodium, 75 mg  K2 ⊘
Use this code for Photofrin.

MED: 100-2,15,50

N **J9999** NOC, antineoplastic drug  N1
Determine if an alternative HCPCS Level II or a CPT code better describes the service being reported. This code should be used only if a more specific code is unavailable.

MED: 100-2,15,50; 100-3,110.2

---

Special Coverage Instructions    Noncovered by Medicare    Carrier Discretion    ☑ Quantity Alert    ● New Code    ○ Recycled/Reinstated    ▲ Revised Code

**2008 HCPCS**    A2-Z6 ASC Payment Indicators    **MED:** Pub 100/NCD References    ⅙ DMEPOS Paid    ⊘ SNF Excluded    P0 PQRI    **J Codes — 93**

## TEMPORARY CODES K0000-K9999

The K codes were established for use by the DME Medicare Administrative Contractors (DME MACs). The K codes are developed when the currently existing permanent national codes for supplies and certain product categories do not include the codes needed to implement a DME MAC medical review policy.

## K CODES ASSIGNED TO DURABLE MEDICAL EQUIPMENT ADMINISTRATIVE CONTRACTORS (DME MACS)

### WHEELCHAIR AND WHEELCHAIR ACCESSORIES

Y K0001 Standard wheelchair ⊘ &

Y K0002 Standard hemi (low seat) wheelchair ⊘ &

Y K0003 Lightweight wheelchair ⊘ &

Y K0004 High strength, lightweight wheelchair ⊘ &

Y K0005 Ultralightweight wheelchair ⊘ &

Y K0006 Heavy-duty wheelchair ⊘ &

Y K0007 Extra heavy-duty wheelchair ⊘ &

Y K0009 Other manual wheelchair/base ⊘

Y K0010 Standard-weight frame motorized/power wheelchair ⊘ &

Y K0011 Standard-weight frame motorized/power wheelchair with programmable control parameters for speed adjustment, tremor dampening, acceleration control and braking ⊘ &

Y K0012 Lightweight portable motorized/power wheelchair ⊘ &

Y K0014 Other motorized/power wheelchair base ⊘

Y ☑ K0015 Detachable, nonadjustable height armrest, each ⊘ &

Y ☑ K0017 Detachable, adjustable height armrest, base, each ⊘ &

Y ☑ K0018 Detachable, adjustable height armrest, upper portion, each ⊘ &

Y ☑ K0019 Arm pad, each ⊘ &

Y ☑ K0020 Fixed, adjustable height armrest, pair ⊘ &

Y ☑ K0037 High mount flip-up footrest, each ⊘ &

Y ☑ K0038 Leg strap, each ⊘ &

Y ☑ K0039 Leg strap, H style, each ⊘ &

Y ☑ K0040 Adjustable angle footplate, each ⊘ &

Y ☑ K0041 Large size footplate, each ⊘ &

Y ☑ K0042 Standard size footplate, each ⊘ &

Y ☑ K0043 Footrest, lower extension tube, each ⊘ &

Y ☑ K0044 Footrest, upper hanger bracket, each ⊘ &

Y K0045 Footrest, complete assembly ⊘ &

Y ☑ K0046 Elevating leg rest, lower extension tube, each ⊘ &

Y ☑ K0047 Elevating leg rest, upper hanger bracket, each ⊘ &

Y K0050 Ratchet assembly ⊘ &

Y ☑ K0051 Cam release assembly, footrest or leg rest, each ⊘ &

Y ☑ K0052 Swingaway, detachable foot rests, each ⊘ &

Y ☑ K0053 Elevating footrests, articulating (telescoping), each ⊘ &

Y ☑ K0056 Seat height less than 17 in. or equal to or greater than 21 in. for a high strength, lightweight, or ultralightweight wheelchair ⊘ &

Y ☑ K0065 Spoke protectors, each ⊘ &

Y ☑ K0069 Rear wheel assembly, complete, with solid tire, spokes or molded, each ⊘ &

Y ☑ K0070 Rear wheel assembly, complete with pneumatic tire, spokes or molded, each ⊘ &

Y ☑ K0071 Front caster assembly, complete, with pneumatic tire, each ⊘ &

Y ☑ K0072 Front caster assembly, complete, with semipneumatic tire, each ⊘ &

Y ☑ K0073 Caster pin lock, each ⊘ &

Y ☑ K0077 Front caster assembly, complete, with solid tire, each ⊘ &

Y K0098 Drive belt for power wheelchair ⊘ &

Y ☑ K0105 IV hanger, each ⊘ &

Y K0108 Wheelchair component or accessory, not otherwise specified ⊘

Y K0195 Elevating legrest, pair (for use with capped rental wheelchair base)
MED: 100-3,230.10

Y K0455 Infusion pump used for uninterrupted parenteral administration of medication, (e.g., epoprostenol or treprostinol) ⊘ &
MED: 100-3,280.14

Y K0462 Temporary replacement for patient owned equipment being repaired, any type ⊘
MED: 100-4,20,40.1

Y ☑ K0552 Supplies for external drug infusion pump, syringe type cartridge, sterile, each ⊘ &
MED: 100-3,280.14

~~K0553~~ ~~Combination oral/nasal mask, used with continuous positive airway pressure device, each~~
See A7027.

~~K0554~~ ~~Oral cushion for combination oral/nasal mask, replacement only, each~~
See A7029.

~~K0555~~ ~~Nasal pillows for combination oral/nasal mask, replacement only, pair~~

Y ☑ K0601 Replacement battery for external infusion pump owned by patient, silver oxide, 1.5 volt, each ⊘ &
AHA: 2Q,'03,7

Y ☑ K0602 Replacement battery for external infusion pump owned by patient, silver oxide, 3 volt, each ⊘ &
AHA: 2Q,'03,7

Y ☑ K0603 Replacement battery for external infusion pump owned by patient, alkaline, 1.5 volt, each ⊘ &
AHA: 2Q,'03,7

Y ☑ K0604 Replacement battery for external infusion pump owned by patient, lithium, 3.6 volt, each ⊘ &
AHA: 2Q,'03,7

Y ☑ K0605 Replacement battery for external infusion pump owned by patient, lithium, 4.5 volt, each ⊘ &
AHA: 2Q,'03,7

Y K0606 Automatic external defibrillator, with integrated electrocardiogram analysis, garment type ⊘ &
AHA: 4Q,'03,4

Y ☑ K0607 Replacement battery for automated external defibrillator, garment type only, each ⊘ &
AHA: 4Q,'03,4

Y ☑ K0608 Replacement garment for use with automated external defibrillator, each ⊘ &
AHA: 4Q,'03,4

| ▨ Special Coverage Instructions | ▨ Noncovered by Medicare | ▨ Carrier Discretion | ☑ Quantity Alert | ● New Code | ○ Recycled/Reinstated | ▲ Revised Code |

**2008 HCPCS** | A2-Z3 ASC Payment Indicators | MED: Pub 100/NCD References | & DMEPOS Paid | ⊘ SNF Excluded | PQRI PQRI | **K Codes — 95**

**Temporary Codes**

**K0609 — K0852**

Ⓨ ☑ **K0609** Replacement electrodes for use with automated external defibrillator, garment type only, each ⊘ �
AHA: 4Q,'03,4

Ⓨ **K0669** Wheelchair accessory, wheelchair seat or back cushion, does not meet specific code criteria or no written coding verification from SADMERC

Ⓨ **K0730** Controlled dose inhalation drug delivery system

Ⓨ **K0733** Power wheelchair accessory, 12 to 24 amp hour sealed lead acid battery, each (e.g. gel cell, absorbed glassmat) ⅙

Ⓨ **K0734** Skin protection wheelchair seat cushion, adjustable, width less than 22 inches, any depth

Ⓨ **K0735** Skin protection wheelchair seat cushion, adjustable, width 22 inches or greater, any depth

Ⓨ **K0736** Skin protection and positioning wheelchair seat cushion, adjustable, width less than 22 inches, any depth

Ⓨ **K0737** Skin protection and positioning wheelchair seat cushion, adjustable, width 22 inches or greater, any depth

Ⓨ **K0738** Portable gaseous oxygen system, rental; home compressor used to fill portable oxygen cylinders; includes portable containers, regulator, flowmeter, humidifier, cannula or mask, and tubing

Ⓨ **K0800** Power operated vehicle, group 1 standard, patient weight capacity up to and including 300 pounds ⅙

Ⓨ **K0801** Power operated vehicle, group 1 heavy duty, patient weight capacity 301 to 450 pounds ⅙

Ⓨ **K0802** Power operated vehicle, group 1 very heavy duty, patient weight capacity 451 to 600 pounds ⅙

Ⓨ **K0806** Power operated vehicle, group 2 standard, patient weight capacity up to and including 300 pounds ⅙

Ⓨ **K0807** Power operated vehicle, group 2 heavy duty, patient weight capacity 301 to 450 pounds ⅙

Ⓨ **K0808** Power operated vehicle, group 2 very heavy duty, patient weight capacity 451 to 600 pounds ⅙

Ⓨ **K0812** Power operated vehicle, not otherwise classified ⅙

Ⓨ **K0813** Power wheelchair, group 1 standard, portable, sling/solid seat and back, patient weight capacity up to and including 300 pounds ⅙

Ⓨ **K0814** Power wheelchair, group 1 standard, portable, captains chair, patient weight capacity up to and including 300 pounds ⅙

Ⓨ **K0815** Power wheelchair, group 1 standard, sling/solid seat and back, patient weight capacity up to and including 300 pounds ⅙

Ⓨ **K0816** Power wheelchair, group 1 standard, captain's chair, patient weight capacity up to and including 300 pounds ⅙

Ⓨ **K0820** Power wheelchair, group 2 standard, portable, sling/solid seat/back, patient weight capacity up to and including 300 pounds ⅙

Ⓨ **K0821** Power wheelchair, group 2 standard, portable, captain's chair, patient weight capacity up to and including 300 pounds ⅙

Ⓨ **K0822** Power wheelchair, group 2 standard, sling/solid seat/back, patient weight capacity up to and including 300 pounds ⅙

Ⓨ **K0823** Power wheelchair, group 2 standard, captain's chair, patient weight capacity up to and including 300 pounds ⅙

Ⓨ **K0824** Power wheelchair, group 2 heavy duty, sling/solid seat/back, patient weight capacity 301 to 450 pounds ⅙

Ⓨ **K0825** Power wheelchair, group 2 heavy duty, captain's chair, patient weight capacity 301 to 450 pounds ⅙

Ⓨ **K0826** Power wheelchair, group 2 very heavy duty, sling/solid seat/back, patient weight capacity 451 to 600 pounds ⅙

Ⓨ **K0827** Power wheelchair, group 2 very heavy duty, captain's chair, patient weight capacity 451 to 600 pounds ⅙

Ⓨ **K0828** Power wheelchair, group 2 extra heavy duty, sling/solid seat/back, patient weight capacity 601 pounds or more ⅙

Ⓨ **K0829** Power wheelchair, group 2 extra heavy duty, captain's chair, patient weight capacity 601 pounds or more ⅙

Ⓨ **K0830** Power wheelchair, group 2 standard, seat elevator, sling/solid seat/back, patient weight capacity up to and including 300 pounds ⅙

Ⓨ **K0831** Power wheelchair, group 2 standard, seat elevator, captain's chair, patient weight capacity up to and including 300 pounds ⅙

Ⓨ **K0835** Power wheelchair, group 2 standard, single power option, sling/solid seat/back, patient weight capacity up to and including 300 pounds ⅙

Ⓨ **K0836** Power wheelchair, group 2 standard, single power option, captain's chair, patient weight capacity up to and including 300 pounds ⅙

Ⓨ **K0837** Power wheelchair, group 2 heavy duty, single power option, sling/solid seat/back, patient weight capacity 301 to 450 pounds ⅙

Ⓨ **K0838** Power wheelchair, group 2 heavy duty, single power option, captain's chair, patient weight capacity 301 to 450 pounds ⅙

Ⓨ **K0839** Power wheelchair, group 2 very heavy duty, single power option, sling/solid seat/back, patient weight capacity 451 to 600 pounds ⅙

Ⓨ **K0840** Power wheelchair, group 2 extra heavy duty, single power option, sling/solid seat/back, patient weight capacity 601 pounds or more ⅙

Ⓨ **K0841** Power wheelchair, group 2 standard, multiple power option, sling/solid seat/back, patient weight capacity up to and including 300 pounds ⅙

Ⓨ **K0842** Power wheelchair, group 2 standard, multiple power option, captain's chair, patient weight capacity up to and including 300 pounds ⅙

Ⓨ **K0843** Power wheelchair, group 2 heavy duty, multiple power option, sling/solid seat/back, patient weight capacity 301 to 450 pounds ⅙

Ⓨ **K0848** Power wheelchair, group 3 standard, sling/solid seat/back, patient weight capacity up to and including 300 pounds ⅙

Ⓨ **K0849** Power wheelchair, group 3 standard, captain's chair, patient weight capacity up to and including 300 pounds ⅙

Ⓨ **K0850** Power wheelchair, group 3 heavy duty, sling/solid seat/back, patient weight capacity 301 to 450 pounds ⅙

Ⓨ **K0851** Power wheelchair, group 3 heavy duty, captain's chair, patient weight capacity 301 to 450 pounds ⅙

Ⓨ **K0852** Power wheelchair, group 3 very heavy duty, sling/solid seat/back, patient weight capacity 451 to 600 pounds ⅙

---

▨ Special Coverage Instructions    ▨ Noncovered by Medicare    ▨ Carrier Discretion     ☑ Quantity Alert   ● New Code   ○ Recycled/Reinstated   ▲ Revised Code

**96 — K Codes**    Ⓐ Age Edit    Ⓜ Maternity Edit   ♀ Female Only   ♂ Male Only   Ⓐ-Ⓨ OPPS Status Indicators    **2008 HCPCS**

Y **K0853** Power wheelchair, group 3 very heavy duty, captain's chair, patient weight capacity, 451 to 600 pounds &

Y **K0854** Power wheelchair, group 3 extra heavy duty, sling/solid seat/back, patient weight capacity 601 pounds or more &

Y **K0855** Power wheelchair, group 3 extra heavy duty, captain's chair, patient weight 601 pounds or more &

Y **K0856** Power wheelchair, group 3 standard, single power option, sling/solid seat/back, patient weight capacity up to and including 300 pounds &

Y **K0857** Power wheelchair, group 3 standard, single power option, captain's chair, patient weight capacity up to and including 300 pounds &

Y **K0858** Power wheelchair, group 3 heavy duty, single power option, sling/solid seat/back, patient weight capacity 301 to 450 pounds &

Y **K0859** Power wheelchair, group 3 heavy duty, single power option, captain's chair, patient weight capacity 301 to 450 pounds &

Y **K0860** Power wheelchair, group 3 very heavy duty, single power option, sling/solid seat/back, patient weight capacity 451 to 600 pounds &

Y **K0861** Power wheelchair, group 3 standard, multiple power option, sling/solid seat/back, patient weight capacity up to and including 300 pounds &

Y **K0862** Power wheelchair, group 3 heavy duty, multiple power option, sling/solid seat/back, patient weight capacity 301 to 450 pounds &

Y **K0863** Power wheelchair, group 3 very heavy duty, multiple power option, sling/solid seat/back, patient weight capacity 451 to 600 pounds &

Y **K0864** Power wheelchair, group 3 extra heavy duty, multiple power option, sling/solid seat/back, patient weight capacity 601 pounds or more &

Y **K0868** Power wheelchair, group 4 standard, sling/solid seat/back, patient weight capacity up to and including 300 pounds &

Y **K0869** Power wheelchair, group 4 standard, captain's chair, patient weight capacity up to and including 300 pounds &

Y **K0870** Power wheelchair, group 4 heavy duty, sling/solid seat/back, patient weight capacity 301 to 450 pounds &

Y **K0871** Power wheelchair, group 4 very heavy duty, sling/solid seat/back, patient weight capacity 451 to 600 pounds &

Y **K0877** Power wheelchair, group 4 standard, single power option, sling/solid seat/back, patient weight capacity up to and including 300 pounds &

Y **K0878** Power wheelchair, group 4 standard, single power option, captain's chair, patient weight capacity up to and including 300 pounds &

Y **K0879** Power wheelchair, group 4 heavy duty, single power option, sling/solid seat/back, patient weight capacity 301 to 450 pounds &

Y **K0880** Power wheelchair, group 4 very heavy duty, single power option, sling/solid seat/back, patient weight 451 to 600 pounds &

Y **K0884** Power wheelchair, group 4 standard multiple power option, sling/solid seat/back, patient weight capacity up to and including 300 pounds &

Y **K0885** Power wheelchair, group 4 standard, multiple power option, captain's chair, weight capacity up to and including 300 pounds &

Y **K0886** Power wheelchair, group 4 heavy duty, multiple power option, sling/solid seat/back, patient weight capacity 301 to 450 pounds &

Y **K0890** Power wheelchair, group 5 pediatric, single power option, sling/solid seat/back, patient weight capacity up to and including 125 pounds &

Y **K0891** Power wheelchair, group 5 pediatric, multiple power option, sling/solid seat/back, patient weight capacity up to and including 125 pounds &

Y **K0898** Power wheelchair, not otherwise classified &

Y **K0899** Power mobility device, not coded by SADMERC or does not meet criteria &

Special Coverage Instructions | Noncovered by Medicare | Carrier Discretion | ☑ Quantity Alert | ● New Code | ○ Recycled/Reinstated | ▲ Revised Code

**2008 HCPCS** | A2-Z3 ASC Payment Indicators | **MED:** Pub 100/NCD References | & DMEPOS Paid | ⊘ SNF Excluded | PQ PQRI | **K Codes — 97**

## ORTHOTIC PROCEDURES AND DEVICES L0000-L4999

L codes include orthotic and prosthetic procedures and devices, as well as scoliosis equipment, orthopedic shoes, and prosthetic implants.

## ORTHOTIC DEVICES - SPINAL

### CERVICAL

Ⓐ **L0112** Cranial cervical orthosis, congenital torticollis type, with or without soft interface material, adjustable range of motion joint, custom fabricated

Ⓐ **L0120** Cervical, flexible, nonadjustable (foam collar)

Ⓐ **L0130** Cervical, flexible, thermoplastic collar, molded to patient

Ⓐ **L0140** Cervical, semi-rigid, adjustable (plastic collar)

Ⓐ **L0150** Cervical, semi-rigid, adjustable molded chin cup (plastic collar with mandibular/occipital piece)

Ⓐ **L0160** Cervical, semi-rigid, wire frame occipital/mandibular support

Ⓐ **L0170** Cervical, collar, molded to patient model

Ⓐ **L0172** Cervical, collar, semi-rigid thermoplastic foam, two piece

Ⓐ **L0174** Cervical, collar, semi-rigid, thermoplastic foam, two piece with thoracic extension

### MULTIPLE POST COLLAR

Ⓐ **L0180** Cervical, multiple post collar, occipital/mandibular supports, adjustable

Ⓐ **L0190** Cervical, multiple post collar, occipital/mandibular supports, adjustable cervical bars (SOMI, Guilford, Taylor types)

Ⓐ **L0200** Cervical, multiple post collar, occipital/mandibular supports, adjustable cervical bars, and thoracic extension

### THORACIC

Ⓐ **L0210** Thoracic, rib belt

Ⓐ **L0220** Thoracic, rib belt, custom fabricated

Ⓐ **L0430** Spinal orthosis, anterior-posterior-lateral control, with interface material, custom fitted (DeWall Posture Protector only)

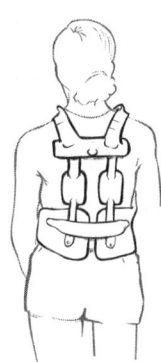

TLSO brace with adjustable straps and pads (L0450). The model at right and similar devices such as the Boston brace are molded polymer over foam and may be bivalve (front and back components)

Thoracic lumbar sacral orthosis (TLSO)

Ⓐ **L0450** TLSO, flexible, provides trunk support, upper thoracic region, produces intracavitary pressure to reduce load on the intervertebral disks with rigid stays or panel(s), includes shoulder straps and closures, prefabricated, includes fitting and adjustment

Ⓐ **L0452** TLSO, flexible, provides trunk support, upper thoracic region, produces intracavitary pressure to reduce load on the intervertebral disks with rigid stays or panel(s), includes shoulder straps and closures, custom fabricated

Ⓐ **L0454** TLSO flexible, provides trunk support, extends from sacrococcygeal junction to above T-9 vertebra, restricts gross trunk motion in the sagittal plane, produces intracavitary pressure to reduce load on the intervertebral disks with rigid stays or panel(s), includes shoulder straps and closures, prefabricated, includes fitting and adjustment

Ⓐ **L0456** TLSO, flexible, provides trunk support, thoracic region, rigid posterior panel and soft anterior apron, extends from the sacrococcygeal junction and terminates just inferior to the scapular spine, restricts gross trunk motion in the sagittal plane, produces intracavitary pressure to reduce load on the intervertebral disks, includes straps and closures, prefabricated, includes fitting and adjustment

Ⓐ **L0458** TLSO, triplanar control, modular segmented spinal system, two rigid plastic shells, posterior extends from the sacrococcygeal junction and terminates just inferior to the scapular spine, anterior extends from the symphysis pubis to the xiphoid, soft liner, restricts gross trunk motion in the sagittal, coronal, and transverse planes, lateral strength is provided by overlapping plastic and stabilizing closures, includes straps and closures, prefabricated, includes fitting and adjustment

Ⓐ **L0460** TLSO, triplanar control, modular segmented spinal system, two rigid plastic shells, posterior extends from the sacrococcygeal junction and terminates just inferior to the scapular spine, anterior extends from the symphysis pubis to the sternal notch, soft liner, restricts gross trunk motion in the sagittal, coronal, and transverse planes, lateral strength is provided by overlapping plastic and stabilizing closures, includes straps and closures, prefabricated, includes fitting and adjustment  &#9855;

Ⓐ **L0462** TLSO, triplanar control, modular segmented spinal system, three rigid plastic shells, posterior extends from the sacrococcygeal junction and terminates just inferior to the scapular spine, anterior extends from the symphysis pubis to the sternal notch, soft liner, restricts gross trunk motion in the sagittal, coronal, and transverse planes, lateral strength is provided by overlapping plastic and stabilizing closures, includes straps and closures, prefabricated, includes fitting and adjustment  &#9855;

Ⓐ **L0464** TLSO, triplanar control, modular segmented spinal system, four rigid plastic shells, posterior extends from sacrococcygeal junction and terminates just inferior to scapular spine, anterior extends from symphysis pubis to the sternal notch, soft liner, restricts gross trunk motion in sagittal, coronal, and transverse planes, lateral strength is provided by overlapping plastic and stabilizing closures, includes straps and closures, prefabricated, includes fitting and adjustment  &#9855;

Ⓐ **L0466** TLSO, sagittal control, rigid posterior frame and flexible soft anterior apron with straps, closures and padding, restricts gross trunk motion in sagittal plane, produces intracavitary pressure to reduce load on intervertebral disks, includes fitting and shaping the frame, prefabricated, includes fitting and adjustment  &#9855;

⬛ Special Coverage Instructions    ⬛ Noncovered by Medicare    ⬛ Carrier Discretion    ☑ Quantity Alert    ● New Code    ○ Recycled/Reinstated    ▲ Revised Code

**2008 HCPCS**    A2-Z3 ASC Payment Indicators    **MED:** Pub 100/NCD References    &#9855; DMEPOS Paid    ⊘ SNF Excluded    PQ PQRI    **L Codes — 99**

Ⓐ **L0468** TLSO, sagittal-coronal control, rigid posterior frame and flexible soft anterior apron with straps, closures and padding, extends from sacrococcygeal junction over scapulae, lateral strength provided by pelvic, thoracic, and lateral frame pieces, restricts gross trunk motion in sagittal, and coronal planes, produces intracavitary pressure to reduce load on intervertebral disks, includes fitting and shaping the frame, prefabricated, includes fitting and adjustment   ሔ

Ⓐ **L0470** TLSO, triplanar control, rigid posterior frame and flexible soft anterior apron with straps, closures and padding, extends from sacrococcygeal junction to scapula, lateral strength provided by pelvic, thoracic, and lateral frame pieces, rotational strength provided by subclavicular extensions, restricts gross trunk motion in sagittal, coronal, and transverse planes, produces intracavitary pressure to reduce load on the intervertebral disks, includes fitting and shaping the frame, prefabricated, includes fitting and adjustment   ሔ

Ⓐ **L0472** TLSO, triplanar control, hyperextension, rigid anterior and lateral frame extends from symphysis pubis to sternal notch with two anterior components (one pubic and one sternal), posterior and lateral pads with straps and closures, limits spinal flexion, restricts gross trunk motion in sagittal, coronal, and transverse planes, includes fitting and shaping the frame, prefabricated, includes fitting and adjustment   ሔ

Ⓐ **L0480** TLSO, triplanar control, one piece rigid plastic shell without interface liner, with multiple straps and closures, posterior extends from sacrococcygeal junction and terminates just inferior to scapular spine, anterior extends from symphysis pubis to sternal notch, anterior or posterior opening, restricts gross trunk motion in sagittal, coronal, and transverse planes, includes a carved plaster or CAD-CAM model, custom fabricated   ሔ

Ⓐ **L0482** TLSO, triplanar control, one piece rigid plastic shell with interface liner, multiple straps and closures, posterior extends from sacrococcygeal junction and terminates just inferior to scapular spine, anterior extends from symphysis pubis to sternal notch, anterior or posterior opening, restricts gross trunk motion in sagittal, coronal, and transverse planes, includes a carved plaster or CAD-CAM model, custom fabricated   ሔ

Ⓐ **L0484** TLSO, triplanar control, two piece rigid plastic shell without interface liner, with multiple straps and closures, posterior extends from sacrococcygeal junction and terminates just inferior to scapular spine, anterior extends from symphysis pubis to sternal notch, lateral strength is enhanced by overlapping plastic, restricts gross trunk motion in the sagittal, coronal, and transverse planes, includes a carved plaster or CAD-CAM model, custom fabricated   ሔ

Ⓐ **L0486** TLSO, triplanar control, two piece rigid plastic shell with interface liner, multiple straps and closures, posterior extends from sacrococcygeal junction and terminates just inferior to scapular spine, anterior extends from symphysis pubis to sternal notch, lateral strength is enhanced by overlapping plastic, restricts gross trunk motion in the sagittal, coronal, and transverse planes, includes a carved plaster or CAD-CAM model, custom fabricated   ሔ

Ⓐ **L0488** TLSO, triplanar control, one piece rigid plastic shell with interface liner, multiple straps and closures, posterior extends from sacrococcygeal junction and terminates just inferior to scapular spine, anterior extends from symphysis pubis to sternal notch, anterior or posterior opening, restricts gross trunk motion in sagittal, coronal, and transverse planes, prefabricated, includes fitting and adjustment   ሔ

Ⓐ **L0490** TLSO, sagittal-coronal control, one piece rigid plastic shell, with overlapping reinforced anterior, with multiple straps and closures, posterior extends from sacrococcygeal junction and terminates at or before the T-9 vertebra, anterior extends from symphysis pubis to xiphoid, anterior opening, restricts gross trunk motion in sagittal and coronal planes, prefabricated, includes fitting and adjustment   ሔ

Ⓐ **L0491** TLSO, sagittal-coronal control, modular segmented spinal System, two rigid plastic shells, posterior extends from the sacrococcygeal junction and terminates just inferior to the scapular spine, anterior extends from the symphysis pubis to the xiphoid, soft liner, restricts gross trunk motion in the sagittal and coronal planes, lateral strength is provided by overlapping plastic and stabilizing closures, includes straps and closures, prefabricated, includes fitting and adjustment

Ⓐ **L0492** TLSO, sagittal-coronal control, modular segmented spinal system, three rigid plastic shells, posterior extends from the sacrococcygeal junction and terminates just inferior to the scapular spine, anterior extends from the symphysis pubis to the xiphoid, soft liner, restricts gross trunk motion in the sagittal and coronal planes, lateral strength is provided by overlapping plastic and stabilizing closures, includes straps and closures, prefabricated, includes fitting and adjustment

## CERVICAL-THORACIC-LUMBAR-SACRAL ORTHOSIS (CTLSO)

Ⓐ **L0621** Sacroiliac orthosis, flexible, provides pelvic-sacral support, reduces motion about the sacroiliac joint, includes straps, closures, may include pendulous abdomen design, prefabricated, includes fitting and adjustment

Ⓐ **L0622** Sacroiliac orthosis, flexible, provides pelvic-sacral support, reduces motion about the sacroiliac joint, includes straps, closures, may include pendulous abdomen design, custom fabricated

Ⓐ **L0623** Sacroiliac orthosis, provides pelvic-sacral support, with rigid or semi-rigid panels over the sacrum and abdomen, reduces motion about the sacroiliac joint, includes straps, closures, may include pendulous abdomen design, prefabricated, includes fitting and adjustment

Ⓐ **L0624** Sacroiliac orthosis, provides pelvic-sacral support, with rigid or semi-rigid panels placed over the sacrum and abdomen, reduces motion about the sacroiliac joint, includes straps, closures, may include pendulous abdomen design, custom fabricated

Ⓐ **L0625** Lumbar orthosis, flexible, provides lumbar support, posterior extends from L-1 to below L-5 vertebra, produces intracavitary pressure to reduce load on the intervertebral discs, includes straps, closures, may include pendulous abdomen design, shoulder straps, stays, prefabricated, includes fitting and adjustment

Special Coverage Instructions    Noncovered by Medicare    Carrier Discretion    ☑ Quantity Alert    ● New Code    ○ Recycled/Reinstated    ▲ Revised Code

**100 — L Codes**    Ⓐ Age Edit    Ⓜ Maternity Edit    ♀ Female Only    ♂ Male Only    Ⓐ-Ⓨ OPPS Status Indicators    **2008 HCPCS**

[A] **L0626** Lumbar orthosis, sagittal control, with rigid posterior panel(s), posterior extends from L-1 to below L-5 vertebra, produces intracavitary pressure to reduce load on the intervertebral discs, includes straps, closures, may include padding, stays, shoulder straps, pendulous abdomen design, prefabricated, includes fitting and adjustment

[A] **L0627** Lumbar orthosis, sagittal control, with rigid anterior and posterior panels, posterior extends from L-1 to below L-5 vertebra, produces intracavitary pressure to reduce load on the intervertebral discs, includes straps, closures, may include padding, shoulder straps, pendulous abdomen design, prefabricated, includes fitting and adjustment

[A] **L0628** Lumbar-sacral orthosis, flexible, provides lumbo-sacral support, posterior extends from sacrococcygeal junction to T-9 vertebra, produces intracavitary pressure to reduce load on the intervertebral discs, includes straps, closures, may include stays, shoulder straps, pendulous abdomen design, prefabricated, includes fitting and adjustment

[A] **L0629** Lumbar-sacral orthosis, flexible, provides lumbo-sacral support, posterior extends from sacrococcygeal junction to T-9 vertebra, produces intracavitary pressure to reduce load on the intervertebral discs, includes straps, closures, may include stays, shoulder straps, pendulous abdomen design, custom fabricated

[A] **L0630** Lumbar-sacral orthosis, sagittal control, with rigid posterior panel(s), posterior extends from sacrococcygeal junction to T-9 vertebra, produces intracavitary pressure to reduce load on the intervertebral discs, includes straps, closures, may include padding, stays, shoulder straps, pendulous abdomen design, prefabricated, includes fitting and adjustment

[A] **L0631** Lumbar-sacral orthosis, sagittal control, with rigid anterior and posterior panels, posterior extends from sacrococcygeal junction to T-9 vertebra, produces intracavitary pressure to reduce load on the intervertebral discs, includes straps, closures, may include padding, shoulder straps, pendulous abdomen design, prefabricated, includes fitting and adjustment

[A] **L0632** LSO, sagittal control, with rigid anterior and posterior panels, posterior extends from sacrococcygeal junction to T-9 vertebra, produces intracavitary pressure to reduce load on the intervertebral discs, includes straps, closures, may include padding, shoulder straps, pendulous abdomen design, custom fabricated

[A] **L0633** LSO, sagittal-coronal control, with rigid posterior frame/panel(s), posterior extends from sacrococcygeal junction to T-9 vertebra, lateral strength provided by rigid lateral frame/panels, produces intracavitary pressure to reduce load on intervertebral discs, includes straps, closures, may include padding, stays, shoulder straps, pendulous abdomen design, prefabricated, includes fitting and adjustment

[A] **L0634** LSO, sagittal-coronal control, with rigid posterior frame/panel(s), posterior extends from sacrococcygeal junction to T-9 vertebra, lateral strength provided by rigid lateral frame/panel(s), produces intracavitary pressure to reduce load on intervertebral discs, includes straps, closures, may include padding, stays, shoulder straps, pendulous abdomen design, custom fabricated

[A] **L0635** LSO, sagittal-coronal control, lumbar flexion, rigid posterior frame/panel(s), lateral articulating design to flex the lumbar spine, posterior extends from sacrococcygeal junction to T-9 vertebra, lateral strength provided by rigid lateral frame/panel(s), produces intracavitary pressure to reduce load on intervertebral discs, includes straps, closures, may include padding, anterior panel, pendulous abdomen design, prefabricated, includes fitting and adjustment

[A] **L0636** LSO, sagittal-coronal control, lumbar flexion, rigid posterior frame/panels, lateral articulating design to flex the lumbar spine, posterior extends from sacrococcygeal junction to T-9 vertebra, lateral strength provided by rigid lateral frame/panels, produces intracavitary pressure to reduce load on intervertebral discs, includes straps, closures, may include padding, anterior panel, pendulous abdomen design, custom fabricated

[A] **L0637** LSO, sagittal-coronal control, with rigid anterior and posterior frame/panels, posterior extends from sacrococcygeal junction to T-9 vertebra, lateral strength provided by rigid lateral frame/panels, produces intracavitary pressure to reduce load on intervertebral discs, includes straps, closures, may include padding, shoulder straps, pendulous abdomen design, prefabricated, includes fitting and adjustment

[A] **L0638** LSO, sagittal-coronal control, with rigid anterior and posterior frame/panels, posterior extends from sacrococcygeal junction to T-9 vertebra, lateral strength provided by rigid lateral frame/panels, produces intracavitary pressure to reduce load on intervertebral discs, includes straps, closures, may include padding, shoulder straps, pendulous abdomen design, custom fabricated

[A] **L0639** LSO, sagittal-coronal control, rigid shell(s)/panel(s), posterior extends from sacrococcygeal junction to T-9 vertebra, anterior extends from symphysis pubis to xyphoid, produces intracavitary pressure to reduce load on the intervertebral discs, overall strength is provided by overlapping rigid material and stabilizing closures, includes straps, closures, may include soft interface, pendulous abdomen design, prefabricated, includes fitting and adjustment

[A] **L0640** LSO, sagittal-coronal control, rigid shell(s)/panel(s), posterior extends from sacrococcygeal junction to T-9 vertebra, anterior extends from symphysis pubis to xyphoid, produces intracavitary pressure to reduce load on the intervertebral discs, overall strength is provided by overlapping rigid material and stabilizing closures, includes straps, closures, may include soft interface, pendulous abdomen design, custom fabricated

## ANTERIOR-POSTERIOR-LATERAL CONTROL

[A] **L0700** CTLSO, anterior-posterior-lateral control, molded to patient model (Minerva type) &

[A] **L0710** CTLSO, anterior-posterior-lateral control, molded to patient model, with interface material (Minerva type) &

## HALO PROCEDURE

[A] **L0810** Halo procedure, cervical halo incorporated into jacket vest &

[A] **L0820** Halo procedure, cervical halo incorporated into plaster body jacket &

[A] **L0830** Halo procedure, cervical halo incorporated into Milwaukee type orthosis &

---

Special Coverage Instructions    Noncovered by Medicare    Carrier Discretion    ☑ Quantity Alert    ● New Code    ○ Recycled/Reinstated    ▲ Revised Code

**2008 HCPCS**    [A2]–[Z6] ASC Payment Indicators    **MED:** Pub 100/NCD References    & DMEPOS Paid    ○ SNF Excluded    [PQ] PQRI    **L Codes — 101**

L0626 — L0830

| A | | L0859 | Addition to halo procedure, magnetic resonance image compatible systems, rings and pins, any material |
|---|---|---|---|
| A | | L0861 | Addition to halo procedure, replacement liner/interface material &#9854; |
| | | ~~L0960~~ | ~~Torso support, postsurgical support, pads for postsurgical support~~ |

### ADDITIONS TO SPINAL ORTHOSIS

| A | | L0970 | TLSO, corset front &#9854; |
|---|---|---|---|
| A | | L0972 | LSO, corset front &#9854; |
| A | | L0974 | TLSO, full corset &#9854; |
| A | | L0976 | LSO, full corset &#9854; |
| A | | L0978 | Axillary crutch extension &#9854; |
| A | ☑ | L0980 | Peroneal straps, pair &#9854; |
| A | ☑ | L0982 | Stocking supporter grips, set of four (4) &#9854; |
| A | ☑ | L0984 | Protective body sock, each &#9854; |
| A | | L0999 | Addition to spinal orthosis, NOS<br>Determine if an alternative HCPCS Level II or a CPT code better describes the service being reported. This code should be used only if a more specific code is unavailable. |

## ORTHOTIC DEVICES - SCOLIOSIS PROCEDURES

The orthotic care of scoliosis differs from other orthotic care in that the treatment is more dynamic in nature and uses continual modification of the orthosis to the patient's changing condition. This coding structure uses the proper names - or eponyms - of the procedures because they have historic and universal acceptance in the profession. It should be recognized that variations to the basic procedures described by the founders/developers are accepted in various medical and orthotic practices throughout the country. All procedures include model of patient when indicated.

### CERVICAL-THORACIC-LUMBAR-SACRAL ORTHOSIS (CTLSO)

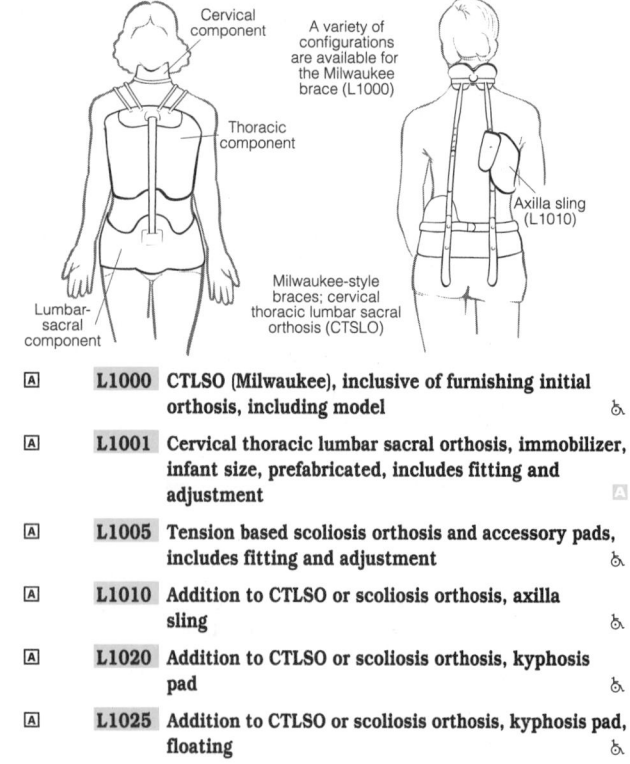

Cervical component

A variety of configurations are available for the Milwaukee brace (L1000)

Thoracic component

Axilla sling (L1010)

Lumbar-sacral component

Milwaukee-style braces; cervical thoracic lumbar sacral orthosis (CTSLO)

| A | | L1000 | CTLSO (Milwaukee), inclusive of furnishing initial orthosis, including model &#9854; |
|---|---|---|---|
| A | | L1001 | Cervical thoracic lumbar sacral orthosis, immobilizer, infant size, prefabricated, includes fitting and adjustment &#9398; |
| A | | L1005 | Tension based scoliosis orthosis and accessory pads, includes fitting and adjustment &#9854; |
| A | | L1010 | Addition to CTLSO or scoliosis orthosis, axilla sling &#9854; |
| A | | L1020 | Addition to CTLSO or scoliosis orthosis, kyphosis pad &#9854; |
| A | | L1025 | Addition to CTLSO or scoliosis orthosis, kyphosis pad, floating &#9854; |

| A | | L1030 | Addition to CTLSO or scoliosis orthosis, lumbar bolster pad |
|---|---|---|---|
| A | | L1040 | Addition to CTLSO or scoliosis orthosis, lumbar or lumbar rib pad &#9854; |
| A | | L1050 | Addition to CTLSO or scoliosis orthosis, sternal pad &#9854; |
| A | | L1060 | Addition to CTLSO or scoliosis orthosis, thoracic pad &#9854; |
| A | | L1070 | Addition to CTLSO or scoliosis orthosis, trapezius sling &#9854; |
| A | | L1080 | Addition to CTLSO or scoliosis orthosis, outrigger &#9854; |
| A | | L1085 | Addition to CTLSO or scoliosis orthosis, outrigger, bilateral with vertical extensions &#9854; |
| A | | L1090 | Addition to CTLSO or scoliosis orthosis, lumbar sling &#9854; |
| A | | L1100 | Addition to CTLSO or scoliosis orthosis, ring flange, plastic or leather &#9854; |
| A | | L1110 | Addition to CTLSO or scoliosis orthosis, ring flange, plastic or leather, molded to patient model &#9854; |
| A | ☑ | L1120 | Addition to CTLSO, scoliosis orthosis, cover for upright, each &#9854; |

### THORACIC-LUMBAR-SACRAL ORTHOSIS (TLSO) (LOW PROFILE)

| A | | L1200 | TLSO, inclusive of furnishing initial orthosis only &#9854; |
|---|---|---|---|
| A | | L1210 | Addition to TLSO, (low profile), lateral thoracic extension &#9854; |
| A | | L1220 | Addition to TLSO, (low profile), anterior thoracic extension &#9854; |
| A | | L1230 | Addition to TLSO, (low profile), Milwaukee type superstructure &#9854; |
| A | | L1240 | Addition to TLSO, (low profile), lumbar derotation pad &#9854; |
| A | | L1250 | Addition to TLSO, (low profile), anterior ASIS pad &#9854; |
| A | | L1260 | Addition to TLSO, (low profile), anterior thoracic derotation pad &#9854; |
| A | | L1270 | Addition to TLSO, (low profile), abdominal pad &#9854; |
| A | ☑ | L1280 | Addition to TLSO, (low profile), rib gusset (elastic), each &#9854; |
| A | | L1290 | Addition to TLSO, (low profile), lateral trochanteric pad &#9854; |

### OTHER SCOLIOSIS PROCEDURES

| A | | L1300 | Other scoliosis procedure, body jacket molded to patient model &#9854; |
|---|---|---|---|
| A | | L1310 | Other scoliosis procedure, postoperative body jacket &#9854; |
| A | | L1499 | Spinal orthosis, not otherwise specified<br>Determine if an alternative HCPCS Level II or a CPT code better describes the service being reported. This code should be used only if a more specific code is unavailable. |

### THORACIC-HIP-KNEE-ANKLE ORTHOSIS (THKAO)

| A | | L1500 | THKAO, mobility frame (Newington, Parapodium types) &#9854; |
|---|---|---|---|
| A | | L1510 | THKAO, standing frame, with or without tray and accessories &#9854; |
| A | | L1520 | THKAO, swivel walker &#9854; |

Special Coverage Instructions    Noncovered by Medicare    Carrier Discretion    ☑ Quantity Alert    ● New Code    ○ Recycled/Reinstated    ▲ Revised Code

**102 — L Codes**    A Age Edit    M Maternity Edit    ♀ Female Only    ♂ Male Only    A-Y OPPS Status Indicators    **2008 HCPCS**

## ORTHOTIC DEVICES - LOWER LIMB

The procedures in L1600-L2999 are considered as "base" or "basic procedures" and may be modified by listing procedure from the "additions" sections and adding them to the base procedures.

### HIP ORTHOSIS (HO) - FLEXIBLE

[A] **L1600** HO, abduction control of hip joints, flexible, Frejka type with cover, prefabricated, includes fitting and adjustment &

[A] **L1610** HO, abduction control of hip joints, flexible, (Frejka cover only), prefabricated, includes fitting and adjustment &

[A] **L1620** HO, abduction control of hip joints, flexible, (Pavlik harness), prefabricated, includes fitting and adjustment &

[A] **L1630** HO, abduction control of hip joints, semi-flexible (Von Rosen type), custom fabricated &

[A] **L1640** HO, abduction control of hip joints, static, pelvic band or spreader bar, thigh cuffs, custom fabricated &

[A] **L1650** HO, abduction control of hip joints, static, adjustable (Ilfled type), prefabricated, includes fitting and adjustment &

[A] **L1652** Hip orthosis, bilateral thigh cuffs with adjustable abductor spreader bar, adult size, prefabricated, includes fitting and adjustment, any type &

[A] **L1660** HO, abduction control of hip joints, static, plastic, prefabricated, includes fitting and adjustment &

[A] **L1680** HO, abduction control of hip joints, dynamic, pelvic control, adjustable hip motion control, thigh cuffs (Rancho hip action type), custom fabricated &

[A] **L1685** HO, abduction control of hip joint, postoperative hip abduction type, custom fabricated &

[A] **L1686** HO, abduction control of hip joint, postoperative hip abduction type, prefabricated, includes fitting and adjustments &

[A] **L1690** Combination, bilateral, lumbo-sacral, hip, femur orthosis providing adduction and internal rotation control, prefabricated, includes fitting and adjustment &

### LEGG PERTHES

[A] **L1700** Legg Perthes orthosis, (Toronto type), custom fabricated &

[A] **L1710** Legg Perthes orthosis, (Newington type), custom fabricated &

[A] **L1720** Legg Perthes orthosis, trilateral, (Tachdijan type), custom fabricated &

[A] **L1730** Legg Perthes orthosis, (Scottish Rite type), custom fabricated &

[A] **L1755** Legg Perthes orthosis, (Patten bottom type), custom fabricated &

### KNEE ORTHOSIS (KO)

[A] **L1800** KO, elastic with stays, prefabricated, includes fitting and adjustment &

[A] **L1810** KO, elastic with joints, prefabricated, includes fitting and adjustment &

[A] **L1815** KO, elastic or other elastic type material with condylar pad(s), prefabricated, includes fitting and adjustment &

[A] **L1820** Knee orthosis, elastic with condylar pads and joints, with or without patellar control, prefabricated, includes fitting and adjustment &

[A] **L1825** KO, elastic knee cap, prefabricated, includes fitting and adjustment &

[A] **L1830** KO, immobilizer, canvas longitudinal, prefabricated, includes fitting and adjustment &

[A] **L1831** Knee orthosis, locking knee joint(s), positional orthosis, prefabricated, includes fitting and adjustment &

[A] **L1832** Knee orthosis, adjustable knee joints (unicentric or polycentric), positional orthosis, rigid support, prefabricated, includes fitting and adjustment &

[A] **L1834** KO, without knee joint, rigid, custom fabricated &

[A] **L1836** Knee orthosis, rigid, without joint(s), includes soft interface material, prefabricated, includes fitting and adjustment &

[A] **L1840** KO, derotation, medial-lateral, anterior cruciate ligament, custom fabricated &

[A] **L1843** Knee orthosis, single upright, thigh and calf, with adjustable flexion and extension joint (unicentric or polycentric), medial-lateral and rotation control, with or without varus/valgus adjustment, prefabricated, includes fitting and adjustment &

[A] **L1844** Knee orthosis, single upright, thigh and calf, with adjustable flexion and extension joint (unicentric or polycentric), medial-lateral and rotation control, with or without varus/valgus adjustment, custom fabricated &

[A] **L1845** Knee orthosis, double upright, thigh and calf, with adjustable flexion and extension joint (unicentric or polycentric), medial-lateral and rotation control, with or without varus/valgus adjustment, prefabricated, includes fitting and adjustment &

[A] **L1846** Knee orthosis, double upright, thigh and calf, with adjustable flexion and extension joint (unicentric or polycentric), medial-lateral and rotation control, with or without varus/valgus adjustment, custom fabricated &

[A] **L1847** KO, double upright with adjustable joint, with inflatable air support chamber(s), prefabricated, includes fitting and adjustment &

[A] **L1850** KO, Swedish type, prefabricated, includes fitting and adjustment &

~~**L1855** KO, molded plastic, thigh and calf sections, with double upright knee joints, custom fabricated~~
See L1846.

~~**L1858** KO, molded plastic, polycentric knee joints, pneumatic knee pads (CTI), custom fabricated~~
See L1846.

[A] **L1860** KO, modification of supracondylar prosthetic socket, custom fabricated (SK) &

~~**L1870** KO, double upright, thigh and calf lacers, with knee joints, custom fabricated~~
See L1846.

~~**L1880** KO, double upright, nonmolded thigh and calf cuffs/lacers with knee joints, custom fabricated~~
See L1846.

### ANKLE-FOOT ORTHOSIS (AFO)

[A] **L1900** AFO, spring wire, dorsiflexion assist calf band, custom fabricated &

Special Coverage Instructions    Noncovered by Medicare    Carrier Discretion    ☑ Quantity Alert    ● New Code    ○ Recycled/Reinstated    ▲ Revised Code

**2008 HCPCS**    N2- Z3 ASC Payment Indicators    **MED:** Pub 100/NCD References    & DMEPOS Paid    ⊘ SNF Excluded    PQ PQRI    **L Codes — 103**

**Orthotic Procedures**

**L1901 — L2114**

[A] **L1901** Ankle orthosis, elastic, prefabricated, includes fitting and adjustment (e.g., neoprene, Lycra)

[A] **L1902** AFO, ankle gauntlet, prefabricated, includes fitting and adjustment &

[A] **L1904** AFO, molded ankle gauntlet, custom fabricated

[A] **L1906** AFO, multiligamentus ankle support, prefabricated, includes fitting and adjustment &

[A] **L1907** AFO, supramalleolar with straps, with or without interface/pads, custom fabricated &

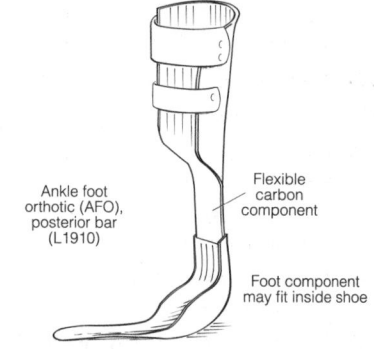

Ankle foot orthotic (AFO), posterior bar (L1910)

Flexible carbon component

Foot component may fit inside shoe

[A] **L1910** AFO, posterior, single bar, clasp attachment to shoe counter, prefabricated, includes fitting and adjustment &

[A] **L1920** AFO, single upright with static or adjustable stop (Phelps or Perlstein type), custom fabricated &

[A] **L1930** AFO, plastic or other material, prefabricated, includes fitting and adjustment &

[A] **L1932** AFO, rigid anterior tibial section, total carbon fiber or equal material, prefabricated, includes fitting and adjustment

[A] **L1940** AFO, plastic or other material, custom-fabricated &

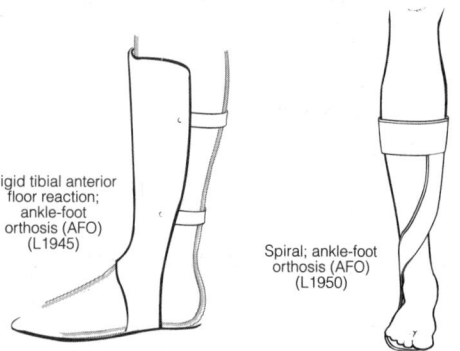

Rigid tibial anterior floor reaction; ankle-foot orthosis (AFO) (L1945)

Spiral; ankle-foot orthosis (AFO) (L1950)

[A] **L1945** AFO, molded to patient model, plastic, rigid anterior tibial section (floor reaction), custom fabricated &

[A] **L1950** AFO, spiral, (Institute of Rehabilitative Medicine type), plastic, custom fabricated &

[A] **L1951** AFO, spiral, (Institute of Rehabilitative Medicine type), plastic or other material, prefabricated, includes fitting and adjustment &

[A] **L1960** AFO, posterior solid ankle, plastic, custom fabricated &

[A] **L1970** AFO, plastic, with ankle joint, custom fabricated &

[A] **L1971** AFO, plastic or other material with ankle joint, prefabricated, includes fitting and adjustment &

[A] **L1980** AFO, single upright free plantar dorsiflexion, solid stirrup, calf band/cuff (single bar BK orthosis), custom fabricated &

[A] **L1990** AFO, double upright free plantar dorsiflexion, solid stirrup, calf band/cuff (double bar BK orthosis), custom fabricated &

## KNEE-ANKLE-FOOT ORTHOSIS (KAFO) - OR ANY COMBINATION

[A] **L2000** KAFO, single upright, free knee, free ankle, solid stirrup, thigh and calf bands/cuffs (single bar AK orthosis), custom fabricated &

[A] **L2005** Knee ankle foot orthosis, any material, single or double upright, stance control, automatic lock and swing phase release, mechanical activation, includes ankle joint, any type, custom fabricated

[A] **L2010** KAFO, single upright, free ankle, solid stirrup, thigh and calf bands/cuffs (single bar AK orthosis), without knee joint, custom fabricated

[A] **L2020** KAFO, double upright, free knee, free ankle, solid stirrup, thigh and calf bands/cuffs (double bar AK orthosis), custom fabricated &

[A] **L2030** KAFO, double upright, free ankle, solid stirrup, thigh and calf bands/cuffs, (double bar AK orthosis), without knee joint, custom fabricated &

[A] **L2034** Knee ankle foot orthosis, full plastic, single upright, with or without free motion knee, medial lateral rotation control, with or without free motion ankle, custom fabricated

[A] **L2035** Knee ankle foot orthosis, full plastic, static (pediatric size), without free motion ankle, prefabricated, includes fitting and adjustment

[A] **L2036** Knee ankle foot orthosis, full plastic, double upright, with or without free motion knee, with or without free motion ankle, custom fabricated

[A] **L2037** Knee ankle foot orthosis, full plastic, single upright, with or without free motion knee, with or without free motion ankle, custom fabricated

[A] **L2038** Knee ankle foot orthosis, full plastic, with or without free motion knee, multi-axis ankle, custom fabricated &

## TORSION CONTROL: HIP-KNEE-ANKLE-FOOT ORTHOSIS (HKAFO)

[A] **L2040** HKAFO, torsion control, bilateral rotation straps, pelvic band/belt, custom fabricated &

[A] **L2050** HKAFO, torsion control, bilateral torsion cables, hip joint, pelvic band/belt, custom fabricated &

[A] **L2060** HKAFO, torsion control, bilateral torsion cables, ball bearing hip joint, pelvic band/ belt, custom fabricated &

[A] **L2070** HKAFO, torsion control, unilateral rotation straps, pelvic band/belt, custom fabricated &

[A] **L2080** HKAFO, torsion control, unilateral torsion cable, hip joint, pelvic band/belt, custom fabricated &

[A] **L2090** HKAFO, torsion control, unilateral torsion cable, ball bearing hip joint, pelvic band/belt, custom fabricated &

[A] **L2106** AFO, fracture orthosis, tibial fracture cast orthosis, thermoplastic type casting material, custom fabricated &

[A] **L2108** AFO, fracture orthosis, tibial fracture cast orthosis, custom fabricated &

[A] **L2112** AFO, fracture orthosis, tibial fracture orthosis, soft, prefabricated, includes fitting and adjustment &

[A] **L2114** AFO, fracture orthosis, tibial fracture orthosis, semi-rigid, prefabricated, includes fitting and adjustment &

---

Special Coverage Instructions    Noncovered by Medicare    Carrier Discretion    ☑ Quantity Alert    ● New Code    ○ Recycled/Reinstated    ▲ Revised Code

Orthotic Procedures

[A] **L2116** AFO, fracture orthosis, tibial fracture orthosis, rigid, prefabricated, includes fitting and adjustment &

[A] **L2126** KAFO, fracture orthosis, femoral fracture cast orthosis, thermoplastic type casting material, custom fabricated &

[A] **L2128** KAFO, fracture orthosis, femoral fracture cast orthosis, custom fabricated &

[A] **L2132** Knee ankle foot orthosis (KAFO), fracture orthosis, femoral fracture cast orthosis, soft, prefabricated, includes fitting and adjustment &

[A] **L2134** Knee ankle foot orthosis (KAFO), fracture orthosis, femoral fracture cast orthosis, semi-rigid, prefabricated, includes fitting and adjustment &

[A] **L2136** KAFO, fracture orthosis, femoral fracture cast orthosis, rigid, prefabricated, includes fitting and adjustment &

## ADDITIONS TO FRACTURE ORTHOSIS

[A] **L2180** Addition to lower extremity fracture orthosis, plastic shoe insert with ankle joints &

[A] **L2182** Addition to lower extremity fracture orthosis, drop lock knee joint &

[A] **L2184** Addition to lower extremity fracture orthosis, limited motion knee joint &

[A] **L2186** Addition to lower extremity fracture orthosis, adjustable motion knee joint, Lerman type &

[A] **L2188** Addition to lower extremity fracture orthosis, quadrilateral brim &

[A] **L2190** Addition to lower extremity fracture orthosis, waist belt &

[A] **L2192** Addition to lower extremity fracture orthosis, hip joint, pelvic band, thigh flange, and pelvic belt &

## ADDITIONS TO LOWER EXTREMITY ORTHOSIS: SHOE-ANKLE-SHIN-KNEE

[A] ☑ **L2200** Addition to lower extremity, limited ankle motion, each joint &

[A] ☑ **L2210** Addition to lower extremity, dorsiflexion assist (plantar flexion resist), each joint &

[A] ☑ **L2220** Addition to lower extremity, dorsiflexion and plantar flexion assist/resist, each joint &

[A] **L2230** Addition to lower extremity, split flat caliper stirrups and plate attachment &

[A] **L2232** Addition to lower extremity orthosis, rocker bottom for total contact ankle foot orthosis, for custom fabricated orthosis only &

[A] **L2240** Addition to lower extremity, round caliper and plate attachment &

[A] **L2250** Addition to lower extremity, foot plate, molded to patient model, stirrup attachment &

[A] **L2260** Addition to lower extremity, reinforced solid stirrup (Scott-Craig type) &

[A] **L2265** Addition to lower extremity, long tongue stirrup &

[A] **L2270** Addition to lower extremity, varus/valgus correction (T) strap, padded/lined or malleolus pad &

[A] **L2275** Addition to lower extremity, varus/valgus correction, plastic modification, padded/lined &

[A] **L2280** Addition to lower extremity, molded inner boot &

[A] **L2300** Addition to lower extremity, abduction bar (bilateral hip involvement), jointed, adjustable &

[A] **L2310** Addition to lower extremity, abduction bar, straight &

[A] **L2320** Addition to lower extremity, non-molded lacer, for custom fabricated orthosis only &

[A] **L2330** Addition to lower extremity, lacer molded to patient model, for custom fabricated orthosis only &

[A] **L2335** Addition to lower extremity, anterior swing band &

[A] **L2340** Addition to lower extremity, pretibial shell, molded to patient model &

[A] **L2350** Addition to lower extremity, prosthetic type, (BK) socket, molded to patient model, (used for PTB, AFO orthoses) &

[A] **L2360** Addition to lower extremity, extended steel shank &

[A] **L2370** Addition to lower extremity, Patten bottom &

[A] **L2375** Addition to lower extremity, torsion control, ankle joint and half solid stirrup &

[A] ☑ **L2380** Addition to lower extremity, torsion control, straight knee joint, each joint &

[A] ☑ **L2385** Addition to lower extremity, straight knee joint, heavy duty, each joint &

[A] **L2387** Addition to lower extremity, polycentric knee joint, for custom fabricated knee ankle foot orthosis, each joint &

[A] ☑ **L2390** Addition to lower extremity, offset knee joint, each joint &

[A] ☑ **L2395** Addition to lower extremity, offset knee joint, heavy duty, each joint &

[A] **L2397** Addition to lower extremity orthosis, suspension sleeve &

## ADDITIONS TO STRAIGHT KNEE OR OFFSET KNEE JOINTS

[A] ☑ **L2405** Addition to knee joint, drop lock, each &

[A] ☑ **L2415** Addition to knee lock with integrated release mechanism (bail, cable, or equal), any material, each joint &

[A] ☑ **L2425** Addition to knee joint, disc or dial lock for adjustable knee flexion, each joint &

[A] ☑ **L2430** Addition to knee joint, ratchet lock for active and progressive knee extension, each joint &

[A] **L2492** Addition to knee joint, lift loop for drop lock ring &

## ADDITIONS: THIGH/WEIGHT BEARING - GLUTEAL/ISCHIAL WEIGHT BEARING

[A] **L2500** Addition to lower extremity, thigh/weight bearing, gluteal/ischial weight bearing, ring &

[A] **L2510** Addition to lower extremity, thigh/weight bearing, quadri-lateral brim, molded to patient model &

[A] **L2520** Addition to lower extremity, thigh/weight bearing, quadri-lateral brim, custom fitted &

[A] **L2525** Addition to lower extremity, thigh/weight bearing, ischial containment/narrow M–L brim molded to patient model &

[A] **L2526** Addition to lower extremity, thigh/weight bearing, ischial containment/narrow M–L brim, custom fitted &

[A] **L2530** Addition to lower extremity, thigh/weight bearing, lacer, nonmolded &

[A] **L2540** Addition to lower extremity, thigh/weight bearing, lacer, molded to patient model &

L2116 — L2540

---

| Special Coverage Instructions | Noncovered by Medicare | Carrier Discretion | ☑ Quantity Alert | ● New Code | ○ Recycled/Reinstated | ▲ Revised Code |

**2008 HCPCS** | [A2]–[Z3] ASC Payment Indicators | **MED:** Pub 100/NCD References | & DMEPOS Paid | ⊘ SNF Excluded | [PQ] PQRI | **L Codes — 105**

**Orthotic Procedures**

**L2550 — L3080**

[A]　　L2550　Addition to lower extremity, thigh/weight bearing, high roll cuff

## ADDITIONS: PELVIC AND THORACIC CONTROL

[A] ☑　L2570　Addition to lower extremity, pelvic control, hip joint, Clevis type, two position joint, each ♿

[A]　　L2580　Addition to lower extremity, pelvic control, pelvic sling ♿

[A] ☑　L2600　Addition to lower extremity, pelvic control, hip joint, Clevis type, or thrust bearing, free, each ♿

[A] ☑　L2610　Addition to lower extremity, pelvic control, hip joint, Clevis or thrust bearing, lock, each ♿

[A] ☑　L2620　Addition to lower extremity, pelvic control, hip joint, heavy-duty, each ♿

[A] ☑　L2622　Addition to lower extremity, pelvic control, hip joint, adjustable flexion, each ♿

[A] ☑　L2624　Addition to lower extremity, pelvic control, hip joint, adjustable flexion, extension, abduction control, each ♿

[A]　　L2627　Addition to lower extremity, pelvic control, plastic, molded to patient model, reciprocating hip joint and cables

[A]　　L2628　Addition to lower extremity, pelvic control, metal frame, reciprocating hip joint and cables

[A]　　L2630　Addition to lower extremity, pelvic control, band and belt, unilateral ♿

[A]　　L2640　Addition to lower extremity, pelvic control, band and belt, bilateral ♿

[A] ☑　L2650　Addition to lower extremity, pelvic and thoracic control, gluteal pad, each ♿

[A]　　L2660　Addition to lower extremity, thoracic control, thoracic band ♿

[A]　　L2670　Addition to lower extremity, thoracic control, paraspinal uprights ♿

[A]　　L2680　Addition to lower extremity, thoracic control, lateral support uprights ♿

## ADDITIONS: GENERAL

[A] ☑　L2750　Addition to lower extremity orthosis, plating chrome or nickel, per bar ♿

[A]　　L2755　Addition to lower extremity orthosis, high strength, lightweight material, all hybrid lamination/prepreg composite, per segment, for custom fabricated orthosis only ♿

[A] ☑　L2760　Addition to lower extremity orthosis, extension, per extension, per bar (for lineal adjustment for growth) ♿

[A] ☑　L2768　Orthotic side bar disconnect device, per bar ♿

[A] ☑　L2770　Addition to lower extremity orthosis, any material, per bar or joint ♿

[A] ☑　L2780　Addition to lower extremity orthosis, noncorrosive finish, per bar ♿

[A] ☑　L2785　Addition to lower extremity orthosis, drop lock retainer, each ♿

[A]　　L2795　Addition to lower extremity orthosis, knee control, full kneecap ♿

[A]　　L2800　Addition to lower extremity orthosis, knee control, knee cap, medial or lateral pull, for use with custom fabricated orthosis only ♿

[A]　　L2810　Addition to lower extremity orthosis, knee control, condylar pad ♿

[A]　　L2820　Addition to lower extremity orthosis, soft interface for molded plastic, below knee section ♿

[A]　　L2830　Addition to lower extremity orthosis, soft interface for molded plastic, above knee section ♿

[A] ☑　L2840　Addition to lower extremity orthosis, tibial length sock, fracture or equal, each ♿

[A] ☑　L2850　Addition to lower extremity orthosis, femoral length sock, fracture or equal, each ♿

[A] ☑　L2860　Addition to lower extremity joint, knee or ankle, concentric adjustable torsion style mechanism, each

[A]　　L2999　Lower extremity orthoses, NOS
Determine if an alternative HCPCS Level II or a CPT code better describes the service being reported. This code should be used only if a more specific code is unavailable.

## ORTHOPEDIC SHOES

### INSERTS

[A] ☑　L3000　Foot insert, removable, molded to patient model, UCB type, Berkeley shell, each
MED: 100-2,15,290

[A] ☑　L3001　Foot insert, removable, molded to patient model, Spenco, each
MED: 100-2,15,290

[A] ☑　L3002　Foot insert, removable, molded to patient model, Plastazote or equal, each
MED: 100-2,15,290

[A] ☑　L3003　Foot insert, removable, molded to patient model, silicone gel, each
MED: 100-2,15,290

[A] ☑　L3010　Foot insert, removable, molded to patient model, longitudinal arch support, each
MED: 100-2,15,290

[A] ☑　L3020　Foot insert, removable, molded to patient model, longitudinal/metatarsal support, each
MED: 100-2,15,290

[A] ☑　L3030　Foot insert, removable, formed to patient foot, each
MED: 100-2,15,290

[A] ☑　L3031　Foot, insert/plate, removable, addition to lower extremity orthosis, high strength, lightweight material, all hybrid lamination/prepreg composite, each

### ARCH SUPPORT, REMOVABLE, PREMOLDED

[A] ☑　L3040　Foot, arch support, removable, premolded, longitudinal, each
MED: 100-2,15,290

[A] ☑　L3050　Foot, arch support, removable, premolded, metatarsal, each
MED: 100-2,15,290

[A] ☑　L3060　Foot, arch support, removable, premolded, longitudinal/metatarsal, each
MED: 100-2,15,290

### ARCH SUPPORT, NONREMOVABLE, ATTACHED TO SHOE

[A] ☑　L3070　Foot, arch support, nonremovable, attached to shoe, longitudinal, each
MED: 100-2,15,290

[A] ☑　L3080　Foot, arch support, nonremovable, attached to shoe, metatarsal, each
MED: 100-2,15,290

---

☑ Special Coverage Instructions　　Noncovered by Medicare　　Carrier Discretion　　☑ Quantity Alert　　● New Code　　○ Recycled/Reinstated　　▲ Revised Code

**106 — L Codes**　　[A] Age Edit　　[M] Maternity Edit　　♀ Female Only　　♂ Male Only　　[A]-[Y] OPPS Status Indicators　　**2008 HCPCS**

[A] ☑ **L3090** Foot, arch support, nonremovable, attached to shoe, longitudinal/metatarsal, each
MED: 100-2,15,290

[A] **L3100** Hallus-valgus night dynamic splint
MED: 100-2,15,290; 100-4,4,240

## ABDUCTION AND ROTATION BARS

A Denis-Browne style splint is a bar that can be applied by strapping or mounted on a shoe. This type of splint generally corrects congenital conditions such as genu varus

Denis-Browne splint

The angle may be adjusted on a plate on the sole of the shoe

[A] **L3140** Foot, abduction rotation bar, including shoes
MED: 100-2,15,290

[A] **L3150** Foot, abduction rotation bar, without shoes
MED: 100-2,15,290

[A] **L3160** Foot, adjustable shoe-styled positioning device

[A] **L3170** Foot, plastic, silicone, or equal, heel stabilizer, each
MED: 100-2,15,290

## ORTHOPEDIC FOOTWEAR

[A] **L3201** Orthopedic shoe, Oxford with supinator or pronator, infant [A]
MED: 100-2,15,290

[A] **L3202** Orthopedic shoe, Oxford with supinator or pronator, child [A]
MED: 100-2,15,290

[A] **L3203** Orthopedic shoe, Oxford with supinator or pronator, junior [A]
MED: 100-2,15,290

[A] **L3204** Orthopedic shoe, hightop with supinator or pronator, infant [A]
MED: 100-2,15,290

[A] **L3206** Orthopedic shoe, hightop with supinator or pronator, child [A]
MED: 100-2,15,290

[A] **L3207** Orthopedic shoe, hightop with supinator or pronator, junior [A]
MED: 100-2,15,290

[A] ☑ **L3208** Surgical boot, each, infant [A]
MED: 100-2,15,100

[A] ☑ **L3209** Surgical boot, each, child [A]
MED: 100-2,15,100

[A] ☑ **L3211** Surgical boot, each, junior [A]
MED: 100-2,15,100

[A] ☑ **L3212** Benesch boot, pair, infant [A]
MED: 100-2,15,100

[A] ☑ **L3213** Benesch boot, pair, child [A]
MED: 100-2,15,100

[A] ☑ **L3214** Benesch boot, pair, junior [A]
MED: 100-2,15,100

[E] ☑ **L3215** Orthopedic footwear, ladies shoe, oxford, each [A]♀

[E] ☑ **L3216** Orthopedic footwear, ladies shoe, depth inlay, each [A]♀

[E] ☑ **L3217** Orthopedic footwear, ladies shoe, hightop, depth inlay, each [A]♀

[E] ☑ **L3219** Orthopedic footwear, mens shoe, oxford, each [A]♂

[E] ☑ **L3221** Orthopedic footwear, mens shoe, depth inlay, each [A]♂

[E] ☑ **L3222** Orthopedic footwear, mens shoe, hightop, depth inlay, each [A]♂

[A] **L3224** Orthopedic footwear, woman's shoe, oxford, used as an integral part of a brace (orthosis) ♀&
MED: 100-2,15,290

[A] **L3225** Orthopedic footwear, man's shoe, oxford, used as an integral part of a brace (orthosis) ♂&
MED: 100-2,15,290

[A] **L3230** Orthopedic footwear, custom shoe, depth inlay, each
MED: 100-2,15,290

[A] ☑ **L3250** Orthopedic footwear, custom molded shoe, removable inner mold, prosthetic shoe, each
MED: 100-2,15,290

[A] ☑ **L3251** Foot, shoe molded to patient model, silicone shoe, each
MED: 100-2,15,290

[A] ☑ **L3252** Foot, shoe molded to patient model, Plastazote (or similar), custom fabricated, each
MED: 100-2,15,290

[A] ☑ **L3253** Foot, molded shoe Plastazote (or similar), custom fitted, each
MED: 100-2,15,290

[A] **L3254** Nonstandard size or width
MED: 100-2,15,290

[A] **L3255** Nonstandard size or length
MED: 100-2,15,290

[A] **L3257** Orthopedic footwear, additional charge for split size
MED: 100-2,15,290

[E] ☑ **L3260** Surgical boot/shoe, each
MED: 100-2,15,100

[A] ☑ **L3265** Plastazote sandal, each

## SHOE MODIFICATION - LIFTS

[A] ☑ **L3300** Lift, elevation, heel, tapered to metatarsals, per inch
MED: 100-2,15,290

[A] ☑ **L3310** Lift, elevation, heel and sole, neoprene, per inch
MED: 100-2,15,290

[A] ☑ **L3320** Lift, elevation, heel and sole, cork, per inch
MED: 100-2,15,290

[A] **L3330** Lift, elevation, metal extension (skate)
MED: 100-2,15,290

[A] ☑ **L3332** Lift, elevation, inside shoe, tapered, up to one-half in.
MED: 100-2,15,290

[A] ☑ **L3334** Lift, elevation, heel, per in.
MED: 100-2,15,290

## SHOE MODIFICATION - WEDGES

[A] **L3340** Heel wedge, SACH
MED: 100-2,15,290

[A] **L3350** Heel wedge
MED: 100-2,15,290

Special Coverage Instructions    Noncovered by Medicare    Carrier Discretion    ☑Quantity Alert    ● New Code    ○ Recycled/Reinstated    ▲ Revised Code

**2008 HCPCS**    [A2][Z3] ASC Payment Indicators    **MED:** Pub 100/NCD References    & DMEPOS Paid    ⊘ SNF Excluded    [PQ]PQRI    **L Codes — 107**

**Orthotic Procedures**

**L3360 — L3675**

[A] **L3360** Sole wedge, outside sole
MED: 100-2,15,290

[A] **L3370** Sole wedge, between sole
MED: 100-2,15,290

[A] **L3380** Clubfoot wedge
MED: 100-2,15,290

[A] **L3390** Outflare wedge
MED: 100-2,15,290

[A] **L3400** Metatarsal bar wedge, rocker
MED: 100-2,15,290

[A] **L3410** Metatarsal bar wedge, between sole
MED: 100-2,15,290

[A] **L3420** Full sole and heel wedge, between sole
MED: 100-2,15,290

## SHOE MODIFICATIONS - HEELS

[A] **L3430** Heel, counter, plastic reinforced
MED: 100-2,15,290

[A] **L3440** Heel, counter, leather reinforced
MED: 100-2,15,290

[A] **L3450** Heel, SACH cushion type
MED: 100-2,15,290

[A] **L3455** Heel, new leather, standard
MED: 100-2,15,290

[A] **L3460** Heel, new rubber, standard
MED: 100-2,15,290

[A] **L3465** Heel, Thomas with wedge
MED: 100-2,15,290

[A] **L3470** Heel, Thomas extended to ball
MED: 100-2,15,290

[A] **L3480** Heel, pad and depression for spur
MED: 100-2,15,290

[A] **L3485** Heel, pad, removable for spur
MED: 100-2,15,290

## MISCELLANEOUS SHOE ADDITIONS

[A] **L3500** Orthopedic shoe addition, insole, leather
MED: 100-2,15,290

[A] **L3510** Orthopedic shoe addition, insole, rubber
MED: 100-2,15,290

[A] **L3520** Orthopedic shoe addition, insole, felt covered with leather
MED: 100-2,15,290

[A] **L3530** Orthopedic shoe addition, sole, half
MED: 100-2,15,290

[A] **L3540** Orthopedic shoe addition, sole, full
MED: 100-2,15,290

[A] **L3550** Orthopedic shoe addition, toe tap, standard
MED: 100-2,15,290

[A] **L3560** Orthopedic shoe addition, toe tap, horseshoe
MED: 100-2,15,290

[A] **L3570** Orthopedic shoe addition, special extension to instep (leather with eyelets)
MED: 100-2,15,290

[A] **L3580** Orthopedic shoe addition, convert instep to Velcro closure
MED: 100-2,15,290

[A] **L3590** Orthopedic shoe addition, convert firm shoe counter to soft counter
MED: 100-2,15,290

[A] **L3595** Orthopedic shoe addition, March bar
MED: 100-2,15,290

## TRANSFER OR REPLACEMENT

[A] **L3600** Transfer of an orthosis from one shoe to another, caliper plate, existing
MED: 100-2,15,290

[A] **L3610** Transfer of an orthosis from one shoe to another, caliper plate, new
MED: 100-2,15,290

[A] **L3620** Transfer of an orthosis from one shoe to another, solid stirrup, existing
MED: 100-2,15,290

[A] **L3630** Transfer of an orthosis from one shoe to another, solid stirrup, new
MED: 100-2,15,290

[A] **L3640** Transfer of an orthosis from one shoe to another, Dennis Browne splint (Riveton), both shoes
MED: 100-2,15,290

[A] **L3649** Orthopedic shoe, modification, addition or transfer, not otherwise specified
Determine if an alternative HCPCS Level II or a CPT code better describes the service being reported. This code should be used only if a more specific code is unavailable.
MED: 100-2,15,290

## ORTHOTIC DEVICES - UPPER LIMB

The procedures in this section are considered as "base" or "basic procedures" and may be modified by listing procedures from the "additions" sections and adding them to the base procedure.

## SHOULDER ORTHOSIS (SO)

[A] **L3650** SO, figure of eight design abduction restrainer, prefabricated, includes fitting and adjustment &

[A] **L3651** SO, single shoulder, elastic, prefabricated, includes fitting and adjustment (e.g., neoprene, Lycra) &

[A] **L3652** SO, double shoulder, elastic, prefabricated, includes fitting and adjustment (e.g., neoprene, Lycra) &

[A] **L3660** SO, figure of eight design abduction restrainer, canvas and webbing, prefabricated, includes fitting and adjustment &

[A] **L3670** SO, acromio/clavicular (canvas and webbing type), prefabricated, includes fitting and adjustment &

[A] **L3671** Shoulder orthosis (SO), shoulder cap design, without joints, may include soft interface, straps, custom fabricated, includes fitting and adjustment

[A] **L3672** SO, abduction positioning (airplane design), thoracic component and support bar, without joints, may inlcude soft interface, straps, custom fabricated, includes fitting and adjustment

[A] **L3673** Shoulder orthosis (SO), abduction positioning (airplane design), thoracic component and support bar, includes nontorsion joint/turnbuckle, may include soft interface, straps, custom fabricated, includes fitting and adjustment

[A] **L3675** SO, vest type abduction restrainer, canvas webbing type, or equal, prefabricated, includes fitting and adjustment &

[Special Coverage Instructions]   [Noncovered by Medicare]   [Carrier Discretion]    ☑ Quantity Alert   ● New Code   ○ Recycled/Reinstated   ▲ Revised Code

**108 — L Codes**   [A] Age Edit   [M] Maternity Edit   ♀ Female Only   ♂ Male Only   [A]-[Y] OPPS Status Indicators    **2008 HCPCS**

E | L3677 | Shoulder orthosis (SO), hard plastic, shoulder stabilizer, prefabricated, includes fitting and adjustment
MED: 100-2,15,120

## ELBOW ORTHOSIS (EO)

A | L3700 | EO, elastic with stays, prefabricated, includes fitting and adjustment &

A | L3701 | Elbow orthosis (EO), elastic, prefabricated, includes fitting and adjustment (e.g., neoprene, Lycra) &

A | L3702 | Elbow orthosis (EO), without joints, may include soft interface, straps, custom fabricated, includes fitting and adjustment

A | L3710 | EO, elastic with metal joints, prefabricated, includes fitting and adjustment &

A | L3720 | Elbow orthosis (EO), double upright with forearm/arm cuffs, free motion, custom fabricated &

A | L3730 | EO, double upright with forearm/arm cuffs, extension/flexion assist, custom fabricated &

A | L3740 | Elbow orthosis (EO), double upright with forearm/arm cuffs, adjustable position Lock with active control, custom fabricated &

A | L3760 | Elbow orthosis (EO), with adjustable position locking joint(s), prefabricated, includes fitting and adjustments, any type &

A | L3762 | Elbow orthosis (EO), rigid, without joints, includes soft interface material, prefabricated, includes fitting and adjustment &

A | L3763 | Elbow wrist hand orthosis (EWHO), rigid, without joints, may include soft interface, straps, custom fabricated, includes fitting and adjustment

A | L3764 | Elbow wrist hand orthosis (EWHO), includes one or more nontorsion joints, elastic bands, turnbuckles, may include soft interface, straps, custom fabricated, includes fitting and adjustment

A | L3765 | Elbow wrist hand finger orthosis (EWHFO), rigid, without joints, may include soft interface, straps, custom fabricated, includes fitting and adjustment

A | L3766 | Elbow wrist hand finger orthosis (EWHFO), includes one or more nontorsion joints, elastic bands, turnbuckles, may include soft interface, straps, custom fabricated, includes fitting and adjustment

## WRIST-HAND-FINGER ORTHOSIS (WHFO)

~~L3800~~ | ~~WHFO, short opponens, no attachments, custom fabricated~~
See L3808.

~~L3805~~ | ~~WHFO, long opponens, no attachment, custom fabricated~~
See L3808.

▲ A | L3806 | WHFO, includes one or more nontorsion joint(s), turnbuckles, elastic bands/springs, may include soft interface material, straps, custom fabricated, includes fitting and adjustment &

A | L3807 | Wrist hand finger orthosis (WHFO), without joint(s), prefabricated, includes fitting and adjustments, any type &

A | L3808 | Wrist hand finger orthosis (WHFO), rigid without joints, may include soft interface material; straps, custom fabricated, includes fitting and adjustment &

## ADDITIONS

~~L3810~~ | ~~WHFO, addition to short and long opponens, thumb abduction (C) bar~~

~~L3815~~ | ~~WHFO, addition to short and long opponens, second M.P. abduction assist~~

~~L3820~~ | ~~WHFO, addition to short and long opponens, I.P. extension assist, with M.P. extension stop~~

~~L3825~~ | ~~WHFO, addition to short and long opponens, M.P. extension stop~~

~~L3830~~ | ~~WHFO, addition to short and long opponens, M.P. extension assist~~

~~L3835~~ | ~~WHFO, addition to short and long opponens, M.P. spring extension assist~~

~~L3840~~ | ~~WHFO, addition to short and long opponens, spring swivel thumb~~

~~L3845~~ | ~~WHFO, addition to short and long opponens, thumb I.P. extension assist, with M.P. stop~~

~~L3850~~ | ~~WHFO, addition to short and long opponens, action wrist, with dorsiflexion assist~~

~~L3855~~ | ~~WHFO, addition to short and long opponens, adjustable M.P. flexion control~~

~~L3860~~ | ~~Wrist hand finger orthosis (WHFO), addition to short and long opponens, adjustable M.P. flexion control and I.P.~~

B ☑ | L3890 | Addition to upper extremity joint, wrist or elbow, concentric adjustable torsion style mechanism, each

## DYNAMIC FLEXOR HINGE, RECIPROCAL WRIST EXTENSION/FLEXION, FINGER FLEXION/EXTENSION

A | L3900 | WHFO, dynamic flexor hinge, reciprocal wrist extension/flexion, finger flexion/extension, wrist or finger driven, custom fabricated &

A | L3901 | WHFO, dynamic flexor hinge, reciprocal wrist extension/flexion, finger flexion/extension, cable driven, custom fabricated &

## EXTERNAL POWER

A | L3904 | WHFO, external powered, electric, custom fabricated &

## OTHER WHFOS - CUSTOM FITTED

A | L3905 | Wrist hand finger orthosis (WHFO), includes one or more nontorsion joints, elastic bands, turnbuckles, may include soft interface, straps, custom fabricated, includes fitting and adjustment

A | L3906 | Wrist hand orthosis (WHO), without joints, may include soft interface, straps, custom fabricated, includes fitting and adjustment &

~~L3907~~ | ~~WHFO, wrist gauntlet with thumb spica, molded to patient model, custom fabricated~~
See L3808.

A | L3908 | WHO, wrist extension control cock-up, nonmolded, prefabricated, includes fitting and adjustment &

A | L3909 | WO, elastic, prefabricated, includes fitting and adjustment (e.g., neoprene, Lycra) &

~~L3910~~ | ~~WHFO, Swanson design, prefabricated, includes fitting and adjustment~~
See L3931.

A | L3911 | Wrist hand finger orthosis (WHFO), elastic, prefabricated, includes fitting and adjustment (e.g., neoprene, Lycra) &

A | L3912 | HFO, flexion glove with elastic finger control, prefabricated, includes fitting and adjustment &

| Special Coverage Instructions | Noncovered by Medicare | Carrier Discretion | ☑ Quantity Alert | ● New Code | ○ Recycled/Reinstated | ▲ Revised Code |

**2008 HCPCS**   A2-Z3 ASC Payment Indicators   **MED:** Pub 100/NCD References   & DMEPOS Paid   ⊘ SNF Excluded   PQ PQRI   **L Codes — 109**

[A]  **L3913**  Hand finger orthosis (HFO), without joints, may include soft interface, straps, custom fabricated, includes fitting and adjustment

[A]  **L3915**  Wrist hand orthosis (WHO), includes one or more nontorsion joint(s), elastic bands, turnbuckles, may include soft interface, straps, prefabricated, includes fitting and adjustment ♿

~~L3916  WHFO, wrist extension cock-up, with outrigger, prefabricated, includes fitting and adjustment~~
See L3931.

[A]  **L3917**  Hand orthosis (HO), metacarpal fracture orthosis, prefabricated, includes fitting and adjustment ♿

~~L3918  HFO, knuckle bender, prefabricated, includes fitting and adjustment~~
See L3929.

[A]  **L3919**  Hand orthosis (HO), without joints, may include soft interface, straps, custom fabricated, includes fitting and adjustment

~~L3920  HFO, knuckle bender, with outrigger, prefabricated, includes fitting and adjustment~~
See L3929.

[A]  **L3921**  Hand finger orthosis (HFO), includes one or more nontorsion joints, elastic bands, turnbuckles, may include soft interface, straps, custom fabricated, includes fitting and adjustment

~~L3922  HFO, knuckle bender, two segment to flex joints, prefabricated, includes fitting and adjustment~~

[A]  **L3923**  Hand finger orthosis (HFO), without joints, may include soft interface, straps, prefabricated, includes fitting and adjustment ♿

~~L3924  WHFO, Oppenheimer, prefabricated, includes fitting and adjustment~~
See L3931.

● [A]  **L3925**  FO, proximal interphalangeal (PIP)/distal interphalangeal (DIP), nontorsion joint/spring, extension/flexion, may include soft interface material, prefabricated, includes fitting and adjustment

~~L3926  WHFO, Thomas suspension, prefabricated, includes fitting and adjustment~~
See L3931.

● [A]  **L3927**  FO, proximal interphalangeal (PIP)/distal interphalangeal (DIP), without joint/spring, extension/flexion (e.g., static or ring type), may include soft interface material, prefabricated, includes fitting and adjustment

~~L3928  HFO, finger extension, with clock spring, prefabricated, includes fitting and adjustment~~
See L3929.

● [A]  **L3929**  HFO, includes one or more nontorsion joint(s), turnbuckles, elastic bands/springs, may include soft interface material, straps, prefabricated, includes fitting and adjustment

~~L3930  WHFO, finger extension, with wrist support, prefabricated, includes fitting and adjustment~~
See L3931.

● [A]  **L3931**  WHFO, includes one or more nontorsion joint(s), turnbuckles, elastic bands/springs, may include soft interface material, straps, prefabricated, includes fitting and adjustment

~~L3932  FO, safety pin, spring wire, prefabricated, includes fitting and adjustment~~
See L3925.

[A]  **L3933**  Finger orthosis (FO), without joints, may include soft interface, custom fabricated, includes fitting and adjustment

~~L3934  FO, safety pin, modified, prefabricated, includes fitting and adjustment~~
See L3925.

[A]  **L3935**  Finger orthosis, nontorsion joint, may include soft interface, custom fabricated, includes fitting and adjustment

~~L3936  WHFO, Palmer, prefabricated, includes fitting and adjustment~~
See L3931.

~~L3938  WHFO, dorsal wrist, prefabricated, includes fitting and adjustment~~
See L3931.

~~L3940  WHFO, dorsal wrist, with outrigger attachment, prefabricated, includes fitting and adjustment~~
SWee L3931.

~~L3942  HFO, reverse knuckle bender, prefabricated, includes fitting and adjustment~~
See L3929.

~~L3944  HFO, reverse knuckle bender, with outrigger, prefabricated, includes fitting and adjustment~~
See L3929.

~~L3946  HFO, composite elastic, prefabricated, includes fitting and adjustment~~

~~L3948  FO, finger knuckle bender, prefabricated, includes fitting and adjustment~~
See L3929.

~~L3950  WHFO, combination Oppenheimer, with knuckle bender and two attachments, prefabricated, includes fitting and adjustment~~
See L3925.

~~L3952  WHFO, combination Oppenheimer, with reverse knuckle and two attachments, prefabricated, includes fitting and adjustment~~
See L3931.

~~L3954  HFO, spreading hand, prefabricated, includes fitting and adjustment~~
See L3923.

[A] ☑  **L3956**  Addition of joint to upper extremity orthosis, any material; per joint ♿

## SHOULDER-ELBOW-WRIST-HAND ORTHOSIS (SEWHO)

## ABDUCTION POSITION, CUSTOM FITTED

[A]  **L3960**  SEWHO, abduction positioning, airplane design, prefabricated, includes fitting and adjustment ♿

[A]  **L3961**  Shoulder elbow wrist hand orthosis (SEWHO), shoulder cap design, without joints, may include soft interface, straps, custom fabricated, includes fitting and adjustment

[A]  **L3962**  SEWHO, abduction positioning, Erb's palsy design, prefabricated, includes fitting and adjustment ♿

[Y]  **L3964**  SEO, mobile arm support attached to wheelchair, balanced, adjustable, prefabricated, includes fitting and adjustment ♿

[Y]  **L3965**  SEO, mobile arm support attached to wheelchair, balanced, adjustable Rancho type, prefabricated, includes fitting and adjustment ♿

░ Special Coverage Instructions    ▪ Noncovered by Medicare    ▪ Carrier Discretion    ☑ Quantity Alert    ● New Code    ○ Recycled/Reinstated    ▲ Revised Code

110 — L Codes    [A] Age Edit    [M] Maternity Edit    ♀ Female Only    ♂ Male Only    [A]-[Y] OPPS Status Indicators    **2008 HCPCS**

Y L3966 SEO, mobile arm support attached to wheelchair, balanced, reclining, prefabricated, includes fitting and adjustment &

A L3967 Shoulder elbow wrist hand orthosis (SEWHO), abduction positioning (airplane design), thoracic component and support bar, without joints, may include soft interface, straps, custom fabricated, includes fitting and adjustment

Y L3968 SEO, mobile arm support attached to wheelchair, balanced, friction arm support (friction dampening to proximal and distal joints), prefabricated, includes fitting and adjustment &

Y L3969 SEO, mobile arm support, monosuspension arm and hand support, overhead elbow forearm hand sling support, yoke type arm suspension support, prefabricated, includes fitting and adjustment &

## ADDITIONS TO MOBILE ARM SUPPORTS

Y L3970 Shoulder elbow orthosis (SEO), addition to mobile arm support, elevating proximal arm &

A L3971 Shoulder elbow wrist hand orthosis (SEWHO), shoulder cap design, includes one or more nontorsion joints, elastic bands, turnbuckles, may include soft interface, straps, custom fabricated, includes fitting and adjustment

Y L3972 Shoulder elbow orthosis (SEO), addition to mobile arm support, offset or lateral rocker arm with elastic balance control &

A L3973 Shoulder elbow wrist hand orthosis (SEWHO), abduction positioning (airplane design), thoracic component and support bar, includes one or more nontorsion joints, elastic bands, turnbuckles, may include soft interface, straps, custom fabricated, includes fitting and adjustment

Y L3974 Shoulder elbow orthosis (SEO), addition to mobile arm support, supinator &

A L3975 Shoulder elbow wrist hand finger orthosis (SEWHO), shoulder cap design, without joints, may include soft interface, straps, custom fabricated, includes fitting and adjustment

A L3976 Shoulder elbow wrist hand finger orthosis (SEWHO), abduction positioning (airplane design), thoracic component and support bar, without joints, may include soft interface, straps, custom fabricated, includes fitting and adjustment

A L3977 Shoulder elbow wrist hand finger orthosis (SEWHO), shoulder cap design, includes one or more nontorsion joints, elastic bands, turnbuckles, may include soft interface, straps, custom fabricated, includes fitting and adjustment

A L3978 Shoulder elbow wrist hand finger orthosis (SEWHO), abduction positioning (airplane design), thoracic component and support bar, includes one or more nontorsion joints, elastic bands, turnbuckles, may include soft interface, straps, custom fabricated, includes fitting and adjustment

## FRACTURE ORTHOSIS

A L3980 Upper extremity fracture orthosis, humeral, prefabricated, includes fitting and adjustment &

A L3982 Upper extremity fracture orthosis, radius/ulnar, prefabricated, includes fitting and adjustment &

A L3984 Upper extremity fracture orthosis, wrist, prefabricated, includes fitting and adjustment &

L3985 ~~Upper extremity fracture orthosis, forearm, hand with wrist hinge, custom fabricated~~
See L3764.

L3986 ~~Upper extremity fracture orthosis, combination of humeral, radius/ulnar, wrist (example: Colles' fracture); custom fabricated~~
See L3763.

A ☑ L3995 Addition to upper extremity orthosis, sock, fracture or equal, each &

A L3999 Upper limb orthosis, NOS

## SPECIFIC REPAIR

A L4000 Replace girdle for spinal orthosis (CTLSO or SO) &

A L4002 Replacement strap, any orthosis, includes all components, any length, any type

A L4010 Replace trilateral socket brim &

A L4020 Replace quadrilateral socket brim, molded to patient model &

A L4030 Replace quadrilateral socket brim, custom fitted &

A L4040 Replace molded thigh lacer, for custom fabricated orthosis only &

A L4045 Replace non-molded thigh lacer, for custom fabricated orthosis only &

A L4050 Replace molded calf lacer, for custom fabricated orthosis only &

A L4055 Replace non-molded calf lacer, for custom fabricated orthosis only &

A L4060 Replace high roll cuff &

A L4070 Replace proximal and distal upright for KAFO &

A L4080 Replace metal bands KAFO, proximal thigh &

A L4090 Replace metal bands KAFO-AFO, calf or distal thigh &

A L4100 Replace leather cuff KAFO, proximal thigh &

A L4110 Replace leather cuff KAFO-AFO, calf or distal thigh &

A L4130 Replace pretibial shell &

## REPAIRS

A ☑ L4205 Repair of orthotic device, labor component, per 15 minutes
MED: 100-2,15,110.2

A L4210 Repair of orthotic device, repair or replace minor parts
MED: 100-2,15,110.2; 100-2,15,120

A L4350 Ankle control orthosis, stirrup style, rigid, includes any type interface (e.g., pneumatic, gel), prefabricated, includes fitting and adjustment &

A L4360 Walking boot, pneumatic, with or without joints, with or without interface material, prefabricated, includes fitting and adjustment &

A L4370 Pneumatic full leg splint, prefabricated, includes fitting and adjustment &
MED: 100-4,4,240

A L4380 Pneumatic knee splint, prefabricated, includes fitting and adjustment &
MED: 100-4,4,240

A L4386 Walking boot, non-pneumatic, with or without joints, with or without interface material, prefabricated, includes fitting and adjustment &

Special Coverage Instructions   Noncovered by Medicare   Carrier Discretion   ☑ Quantity Alert   ● New Code   ○ Recycled/Reinstated   ▲ Revised Code

2008 HCPCS   A2-Z3 ASC Payment Indicators   MED: Pub 100/NCD References   & DMEPOS Paid   ⊘ SNF Excluded   PQ PQRI   L Codes — 111

**Prosthetic Procedures**

**L4392 — L5420**

[A] **L4392** Replacement, soft interface material, static AFO &

[A] **L4394** Replace soft interface material, foot drop splint &

[A] **L4396** Static ankle foot orthosis, including soft interface material, adjustable for fit, for positioning, pressure reduction, may be used for minimal ambulation, prefabricated, includes fitting and adjustment &

[A] **L4398** Foot drop splint, recumbent positioning device, prefabricated, includes fitting and adjustment &
MED: 100-4,4,240

## PROSTHETIC PROCEDURES L5000-L9999

### LOWER LIMB

The procedures in this section are considered as "base" or "basic procedures" and may be modified by listing items/procedures or special materials from the "additions" sections and adding them to the base procedure.

### PARTIAL FOOT

[A] **L5000** Partial foot, shoe insert with longitudinal arch, toe filler
MED: 100-2,15,290; 100-4,3,10.4

[A] **L5010** Partial foot, molded socket, ankle height, with toe filler
MED: 100-2,15,290; 100-4,3,10.4

[A] **L5020** Partial foot, molded socket, tibial tubercle height, with toe filler
MED: 100-2,15,290; 100-4,3,10.4

### ANKLE

[A] **L5050** Ankle, Symes, molded socket, SACH foot ⊘ &
MED: 100-4,3,10.4

[A] **L5060** Ankle, Symes, metal frame, molded leather socket, articulated ankle/foot ⊘ &
MED: 100-4,3,10.4

### BELOW KNEE

[A] **L5100** Below knee, molded socket, shin, SACH foot ⊘ &
MED: 100-4,3,10.4

[A] **L5105** Below knee, plastic socket, joints and thigh lacer, SACH foot ⊘ &
MED: 100-4,3,10.4

### KNEE DISARTICULATION

[A] **L5150** Knee disarticulation (or through knee), molded socket, external knee joints, shin, SACH foot ⊘ &
MED: 100-4,3,10.4

[A] **L5160** Knee disarticulation (or through knee), molded socket, bent knee configuration, external knee joints, shin, SACH foot ⊘ &
MED: 100-4,3,10.4

### ABOVE KNEE

[A] **L5200** Above knee, molded socket, single axis constant friction knee, shin, SACH foot ⊘ &
MED: 100-4,3,10.4

[A] ☑ **L5210** Above knee, short prosthesis, no knee joint (stubbies), with foot blocks, no ankle joints, each ⊘ &
MED: 100-4,3,10.4

[A] ☑ **L5220** Above knee, short prosthesis, no knee joint (stubbies), with articulated ankle/foot, dynamically aligned, each ⊘ &
MED: 100-4,3,10.4

[A] **L5230** Above knee, for proximal femoral focal deficiency, constant friction knee, shin, SACH foot ⊘ &
MED: 100-4,3,10.4

### HIP DISARTICULATION

[A] **L5250** Hip disarticulation, Canadian type; molded socket, hip joint, single axis constant friction knee, shin, SACH foot ⊘ &
MED: 100-4,3,10.4

[A] **L5270** Hip disarticulation, tilt table type; molded socket, locking hip joint, single axis constant friction knee, shin, SACH foot ⊘ &
MED: 100-4,3,10.4

### HEMIPELVECTOMY

[A] **L5280** Hemipelvectomy, Canadian type; molded socket, hip joint, single axis constant friction knee, shin, SACH foot ⊘ &
MED: 100-4,3,10.4

[A] **L5301** Below knee, molded socket, shin, SACH foot, endoskeletal system ⊘ &
MED: 100-4,3,10.4

[A] **L5311** Knee disarticulation (or through knee), molded socket, external knee joints, shin, SACH foot, endoskeletal system ⊘ &
MED: 100-4,3,10.4

[A] **L5321** Above knee, molded socket, open end, SACH foot, endoskeletal system, single axis knee ⊘ &
MED: 100-4,3,10.4

[A] **L5331** Hip disarticulation, Canadian type, molded socket, endoskeletal system, hip joint, single axis knee, SACH foot ⊘ &
MED: 100-4,3,10.4

[A] **L5341** Hemipelvectomy, Canadian type, molded socket, endoskeletal system, hip joint, single axis knee, SACH foot ⊘ &
MED: 100-4,3,10.4

### IMMEDIATE POSTSURGICAL OR EARLY FITTING PROCEDURES

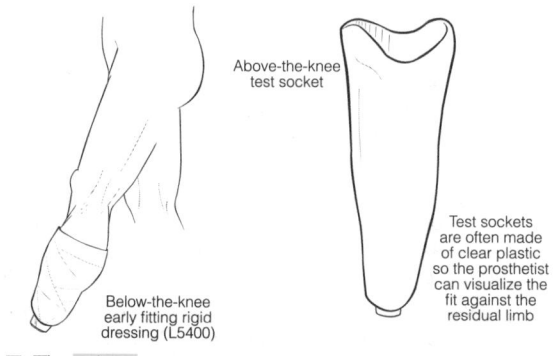

Above-the-knee test socket

Test sockets are often made of clear plastic so the prosthetist can visualize the fit against the residual limb

Below-the-knee early fitting rigid dressing (L5400)

[A] ☑ **L5400** Immediate postsurgical or early fitting, application of initial rigid dressing, including fitting, alignment, suspension, and one cast change, below knee

[A] ☑ **L5410** Immediate postsurgical or early fitting, application of initial rigid dressing, including fitting, alignment and suspension, below knee, each additional cast change and realignment ⊘ &

[A] ☑ **L5420** Immediate postsurgical or early fitting, application of initial rigid dressing, including fitting, alignment and suspension and one cast change AK or knee disarticulation ⊘ &

Special Coverage Instructions    Noncovered by Medicare    Carrier Discretion    ☑ Quantity Alert   ● New Code   ○ Recycled/Reinstated   ▲ Revised Code

112 — L Codes    [A] Age Edit    [M] Maternity Edit   ♀ Female Only   ♂ Male Only   [A]-[Y] OPPS Status Indicators    2008 HCPCS

A ☑ **L5430** Immediate postsurgical or early fitting, application of initial rigid dressing, including fitting, alignment and suspension, AK or knee disarticulation, each additional cast change and realignment ⊘ &

A **L5450** Immediate postsurgical or early fitting, application of nonweight bearing rigid dressing, below knee ⊘ &

A **L5460** Immediate postsurgical or early fitting, application of nonweight bearing rigid dressing, above knee ⊘ &

## INITIAL PROSTHESIS

A **L5500** Initial, below knee PTB type socket, nonalignable system, pylon, no cover, SACH foot, plaster socket, direct formed ⊘ &
MED: 100-2,1,40; 100-4,3,10.4

A **L5505** Initial, above knee — knee disarticulation, ischial level socket, nonalignable system, pylon, no cover, SACH foot plaster socket, direct formed ⊘ &
MED: 100-2,1,40; 100-4,3,10.4

## PREPARATORY PROSTHESIS

A **L5510** Preparatory, below knee PTB type socket, nonalignable system, pylon, no cover, SACH foot, plaster socket, molded to model ⊘ &

A **L5520** Preparatory, below knee PTB type socket, nonalignable system, pylon, no cover, SACH foot, thermoplastic or equal, direct formed ⊘ &

A **L5530** Preparatory, below knee PTB type socket, nonalignable system, pylon, no cover, SACH foot, thermoplastic or equal, molded to model ⊘ &

A **L5535** Preparatory, below knee PTB type socket, nonalignable system, pylon, no cover, SACH foot, prefabricated, adjustable open end socket ⊘ &

A **L5540** Preparatory, below knee PTB type socket, nonalignable system, pylon, no cover, SACH foot, laminated socket, molded to model ⊘ &

A **L5560** Preparatory, above knee — knee disarticulation, ischial level socket, nonalignable system, pylon, no cover, SACH foot, plaster socket, molded to model ⊘ &

A **L5570** Preparatory, above knee — knee disarticulation, ischial level socket, nonalignable system, pylon, no cover, SACH foot, thermoplastic or equal, direct formed ⊘ &

A **L5580** Preparatory, above knee — knee disarticulation, ischial level socket, nonalignable system, pylon, no cover, SACH foot, thermoplastic or equal, molded to model ⊘ &

A **L5585** Preparatory, above knee — knee disarticulation, ischial level socket, nonalignable system, pylon, no cover, SACH foot, prefabricated adjustable open end socket ⊘ &

A **L5590** Preparatory, above knee — knee disarticulation, ischial level socket, nonalignable system, pylon, no cover, SACH foot, laminated socket, molded to model ⊘ &

A **L5595** Preparatory, hip disarticulation — hemipelvectomy, pylon, no cover, SACH foot, thermoplastic or equal, molded to patient model ⊘ &

A **L5600** Preparatory, hip disarticulation — hemipelvectomy, pylon, no cover, SACH foot, laminated socket, molded to patient model ⊘ &

## ADDITIONS: LOWER EXTREMITY

A **L5610** Addition to lower extremity, endoskeletal system, above knee, hydracadence system ⊘ &

A **L5611** Addition to lower extremity, endoskeletal system, above knee — knee disarticulation, 4-bar linkage, with friction swing phase control ⊘ &

A **L5613** Addition to lower extremity, endoskeletal system, above knee — knee disarticulation, 4-bar linkage, with hydraulic swing phase control ⊘ &

A **L5614** Addition to lower extremity, endoskeletal system, above knee — knee disarticulation, 4-bar linkage, with pneumatic swing phase control ⊘ &

A **L5616** Addition to lower extremity, endoskeletal system, above knee, universal multiplex system, friction swing phase control ⊘ &

A ☑ **L5617** Addition to lower extremity, quick change self-aligning unit, above or below knee, each ⊘ &

## ADDITIONS: TEST SOCKETS

A **L5618** Addition to lower extremity, test socket, Symes ⊘ &

A **L5620** Addition to lower extremity, test socket, below knee ⊘ &

A **L5622** Addition to lower extremity, test socket, knee disarticulation ⊘ &

A **L5624** Addition to lower extremity, test socket, above knee ⊘ &

A **L5626** Addition to lower extremity, test socket, hip disarticulation ⊘ &

A **L5628** Addition to lower extremity, test socket, hemipelvectomy ⊘ &

A **L5629** Addition to lower extremity, below knee, acrylic socket ⊘ &

## ADDITIONS: SOCKET VARIATIONS

A **L5630** Addition to lower extremity, Symes type, expandable wall socket ⊘ &

A **L5631** Addition to lower extremity, above knee or knee disarticulation, acrylic socket ⊘ &

A **L5632** Addition to lower extremity, Symes type, PTB brim design socket ⊘ &

A **L5634** Addition to lower extremity, Symes type, posterior opening (Canadian) socket ⊘ &

A **L5636** Addition to lower extremity, Symes type, medial opening socket ⊘ &

A **L5637** Addition to lower extremity, below knee, total contact ⊘ &

A **L5638** Addition to lower extremity, below knee, leather socket ⊘ &

A **L5639** Addition to lower extremity, below knee, wood socket ⊘ &

A **L5640** Addition to lower extremity, knee disarticulation, leather socket ⊘ &

A **L5642** Addition to lower extremity, above knee, leather socket ⊘ &

A **L5643** Addition to lower extremity, hip disarticulation, flexible inner socket, external frame ⊘ &

A **L5644** Addition to lower extremity, above knee, wood socket ⊘ &

A **L5645** Addition to lower extremity, below knee, flexible inner socket, external frame ⊘ &

A **L5646** Addition to lower extremity, below knee, air, fluid, gel or equal, cushion socket ⊘ &

▨ Special Coverage Instructions   ▨ Noncovered by Medicare   ▨ Carrier Discretion   ☑ Quantity Alert   ● New Code   ○ Recycled/Reinstated   ▲ Revised Code

**2008 HCPCS**   ▣-▣ ASC Payment Indicators   **MED:** Pub 100/NCD References   & DMEPOS Paid   ⊘ SNF Excluded   ᴾᵠ PQRI   **L Codes — 113**

**Prosthetic Procedures**

**L5647 — L5704**

[A] **L5647** Addition to lower extremity, below knee, suction socket ⊘&

[A] **L5648** Addition to lower extremity, above knee, air, fluid, gel or equal, cushion socket ⊘&

[A] **L5649** Addition to lower extremity, ischial containment/narrow M-L socket ⊘&

[A] **L5650** Addition to lower extremity, total contact, above knee or knee disarticulation socket ⊘&

[A] **L5651** Addition to lower extremity, above knee, flexible inner socket, external frame ⊘&

[A] **L5652** Addition to lower extremity, suction suspension, above knee or knee disarticulation socket ⊘&

[A] **L5653** Addition to lower extremity, knee disarticulation, expandable wall socket ⊘&

## ADDITIONS: SOCKET INSERT AND SUSPENSION

[A] **L5654** Addition to lower extremity, socket insert, Symes (Kemblo, Pelite, Aliplast, Plastazote or equal) ⊘&

[A] **L5655** Addition to lower extremity, socket insert, below knee (Kemblo, Pelite, Aliplast, Plastazote or equal) ⊘&

[A] **L5656** Addition to lower extremity, socket insert, knee disarticulation (Kemblo, Pelite, Aliplast, Plastazote or equal) ⊘&

[A] **L5658** Addition to lower extremity, socket insert, above knee (Kemblo, Pelite, Aliplast, Plastazote or equal) ⊘&

[A] **L5661** Addition to lower extremity, socket insert, multidurometer, Symes ⊘&

[A] **L5665** Addition to lower extremity, socket insert, multidurometer, below knee ⊘&

[A] **L5666** Addition to lower extremity, below knee, cuff suspension ⊘&

[A] **L5668** Addition to lower extremity, below knee, molded distal cushion ⊘&

As the suspension sleeve is donned, air is driven out through a valve

The valve is closed upon donning and a suction fit is formed around the residual limb

Residual limb

Sealing membrane

Sleeve

Open valve

Closed valve

[A] **L5670** Addition to lower extremity, below knee, molded supracondylar suspension (PTS or similar) ⊘&

[A] **L5671** Addition to lower extremity, below knee/above knee suspension locking mechanism (shuttle, lanyard or equal), excludes socket insert ⊘&

[A] **L5672** Addition to lower extremity, below knee, removable medial brim suspension ⊘&

[A] **L5673** Addition to lower extremity, below knee/above knee, custom fabricated from existing mold or prefabricated, socket insert, silicone gel, elastomeric or equal, for use with locking mechanism ⊘&

[A] ☑ **L5676** Addition to lower extremity, below knee, knee joints, single axis, pair ⊘&

[A] ☑ **L5677** Addition to lower extremity, below knee, knee joints, polycentric, pair ⊘&

[A] ☑ **L5678** Addition to lower extremity, below knee joint covers, pair ⊘&

[A] **L5679** Addition to lower extremity, below knee/above knee, custom fabricated from existing mold or prefabricated, socket insert, silicone gel, elastomeric or equal, not for use with locking mechanism ⊘&

[A] **L5680** Addition to lower extremity, below knee, thigh lacer, nonmolded ⊘&

[A] **L5681** Addition to lower extremity, below knee/above knee, custom fabricated socket insert for congenital or atypical traumatic amputee, silicone gel, elastomeric or equal, for use with or without locking mechanism, initial only (for other than initial, use code L5673 or L5679) ⊘&

[A] **L5682** Addition to lower extremity, below knee, thigh lacer, gluteal/ischial, molded ⊘&

[A] **L5683** Addition to lower extremity, below knee/above knee, custom fabricated socket insert for other than congenital or atypical traumatic amputee, silicone gel, elastomeric or equal, for use with or without locking mechanism, initial only (for other than initial, use code L5673 or L5679) ⊘&

[A] **L5684** Addition to lower extremity, below knee, fork strap ⊘&

[A] **L5685** Addition to lower extremity prosthesis, below knee, suspension/sealing sleeve, with or without valve, any material, each ⊘

[A] **L5686** Addition to lower extremity, below knee, back check (extension control) ⊘&

[A] **L5688** Addition to lower extremity, below knee, waist belt, webbing ⊘&

[A] **L5690** Addition to lower extremity, below knee, waist belt, padded and lined ⊘&

[A] **L5692** Addition to lower extremity, above knee, pelvic control belt, light ⊘&

[A] **L5694** Addition to lower extremity, above knee, pelvic control belt, padded and lined ⊘&

[A] ☑ **L5695** Addition to lower extremity, above knee, pelvic control, sleeve suspension, neoprene or equal, each ⊘

[A] **L5696** Addition to lower extremity, above knee or knee disarticulation, pelvic joint ⊘

[A] **L5697** Addition to lower extremity, above knee or knee disarticulation, pelvic band ⊘

[A] **L5698** Addition to lower extremity, above knee or knee disarticulation, Silesian bandage ⊘

[A] **L5699** All lower extremity prostheses, shoulder harness ⊘

## REPLACEMENTS

[A] **L5700** Replacement, socket, below knee, molded to patient model ⊘

[A] **L5701** Replacement, socket, above knee/knee disarticulation, including attachment plate, molded to patient model ⊘

[A] **L5702** Replacement, socket, hip disarticulation, including hip joint, molded to patient model ⊘

[A] **L5703** Ankle, Symes, molded to patient model, socket without solid ankle cushion heel (SACH) foot, replacement only ⊘

[A] **L5704** Custom shaped protective cover, below knee ⊘

▨ Special Coverage Instructions    ▨ Noncovered by Medicare    ▨ Carrier Discretion    ☑ Quantity Alert    ● New Code    ○ Recycled/Reinstated    ▲ Revised Code

**114 — L Codes**    [A] Age Edit    [M] Maternity Edit    ♀ Female Only    ♂ Male Only    [A]-[Y] OPPS Status Indicators    **2008 HCPCS**

[A] **L5705** Custom shaped protective cover, above knee ⊘

[A] **L5706** Custom shaped protective cover, knee disarticulation ⊘

[A] **L5707** Custom shaped protective cover, hip disarticulation ⊘

## ADDITIONS: EXOSKELETAL KNEE-SHIN SYSTEM

[A] **L5710** Addition, exoskeletal knee-shin system, single axis, manual lock ⊘

[A] **L5711** Addition, exoskeletal knee-shin system, single axis, manual lock, ultra-light material ⊘

[A] **L5712** Addition, exoskeletal knee-shin system, single axis, friction swing and stance phase control (safety knee) ⊘

[A] **L5714** Addition, exoskeletal knee-shin system, single axis, variable friction swing phase control ⊘

[A] **L5716** Addition, exoskeletal knee-shin system, polycentric, mechanical stance phase lock ⊘

[A] **L5718** Addition, exoskeletal knee-shin system, polycentric, friction swing and stance phase control ⊘

[A] **L5722** Addition, exoskeletal knee-shin system, single axis, pneumatic swing, friction stance phase control ⊘

[A] **L5724** Addition, exoskeletal knee-shin system, single axis, fluid swing phase control ⊘

[A] **L5726** Addition, exoskeletal knee-shin system, single axis, external joints, fluid swing phase control ⊘

[A] **L5728** Addition, exoskeletal knee-shin system, single axis, fluid swing and stance phase control ⊘

[A] **L5780** Addition, exoskeletal knee-shin system, single axis, pneumatic/hydra pneumatic swing phase control ⊘

[A] **L5781** Addition to lower limb prosthesis, vacuum pump, residual limb volume management and moisture evacuation system ⊘

[A] **L5782** Addition to lower limb prosthesis, vacuum pump, residual limb volume management and moisture evacuation system, heavy duty ⊘

## COMPONENT MODIFICATION

[A] **L5785** Addition, exoskeletal system, below knee, ultra-light material (titanium, carbon fiber or equal) ⊘

[A] **L5790** Addition, exoskeletal system, above knee, ultra-light material (titanium, carbon fiber or equal) ⊘

[A] **L5795** Addition, exoskeletal system, hip disarticulation, ultra-light material (titanium, carbon fiber or equal) ⊘

## ADDITIONS: ENDOSKELETAL KNEE-SHIN SYSTEM

[A] **L5810** Addition, endoskeletal knee-shin system, single axis, manual lock ⊘

[A] **L5811** Addition, endoskeletal knee-shin system, single axis, manual lock, ultra-light material ⊘

[A] **L5812** Addition, endoskeletal knee-shin system, single axis, friction swing and stance phase control (safety knee) ⊘

[A] **L5814** Addition, endoskeletal knee-shin system, polycentric, hydraulic swing phase control, mechanical stance phase lock ⊘

[A] **L5816** Addition, endoskeletal knee-shin system, polycentric, mechanical stance phase lock ⊘

[A] **L5818** Addition, endoskeletal knee-shin system, polycentric, friction swing and stance phase control ⊘

[A] **L5822** Addition, endoskeletal knee-shin system, single axis, pneumatic swing, friction stance phase control ⊘

[A] **L5824** Addition, endoskeletal knee-shin system, single axis, fluid swing phase control ⊘

[A] **L5826** Addition, endoskeletal knee-shin system, single axis, hydraulic swing phase control, with miniature high activity frame ⊘

[A] **L5828** Addition, endoskeletal knee-shin system, single axis, fluid swing and stance phase control ⊘

[A] **L5830** Addition, endoskeletal knee-shin system, single axis, pneumatic/swing phase control ⊘

[A] **L5840** Addition, endoskeletal knee-shin system, 4-bar linkage or multiaxial, pneumatic swing phase control ⊘

[A] **L5845** Addition, endoskeletal knee-shin system, stance flexion feature, adjustable ⊘

[A] **L5848** Addition to endoskeletal knee-shin system, fluid stance extension, dampening feature, with or without adjustability ⊘

[A] **L5850** Addition, endoskeletal system, above knee or hip disarticulation, knee extension assist ⊘

[A] **L5855** Addition, endoskeletal system, hip disarticulation, mechanical hip extension assist ⊘

[A] **L5856** Addition to lower extremity prosthesis, endoskeletal knee-shin system, microprocessor control feature, swing and stance phase, includes electronic sensor(s), any type ⊘

[A] **L5857** Addition to lower extremity prosthesis, endoskeletal knee-shin system, microprocessor control feature, swing phase only, includes electronic sensor(s), any type ⊘

[A] **L5858** Addition to lower extremity prosthesis, endoskeletal knee shin system, microprocessor control feature, stance phase only, includes electronic sensor(s), any type ⊘

[A] **L5910** Addition, endoskeletal system, below knee, alignable system ⊘

[A] **L5920** Addition, endoskeletal system, above knee or hip disarticulation, alignable system ⊘

[A] **L5925** Addition, endoskeletal system, above knee, knee disarticulation or hip disarticulation, manual lock ⊘

[A] **L5930** Addition, endoskeletal system, high activity knee control frame ⊘

[A] **L5940** Addition, endoskeletal system, below knee, ultra-light material (titanium, carbon fiber or equal) ⊘

[A] **L5950** Addition, endoskeletal system, above knee, ultra-light material (titanium, carbon fiber or equal) ⊘

[A] **L5960** Addition, endoskeletal system, hip disarticulation, ultra-light material (titanium, carbon fiber or equal) ⊘

[A] **L5962** Addition, endoskeletal system, below knee, flexible protective outer surface covering system ⊘

[A] **L5964** Addition, endoskeletal system, above knee, flexible protective outer surface covering system ⊘

[A] **L5966** Addition, endoskeletal system, hip disarticulation, flexible protective outer surface covering system ⊘

[A] **L5968** Addition to lower limb prosthesis, multiaxial ankle with swing phase active dorsiflexion feature ⊘

[A] **L5970** All lower extremity prostheses, foot, external keel, SACH foot ⊘

---

Special Coverage Instructions    Noncovered by Medicare    Carrier Discretion    ☑ Quantity Alert    ● New Code    ○ Recycled/Reinstated    ▲ Revised Code

[A] **L5971** All lower extremity prosthesis, solid ankle cushion heel (SACH) foot, replacement only ⊘

[A] **L5972** All lower extremity prostheses, flexible keel foot (SAFE, STEN, Bock Dynamic or equal) ⊘

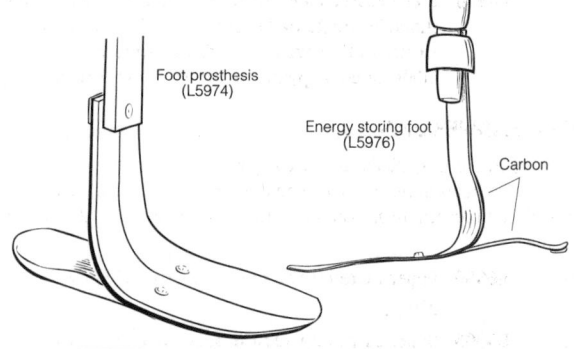

Foot prosthesis
(L5974)

Energy storing foot
(L5976)

Carbon

[A] **L5974** All lower extremity prostheses, foot, single axis ankle/foot ⊘

[A] **L5975** All lower extremity prosthesis, combination single axis ankle and flexible keel foot ⊘

[A] **L5976** All lower extremity prostheses, energy storing foot (Seattle Carbon Copy II or equal) ⊘

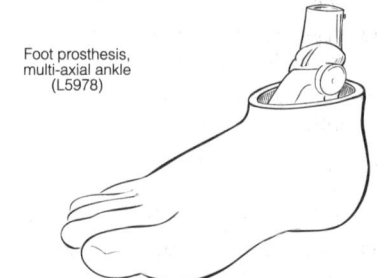

Foot prosthesis,
multi-axial ankle
(L5978)

[A] **L5978** All lower extremity prostheses, foot, multiaxial ankle/foot ⊘

[A] **L5979** All lower extremity prostheses, multiaxial ankle, dynamic response foot, one piece system ⊘

[A] **L5980** All lower extremity prostheses, flex-foot system ⊘

[A] **L5981** All lower extremity prostheses, flex-walk system or equal ⊘

[A] **L5982** All exoskeletal lower extremity prostheses, axial rotation unit ⊘

[A] **L5984** All endoskeletal lower extremity prosthesis, axial rotation unit, with or without adjustability ⊘

[A] **L5985** All endoskeletal lower extremity prostheses, dynamic prosthetic pylon ⊘

[A] **L5986** All lower extremity prostheses, multiaxial rotation unit (MCP or equal) ⊘

[A] **L5987** All lower extremity prosthesis, shank foot system with vertical loading pylon ⊘

[A] **L5988** Addition to lower limb prosthesis, vertical shock reducing pylon feature ⊘

[A] **L5990** Addition to lower extremity prosthesis, user adjustable heel height ⊘

[A] **L5993** Addition to lower extremity prosthesis, heavy duty feature, foot only, (for patient weight greater than 300 lbs) ⊘ ⅖

[A] **L5994** Addition to lower extremity prosthesis, heavy duty feature, knee only, (for patient weight greater than 300 lbs) ⊘

[A] **L5995** Addition to lower extremity prosthesis, heavy duty feature, other than foot or knee, (for patient weight greater than 300 lbs) ⊘

[A] **L5999** Lower extremity prosthesis, not otherwise specified Determine if an alternative HCPCS Level II or a CPT code better describes the service being reported. This code should be used only if a more specific code is unavailable.

## UPPER LIMB

The procedures in L6000-L6590 are considered as "base" or "basic procedures" and may be modified by listing procedures from the "addition" sections. The base procedures include only standard friction wrist and control cable system unless otherwise specified.

### PARTIAL HAND

[A] **L6000** Partial hand, Robin-Aids, thumb remaining (or equal)

[A] **L6010** Partial hand, Robin-Aids, little and/or ring finger remaining (or equal)

[A] **L6020** Partial hand, Robin-Aids, no finger remaining (or equal)

[A] **L6025** Transcarpal/metacarpal or partial hand disarticulation prosthesis, external power, self-suspended, inner socket with removable forearm section, electrodes and cables, two batteries, charger, myoelectric control of terminal device

### WRIST DISARTICULATION

[A] **L6050** Wrist disarticulation, molded socket, flexible elbow hinges, triceps pad ⊘

[A] **L6055** Wrist disarticulation, molded socket with expandable interface, flexible elbow hinges, triceps pad ⊘

### BELOW ELBOW

[A] **L6100** Below elbow, molded socket, flexible elbow hinge, triceps pad ⊘

[A] **L6110** Below elbow, molded socket (Muenster or Northwestern suspension types) ⊘

[A] **L6120** Below elbow, molded double wall split socket, step-up hinges, half cuff ⊘

[A] **L6130** Below elbow, molded double wall split socket, stump activated locking hinge, half cuff ⊘

### ELBOW DISARTICULATION

[A] **L6200** Elbow disarticulation, molded socket, outside locking hinge, forearm ⊘

[A] **L6205** Elbow disarticulation, molded socket with expandable interface, outside locking hinges, forearm ⊘ ⅖

### ABOVE ELBOW

[A] **L6250** Above elbow, molded double wall socket, internal locking elbow, forearm ⊘ ⅖

### SHOULDER DISARTICULATION

[A] **L6300** Shoulder disarticulation, molded socket, shoulder bulkhead, humeral section, internal locking elbow, forearm ⊘ ⅖

[A] **L6310** Shoulder disarticulation, passive restoration (complete prosthesis) ⊘ ⅖

[A] **L6320** Shoulder disarticulation, passive restoration (shoulder cap only) ⊘ ⅖

---

Special Coverage Instructions    Noncovered by Medicare    Carrier Discretion    ☑ Quantity Alert    ● New Code    ○ Recycled/Reinstated    ▲ Revised Code

**116 — L Codes**    [A] Age Edit    [M] Maternity Edit    ♀ Female Only    ♂ Male Only    [A]-[Y] OPPS Status Indicators    **2008 HCPCS**

## INTERSCAPULAR THORACIC

[A] **L6350** Interscapular thoracic, molded socket, shoulder bulkhead, humeral section, internal locking elbow, forearm ⊘ ⅋

[A] **L6360** Interscapular thoracic, passive restoration (complete prosthesis) ⊘ ⅋

[A] **L6370** Interscapular thoracic, passive restoration (shoulder cap only) ⊘ ⅋

## IMMEDIATE AND EARLY POSTSURGICAL PROCEDURES

[A] **L6380** Immediate postsurgical or early fitting, application of initial rigid dressing, including fitting alignment and suspension of components, and one cast change, wrist disarticulation or below elbow ⅋

[A] ☑ **L6382** Immediate postsurgical or early fitting, application of initial rigid dressing including fitting alignment and suspension of components, and one cast change, elbow disarticulation or above elbow ⅋

[A] ☑ **L6384** Immediate postsurgical or early fitting, application of initial rigid dressing including fitting alignment and suspension of components, and one cast change, shoulder disarticulation or interscapular thoracic ⅋

[A] ☑ **L6386** Immediate postsurgical or early fitting, each additional cast change and realignment ⅋

[A] **L6388** Immediate postsurgical or early fitting, application of rigid dressing only ⅋

## ENDOSKELETAL: BELOW ELBOW

[A] **L6400** Below elbow, molded socket, endoskeletal system, including soft prosthetic tissue shaping ⊘ ⅋

## ENDOSKELETAL: ELBOW DISARTICULATION

[A] **L6450** Elbow disarticulation, molded socket, endoskeletal system, including soft prosthetic tissue shaping ⊘ ⅋

## ENDOSKELETAL: ABOVE ELBOW

[A] **L6500** Above elbow, molded socket, endoskeletal system, including soft prosthetic tissue shaping ⊘ ⅋

## ENDOSKELETAL: SHOULDER DISARTICULATION

[A] **L6550** Shoulder disarticulation, molded socket, endoskeletal system, including soft prosthetic tissue shaping ⊘ ⅋

## ENDOSKELETAL: INTERSCAPULAR THORACIC

[A] **L6570** Interscapular thoracic, molded socket, endoskeletal system, including soft prosthetic tissue shaping ⊘ ⅋

[A] **L6580** Preparatory, wrist disarticulation or below elbow, single wall plastic socket, friction wrist, flexible elbow hinges, figure of eight harness, humeral cuff, Bowden cable control, USMC or equal pylon, no cover, molded to patient model ⊘ ⅋

[A] **L6582** Preparatory, wrist disarticulation or below elbow, single wall socket, friction wrist, flexible elbow hinges, figure of eight harness, humeral cuff, Bowden cable control, USMC or equal pylon, no cover, direct formed ⊘ ⅋

[A] **L6584** Preparatory, elbow disarticulation or above elbow, single wall plastic socket, friction wrist, locking elbow, figure of eight harness, fair lead cable control, USMC or equal pylon, no cover, molded to patient model ⊘ ⅋

[A] **L6586** Preparatory, elbow disarticulation or above elbow, single wall socket, friction wrist, locking elbow, figure of eight harness, fair lead cable control, USMC or equal pylon, no cover, direct formed ⊘ ⅋

[A] **L6588** Preparatory, shoulder disarticulation or interscapular thoracic, single wall plastic socket, shoulder joint, locking elbow, friction wrist, chest strap, fair lead cable control, USMC or equal pylon, no cover, molded to patient model ⊘ ⅋

[A] **L6590** Preparatory, shoulder disarticulation or interscapular thoracic, single wall socket, shoulder joint, locking elbow, friction wrist, chest strap, fair lead cable control, USMC or equal pylon, no cover, direct formed ⊘ ⅋

## ADDITIONS: UPPER LIMB

The following procedures/modifications/components may be added to other base procedures. The items in this section should reflect the additional complexity of each modification procedure, in addition to the base procedure, at the time of the original order.

[A] ☑ **L6600** Upper extremity additions, polycentric hinge, pair ⊘ ⅋

[A] ☑ **L6605** Upper extremity additions, single pivot hinge, pair ⊘ ⅋

[A] ☑ **L6610** Upper extremity additions, flexible metal hinge, pair ⊘ ⅋

[A] **L6611** Addition to upper extremity prosthesis, external powered, additional switch, any type ⊘ ⅋

[A] **L6615** Upper extremity addition, disconnect locking wrist unit ⊘ ⅋

[A] ☑ **L6616** Upper extremity addition, additional disconnect insert for locking wrist unit, each ⊘ ⅋

[A] **L6620** Upper extremity addition, flexion/extension wrist unit, with or without friction ⊘ ⅋

[A] **L6621** Upper extremity prosthesis addition, flexion/extension wrist with or without friction, for use with external powered terminal device ⊘

[A] **L6623** Upper extremity addition, spring assisted rotational wrist unit with latch release ⊘ ⅋

[A] **L6624** Upper extremity addition, flexion/extension and rotation wrist unit ⊘ ⅋

[A] **L6625** Upper extremity addition, rotation wrist unit with cable lock ⊘ ⅋

[A] **L6628** Upper extremity addition, quick disconnect hook adapter, Otto Bock or equal ⊘ ⅋

[A] **L6629** Upper extremity addition, quick disconnect lamination collar with coupling piece, Otto Bock or equal ⊘ ⅋

[A] **L6630** Upper extremity addition, stainless steel, any wrist ⊘ ⅋

[A] ☑ **L6632** Upper extremity addition, latex suspension sleeve, each ⊘ ⅋

[A] **L6635** Upper extremity addition, lift assist for elbow ⊘ ⅋

[A] **L6637** Upper extremity addition, nudge control elbow lock ⊘ ⅋

[A] **L6638** Upper extremity addition to prosthesis, electric locking feature, only for use with manually powered elbow ⊘ ⅋

[A] **L6639** Upper extremity addition, heavy duty feature, any elbow ⊘ ⅋

[A] ☑ **L6640** Upper extremity additions, shoulder abduction joint, pair ⊘ ⅋

[A] **L6641** Upper extremity addition, excursion amplifier, pulley type ⊘ ⅋

[A] **L6642** Upper extremity addition, excursion amplifier, lever type ⊘ ⅋

L6350 — L6642

Special Coverage Instructions | Noncovered by Medicare | Carrier Discretion | ☑ Quantity Alert | ● New Code | ○ Recycled/Reinstated | ▲ Revised Code

**2008 HCPCS** | A2–Z3 ASC Payment Indicators | **MED:** Pub 100/NCD References | ⅋ DMEPOS Paid | ⊘ SNF Excluded | P0 PQRI | **L Codes — 117**

**Prosthetic Procedures**

**L6645 — L6895**

[A] ☑ **L6645** Upper extremity addition, shoulder flexion-abduction joint, each ⊘ ♿

[A] **L6646** Upper extremity addition, shoulder joint, multipositional locking, flexion, adjustable abduction friction control, for use with body powered or external powered system ⊘ ♿

[A] **L6647** Upper extremity addition, shoulder lock mechanism, body powered actuator ⊘ ♿

[A] **L6648** Upper extremity addition, shoulder lock mechanism, external powered actuator ⊘ ♿

[A] ☑ **L6650** Upper extremity addition, shoulder universal joint, each ⊘ ♿

[A] **L6655** Upper extremity addition, standard control cable, extra ⊘ ♿

[A] **L6660** Upper extremity addition, heavy duty control cable ⊘ ♿

[A] **L6665** Upper extremity addition, Teflon, or equal, cable lining ⊘ ♿

[A] **L6670** Upper extremity addition, hook to hand, cable adapter ⊘ ♿

[A] **L6672** Upper extremity addition, harness, chest or shoulder, saddle type ⊘ ♿

[A] **L6675** Upper extremity addition, harness, (e.g. figure of eight type), single cable design ⊘ ♿

[A] **L6676** Upper extremity addition, harness, (e.g. figure of eight type), dual cable design ⊘ ♿

[A] **L6677** Upper extremity addition, harness, triple control, simultaneous operation of terminal device and elbow ⊘

[A] **L6680** Upper extremity addition, test socket, wrist disarticulation or below elbow ⊘ ♿

[A] **L6682** Upper extremity addition, test socket, elbow disarticulation or above elbow ⊘ ♿

[A] **L6684** Upper extremity addition, test socket, shoulder disarticulation or interscapular thoracic ⊘ ♿

[A] **L6686** Upper extremity addition, suction socket ⊘ ♿

[A] **L6687** Upper extremity addition, frame type socket, below elbow or wrist disarticulation ⊘ ♿

[A] **L6688** Upper extremity addition, frame type socket, above elbow or elbow disarticulation ⊘ ♿

[A] **L6689** Upper extremity addition, frame type socket, shoulder disarticulation ⊘ ♿

[A] **L6690** Upper extremity addition, frame type socket, interscapular-thoracic ⊘ ♿

[A] ☑ **L6691** Upper extremity addition, removable insert, each ⊘ ♿

[A] ☑ **L6692** Upper extremity addition, silicone gel insert or equal, each ⊘ ♿

[A] **L6693** Upper extremity addition, locking elbow, forearm counterbalance ⊘ ♿

[A] **L6694** Addition to upper extremity prosthesis, below elbow/above elbow, custom fabricated from existing mold or prefabricated, socket insert, silicone gel, elastomeric or equal, for use with locking mechanism ⊘

[A] **L6695** Addition to upper extremity prosthesis, below elbow/above elbow, custom fabricated from existing mold or prefabricated, socket insert, silicone gel, elastomeric or equal, not for use with locking mechanism ⊘

[A] **L6696** Addition to upper extremity prosthesis, below elbow/above elbow, custom fabricated socket insert for congenital or atypical traumatic amputee, silicone gel, elastomeric or equal, for use with or without locking mechanism, initial only (for other than initial, use code L6694 or L6695) ⊘

[A] **L6697** Addition to upper extremity prosthesis, below elbow/above elbow, custom fabricated socket insert for other than congenital or atypical traumatic amputee, silicone gel, elastomeric or equal, for use with or without locking mechanism, initial only (for other than initial, use code L6694 or L6695) ⊘

[A] **L6698** Addition to upper extremity prosthesis, below elbow/above elbow, lock mechanism, excludes socket insert ⊘

## TERMINAL DEVICES

### HOOKS

[A] **L6703** Terminal device, passive hand/mitt, any material, any size ⊘

[A] **L6704** Terminal device, sport/recreational/work attachment, any material, any size ⊘

[A] **L6706** Terminal device, hook, mechanical, voluntary opening, any material, any size, lined or unlined ⊘

[A] **L6707** Terminal device, hook, mechanical, voluntary closing, any material, any size, lined or unlined ⊘

[A] **L6708** Terminal device, hand, mechanical, voluntary opening, any material, any size ⊘

[A] **L6709** Terminal device, hand, mechanical, voluntary closing, any material, any size ⊘

[A] **L6805** Addition to terminal device, modifier wrist unit ⊘ ♿

MED: 100-2,15,120; 100-4,3,10.4

[A] **L6810** Addition to terminal device, precision pinch device ⊘ ♿

MED: 100-2,15,120; 100-4,3,10.4

### HANDS

[A] **L6881** Automatic grasp feature, addition to upper limb electric prosthetic terminal device ⊘ ♿

[A] **L6882** Microprocessor control feature, addition to upper limb prosthetic terminal device ⊘ ♿

MED: 100-2,15,120; 100-4,3,10.4

[A] **L6883** Replacement socket, below elbow/wrist disarticulation, molded to patient model, for use with or without external power

[A] **L6884** Replacement socket, above elbow/elbow disarticulation, molded to patient model, for use with or without external power

[A] **L6885** Replacement socket, shoulder disarticulation/interscapular thoracic, molded to patient model, for use with or without external power

### GLOVES FOR ABOVE HANDS

[A] **L6890** Addition to upper extremity prosthesis, glove for terminal device, any material, prefabricated, includes fitting and adjustment ♿

[A] **L6895** Addition to upper extremity prosthesis, glove for terminal device, any material, custom fabricated ♿

---

Special Coverage Instructions    Noncovered by Medicare    Carrier Discretion    ☑ Quantity Alert    ● New Code    ○ Recycled/Reinstated    ▲ Revised Code

**118 — L Codes**    [A] Age Edit    [M] Maternity Edit    ♀ Female Only    ♂ Male Only    [A-Y] OPPS Status Indicators    **2008 HCPCS**

## HAND RESTORATION

[A] **L6900** Hand restoration (casts, shading and measurements included), partial hand, with glove, thumb or one finger remaining ♿

[A] **L6905** Hand restoration (casts, shading and measurements included), partial hand, with glove, multiple fingers remaining ♿

[A] **L6910** Hand restoration (casts, shading and measurements included), partial hand, with glove, no fingers remaining ♿

[A] **L6915** Hand restoration (shading and measurements included), replacement glove for above ♿

## EXTERNAL POWER

### BASE DEVICES

[A] **L6920** Wrist disarticulation, external power, self-suspended inner socket, removable forearm shell, Otto Bock or equal switch, cables, two batteries and one charger, switch control of terminal device ⊘♿

[A] **L6925** Wrist disarticulation, external power, self-suspended inner socket, removable forearm shell, Otto Bock or equal electrodes, cables, two batteries and one charger, myoelectronic control of terminal device ⊘♿

[A] **L6930** Below elbow, external power, self-suspended inner socket, removable forearm shell, Otto Bock or equal switch, cables, two batteries and one charger, switch control of terminal device ⊘♿

[A] **L6935** Below elbow, external power, self-suspended inner socket, removable forearm shell, Otto Bock or equal electrodes, cables, two batteries and one charger, myoelectronic control of terminal device ⊘♿

[A] **L6940** Elbow disarticulation, external power, molded inner socket, removable humeral shell, outside locking hinges, forearm, Otto Bock or equal switch, cables, two batteries and one charger, switch control of terminal device ⊘♿

[A] **L6945** Elbow disarticulation, external power, molded inner socket, removable humeral shell, outside locking hinges, forearm, Otto Bock or equal electrodes, cables, two batteries and one charger, myoelectronic control of terminal device ⊘♿

[A] **L6950** Above elbow, external power, molded inner socket, removable humeral shell, internal locking elbow, forearm, Otto Bock or equal switch, cables, two batteries and one charger, switch control of terminal device ⊘♿

[A] **L6955** Above elbow, external power, molded inner socket, removable humeral shell, internal locking elbow, forearm, Otto Bock or equal electrodes, cables, two batteries and one charger, myoelectronic control of terminal device ⊘♿

[A] **L6960** Shoulder disarticulation, external power, molded inner socket, removable shoulder shell, shoulder bulkhead, humeral section, mechanical elbow, forearm, Otto Bock or equal switch, cables, two batteries and one charger, switch control of terminal device ⊘♿

[A] **L6965** Shoulder disarticulation, external power, molded inner socket, removable shoulder shell, shoulder bulkhead, humeral section, mechanical elbow, forearm, Otto Bock or equal electrodes, cables, two batteries and one charger, myoelectronic control of terminal device ⊘♿

[A] **L6970** Interscapular-thoracic, external power, molded inner socket, removable shoulder shell, shoulder bulkhead, humeral section, mechanical elbow, forearm, Otto Bock or equal switch, cables, two batteries and one charger, switch control of terminal device ⊘♿

[A] **L6975** Interscapular-thoracic, external power, molded inner socket, removable shoulder shell, shoulder bulkhead, humeral section, mechanical elbow, forearm, Otto Bock or equal electrodes, cables, two batteries and one charger, myoelectronic control of terminal device ⊘♿

[A] **L7007** Electric hand, switch or myoelectric controlled, adult [A]

[A] **L7008** Electric hand, switch or myoelectric, controlled, pediatric [A]

[A] **L7009** Electric hook, switch or myoelectric controlled, adult [A]

[A] **L7040** Prehensile actuator, switch controlled ⊘♿

[A] **L7045** Electric hook, switch or myoelectric controlled, pediatric ⊘♿

### ELBOW

[A] **L7170** Electronic elbow, Hosmer or equal, switch controlled ⊘♿

[A] **L7180** Electronic elbow, microprocessor sequential control of elbow and terminal device ⊘♿

[A] **L7181** Electronic elbow, microprocessor simultaneous control of elbow and terminal device ⊘

[A] **L7185** Electronic elbow, adolescent, Variety Village or equal, switch controlled ⊘♿

[A] **L7186** Electronic elbow, child, Variety Village or equal, switch controlled ⊘♿

[A] **L7190** Electronic elbow, adolescent, Variety Village or equal, myoelectronically controlled ⊘♿

[A] **L7191** Electronic elbow, child, Variety Village or equal, myoelectronically controlled ⊘♿

[A] **L7260** Electronic wrist rotator, Otto Bock or equal ⊘♿

[A] **L7261** Electronic wrist rotator, for Utah arm ⊘♿

[A] **L7266** Servo control, Steeper or equal ⊘♿

[A] **L7272** Analogue control, UNB or equal ⊘♿

[A] **L7274** Proportional control, 6–12 volt, Liberty, Utah or equal ⊘♿

### BATTERY COMPONENTS

▲ [A] ☑ **L7360** Six volt battery, each ♿

▲ [A] ☑ **L7362** Battery charger, six volt, each ⊘♿

▲ [A] ☑ **L7364** Twelve volt battery, each ♿

▲ [A] ☑ **L7366** Battery charger, twelve volt, each ⊘♿

[A] **L7367** Lithium ion battery, replacement ⊘♿

[A] **L7368** Lithium ion battery charger ⊘♿

[A] **L7400** Addition to upper extremity prosthesis, below elbow/wrist disarticulation, ultralight material (titanium, carbon fiber or equal) ⊘

[A] **L7401** Addition to upper extremity prosthesis, above elbow disarticulation, ultralight material (titanium, carbon fiber or equal) ⊘

[A] **L7402** Addition to upper extremity prosthesis, shoulder disarticulation/interscapular thoracic, ultralight material (titanium, carbon fiber or equal) ⊘

---

Special Coverage Instructions   Noncovered by Medicare   Carrier Discretion   ☑ Quantity Alert   ● New Code   ○ Recycled/Reinstated   ▲ Revised Code

**2008 HCPCS**   [A2–Z3] ASC Payment Indicators   **MED:** Pub 100/NCD References   ♿ DMEPOS Paid   ⊘ SNF Excluded   [PQ] PQRI   **L Codes — 119**

**Prosthetic Procedures**

**L7403 — L8417**

| | | | |
|---|---|---|---|
| Ⓐ | **L7403** | Addition to upper extremity prosthesis, below elbow/wrist disarticulation, acrylic material | ⊘ |
| Ⓐ | **L7404** | Addition to upper extremity prosthesis, above elbow disarticulation, acrylic material | ⊘ |
| Ⓐ | **L7405** | Addition to upper extremity prosthesis, shoulder disarticulation/interscapular thoracic, acrylic material | ⊘ |
| Ⓐ | **L7499** | Upper extremity prosthesis, NOS | |

## REPAIRS

| | | |
|---|---|---|
| Ⓐ | **L7500** | Repair of prosthetic device, hourly rate (excludes V5335 repair of oral or laryngeal prosthesis or artificial larynx) |

Medicare jurisdiction: local contractor if repair or implanted prosthetic device.

MED: 100-2,15,110.2; 100-2,15,120; 100-4,32,100

| | | |
|---|---|---|
| Ⓐ | **L7510** | Repair of prosthetic device, repair or replace minor parts |

Medicare jurisdiction: local contractor if repair of implanted prosthetic device.

MED: 100-2,15,110.2; 100-2,15,120; 100-4,32,100

| | | |
|---|---|---|
| Ⓐ ☑ | **L7520** | Repair prosthetic device, labor component, per 15 minutes |

Medicare jurisdiction: local contractor if repair of implanted prosthetic device.

| | | |
|---|---|---|
| Ⓔ ☑ | **L7600** | Prosthetic donning sleeve, any material, each |

## TERMINAL DEVICES

| | | |
|---|---|---|
| ● Ⓐ | **L7611** | Terminal device, hook, mechanical, voluntary opening, any material, any size, lined or unlined, pediatric |
| ● Ⓐ | **L7612** | Terminal device, hook, mechanical, voluntary closing, any material, any size, lined or unlined, pediatric |
| ● Ⓐ | **L7613** | Terminal device, hand, mechanical, voluntary opening, any material, any size, pediatric |
| ● Ⓐ | **L7614** | Terminal device, hand, mechanical, voluntary closing, any material, any size, pediatric |
| ● Ⓐ | **L7621** | Terminal device, hook or hand, heavy duty, mechanical, voluntary opening, any material, any size, lined or unlined |
| ● Ⓐ | **L7622** | Terminal device, hook or hand, heavy duty, mechanical, voluntary closing, any material, any size, lined or unlined |

## GENERAL

| | | | |
|---|---|---|---|
| Ⓐ | **L7900** | Male vacuum erection system | Ⓐ ♂ ♿ |

## PROSTHESIS

| | | | |
|---|---|---|---|
| Ⓐ | **L8000** | Breast prosthesis, mastectomy bra | Ⓐ ♀ ♿ |

MED: 100-2,15,120

| | | | |
|---|---|---|---|
| Ⓐ | **L8001** | Breast prosthesis, mastectomy bra, with integrated breast prosthesis form, unilateral | Ⓐ ♀ ♿ |

MED: 100-2,15,120

| | | | |
|---|---|---|---|
| Ⓐ | **L8002** | Breast prosthesis, mastectomy bra, with integrated breast prosthesis form, bilateral | Ⓐ ♀ ♿ |

MED: 100-2,15,120

| | | | |
|---|---|---|---|
| Ⓐ | **L8010** | Breast prosthesis, mastectomy sleeve | Ⓐ ♀ |

MED: 100-2,15,120

| | | | |
|---|---|---|---|
| Ⓐ | **L8015** | External breast prosthesis garment, with mastectomy form, post-mastectomy | Ⓐ ♀ ♿ |

MED: 100-2,15,120

| | | | |
|---|---|---|---|
| Ⓐ | **L8020** | Breast prosthesis, mastectomy form | Ⓐ ♀ ♿ |

MED: 100-2,15,120

| | | | |
|---|---|---|---|
| Ⓐ | **L8030** | Breast prosthesis, silicone or equal | Ⓐ ♀ ♿ |

MED: 100-2,15,120

| | | | |
|---|---|---|---|
| Ⓐ | **L8035** | Custom breast prosthesis, post mastectomy, molded to patient model | Ⓐ ♀ ♿ |

MED: 100-2,15,120

| | | | |
|---|---|---|---|
| Ⓐ | **L8039** | Breast prosthesis, NOS | Ⓐ ♀ |

Orbital and midfacial prosthesis (L8041-L8042)

Nasal prosthesis (L8040)

Frontal bone

Nasal bone

Maxilla

Zygoma

(L8043-L8044)

Facial prosthetics are typically custom manufactured from polymers and carefully matched to the original features. The maxilla, zygoma, frontal, and nasal bones are often involved, either singly or in combination (L8040-L8044)

| | | | |
|---|---|---|---|
| Ⓐ | **L8040** | Nasal prosthesis, provided by a nonphysician | ♿ |
| Ⓐ | **L8041** | Midfacial prosthesis, provided by a nonphysician | ♿ |
| Ⓐ | **L8042** | Orbital prosthesis, provided by a nonphysician | ♿ |
| Ⓐ | **L8043** | Upper facial prosthesis, provided by a nonphysician | ♿ |
| Ⓐ | **L8044** | Hemi-facial prosthesis, provided by a nonphysician | ♿ |
| Ⓐ | **L8045** | Auricular prosthesis, provided by a nonphysician | ♿ |
| Ⓐ | **L8046** | Partial facial prosthesis, provided by a nonphysician | ♿ |
| Ⓐ | **L8047** | Nasal septal prosthesis, provided by a nonphysician | ♿ |
| Ⓐ | **L8048** | Unspecified maxillofacial prosthesis, by report, provided by a nonphysician | |
| Ⓐ | **L8049** | Repair or modification of maxillofacial prosthesis, labor component, 15 minute increments, provided by a nonphysician | |

## TRUSSES

| | | | |
|---|---|---|---|
| Ⓐ | **L8300** | Truss, single with standard pad | ♿ |

MED: 100-2,15,120; 100-3,280.11; 100-3,280.12; 100-4,4,240

| | | | |
|---|---|---|---|
| Ⓐ | **L8310** | Truss, double with standard pads | ♿ |

MED: 100-2,15,120; 100-3,280.11; 100-3,280.12; 100-4,4,240

| | | | |
|---|---|---|---|
| Ⓐ | **L8320** | Truss, addition to standard pad, water pad | ♿ |

MED: 100-2,15,120; 100-3,280.11; 100-3,280.12; 100-4,4,240

| | | | |
|---|---|---|---|
| Ⓐ | **L8330** | Truss, addition to standard pad, scrotal pad | ♂ ♿ |

MED: 100-2,15,120; 100-3,280.11; 100-3,280.12; 100-4,4,240

## PROSTHETIC SOCKS

| | | | |
|---|---|---|---|
| Ⓐ ☑ | **L8400** | Prosthetic sheath, below knee, each | ♿ |

MED: 100-2,15,120

| | | | |
|---|---|---|---|
| Ⓐ ☑ | **L8410** | Prosthetic sheath, above knee, each | ♿ |

MED: 100-2,15,120

| | | | |
|---|---|---|---|
| Ⓐ ☑ | **L8415** | Prosthetic sheath, upper limb, each | ♿ |

MED: 100-2,15,120

| | | | |
|---|---|---|---|
| Ⓐ ☑ | **L8417** | Prosthetic sheath/sock, including a gel cushion layer, below knee or above knee, each | ♿ |

---

Special Coverage Instructions    Noncovered by Medicare    Carrier Discretion    ☑ Quantity Alert    ● New Code    ○ Recycled/Reinstated    ▲ Revised Code

**120 — L Codes**    Ⓐ Age Edit    Ⓜ Maternity Edit    ♀ Female Only    ♂ Male Only    Ⓐ-ⓨ OPPS Status Indicators    **2008 HCPCS**

[A] ☑ **L8420** Prosthetic sock, multiple ply, below knee, each &
MED: 100-2,15,120

[A] ☑ **L8430** Prosthetic sock, multiple ply, above knee, each &
MED: 100-2,15,120

[A] ☑ **L8435** Prosthetic sock, multiple ply, upper limb, each &
MED: 100-2,15,120

[A] ☑ **L8440** Prosthetic shrinker, below knee, each &
MED: 100-2,15,120

[A] ☑ **L8460** Prosthetic shrinker, above knee, each &
MED: 100-2,15,120

[A] ☑ **L8465** Prosthetic shrinker, upper limb, each &
MED: 100-2,15,120

[A] ☑ **L8470** Prosthetic sock, single ply, fitting, below knee, each &
MED: 100-2,15,120

[A] ☑ **L8480** Prosthetic sock, single ply, fitting, above knee, each &
MED: 100-2,15,120

[A] ☑ **L8485** Prosthetic sock, single ply, fitting, upper limb, each &
MED: 100-2,15,120

[A] **L8499** Unlisted procedure for miscellaneous prosthetic services
Determine if an alternative HCPCS Level II or a CPT code better describes the service being reported. This code should be used only if a more specific code is unavailable.

## PROSTHETIC IMPLANTS

### INTEGUMENTARY SYSTEM

[A] **L8500** Artificial larynx, any type &
MED: 100-2,15,120; 100-3,50.2; 100-4,4,240

[A] **L8501** Tracheostomy speaking valve &
MED: 100-3,50.4

[A] **L8505** Artificial larynx replacement battery/accessory, any type

[A] ☑ **L8507** Tracheo-esophageal voice prosthesis, patient inserted, any type, each &

[A] **L8509** Tracheo-esophageal voice prosthesis, inserted by a licensed health care provider, any type &

[A] **L8510** Voice amplifier &
MED: 100-3,50.2

[A] ☑ **L8511** Insert for indwelling tracheoesophageal prosthesis, with or without valve, replacement only, each &

[A] ☑ **L8512** Gelatin capsules or equivalent, for use with tracheoesophageal voice prosthesis, replacement only, per 10 &

[A] ☑ **L8513** Cleaning device used with tracheoesophageal voice prosthesis, pipet, brush, or equal, replacement only, each &

[A] ☑ **L8514** Tracheoesophageal puncture dilator, replacement only, each &

[A] ☑ **L8515** Gelatin capsule, application device for use with tracheoesophageal voice prosthesis, each

Pectoralis muscle
Rib bones
Prosthesis
Gel-type prosthesis

[N] **L8600** Implantable breast prosthesis, silicone or equal [A] ♀ [N1] &
Medicare covers implants inserted in post-mastectomy reconstruction in a breast cancer patient. Always report concurrent to the implant procedure. Medicare jurisdiction: local contractor.
MED: 100-2,15,120; 100-3,140.2; 100-4,4,190; 100-4,4,240

[N] ☑ **L8603** Injectable bulking agent, collagen implant, urinary tract, 2.5 ml syringe, includes shipping and necessary supplies [N1] &
Medicare covers up to five separate collagen implant treatments in patients with intrinsic sphincter deficiency. Who have passed a collagen sensitivity test. Medicare jurisdiction: local contractor.
MED: 100-3,230.10; 100-4,4,190

[N] ☑ **L8606** Injectable bulking agent, synthetic implant, urinary tract, 1 ml syringe, includes shipping and necessary supplies [N1] &
MED: 100-3,230.10

[N] **L8609** Artificial cornea [N1]

### HEAD: SKULL, FACIAL BONES, AND TEMPOROMANDIBULAR JOINT

[N] **L8610** Ocular implant [N1] &
Medicare jurisdiction: local contractor.
MED: 100-2,15,120; 100-4,4,190; 100-4,4,240

[N] **L8612** Aqueous shunt [N1] &
Medicare jurisdiction: local contractor.
See code(s): Q0074
MED: 100-2,15,120; 100-4,4,190; 100-4,4,240

[N] **L8613** Ossicula implant [N1] &
Medicare jurisdiction: local contractor.
MED: 100-2,15,120; 100-4,4,190; 100-4,4,240

[N] **L8614** Cochlear device, includes all internal and external components [N1] &
A cochlear implant is covered by Medicare when the patient has bilateral sensorineural deafness. Medicare jurisdiction: local contractor.
MED: 100-2,15,120; 100-3,50.3; 100-4,4,190; 100-4,4,240; 100-4,32,100
AHA: 4Q,'03,8; 3Q,'02,5

[A] **L8615** Headset/headpiece for use with cochlear implant device, replacement

[A] **L8616** Microphone for use with cochlear implant device, replacement

[A] **L8617** Transmitting coil for use with cochlear implant device, replacement

[A] **L8618** Transmitter cable for use with cochlear implant device, replacement

[A] **L8619** Cochlear implant external speech processor, replacement &
Medicare jurisdiction: local contractor.
MED: 100-3,50.3; 100-4,32,100

---

Special Coverage Instructions    Noncovered by Medicare    Carrier Discretion    ☑ Quantity Alert    ● New Code    ○ Recycled/Reinstated    ▲ Revised Code

**2008 HCPCS**    [A2]-[Z3] ASC Payment Indicators    **MED:** Pub 100/NCD References    & DMEPOS Paid    ⊘ SNF Excluded    [PQ] PQRI    **L Codes — 121**

**Prosthetic Procedures**

A ☑ **L8621** Zinc air battery for use with cochlear implant device, replacement, each

A ☑ **L8622** Alkaline battery for use with cochlear implant device, any size, replacement, each

A ☑ **L8623** Lithium ion battery for use with cochlear implant device speech processor, other than ear level, replacement, each ♿

A ☑ **L8624** Lithium ion battery for use with cochlear implant device speech processor, ear level, replacement, each ♿

## UPPER EXTREMITY

Bone is cut at the MP joint (arthroplasty)

Bone may be hollowed out in both metacarpal and phalangeal sides in preparation for a prosthesis

Prosthetic joint implant

Prosthesis in place

Metacarpophalangeal prosthetic implant

N **L8630** Metacarpophalangeal joint implant ℕ♿
Medicare jurisdiction: local contractor.
MED: 100-2,15,120; 100-4,4,190; 100-4,4,240

N **L8631** Metacarpal phalangeal joint replacement, two or more pieces, metal (e.g., stainless steel or cobalt chrome), ceramic-like material (e.g., pyrocarbon), for surgical implantation (all sizes, includes entire system) ℕ♿
MED: 100-2,15,120; 100-4,4,240

## LOWER EXTREMITY - JOINT: KNEE, ANKLE, TOE

N **L8641** Metatarsal joint implant ℕ♿
Medicare jurisdiction: local contractor.
MED: 100-2,15,120; 100-4,4,190; 100-4,4,240

N **L8642** Hallux implant ℕ♿
Medicare jurisdiction: local contractor.
See code(s): Q0073
MED: 100-2,15,120; 100-4,4,190; 100-4,4,240

## MISCELLANEOUS MUSCULAR-SKELETAL

N ☑ **L8658** Interphalangeal joint spacer, silicone or equal, each ℕ♿
Medicare jurisdiction: local contractor.
MED: 100-2,15,120; 100-4,4,190; 100-4,4,240

N **L8659** Interphalangeal finger joint replacement, 2 or more pieces, metal (e.g., stainless steel or cobalt chrome), ceramic-like material (e.g., pyrocarbon) for surgical implantation, any size ℕ♿
MED: 100-2,15,120; 100-4,4,240

## CARDIOVASCULAR SYSTEM

N **L8670** Vascular graft material, synthetic, implant ℕ♿
Medicare jurisdiction: local contractor.
MED: 100-2,15,120; 100-4,4,190; 100-4,4,240

## GENERAL

B ☑ **L8680** Implantable neurostimulator electrode, each
MED: 100-4,32,50

A **L8681** Patient programmer (external) for use with implantable programmable neurostimulator pulse generator

N **L8682** Implantable neurostimulator radiofrequency receiver ℕ

A **L8683** Radiofrequency transmitter (external) for use with implantable neurostimulator radiofrequency receiver

A **L8684** Radiofrequency transmitter (external) for use with implantable sacral root neurostimulator receiver for bowel and bladder management, replacement

B **L8685** Implantable neurostimulator pulse generator, single array, rechargeable, includes extension
MED: 100-4,32,50

B **L8686** Implantable neurostimulator pulse generator, single array, non-rechargeable, includes extension
MED: 100-4,32,50

B **L8687** Implantable neurostimulator pulse generator, dual array, rechargeable, includes extension
MED: 100-4,32,50

B **L8688** Implantable neurostimulator pulse generator, dual array, non-rechargeable, includes extension
MED: 100-4,32,50

A **L8689** External recharging system for battery (internal) for use with implantable neurostimulator

H **L8690** Auditory osseointegrated device, includes all internal and external components J7

A **L8691** Auditory osseointegrated device, external sound processor, replacement

A **L8695** External recharging system for battery (external) for use with implantable neurostimulator

N **L8699** Prosthetic implant, not otherwise specified ℕ
Determine if an alternative HCPCS Level II or a CPT code better describes the service being reported. This code should be used only if a more specific code is unavailable. Medicare jurisdiction: local contractor.
MED: 100-4,4,190

A **L9900** Orthotic and prosthetic supply, accessory, and/or service component of another HCPCS L code

---

Special Coverage Instructions    Noncovered by Medicare    Carrier Discretion    ☑ Quantity Alert    ● New Code    ○ Recycled/Reinstated    ▲ Revised Code

122 — L Codes    A Age Edit    M Maternity Edit    ♀ Female Only    ♂ Male Only    A-Y OPPS Status Indicators    **2008 HCPCS**

## MEDICAL SERVICES M0000-M0301

### OTHER MEDICAL SERVICES

M codes include office services, cellular therapy, prolotherapy, intragastric hypothermia, IV chelation therapy, and fabric wrapping of an abdominal aneurysm.

◻ **M0064** Brief office visit for the sole purpose of monitoring or changing drug prescriptions used in the treatment of mental psychoneurotic and personality disorders ⊘

MED: 100-4,12,210.1

E **M0075** Cellular therapy

The therapeutic efficacy of injecting foreign proteins has not been established.

MED: 100-3,30.8

E **M0076** Prolotherapy

The therapeutic efficacy of prolotherapy and joint sclerotherapy has not been established.

MED: 100-3,150.7

E **M0100** Intragastric hypothermia using gastric freezing

Code with caution: This procedure is considered obsolete.

MED: 100-3,100.6

### CARDIOVASCULAR SERVICES

E **M0300** IV chelation therapy (chemical endarterectomy)

Chelation therapy is considered experimental in the United States.

MED: 100-3,20.21

E **M0301** Fabric wrapping of abdominal aneurysm

Code with caution: This procedure has largely been replaced with more effective treatment modalities. Submit documentation.

MED: 100-3,20.23

Special Coverage Instructions    Noncovered by Medicare    Carrier Discretion    ☑ Quantity Alert    ● New Code    ○ Recycled/Reinstated    ▲ Revised Code

**2008 HCPCS**    A2- A3 ASC Payment Indicators    **MED:** Pub 100/NCD References    & DMEPOS Paid    ⊘ SNF Excluded    PQ PQRI    **M Codes — 123**

## PATHOLOGY AND LABORATORY SERVICES P0000-P9999

P codes include chemistry, toxicology, and microbiology tests, screening Papanicolaou procedures, and various blood products.

## CHEMISTRY AND TOXICOLOGY TESTS

[A] **P2028** Cephalin floculation, blood
Code with caution: This test is considered obsolete. Submit documentation.
MED: 100-3,300.1

[A] **P2029** Congo red, blood
Code with caution: This test is considered obsolete. Submit documentation.
MED: 100-3,300.1

[E] **P2031** Hair analysis (excluding arsenic)
For hair analysis for arsenic, see CPT codes 83015, 82175.
MED: 100-3,190.6

[A] **P2033** Thymol turbidity, blood
Code with caution: This test is considered obsolete. Submit documentation.
MED: 100-3,300.1

[A] **P2038** Mucoprotein, blood (seromucoid) (medical necessity procedure)
Code with caution: This test is considered obsolete. Submit documentation.
MED: 100-3,300.1

## PATHOLOGY SCREENING TESTS

[A] **P3000** Screening Papanicolaou smear, cervical or vaginal, up to three smears, by technician under physician supervision [A] ♀ ⊘
One Pap test is covered by Medicare every two years, unless the physician suspects cervical abnormalities and shortens the interval. See also G0123-G0124.
MED: 100-2,6,10; 100-3,190.2; 100-4,4,240

[B] **P3001** Screening Papanicolaou smear, cervical or vaginal, up to three smears, requiring interpretation by physician [A] ♀ ⊘
One Pap test is covered by Medicare every two years, unless the physician suspects cervical abnormalities and shortens the interval. See also G0123-G0124.
MED: 100-2,6,10; 100-3,190.2; 100-4,4,240

## MICROBIOLOGY TESTS

[E] **P7001** Culture, bacterial, urine; quantitative, sensitivity study

## MISCELLANEOUS

[K] ☑ **P9010** Blood (whole), for transfusion, per unit
MED: 100-1,3,20.5; 100-2,1,10; 100-4,3,40.2.2

[K] ☑ **P9011** Blood, split unit
MED: 100-1,3,20.5; 100-2,1,10; 100-4,3,40.2.2

[K] ☑ **P9012** Cryoprecipitate, each unit
MED: 100-1,3,20.5; 100-2,1,10; 100-4,3,40.2.2

[K] ☑ **P9016** Red blood cells, leukocytes reduced, each unit
MED: 100-1,3,20.5; 100-2,1,10; 100-4,3,40.2.2

[K] ☑ **P9017** Fresh frozen plasma (single donor), frozen within 8 hours of collection, each unit
MED: 100-1,3,20.5; 100-2,1,10; 100-4,3,40.2.2

[K] ☑ **P9019** Platelets, each unit
MED: 100-1,3,20.5; 100-2,1,10; 100-4,3,40.2.2

[K] ☑ **P9020** Platelet rich plasma, each unit
MED: 100-1,3,20.5; 100-4,3,40.2.2

[K] ☑ **P9021** Red blood cells, each unit
MED: 100-1,3,20.5; 100-2,1,10; 100-4,3,40.2.2

[K] ☑ **P9022** Red blood cells, washed, each unit
MED: 100-1,3,20.5; 100-2,1,10; 100-4,3,40.2.2

[K] ☑ **P9023** Plasma, pooled multiple donor, solvent/detergent treated, frozen, each unit
MED: 100-1,3,20.5; 100-2,1,10; 100-4,3,40.2.2

[K] ☑ **P9031** Platelets, leukocytes reduced, each unit
MED: 100-1,3,20.5; 100-1,3,20.5.2; 100-1,3,20.5.3; 100-2,1,10; 100-4,3,40.2.2

[K] ☑ **P9032** Platelets, irradiated, each unit
MED: 100-1,3,20.5; 100-1,3,20.5.2; 100-1,3,20.5.3; 100-2,1,10; 100-4,3,40.2.2

[K] ☑ **P9033** Platelets, leukocytes reduced, irradiated, each unit
MED: 100-1,3,20.5; 100-1,3,20.5.2; 100-1,3,20.5.3; 100-2,1,10; 100-4,3,40.2.2

[K] ☑ **P9034** Platelets, pheresis, each unit
MED: 100-1,3,20.5; 100-1,3,20.5.2; 100-1,3,20.5.3; 100-2,1,10; 100-4,3,40.2.2

[K] ☑ **P9035** Platelets, pheresis, leukocytes reduced, each unit
MED: 100-1,3,20.5; 100-1,3,20.5.2; 100-1,3,20.5.3; 100-2,1,10; 100-4,3,40.2.2

[K] ☑ **P9036** Platelets, pheresis, irradiated, each unit
MED: 100-1,3,20.5; 100-1,3,20.5.2; 100-1,3,20.5.3; 100-2,1,10; 100-4,3,40.2.2

[K] ☑ **P9037** Platelets, pheresis, leukocytes reduced, irradiated, each unit
MED: 100-1,3,20.5; 100-1,3,20.5.2; 100-1,3,20.5.3; 100-2,1,10; 100-4,3,40.2.2

[K] ☑ **P9038** Red blood cells, irradiated, each unit
MED: 100-1,3,20.5; 100-1,3,20.5.2; 100-1,3,20.5.3; 100-2,1,10; 100-4,3,40.2.2

[K] ☑ **P9039** Red blood cells, deglycerolized, each unit
MED: 100-1,3,20.5; 100-1,3,20.5.2; 100-1,3,20.5.3; 100-2,1,10; 100-4,3,40.2.2

[K] ☑ **P9040** Red blood cells, leukocytes reduced, irradiated, each unit
MED: 100-1,3,20.5; 100-1,3,20.5.2; 100-1,3,20.5.3; 100-2,1,10; 100-4,3,40.2.2

[K] ☑ **P9041** Infusion, albumin (human), 5%, 50 ml [K2]
Not considered a blood product for OPPS effective July 1, 2005.
MED: 100-2,1,10; 100-4,3,40.2.2

[K] ☑ **P9043** Infusion, plasma protein fraction (human), 5%, 50 ml
MED: 100-1,3,20.5; 100-2,1,10; 100-4,3,40.2.2

[K] ☑ **P9044** Plasma, cryoprecipitate reduced, each unit
MED: 100-1,3,20.5; 100-2,1,10; 100-4,3,40.2.2

[K] ☑ **P9045** Infusion, albumin (human), 5%, 250 ml [K2]
Not considered a blood product for OPPS effective July 1, 2005.
MED: 100-2,1,10; 100-4,3,40.2.2

[K] ☑ **P9046** Infusion, albumin (human), 25%, 20 ml [K2]
Not considered a blood product for OPPS effective July 1, 2005.
MED: 100-2,1,10; 100-4,3,40.2.2

[K] ☑ **P9047** Infusion, albumin (human), 25%, 50 ml [K2]
Not considered a blood product for OPPS effective July 1, 2005.
MED: 100-2,1,10; 100-4,3,40.2.2

---

Special Coverage Instructions    Noncovered by Medicare    Carrier Discretion    ☑ Quantity Alert    ● New Code    ○ Recycled/Reinstated    ▲ Revised Code

K ☑ **P9048** Infusion, plasma protein fraction (human), 5%, 250 ml
MED: 100-2,1,10; 100-4,3,40.2.2

K ☑ **P9050** Granulocytes, pheresis, each unit
MED: 100-2,1,10; 100-4,3,40.2.2

K ☑ **P9051** Whole blood or red blood cells, leukocytes reduced, CMV-negative, each unit
MED: 100-2,1,10; 100-4,3,40.2.2

K ☑ **P9052** Platelets, HLA-matched leukocytes reduced, apheresis/pheresis, each unit
MED: 100-2,1,10; 100-4,3,40.2.2

K ☑ **P9053** Platelets, pheresis, leukocytes reduced, CMV-negative, irradiated, each unit
MED: 100-2,1,10; 100-4,3,40.2.2

K ☑ **P9054** Whole blood or red blood cells, leukocytes reduced, frozen, deglycerol, washed, each unit
MED: 100-2,1,10; 100-4,3,40.2.2

K ☑ **P9055** Platelets, leukocytes reduced, CMV-negative, apheresis/pheresis, each unit
MED: 100-2,1,10; 100-4,3,40.2.2

K ☑ **P9056** Whole blood, leukocytes reduced, irradiated, each unit
MED: 100-2,1,10; 100-4,3,40.2.2

K ☑ **P9057** Red blood cells, frozen/deglycerolized/washed, leukocytes reduced, irradiated, each unit
MED: 100-2,1,10; 100-4,3,40.2.2

K ☑ **P9058** Red blood cells, leukocytes reduced, CMV-negative, irradiated, each unit
MED: 100-2,1,10; 100-4,3,40.2.2

K ☑ **P9059** Fresh frozen plasma between 8-24 hours of collection, each unit
MED: 100-2,1,10; 100-4,3,40.2.2

K ☑ **P9060** Fresh frozen plasma, donor retested, each unit
MED: 100-2,1,10; 100-4,3,40.2.2

A ☑ **P9603** Travel allowance, one way in connection with medically necessary laboratory specimen collection drawn from homebound or nursing homebound patient; prorated miles actually travelled.
MED: 100-4,16,60

A ☑ **P9604** Travel allowance, one way in connection with medically necessary laboratory specimen collection drawn from homebound or nursing homebound patient; prorated trip charge.
MED: 100-4,16,60

A **P9612** Catheterization for collection of specimen, single patient, all places of service
MED: 100-4,16,60

N **P9615** Catheterization for collection of specimen(s) (multiple patients)
MED: 100-4,16,60

Special Coverage Instructions          Noncovered by Medicare          Carrier Discretion          ☑ Quantity Alert     ● New Code     ○ Recycled/Reinstated     ▲ Revised Code

**126 — P Codes**          A Age Edit          M Maternity Edit     ♀ Female Only     ♂ Male Only     A-Y OPPS Status Indicators          **2008 HCPCS**

## Q CODES (TEMPORARY) Q0000-Q9999

New temporary Q codes to pay health care providers for the supplies used in creating casts were established to replace the removal of the practice expense for all HCPCS codes, including the CPT codes for fracture management and for casts and splints. Coders should continue to use the appropriate CPT code to report the work and practice expenses involved with creating the cast or splint; the temporary Q codes replace less specific coding for the casting and splinting supplies.

**X** **Q0035** Cardiokymography

Covered only in conjunction with electrocardiographic stress testing in male patients with atypical angina or nonischemic chest pain, or female patients with angina.

MED: 100-3,20.24

**B** **Q0081** Infusion therapy, using other than chemotherapeutic drugs, per visit

MED: 100-3,280.14

AHA: 1Q,'02,7; 4Q,'02,7

**B** ☑ **Q0083** Chemotherapy administration by other than infusion technique only (e.g., subcutaneous, intramuscular, push), per visit ⊘

**B** ☑ **Q0084** Chemotherapy administration by infusion technique only, per visit ⊘

MED: 100-3,280.14

**B** ☑ **Q0085** Chemotherapy administration by both infusion technique and other technique(s) (e.g., subcutaneous, intramuscular, push), per visit ⊘

**T** **Q0091** Screening Papanicolaou smear; obtaining, preparing and conveyance of cervical or vaginal smear to laboratory Ⓐ♀⊘

One pap test is covered by Medicare every two years for low risk patients and every one year for high risk patients. Q0091 can be reported with an E/M code when a separately identifiable E/M service is provided.

MED: 100-3, 190.2

MED: 100-3,190.2

AHA: 4Q,'02,8

**N** **Q0092** Set-up portable x-ray equipment

MED: 100-4,13,90; 100-4,13,90.4

**A** **Q0111** Wet mounts, including preparations of vaginal, cervical or skin specimens

**A** **Q0112** All potassium hydroxide (KOH) preparations

**A** **Q0113** Pinworm examination

**A** **Q0114** Fern test ♀

**A** **Q0115** Post-coital direct, qualitative examinations of vaginal or cervical mucous Ⓐ♀

**E** ☑ **Q0144** Azithromycin dihydrate, oral, capsules/powder, 1 gm

Use this code for Zithromax, Zithromax Z-PAK.

**N** ☑ **Q0163** Diphenhydramine HCl, 50 mg, oral, FDA approved prescription anti-emetic, for use as a complete therapeutic substitute for an IV anti-emetic at time of chemotherapy treatment not to exceed a 48-hour dosage regimen N1

See also J1200. Medicare covers at the time of chemotherapy if regimen doesn't exceed 48 hours. Submit on the same claim as the chemotherapy. Use this code for Truxadryl.

MED: 100-2,6,10; 100-4,4,240; 100-4,17,80.2

AHA: 1Q,'02,2

**N** ☑ **Q0164** Prochlorperazine maleate, 5 mg, oral, FDA approved prescription anti-emetic, for use as a complete therapeutic substitute for an IV anti-emetic at the time of chemotherapy treatment, not to exceed a 48-hour dosage regimen N1

Medicare covers at the time of chemotherapy if regimen doesn't exceed 48 hours. Submit on the same claim as the chemotherapy. Medicare jurisdiction: DME Medicare Administrative Contractor (DME MAC). Use this code for Compazine.

MED: 100-2,6,10; 100-4,4,240; 100-4,17,80.2

**B** ☑ **Q0165** Prochlorperazine maleate, 10 mg, oral, FDA approved prescription anti-emetic, for use as a complete therapeutic substitute for an IV anti-emetic at the time of chemotherapy treatment, not to exceed a 48-hour dosage regimen

Medicare covers at the time of chemotherapy if regimen doesn't exceed 48 hours. Submit on the same claim as the chemotherapy. Medicare jurisdiction: DME Medicare Administrative Contractor (DME MAC). Use this code for Compazine.

MED: 100-2,6,10; 100-4,4,240; 100-4,17,80.2

**K** ☑ **Q0166** Granisetron HCl, 1 mg, oral, FDA approved prescription anti-emetic, for use as a complete therapeutic substitute for an IV anti-emetic at the time of chemotherapy treatment, not to exceed a 24-hour dosage regimen K2

Medicare covers at the time of chemotherapy if regimen doesn't exceed 48 hours. Submit on the same claim as the chemotherapy. Medicare jurisdiction: DME Medicare Administrative Contractor (DME MAC). Use this code for Kytril.

MED: 100-2,6,10; 100-4,4,240; 100-4,17,80.2

**N** ☑ **Q0167** Dronabinol, 2.5 mg, oral, FDA approved prescription anti-emetic, for use as a complete therapeutic substitute for an IV anti-emetic at the time of chemotherapy treatment, not to exceed a 48-hour dosage regimen N1

Medicare covers at the time of chemotherapy if regimen doesn't exceed 48 hours. Submit on the same claim as the chemotherapy. Medicare jurisdiction: DME Medicare Administrative Contractor (DME MAC). Use this code for Marinol.

MED: 100-2,6,10; 100-4,4,240; 100-4,17,80.2

**B** ☑ **Q0168** Dronabinol, 5 mg, oral, FDA approved prescription anti-emetic, for use as a complete therapeutic substitute for an IV anti-emetic at the time of chemotherapy treatment, not to exceed a 48-hour dosage regimen

Medicare jurisdiction: DME Medicare Administrative Contractor (DME MAC). Use this code for Marinol.

MED: 100-2,6,10; 100-4,4,240; 100-4,17,80.2

**N** ☑ **Q0169** Promethazine HCl, 12.5 mg, oral, FDA approved prescription anti-emetic, for use as a complete therapeutic substitute for an IV anti-emetic at the time of chemotherapy treatment, not to exceed a 48-hour dosage regimen N1

Medicare covers at the time of chemotherapy if regimen doesn't exceed 48 hours. Submit on the same claim as the chemotherapy. Medicare jurisdiction: DME Medicare Administrative Contractor (DME MAC). Use this code for Phenergan, Amergan.

MED: 100-2,6,10; 100-4,4,240; 100-4,17,80.2

Special Coverage Instructions | Noncovered by Medicare | Carrier Discretion | ☑ Quantity Alert | ● New Code | ○ Recycled/Reinstated | ▲ Revised Code

**2008 HCPCS** | A2-Z3 ASC Payment Indicators | **MED:** Pub 100/NCD References | & DMEPOS Paid | ⊘ SNF Excluded | PQRI | **Q Codes — 127**

Q Codes (Temporary)

Q0170 — Q0480

B ☑ **Q0170** Promethazine HCl, 25 mg, oral, FDA approved prescription anti-emetic, for use as a complete therapeutic substitute for an IV anti-emetic at the time of chemotherapy treatment, not to exceed a 48-hour dosage regimen

Medicare covers at the time of chemotherapy if regimen doesn't exceed 48 hours. Submit on the same claim as the chemotherapy. Medicare jurisdiction: DME Medicare Administrative Contractor (DME MAC). Use this code for Phenergan, Amergan.

MED: 100-2,6,10; 100-4,4,240; 100-4,17,80.2

N ☑ **Q0171** Chlorpromazine HCl, 10 mg, oral, FDA approved prescription anti-emetic, for use as a complete therapeutic substitute for an IV anti-emetic at the time of chemotherapy treatment, not to exceed a 48-hour dosage regimen N1

Medicare covers at the time of chemotherapy if regimen doesn't exceed 48 hours. Submit on the same claim as the chemotherapy. Medicare jurisdiction: DME Medicare Administrative Contractor (DME MAC). Use this code for Thorazine.

MED: 100-2,6,10; 100-4,4,240; 100-4,17,80.2

B ☑ **Q0172** Chlorpromazine HCl, 25 mg, oral, FDA approved prescription anti-emetic, for use as a complete therapeutic substitute for an IV anti-emetic at the time of chemotherapy treatment, not to exceed a 48-hour dosage regimen

Medicare covers at the time of chemotherapy if regimen doesn't exceed 48 hours. Submit on the same claim as the chemotherapy. Medicare jurisdiction: DME Medicare Administrative Contractor (DME MAC). Use this code for Thorazine.

MED: 100-2,6,10; 100-4,4,240; 100-4,17,80.2

N ☑ **Q0173** Trimethobenzamide HCl, 250 mg, oral, FDA approved prescription anti-emetic, for use as a complete therapeutic substitute for an IV anti-emetic at the time of chemotherapy treatment, not to exceed a 48-hour dosage regimen N1

Medicare covers at the time of chemotherapy if regimen doesn't exceed 48 hours. Submit on the same claim as the chemotherapy. Medicare jurisdiction: DME Medicare Administrative Contractor (DME MAC). Use this code for Tebamide, T-Gen, Ticon, Tigan, Triban, Thimazide.

MED: 100-2,6,10; 100-4,4,240; 100-4,17,80.2

N ☑ **Q0174** Thiethylperazine maleate, 10 mg, oral, FDA approved prescription anti-emetic, for use as a complete therapeutic substitute for an IV anti-emetic at the time of chemotherapy treatment, not to exceed a 48-hour dosage regimen N1

Medicare covers at the time of chemotherapy if regimen doesn't exceed 48 hours. Submit on the same claim as the chemotherapy. Medicare jurisdiction: DME Medicare Administrative Contractor (DME MAC). Use this code for Torecan.

MED: 100-2,6,10; 100-4,4,240; 100-4,17,80.2

N ☑ **Q0175** Perphenazine, 4 mg, oral, FDA approved prescription anti-emetic, for use as a complete therapeutic substitute for an IV anti-emetic at the time of chemotherapy treatment, not to exceed a 48-hour dosage regimen N1

Medicare covers at the time of chemotherapy if regimen doesn't exceed 48 hours. Submit on the same claim as the chemotherapy. Medicare jurisdiction: DME Medicare Administrative Contractor (DME MAC). Use this code for Trilifon.

MED: 100-2,6,10; 100-4,4,240; 100-4,17,80.2

B ☑ **Q0176** Perphenazine, 8 mg, oral, FDA approved prescription anti-emetic, for use as a complete therapeutic substitute for an IV anti-emetic at the time of chemotherapy treatment, not to exceed a 48-hour dosage regimen

Medicare covers at the time of chemotherapy if regimen doesn't exceed 48 hours. Submit on the same claim as the chemotherapy. Medicare jurisdiction: DME Medicare Administrative Contractor (DME MAC). Use this code for Trilifon.

MED: 100-2,6,10; 100-4,4,240; 100-4,17,80.2

N ☑ **Q0177** Hydroxyzine pamoate, 25 mg, oral, FDA approved prescription anti-emetic, for use as a complete therapeutic substitute for an IV anti-emetic at the time of chemotherapy treatment, not to exceed a 48-hour dosage regimen N1

Medicare covers at the time of chemotherapy if regimen doesn't exceed 48 hours. Submit on the same claim as the chemotherapy. Medicare jurisdiction: DME Medicare Administrative Contractor (DME MAC). Use this code for Vistaril.

MED: 100-2,6,10; 100-4,4,240; 100-4,17,80.2

B ☑ **Q0178** Hydroxyzine pamoate, 50 mg, oral, FDA approved prescription anti-emetic, for use as a complete therapeutic substitute for an IV anti-emetic at the time of chemotherapy treatment, not to exceed a 48-hour dosage regimen

Medicare covers at the time of chemotherapy if regimen doesn't exceed 48 hours. Submit on the same claim as the chemotherapy.

MED: 100-2,6,10; 100-4,4,240; 100-4,17,80.2

K ☑ **Q0179** Ondansetron HCl 8 mg, oral, FDA approved prescription anti-emetic, for use as a complete therapeutic substitute for an IV anti-emetic at the time of chemotherapy treatment, not to exceed a 48-hour dosage regimen K2

Medicare covers at the time of chemotherapy if regimen doesn't exceed 48 hours. Submit on the same claim as the chemotherapy. Medicare jurisdiction: DME Medicare Administrative Contractor (DME MAC). Use this code for Zofran.

MED: 100-2,6,10; 100-4,4,240; 100-4,17,80.2

K ☑ **Q0180** Dolasetron mesylate, 100 mg, oral, FDA approved prescription anti-emetic, for use as a complete therapeutic substitute for an IV anti-emetic at the time of chemotherapy treatment, not to exceed a 24-hour dosage regimen K2

Medicare covers at the time of chemotherapy if regimen doesn't exceed 24 hours. Submit on the same claim as the chemotherapy. Medicare jurisdiction: DME Medicare Administrative Contractor (DME MAC). Use this code for Anzemet.

MED: 100-2,6,10; 100-4,4,240; 100-4,17,80.2

E ☑ **Q0181** Unspecified oral dosage form, FDA approved prescription anti-emetic, for use as a complete therapeutic substitute for an IV anti-emetic at the time of chemotherapy treatment, not to exceed a 48-hour dosage regimen

Medicare covers at the time of chemotherapy if regimen doesn't exceed 48-hours. Submit on the same claim as the chemotherapy. Medicare jurisdiction: DME Medicare Administrative Contractor (DME MAC).

MED: 100-2,6,10; 100-4,4,240; 100-4,17,80.2

A **Q0480** Driver for use with pneumatic ventricular assist device, replacement only ♿

AHA: 3Q,'05,2

---

Special Coverage Instructions   Noncovered by Medicare   Carrier Discretion   ☑ Quantity Alert   ● New Code   ○ Recycled/Reinstated   ▲ Revised Code

Q Codes (Temporary)

Q0481 — Q3025

[A]  **Q0481** Microprocessor control unit for use with electric ventricular assist device, replacement only  &
AHA: 3Q,'05,2

[A]  **Q0482** Microprocessor control unit for use with electric/pneumatic combination ventricular assist device, replacement only  &
AHA: 3Q,'05,2

[A]  **Q0483** Monitor/display module for use with electric ventricular assist device, replacement only  &
AHA: 3Q,'05,2

[A]  **Q0484** Monitor/display module for use with electric or electric/pneumatic ventricular assist device, replacement only  &
AHA: 3Q,'05,2

[A]  **Q0485** Monitor control cable for use with electric ventricular assist device, replacement only  &
AHA: 3Q,'05,2

[A]  **Q0486** Monitor control cable for use with electric/pneumatic ventricular assist device, replacement only  &
AHA: 3Q,'05,2

[A]  **Q0487** Leads (pneumatic/electrical) for use with any type electric/pneumatic ventricular assist device, replacement only  &
AHA: 3Q,'05,2

[A]  **Q0488** Power pack base for use with electric ventricular assist device, replacement only  &
AHA: 3Q,'05,2

[A]  **Q0489** Power pack base for use with electric/pneumatic ventricular assist device, replacement only  &
AHA: 3Q,'05,2

[A]  **Q0490** Emergency power source for use with electric ventricular assist device, replacement only  &
AHA: 3Q,'05,2

[A]  **Q0491** Emergency power source for use with electric/pneumatic ventricular assist device, replacement only  &
AHA: 3Q,'05,2

[A]  **Q0492** Emergency power supply cable for use with electric ventricular assist device, replacement only  &
AHA: 3Q,'05,2

[A]  **Q0493** Emergency power supply cable for use with electric/pneumatic ventricular assist device, replacement only  &
AHA: 3Q,'05,2

[A]  **Q0494** Emergency hand pump for use with electric or electric/pneumatic ventricular assist device, replacement only  &
AHA: 3Q,'05,2

[A]  **Q0495** Battery/power pack charger for use with electric or electric/pneumatic ventricular assist device, replacement only  &
AHA: 3Q,'05,2

[A]  **Q0496** Battery for use with electric or electric/pneumatic ventricular assist device, replacement only  &
AHA: 3Q,'05,2

[A]  **Q0497** Battery clips for use with electric or electric/pneumatic ventricular assist device, replacement only  &
AHA: 3Q,'05,2

[A]  **Q0498** Holster for use with electric or electric/pneumatic ventricular assist device, replacement only  &
AHA: 3Q,'05,2

[A]  **Q0499** Belt/vest for use with electric or electric/pneumatic ventricular assist device, replacement only  &
AHA: 3Q,'05,2

[A] ☑ **Q0500** Filters for use with electric or electric/pneumatic ventricular assist device, replacement only  &
The base unit for this code is for each filter.
AHA: 3Q,'05,2

[A]  **Q0501** Shower cover for use with electric or electric/pneumatic ventricular assist device, replacement only  &
AHA: 3Q,'05,2

[A]  **Q0502** Mobility cart for pneumatic ventricular assist device, replacement only  &
AHA: 3Q,'05,2

[A] ☑ **Q0503** Battery for pneumatic ventricular assist device, replacement only, each  &
AHA: 3Q,'05,2

[A]  **Q0504** Power adapter for pneumatic ventricular assist device, replacement only, vehicle type  &
AHA: 3Q,'05,2

[A]  **Q0505** Miscellaneous supply or accessory for use with ventricular assist device
AHA: 3Q,'05,2

[B]  **Q0510** Pharmacy supply fee for initial immunosuppressive drug(s), first month following transplant
MED: 100-4,4,240

[B]  **Q0511** Pharmacy supply fee for oral anti-cancer, oral anti-emetic, or immunosuppressive drug(s); for the first prescription In a 30-day period
MED: 100-4,4,240

[B]  **Q0512** Pharmacy supply fee for oral anti-cancer, oral anti-emetic, or immunosuppressive drug(s); for a subsequent prescription in a 30-day period
MED: 100-4,4,240

[B]  **Q0513** Pharmacy dispensing fee for inhalation drug(s); per 30 days

[B]  **Q0514** Pharmacy dispensing fee for inhalation drug(s); per 90 days

[K] ☑ **Q0515** Injection, sermorelin acetate, 1 mcg  K2
MED: 100-2,15,50; 100-4,4,230.1

[N]  **Q1003** New technology, intraocular lens, category 3 (reduced spherical aberration) as defined in Federal Register notice, Vol. 65, dated May 3, 2000  L6 ⊘

[E]  **Q1004** New technology intraocular lens category 4 as defined in Federal Register notice

[E]  **Q1005** New technology intraocular lens category 5 as defined in Federal Register notice

[N] ☑ **Q2004** Irrigation solution for treatment of bladder calculi, for example renacidin, per 500 ml  M1
MED: 100-2,15,50

[K] ☑ **Q2009** Injection, fosphenytoin, 50 mg  K2
Use this code for Cerebyx.

[K] ☑ **Q2017** Injection, teniposide, 50 mg  K2
Use this code for Vumon.
MED: 100-2,15,50

[B] ☑ **Q3001** Radioelements for brachytherapy, any type, each  ⊘
MED: 100-4,12,70; 100-4,13,20; 100-4,13,90

[A]  **Q3014** Telehealth originating site facility fee
MED: 100-4,12,190

[K] ☑ **Q3025** Injection, interferon beta-1A, 11 mcg for intramuscular use  K2
Use this code for Avonex, Rebif. See also J1825.
MED: 100-2,15,50

Special Coverage Instructions  Noncovered by Medicare  Carrier Discretion  ☑ Quantity Alert  ● New Code  ○ Recycled/Reinstated  ▲ Revised Code

**2008 HCPCS**  N2–Z3 ASC Payment Indicators  **MED:** Pub 100/NCD References  & DMEPOS Paid  ⊘ SNF Excluded  PQ PQRI  **Q Codes — 129**

**Q Codes (Temporary)**

**Q3026 — Q4038**

E ☑ **Q3026** Injection, interferon beta-1A, 11 mcg for subcutaneous use
A
Use this code for Avonex Rebif. See also J1825.

N **Q3031** Collagen skin test
MED: 100-3,230.10

B **Q4001** Casting supplies, body cast adult, with or without head, plaster A
MED: 100-4,4,240; 100-4,20,170

B **Q4002** Cast supplies, body cast adult, with or without head, fiberglass A
MED: 100-4,4,240; 100-4,20,170

B **Q4003** Cast supplies, shoulder cast, adult (11 years +), plaster A
MED: 100-4,4,240; 100-4,20,170

B **Q4004** Cast supplies, shoulder cast, adult (11 years +), fiberglass A
MED: 100-4,4,240; 100-4,20,170

B **Q4005** Cast supplies, long arm cast, adult (11 years +), plaster A
MED: 100-4,4,240; 100-4,20,170

B **Q4006** Cast supplies, long arm cast, adult (11 years +), fiberglass A
MED: 100-4,4,240; 100-4,20,170

B **Q4007** Cast supplies, long arm cast, pediatric (0–10 years), plaster A
MED: 100-4,4,240; 100-4,20,170

B **Q4008** Cast supplies, long arm cast, pediatric (0–10 years), fiberglass A
MED: 100-4,4,240; 100-4,20,170

B **Q4009** Cast supplies, short arm cast, adult (11 years +), plaster A
MED: 100-4,4,240; 100-4,20,170

B **Q4010** Cast supplies, short arm cast, adult (11 years +), fiberglass A
MED: 100-4,4,240; 100-4,20,170

B **Q4011** Cast supplies, short arm cast, pediatric (0–10 years), plaster A
MED: 100-4,4,240; 100-4,20,170

B **Q4012** Cast supplies, short arm cast, pediatric (0–10 years), fiberglass A
MED: 100-4,4,240; 100-4,20,170

B **Q4013** Cast supplies, gauntlet cast (includes lower forearm and hand), adult (11 years +), plaster A
MED: 100-4,4,240; 100-4,20,170

B **Q4014** Cast supplies, gauntlet cast (includes lower forearm and hand), adult (11 years +), fiberglass A
MED: 100-4,4,240; 100-4,20,170

B **Q4015** Cast supplies, gauntlet cast (includes lower forearm and hand), pediatric (0–10 years), plaster A
MED: 100-4,4,240; 100-4,20,170

B **Q4016** Cast supplies, gauntlet cast (includes lower forearm and hand), pediatric (0–10 years), fiberglass A
MED: 100-4,4,240; 100-4,20,170

B **Q4017** Cast supplies, long arm splint, adult (11 years +), plaster A
MED: 100-4,4,240; 100-4,20,170

B **Q4018** Cast supplies, long arm splint, adult (11 years +), fiberglass A
MED: 100-4,4,240; 100-4,20,170

B **Q4019** Cast supplies, long arm splint, pediatric (0–10 years), plaster A
MED: 100-4,4,240; 100-4,20,170

B **Q4020** Cast supplies, long arm splint, pediatric (0–10 years), fiberglass A
MED: 100-4,4,240; 100-4,20,170

B **Q4021** Cast supplies, short arm splint, adult (11 years +), plaster A
MED: 100-4,4,240; 100-4,20,170

B **Q4022** Cast supplies, short arm splint, adult (11 years +), fiberglass A
MED: 100-4,4,240; 100-4,20,170

B **Q4023** Cast supplies, short arm splint, pediatric (0–10 years), plaster A
MED: 100-4,4,240; 100-4,20,170

B **Q4024** Cast supplies, short arm splint, pediatric (0–10 years), fiberglass A
MED: 100-4,4,240; 100-4,20,170

B **Q4025** Cast supplies, hip spica (one or both legs), adult (11 years +), plaster A
MED: 100-4,4,240; 100-4,20,170

B **Q4026** Cast supplies, hip spica (one or both legs), adult (11 years +), fiberglass A
MED: 100-4,4,240; 100-4,20,170

B **Q4027** Cast supplies, hip spica (one or both legs), pediatric (0–10 years), plaster A
MED: 100-4,4,240; 100-4,20,170

B **Q4028** Cast supplies, hip spica (one or both legs), pediatric (0–10 years), fiberglass A
MED: 100-4,4,240; 100-4,20,170

B **Q4029** Cast supplies, long leg cast, adult (11 years +), plaster A
MED: 100-4,4,240; 100-4,20,170

B **Q4030** Cast supplies, long leg cast, adult (11 years +), fiberglass A
MED: 100-4,4,240; 100-4,20,170

B **Q4031** Cast supplies, long leg cast, pediatric (0–10 years), plaster A
MED: 100-4,4,240; 100-4,20,170

B **Q4032** Cast supplies, long leg cast, pediatric (0–10 years), fiberglass A
MED: 100-4,4,240; 100-4,20,170

B **Q4033** Cast supplies, long leg cylinder cast, adult (11 years +), plaster A
MED: 100-4,4,240; 100-4,20,170

B **Q4034** Cast supplies, long leg cylinder cast, adult (11 years +), fiberglass A
MED: 100-4,4,240; 100-4,20,170

B **Q4035** Cast supplies, long leg cylinder cast, pediatric (0–10 years), plaster A
MED: 100-4,4,240; 100-4,20,170

B **Q4036** Cast supplies, long leg cylinder cast, pediatric (0–10 years), fiberglass A
MED: 100-4,4,240; 100-4,20,170

B **Q4037** Cast supplies, short leg cast, adult (11 years +), plaster A
MED: 100-4,4,240; 100-4,20,170

B **Q4038** Cast supplies, short leg cast, adult (11 years +), fiberglass A
MED: 100-4,4,240; 100-4,20,170

---

Special Coverage Instructions    Noncovered by Medicare    Carrier Discretion    ☑ Quantity Alert    ● New Code    ○ Recycled/Reinstated    ▲ Revised Code

B    **Q4039** Cast supplies, short leg cast, pediatric (0–10 years), plaster   A
MED: 100-4,4,240; 100-4,20,170

B    **Q4040** Cast supplies, short leg cast, pediatric (0–10 years), fiberglass   A
MED: 100-4,4,240; 100-4,20,170

B    **Q4041** Cast supplies, long leg splint, adult (11 years +), plaster   A
MED: 100-4,4,240; 100-4,20,170

B    **Q4042** Cast supplies, long leg splint, adult (11 years +), fiberglass   A
MED: 100-4,4,240; 100-4,20,170

B    **Q4043** Cast supplies, long leg splint, pediatric (0–10 years), plaster   A
MED: 100-4,4,240; 100-4,20,170

B    **Q4044** Cast supplies, long leg splint, pediatric (0–10 years), fiberglass   A
MED: 100-4,4,240; 100-4,20,170

B    **Q4045** Cast supplies, short leg splint, adult (11 years +), plaster   A
MED: 100-4,4,240; 100-4,20,170

B    **Q4046** Cast supplies, short leg splint, adult (11 years +), fiberglass   A
MED: 100-4,4,240; 100-4,20,170

B    **Q4047** Cast supplies, short leg splint, pediatric (0–10 years), plaster   A
MED: 100-4,4,240; 100-4,20,170

B    **Q4048** Cast supplies, short leg splint, pediatric (0–10 years), fiberglass   A
MED: 100-4,4,240; 100-4,20,170

B    **Q4049** Finger splint, static
MED: 100-4,4,240; 100-4,20,170

B    **Q4050** Cast supplies, for unlisted types and materials of casts
MED: 100-4,4,240; 100-4,20,170

B    **Q4051** Splint supplies, miscellaneous (includes thermoplastics, strapping, fasteners, padding and other supplies)
MED: 100-4,4,240; 100-4,20,170

~~Q4079~~ ~~Injection, natalizumab, 1 mg~~
AHA: 2Q,'05,11

▲ Y ☑   **Q4080** Iloprost, inhalation solution, FDA-approved final product, noncompounded, administered through DME, unit dose form, 20 mcg
AHA: 3Q,'05,7

A ☑   **Q4081** Injection, epoetin alfa, 100 units (for ESRD on dialysis)

B    **Q4082** Drug or biological, not otherwise classified, Part B drug competitive acquisition program (CAP)

~~Q4083~~ ~~Hyaluronan or derivative, Hyalgan or Supartz, for intra-articular injection, per dose~~
See J2321.

~~Q4084~~ ~~Hyaluronan or derivative, Synvisc, for intra-articular injection, per dose~~
See J7321.

~~Q4085~~ ~~Hyaluronan or derivative, Euflexxa, for intra-articular injection, per dose~~

~~Q4086~~ ~~Hyaluronan or derivative, Orthovisc, for intra-articular injection, per dose~~
See J7324.

~~Q4087~~ ~~Injection, immune globulin, (Octagam), intravenous, non-lyophilized, (e.g. liquid), 500 mg~~
See J1568.

~~Q4088~~ ~~Injection, immune globulin, (Gammagard liquid), intravenous, non-lyophilized, (e.g. liquid), 500 mg~~
See J1569.

~~Q4089~~ ~~Injection, Rho(D) immune globulin (human), (Rhophylac), intramuscular or intravenous, 100 IU~~
See J2791.

~~Q4090~~ ~~Injection, hepatitis B immune globulin (HepaGam B), intramuscular, 0.5 ml~~
See J1571.

~~Q4091~~ ~~Injection, immune globulin, (Flebogamma), intravenous, non-lyophilized, (e.g. liquid), 500 mg~~
See J1572.

~~Q4092~~ ~~Injection, immune globulin, (Gamunex), intravenous, non-lyophilized, (e.g. liquid), 500 mg~~
See J1561.

~~Q4093~~ ~~Albuterol, all formulations including separated isomers, inhalation solution, FDA-approved final product, non-compounded, administered through DME, concentrated form, per 1 mg (Albuterol) or per 0.5 mg (Levalbuterol)~~
See J7602.

~~Q4094~~ ~~Albuterol, all formulations including separated isomers, inhalation solution, FDA-approved final product, non-compounded, administered through DME, unit dose, per 1 mg (Albuterol) or per 0.5 mg (Levalbuterol)~~
See J7603.

~~Q4095~~ ~~Injection, zoledronic acid (Reclast), 1 mg~~
See J3488.

B    **Q5001** Hospice care provided in patient's home/residence

B    **Q5002** Hospice care provided in assisted living facility

B    **Q5003** Hospice care provided in nursing long-term care facility (LTC) or nonskilled nursing facility (NF)

B    **Q5004** Hospice care provided in skilled nursing facility (SNF)

B    **Q5005** Hospice care provided in inpatient hospital

B    **Q5006** Hospice care provided in inpatient hospice facility

B    **Q5007** Hospice care provided in long term care facility

B    **Q5008** Hospice care provided in inpatient psychiatric facility

B    **Q5009** Hospice care provided in place not otherwise specified (NOS)

~~Q9945~~ ~~Low osmolar contrast material, up to 149 mg/ml iodine concentration, per ml~~
See Q9965.
MED: 100-4,13,20; 100-4,13,90

~~Q9946~~ ~~Low osmolar contrast material, 150–199 mg/ml iodine concentration, per ml~~
See Q9965.
MED: 100-4,12,70; 100-4,13,20; 100-4,13,90

~~Q9947~~ ~~Low osmolar contrast material, 200–249 mg/ml iodine concentration, per ml~~
See Q9966.
MED: 100-4,12,70; 100-4,13,20; 100-4,13,90

---

Special Coverage Instructions    Noncovered by Medicare    Carrier Discretion    ☑ Quantity Alert    ● New Code    ○ Recycled/Reinstated    ▲ Revised Code

~~Q9948 Low osmolar contrast material, 250–299 mg/ml iodine concentration, per ml~~
See Q9966.

MED: 100-4,12,70; 100-4,13,20; 100-4,13,90

~~Q9949 Low osmolar contrast material, 300–349 mg/ml iodine concentration, per ml~~
See Q9967.

MED: 100-4,12,70; 100-4,13,20; 100-4,13,90

~~Q9950 Low osmolar contrast material, 350–399 mg/ml iodine concentration, per ml~~
See Q9967.

MED: 100-4,12,70; 100-4,13,20; 100-4,13,90

N ☑ **Q9951** Low osmolar contrast material, 400 or greater mg/ml iodine concentration, per ml N1
MED: 100-4,12,70; 100-4,13,20; 100-4,13,90

~~Q9952 Injection, gadolinium-based magnetic resonance contrast agent, per ml~~
See A9576-A9579.

MED: 100-4,12,70; 100-4,13,20; 100-4,13,90

N ☑ **Q9953** Injection, iron-based magnetic resonance contrast agent, per ml N1
MED: 100-4,12,70; 100-4,13,20; 100-4,13,90

N ☑ **Q9954** Oral magnetic resonance contrast agent, per 100 ml N1
MED: 100-4,12,70; 100-4,13,20; 100-4,13,90

N ☑ **Q9955** Injection, perflexane lipid microspheres, per ml N1
MED: 100-4,4,230.1

N ☑ **Q9956** Injection, octafluoropropane microspheres, per ml N1
MED: 100-4,4,230.1

N ☑ **Q9957** Injection, perflutren lipid microspheres, per ml N1
MED: 100-4,4,230.1

N ☑ **Q9958** High osmolar contrast material, up to 149 mg/ml iodine concentration, per ml N1
MED: 100-4,12,70; 100-4,13,20; 100-4,13,90
AHA: 3Q,'05,7

N ☑ **Q9959** High osmolar contrast material, 150–199 mg/ml iodine concentration, per ml N1
MED: 100-4,12,70; 100-4,13,20; 100-4,13,90
AHA: 3Q,'05,7

N ☑ **Q9960** High osmolar contrast material, 200–249 mg/ml iodine concentration, per ml N1
MED: 100-4,12,70; 100-4,13,20; 100-4,13,90
AHA: 3Q,'05,7

N ☑ **Q9961** High osmolar contrast material, 250–299 mg/ml iodine concentration, per ml N1
MED: 100-4,12,70; 100-4,13,20; 100-4,13,90
AHA: 3Q,'05,7

N ☑ **Q9962** High osmolar contrast material, 300–349 mg/ml iodine concentration, per ml N1
MED: 100-4,12,70; 100-4,13,20; 100-4,13,90
AHA: 3Q,'05,7

N ☑ **Q9963** High osmolar contrast material, 350–399 mg/ml iodine concentration, per ml N1
MED: 100-4,12,70; 100-4,13,20; 100-4,13,90
AHA: 3Q,'05,7

N ☑ **Q9964** High osmolar contrast material, 400 or greater mg/ml iodine concentration, per ml N1
MED: 100-4,12,70; 100-4,13,20; 100-4,13,90
AHA: 3Q,'05,7

● N ☑ **Q9965** Low osmolar contrast material, 100–199 mg/ml iodine concentration, per ml N1
Use this code for Omnipaque 140, Omnipaque 180, Optiray 160.

● N ☑ **Q9966** Low osmolar contrast material, 200–299 mg/ml iodine concentration, per ml N1
Use this code for Omnipaque 240, Optiray 240.

● N ☑ **Q9967** Low osmolar contrast material, 300–399 mg/ml iodine concentration, per ml N1
Use this code for Omnipaque 300, Omnipaque 350, Optiray, Optiray 300, Optiray 320, Oxilan 300, Oxilan 350.

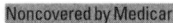 Special Coverage Instructions  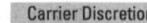 Noncovered by Medicare  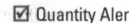 Carrier Discretion  ☑ Quantity Alert  ● New Code  ○ Recycled/Reinstated  ▲ Revised Code

132 — Q Codes   A Age Edit   M Maternity Edit   ♀ Female Only   ♂ Male Only   A-Y OPPS Status Indicators   **2008 HCPCS**

## DIAGNOSTIC RADIOLOGY SERVICES R0000-R5999

R codes are used for the transportation of portable x-ray and/or EKG equipment.

B ☑ **R0070** Transportation of portable x-ray equipment and personnel to home or nursing home, per trip to facility or location, one patient seen

Only a single, reasonable transportation charge is allowed for each trip the portable x-ray supplier makes to a location. When more than one patient is x-rayed at the same location, prorate the single allowable transport charge among all patients.

MED: 100-4,13,90; 100-4,13,90.3

B ☑ **R0075** Transportation of portable x-ray equipment and personnel to home or nursing home, per trip to facility or location, more than one patient seen

Only a single, reasonable transportation charge is allowed for each trip the portable x-ray supplier makes to a location. When more than one patient is x-rayed at the same location, prorate the single allowable transport charge among all patients.

MED: 100-4,13,90; 100-4,13,90.3

B ☑ **R0076** Transportation of portable EKG to facility or location, per patient

Only a single, reasonable transportation charge is allowed for each trip the portable EKG supplier makes to a location. When more than one patient is tested at the same location, prorate the single allowable transport charge among all patients.

MED: 100-1,5,90.2; 100-2,15,80.1; 100-3,20.15; 100-4,13,90; 100-4,13,90.3; 100-4,16,10; 100-4,16,10.1; 100-4,16,110.4

Special Coverage Instructions    Noncovered by Medicare    Carrier Discretion    ☑ Quantity Alert    ● New Code    ○ Recycled/Reinstated    ▲ Revised Code

**2008 HCPCS**    A2-Z3 ASC Payment Indicators    **MED:** Pub 100/NCD References    ⅀ DMEPOS Paid    ⊘ SNF Excluded    PQ PQRI    **R Codes — 133**

## TEMPORARY NATIONAL CODES (NON-MEDICARE)
## S0000-S9999

The S codes are used by the Blue Cross/Blue Shield Association (BCBSA) and the Health Insurance Association of America (HIAA) to report drugs, services, and supplies for which there are no national codes but for which codes are needed by the private sector to implement policies, programs, or claims processing. They are for the purpose of meeting the particular needs of the private sector. These codes are also used by the Medicaid program, but they are not payable by Medicare.

☑ **S0012** Butorphanol tartrate, nasal spray, 25 mg
Use this code for Stadol NS.

☑ **S0014** Tacrine HCl, 10 mg
Use this code for Cognex.

☑ **S0017** Injection, aminocaproic acid, 5 g
Use this code for Amicar.

☑ **S0020** Injection, bupivicaine HCl, 30 ml
Use this code for Marcaine, Sensorcaine.

☑ **S0021** Injection, cefoperazone sodium, 1 g
Use this code for Cefobid.

☑ **S0023** Injection, cimetidine HCl, 300 mg
Use this code for Tagamet HCl.

☑ **S0028** Injection, famotidine, 20 mg
Use this code for Pepcid.

☑ **S0030** Injection, metronidazole, 500 mg
Use this code for Flagyl IV RTU.

☑ **S0032** Injection, nafcillin sodium, 2 g
Use this code for Nallpen, Unipen.

☑ **S0034** Injection, ofloxacin, 400 mg
Use this code for Floxin IV.

☑ **S0039** Injection, sulfamethoxazole and trimethoprim, 10 ml
Use this code for Bactrim IV, Septra IV, SMZ-TMP, Sulfutrim.

☑ **S0040** Injection, ticarcillin disodium and clavulanate potassium, 3.1 g
Use this code for Timentin.

☑ **S0073** Injection, aztreonam, 500 mg
Use this code for Azactam.

☑ **S0074** Injection, cefotetan disodium, 500 mg
Use this code for Cefotan.

☑ **S0077** Injection, clindamycin phosphate, 300 mg
Use this code for Cleocin Phosphate.

☑ **S0078** Injection, fosphenytoin sodium, 750 mg
Use this code for Cerebryx.

☑ **S0080** Injection, pentamidine isethionate, 300 mg
Use this code for NebuPent, Pentam 300, Pentacarinat. See also code J2545.

☑ **S0081** Injection, piperacillin sodium, 500 mg
Use this code for Pipracil.

☑ **S0088** Imatinib injection, 100 mg
Use this code for Gleevec.

☑ **S0090** Sildenafil citrate, 25 mg    Ⓐ
Use this code for Viagra.

☑ **S0091** Granisetron HCl, 1 mg (for circumstances falling under the Medicare statute, use Q0166)
Use this code for Kytril.

☑ **S0092** Injection, hydromorphone HCl, 250 mg (loading dose for infusion pump)
Use this code for Dilaudid, Hydromophone. See also J1170.

☑ **S0093** Injection, morphine sulfate, 500 mg (loading dose for infusion pump)
Use this code for Duramorph, MS Contin, Morphine Sulfate. See also J2270, J2271, J2275.

☑ **S0104** Zidovudine, oral, 100 mg
See also J3485 for Retrovir.

☑ **S0106** Bupropion HCl sustained release tablet, 150 mg, per bottle of 60 tablets
Use this code for Wellbutrin SR tablets.

☑ **S0108** Mercaptopurine, oral, 50 mg
Use this code for Purinethol oral.

☑ **S0109** Methadone, oral, 5 mg
Use this code for Dolophine.

☑ **S0117** Tretinoin, topical, 5 g

☑ **S0122** Injection, menotropins, 75 IU
Use this code for Humegon, Pergonal, Repronex.

☑ **S0126** Injection, follitropin alfa, 75 IU
Use this code for Gonal-F.

☑ **S0128** Injection, follitropin beta, 75 IU    ♀
Use this code for Follistim.

☑ **S0132** Injection, ganirelix acetate, 250 mcg    ♀
Use this code for Antagon.

☑ **S0136** Clozapine, 25 mg
Use this code for Clozaril.

☑ **S0137** Didanosine (ddI), 25 mg
Use this code for Videx.

☑ **S0138** Finasteride, 5 mg    ♂
Use this code for Propecia (oral), Proscar (oral).

☑ **S0139** Minoxidil, 10 mg
Use this code for Loniten (oral).

☑ **S0140** Saquinavir, 200 mg
Use this code for Fortovase (oral), Invirase (oral).

☑ **S0141** Zalcitabine (ddC), 0.375 mg
Use this code for Hivid (oral).

☑ **S0142** Colistimethate sodium, inhalation solution administrated through DME, concentrated form, per mg

☑ **S0143** Aztreonam, inhalation solution administered through DME, concentrated form, per g

☑ **S0145** Injection, pegylated interferon alfa-2a, 180 mcg per ml
Use this code for Pegasys.

☑ **S0146** Injection, pegylated interferon alfa-2b, 10 mcg per 0.5 ml

~~**S0147** Injection, alglucosidase alfa, 20 mg~~
See J0220.

☑ **S0155** Sterile dilutant for epoprostenol, 50 ml
Use this code for Flolan.

☑ **S0156** Exemestane, 25 mg
Use this code for Aromasin.

☑ **S0157** Becaplermin gel 0.01%, 0.5 gm
Use this code for Regraex Gel.

☑ **S0160** Dextroamphetamine sulfate, 5 mg

---

Special Coverage Instructions    Noncovered by Medicare    Carrier Discretion    ☑ Quantity Alert    ● New Code    ○ Recycled/Reinstated    ▲ Revised Code

**Temporary National Codes (Non-Medicare)**

**S0161 — S0320**

▲ ☑ **S0161** Calcitrol, 0.25 mg

☑ **S0162** Injection, efalizumab, 125 mg
Use this code for Raptiva.

☑ **S0164** Injection, pantoprazole sodium, 40 mg
Use this code for Protonix IV.

☑ **S0166** Injection, olanzapine, 2.5 mg
Use this code for Zyprexa.

~~S0167~~ ~~Injection, apomorphine HCl, 1 mg~~

☑ **S0170** Anastrozole, oral, 1mg
Use this code for Arimidex.

☑ **S0171** Injection, bumetanide, 0.5 mg
Use this code for Bumex.

☑ **S0172** Chlorambucil, oral, 2 mg
Use this code for Leukeran.

☑ **S0174** Dolasetron mesylate, oral 50 mg (for circumstances falling under the Medicare statute, use Q0180)
Use this code for Anzemet.

☑ **S0175** Flutamide, oral, 125 mg
Use this code for Eulexin.

☑ **S0176** Hydroxyurea, oral, 500 mg
Use this code for Droxia, Hydrea, Mylocel.

☑ **S0177** Levamisole HCl, oral, 50 mg
Use this code for Ergamisol.

☑ **S0178** Lomustine, oral, 10 mg
Use this code for Ceenu.
MED: 100-4,17,80.2

☑ **S0179** Megestrol acetate, oral, 20 mg
Use this code for Megace.

~~S0180~~ ~~Etonogestrel (contraceptive) implant system, including implant and supplies~~
See J7307.

☑ **S0181** Ondansetron HCl, oral, 4 mg (for circumstances falling under the Medicare statute, use Q0179)
Use this code for Zofran.

☑ **S0182** Procarbazine HCl, oral, 50 mg
Use this code for Matulane.

☑ **S0183** Prochlorperazine maleate, oral, 5 mg (for circumstances falling under the Medicare statute, use Q0164-Q0165)
Use this code for Compazine.

☑ **S0187** Tamoxifen citrate, oral, 10 mg
Use this code for Nolvadex.

☑ **S0189** Testosterone pellet, 75 mg

☑ **S0190** Mitepristone, oral, 200 mg ♀
Use this code for Mifoprex 200 mg oral.

☑ **S0191** Misoprostol, oral, 200 mcg

☑ **S0194** Dialysis/stress vitamin supplement, oral, 100 capsules

**S0195** Pneumococcal conjugate vaccine, polyvalent, intramuscular, for children from five years to nine years of age who have not previously received the vaccine Ⓐ
Use this code for Pneumovax II.

☑ **S0196** Injectable poly-l-lactic acid, restorative implant, 1 ml, face (deep dermis, subcutaneous layers)

☑ **S0197** Prenatal vitamins, 30-day supply Ⓜ ♀

**S0199** Medically induced abortion by oral ingestion of medication including all associated services and supplies (e.g., patient counseling, office visits, confirmation of pregnancy by HCG, ultrasound to confirm duration of pregnancy, ultrasound to confirm completion of abortion) except drugs ♀

**S0201** Partial hospitalization services, less than 24 hours, per diem

**S0207** Paramedic intercept, nonhospital based ALS service (nonvoluntary), nontransport

**S0208** Paramedic intercept, hospital-based ALS service (nonvoluntary), nontransport

**S0209** Wheelchair van, mileage, per mile

☑ **S0215** Nonemergency transportation; mileage, per mile
See also codes A0021-A0999 for transportation.

☑ **S0220** Medical conference by a physician with interdisciplinary team of health professionals or representatives of community agencies to coordinate activities of patient care (patient is present); approximately 30 minutes

☑ **S0221** Medical conference by a physician with interdisciplinary team of health professionals or representatives of community agencies to coordinate activities of patient care (patient is present); approximately 60 minutes

**S0250** Comprehensive geriatric assessment and treatment planning performed by assessment team Ⓐ

**S0255** Hospice referral visit (advising patient and family of care options) performed by nurse, social worker, or other designated staff

**S0257** Counseling and discussion regarding advance directives or end of life care planning and decisions, with patient and/or surrogate (list separately in addition to code for appropriate evaluation and management service)

**S0260** History and physical (outpatient or office) related to surgical procedure (list separately in addition to code for appropriate evaluation and management service)

☑ **S0265** Genetic counseling, under physician supervision, each 15 minutes

● ☑ **S0270** Physician management of patient home care, standard monthly case rate (per 30 days)

● ☑ **S0271** Physician management of patient home care, hospice monthly case rate (per 30 days)

● ☑ **S0272** Physician management of patient home care, episodic care monthly case rate (per 30 days)

● **S0273** Physician visit at member's home, outside of a capitation arrangement

● **S0274** Nurse practitioner visit at member's home, outside of a capitation arrangement

**S0302** Completed early periodic screening diagnosis and treatment (EPSDT) service (list in addition to code for appropriate evaluation and management service)

**S0310** Hospitalist services (list separately in addition to code for appropriate evaluation and management service)

**S0315** Disease management program; initial assessment and initiation of the program

**S0316** Disease management program, follow-up/reassessment

☑ **S0317** Disease management program; per diem

**S0320** Telephone calls by a registered nurse to a disease management program member for monitoring purposes; per month

Special Coverage Instructions    Noncovered by Medicare    Carrier Discretion    ☑ Quantity Alert    ● New Code    ○ Recycled/Reinstated    ▲ Revised Code

136 — S Codes    Ⓐ Age Edit    Ⓜ Maternity Edit    ♀ Female Only    ♂ Male Only    Ⓐ-Ⓥ OPPS Status Indicators    2008 HCPCS

☑ **S0340** Lifestyle modification program for management of coronary artery disease, including all supportive services; first quarter/stage

**S0341** Lifestyle modification program for management of coronary artery disease, including all supportive services; second or third quarter/stage

**S0342** Lifestyle modification program for management of coronary artery disease, including all supportive services; fourth quarter/stage

☑ **S0345** Electrocardiographic monitoring utilizing a home computerized telemetry station with automatic activation and real-time notification of monitoring station, 24-hour attended monitoring, including recording, monitoring, receipt of transmissions, analysis, and physician review and interpretation; per 24-hour period

☑ **S0346** Electrocardiographic monitoring utilizing a home computerized telemetry station with automatic activation and real-time notification of monitoring station, 24-hour attended monitoring, including recording, monitoring, receipt of transmissions, and analysis; per 24-hour period

☑ **S0347** Electrocardiographic monitoring utilizing a home computerized telemetry station with automatic activation and real-time notification of monitoring station, 24-hour attended monitoring, including physician review and interpretation; 24-hour period

**S0390** Routine foot care; removal and/or trimming of corns, calluses and/or nails and preventive maintenance in specific medical conditions (e.g., diabetes), per visit

**S0395** Impression casting of a foot performed by a practitioner other than the manufacturer of the orthotic

**S0400** Global fee for extracorporeal shock wave lithotripsy treatment of kidney stone(s)

☑ **S0500** Disposable contact lens, per lens

☑ **S0504** Single vision prescription lens (safety, athletic, or sunglass), per lens

☑ **S0506** Bifocal vision prescription lens (safety, athletic, or sunglass), per lens

☑ **S0508** Trifocal vision prescription lens (safety, athletic, or sunglass), per lens

☑ **S0510** Nonprescription lens (safety, athletic, or sunglass), per lens

☑ **S0512** Daily wear specialty contact lens, per lens

☑ **S0514** Color contact lens, per lens

**S0515** Scleral lens, liquid bandage device, per lens

**S0516** Safety eyeglass frames

**S0518** Sunglasses frames

**S0580** Polycarbonate lens (list this code in addition to the basic code for the lens)

**S0581** Nonstandard lens (list this code in addition to the basic code for the lens)

**S0590** Integral lens service, miscellaneous services reported separately

**S0592** Comprehensive contact lens evaluation

**S0595** Dispensing new spectacle lenses for patient supplied frame

**S0601** Screening proctoscopy ♂
MED: 100-4,4,240

**S0605** Digital rectal examination, annual

**S0610** Annual gynecological examination; new patient ♀
MED: 100-4,4,240

**S0612** Annual gynecological examination; established patient ♀
MED: 100-4,4,240

**S0613** Annual gynecological examination, clinical breast examination without pelvic examination ♀

**S0618** Audiometry for hearing aid evaluation to determine the level and degree of hearing loss

**S0620** Routine ophthalmological examination including refraction; new patient

**S0621** Routine ophthalmological examination including refraction; established patient

**S0622** Physical exam for college, new or established patient (list separately in addition to appropriate evaluation and management code) Ⓐ

**S0625** Retinal telescreening by digital imaging of multiple different fundus areas to screen for vision-threatening conditions, including imaging, interpretation and report

**S0630** Removal of sutures by a physician other than the physician who originally closed the wound

**S0800** Laser in situ keratomileusis (LASIK)

**S0810** Photorefractive keratectomy (PRK)

**S0812** Phototherapeutic keratectomy (PTK)

~~**S0820** Computerized corneal topography, unilateral~~

**S1001** Deluxe item, patient aware (list in addition to code for basic item)
MED: 100-2,1,10.1.4

**S1002** Customized item (list in addition to code for basic item)

**S1015** IV tubing extension set

**S1016** Non-PVC (polyvinyl chloride) intravenous administration set, for use with drugs that are not stable in PVC e.g., Paclitaxel

~~**S1025** Inhaled nitric oxide for the treatment of hypoxic respiratory failure in the neonate; per diem~~

**S1030** Continuous noninvasive glucose monitoring device, purchase (for physician interpretation of data, use CPT code)

**S1031** Continuous noninvasive glucose monitoring device, rental, including sensor, sensor replacement, and download to monitor (for physician interpretation of data, use CPT code)

**S1040** Cranial remolding orthosis, pediatric, rigid, with soft interface material, custom fabricated, includes fitting and adjustment(s)

**S2053** Transplantation of small intestine, and liver allografts

**S2054** Transplantation of multivisceral organs

**S2055** Harvesting of donor multivisceral organs, with preparation and maintenance of allografts; from cadaver donor

**S2060** Lobar lung transplantation

**S2061** Donor lobectomy (lung) for transplantation, living donor

**S2065** Simultaneous pancreas kidney transplantation

---

| Special Coverage Instructions | Noncovered by Medicare | Carrier Discretion | ☑ Quantity Alert | ● New Code | ○ Recycled/Reinstated | ▲ Revised Code |

Temporary National Codes (Non-Medicare)

S2066 — S2350

● **S2066** Breast reconstruction with gluteal artery perforator (GAP) flap, including harvesting of the flap, microvascular transfer, closure of donor site and shaping the flap into a breast, unilateral ♀

● **S2067** Breast reconstruction of a single breast with "stacked" deep inferior epigastric perforator (DIEP) flap(s) and/or gluteal artery perforator (GAP) flap(s), including harvesting of the flap(s), microvascular transfer, closure of donor site(s) and shaping the flap into a breast, unilateral ♀

▲ **S2068** Breast reconstruction with deep inferior epigastric perforator (DIEP) flap or superficial inferior epigastric artery (SIEA) flap, including harvesting of the flap, microvascular transfer, closure of donor site and shaping the flap into a breast, unilateral ♀

**S2070** Cystourethroscopy, with ureteroscopy and/or pyeloscopy; with endoscopic laser treatment of ureteral calculi (includes ureteral catheterization)

**S2075** Laparoscopy, surgical; repair incisional or ventral hernia

**S2076** Laparoscopy, surgical; repair umbilical hernia

**S2077** Laparoscopy, surgical; implantation of mesh or other prosthesis for incisional or ventral hernia repair (List separately in addition to code for the incisional or ventral hernia repair) ♀

~~**S2078** Laparoscopic supracervical hysterectomy (subtotal hysterectomy), with or without removal of tube(s), with or without removal of ovary(s)~~

**S2079** Laparoscopic esophagomyotomy (Heller type)

**S2080** Laser-assisted uvulopalatoplasty (LAUP)

**S2083** Adjustment of gastric band diameter via subcutaneous port by injection or aspiration of saline

**S2095** Transcatheter occlusion or embolization for tumor destruction, percutaneous, any method, using yttrium-90 microspheres

**S2102** Islet cell tissue transplant from pancreas; allogeneic

**S2103** Adrenal tissue transplant to brain

**S2107** Adoptive immunotherapy, i.e., development of specific antitumor reactivity (e.g., tumor-infiltrating lymphocyte therapy) per course of treatment

**S2112** Arthroscopy, knee, surgical for harvesting of cartilage (chondrocyte cells)

~~**S2114** Arthroscopy, shoulder, surgical; tenodesis of biceps~~
See CPT code 29828.

**S2115** Osteotomy, periacetabular, with internal fixation

**S2117** Arthroereisis, subtalar

**S2120** Low density lipoprotein ( LDL) apheresis using heparin-induced extracorporeal LDLl precipitation

**S2135** Neurolysis, by injection, of metatarsal neuroma/interdigital neuritis, any interspace of the foot

**S2140** Cord blood harvesting for transplantation, allogeneic

**S2142** Cord blood-derived stem-cell transplantation, allogeneic

**S2150** Bone marrow or blood-derived stem cells (peripheral or umbilical), allogeneic or autologous, harvesting, transplantation, and related complications; including: pheresis and cell preparation/storage; marrow ablative therapy; drugs, supplies, hospitalization with outpatient follow-up; medical/surgical, diagnostic, emergency, and rehabilitative services; and the number of days of pre- and post-transplant care in the global definition

**S2152** Solid organ(s), complete or segmental, single organ or combination of organs; deceased or living donor (s), procurement, transplantation, and related complications; including: drugs; supplies; hospitalization with outpatient follow-up; medical/surgical, diagnostic, emergency, and Rehabilitative services, and the number of days of pre- and post-transplant care in the global definition

**S2202** Echosclerotherapy

**S2205** Minimally invasive direct coronary artery bypass surgery involving mini-thoracotomy or mini-sternotomy surgery, performed under direct vision; using arterial graft(s), single coronary arterial graft

**S2206** Minimally invasive direct coronary artery bypass surgery involving mini-thoracotomy or mini-sternotomy surgery, performed under direct vision; using arterial graft(s), two coronary arterial grafts

**S2207** Minimally invasive direct coronary artery bypass surgery involving mini-thoracotomy or mini-sternotomy surgery, performed under direct vision; using venous graft only, single coronary venous graft

**S2208** Minimally invasive direct coronary artery bypass surgery involving mini-thoracotomy or mini-sternotomy surgery, performed under direct vision; using single arterial and venous graft(s), single venous graft

**S2209** Minimally invasive direct coronary artery bypass surgery involving mini-thoracotomy or mini-sternotomy surgery, performed under direct vision; using two arterial grafts and single venous graft

~~**S2213** Implantation of gastric electrical stimulation device~~

**S2225** Myringotomy, laser-assisted

**S2230** Implantation of magnetic component of semi-implantable hearing device on ossicles in middle ear

**S2235** Implantation of auditory brain stem implant

~~**S2250** Uterine artery embolization for uterine fibroids~~

**S2260** Induced abortion, 17 to 24 weeks Ⓜ ♀

**S2265** Induced abortion, 25 to 28 weeks Ⓜ ♀

**S2266** Induced abortion, 29 to 31 weeks Ⓜ ♀

**S2267** Induced abortion, 32 weeks or greater Ⓜ ♀

**S2300** Arthroscopy, shoulder, surgical; with thermally-induced capsulorrhaphy

**S2325** Hip core decompression

**S2340** Chemodenervation of abductor muscle(s) of vocal cord

**S2341** Chemodenervation of adductor muscle(s) of vocal cord

**S2342** Nasal endoscopy for postoperative debridement following functional endoscopic sinus surgery, nasal and/or sinus cavity(s), unilateral or bilateral

**S2344** Nasal/sinus endoscopy, surgical; with enlargement of sinus ostium opening using inflatable device (i.e., balloon sinuplasty)

**S2348** Decompression procedure, percutaneous, of nucleus pulposus of intervertebral disc, using radiofrequency energy, single or multiple levels, lumbar

**S2350** Diskectomy, anterior, with decompression of spinal cord and/or nerve root(s), including osteophytectomy; lumbar, single interspace

---

▨ Special Coverage Instructions    ▨ Noncovered by Medicare    ▨ Carrier Discretion    ☑ Quantity Alert    ● New Code    ○ Recycled/Reinstated    ▲ Revised Code

138 — S Codes    Ⓐ Age Edit    Ⓜ Maternity Edit    ♀ Female Only    ♂ Male Only    Ⓐ-Ⓨ OPPS Status Indicators    **2008 HCPCS**

**S2351** Diskectomy, anterior, with decompression of spinal cord and/or nerve root(s), including osteophytectomy; lumbar, each additional interspace (list separately in addition to code for primary procedure)

**S2360** Percutaneous vertebroplasty, one vertebral body, unilateral or bilateral injection; cervical

**S2361** Each additional cervical vertebral body (list separately in addition to code for primary procedure)

**S2400** Repair, congenital diaphragmatic hernia in the fetus using temporary tracheal occlusion, procedure performed in utero ⓜ♀
Repair, congenital diaphragmatic hernia in the fetus using temporary tracheal occlusion, procedure performed in utero.

**S2401** Repair, urinary tract obstruction in the fetus, procedure performed in utero ⓜ♀

**S2402** Repair, congenital cystic adenomatoid malformation in the fetus, procedure performed in utero ⓜ♀

**S2403** Repair, extralobar pulmonary sequestration in the fetus, procedure performed in utero ⓜ♀

**S2404** Repair, myelomeningocele in the fetus, procedure performed in utero ⓜ♀

**S2405** Repair of sacrococcygeal teratoma in the fetus, procedure performed in utero ⓜ♀

**S2409** Repair, congenital malformation of fetus, procedure performed in utero, not otherwise classified ⓜ♀

**S2411** Fetoscopic laser therapy for treatment of twin-to-twin transfusion syndrome ⓜ♀

**S2900** Surgical techniques requiring use of robotic surgical system (list separately in addition to code for primary procedure)

**S3000** Diabetic indicator; retinal eye exam, dilated, bilateral

**S3005** Performance measurement, evaluation of patient self assessment, depression

**S3600** STAT laboratory request (situations other than S3601)

**S3601** Emergency STAT laboratory charge for patient who is homebound or residing in a nursing facility

**S3618** Blood chemistry for free beta human chorionic gonadotropin (hCG)
See CPT code 84704.

**S3620** Newborn metabolic screening panel, includes test kit, postage and the laboratory tests specified by the state for inclusion in this panel (e.g., galactose; hemoglobin, electrophoresis; hydroxyprogesterone, 17-d; phenylanine (PKU); and thyroxine, total) Ⓐ

**S3625** Maternal serum triple marker screen including alpha-fetoprotein (APF), estriol, and human chorionic gonadotropin (hCG) ⓜ♀

**S3626** Maternal serum quadruple marker screen including alpha-fetoprotein (AFP), estriol, human chorionic gonadotropin hCG) and inhibin A

**S3630** Eosinophil count, blood, direct

**S3645** HIV-1 antibody testing of oral mucosal transudate

**S3650** Saliva test, hormone level; during menopause Ⓐ♀

**S3652** Saliva test, hormone level; to assess preterm labor risk ⓜ♀

**S3655** Antisperm antibodies test (immunobead) Ⓐ♀

**S3708** Gastrointestinal fat absorption study

● **S3800** Genetic testing for amyotrophic lateral sclerosis (ALS)

**S3818** Complete gene sequence analysis; BRCA1 gene

**S3819** Complete gene sequence analysis; BRCA2 gene

**S3820** Complete BRCA1 and BRCA2 gene sequence analysis for susceptibility to breast and ovarian cancer ♀

**S3822** Single mutation analysis (in individual with a known BRCA1 or BRCA2 mutation in the family) for susceptibility to breast and ovarian cancer ♀

**S3823** Three-mutation BRCA1 and BRCA2 analysis for susceptibility to breast and ovarian cancer in Ashkenazi individuals ♀

**S3828** Complete gene sequence analysis; MLH1 gene

**S3829** Complete gene sequence analysis; MLH2 gene

**S3830** Complete MLH1 and MLH2 gene sequence analysis for hereditary nonpolyposis colorectal cancer (HNPCC) genetic testing

**S3831** Single-mutation analysis (in individual with a known MLH1 and MLH2 mutation in the family) for hereditary nonpolyposis colorectal cancer (HNPCC) genetic testing

**S3833** Complete APC gene sequence analysis for susceptibility to familial adenomatous polyposis (FAP) and attenuated fap

**S3834** Single-mutation analysis (in individual with a known APC mutation in the family) for susceptibility to familial adenomatous polyposis (FAP) and attenuated FAP

**S3835** Complete gene sequence analysis for cystic fibrosis genetic testing

**S3837** Complete gene sequence analysis for hemochromatosis genetic testing

**S3840** DNA analysis for germline mutations of the RET proto-oncogene for susceptibility to multiple endocrine neoplasia type 2

**S3841** Genetic testing for retinoblastoma

**S3842** Genetic testing for Von Hippel-Lindau disease

**S3843** DNA analysis of the F5 gene for susceptibility to factor V Leiden thrombophilia

**S3844** DNA analysis of the connexin 26 gene (GJB2) for susceptibility to congenital, profound deafness

**S3845** Genetic testing for alpha-thalassemia

**S3846** Genetic testing for hemoglobin E beta-thalassemia

**S3847** Genetic testing for Tay-Sachs disease

**S3848** Genetic testing for Gaucher disease

**S3849** Genetic testing for Niemann-Pick disease

**S3850** Genetic testing for sickle cell anemia

**S3851** Genetic testing for Canavan disease

**S3852** DNA analysis for APOE epilson 4 allele for susceptibility to Alzheimer's disease

**S3853** Genetic testing for myotonic muscular dystrophy

**S3854** Gene expression profiling panel for use in the management of breast cancer treatment

**S3855** Genetic testing for detection of mutations in the presenilin - 1 gene

**S3890** DNA analysis, fecal, for colorectal cancer screening

**S3900** Surface electromyography (EMG)

**S3902** Ballistocardiogram

**S3904** Masters two step

---

● **S3905** Noninvasive electrodiagnostic testing with automatic computerized hand-held device to stimulate and measure neuromuscular signals in diagnosing and evaluating systemic and entrapment neuropathies

**S4005** Interim labor facility global (labor occurring but not resulting in delivery) Ⓜ ♀

**S4011** In vitro fertilization; including but not limited to identification and incubation of mature oocytes, fertilization with sperm, incubation of embryo(s), and subsequent visualization for determination of development Ⓜ ♀

**S4013** Complete cycle, gamete intrafallopian transfer (GIFT), case rate Ⓜ ♀

**S4014** Complete cycle, zygote intrafallopian transfer (ZIFT), case rate Ⓜ ♀

**S4015** Complete in vitro fertilization cycle, not otherwise specified, case rate Ⓜ ♀

**S4016** Frozen in vitro fertilization cycle, case rate ♀

**S4017** Incomplete cycle, treatment cancelled prior to stimulation, case rate ♀

**S4018** Frozen embryo transfer procedure cancelled before transfer, case rate ♀

**S4020** In vitro fertilization procedure cancelled before aspiration, case rate ♀

**S4021** In vitro fertilization procedure cancelled after aspiration, case rate ♀

**S4022** Assisted oocyte fertilization, case rate ♀

**S4023** Donor egg cycle, incomplete, case rate ♀

**S4025** Donor services for in vitro fertilization (sperm or embryo), case rate Ⓐ

**S4026** Procurement of donor sperm from sperm bank Ⓐ

**S4027** Storage of previously frozen embryos

**S4028** Microsurgical epididymal sperm aspiration (MESA) Ⓐ ♂

**S4030** Sperm procurement and cryopreservation services; initial visit Ⓐ ♂

**S4031** Sperm procurement and cryopreservation services; subsequent visit Ⓐ ♂

**S4035** Stimulated intrauterine insemination (IUI), case rate ♀

**S4037** Cryopreserved embryo transfer, case rate

**S4040** Monitoring and storage of cryopreserved embryos, per 30 days

**S4042** Management of ovulation induction (interpretation of diagnostic tests and studies, non-face-to-face medical management of the patient), per cycle

**S4981** Insertion of levonorgestrel-releasing intrauterine system ♀

**S4989** Contraceptive intrauterine device (e.g., Progestacert IUD), including implants and supplies ♀

☑ **S4990** Nicotine patches, legend

☑ **S4991** Nicotine patches, non-legend

**S4993** Contraceptive pills for birth control ♀

**S4995** Smoking cessation gum

☑ **S5000** Prescription drug, generic

☑ **S5001** Prescription drug, brand name

▲ ☑ **S5010** 5% dextrose and 0.45% normal saline, 1000 ml

☑ **S5011** 5% dextrose in lactated ringer's, 1000 ml

☑ **S5012** 5% dextrose with potassium chloride, 1000 ml

▲ ☑ **S5013** 5% dextrose/0.45% normal saline with potassium chloride and magnesium sulfate, 1000 ml

☑ **S5014** 5% dextrose/45% normal saline with potassium chloride and magnesium sulfate, 1500 ml

**S5035** Home infusion therapy, routine service of infusion device (e.g., pump maintenance)

**S5036** Home infusion therapy, repair of infusion device (e.g., pump repair)

☑ **S5100** Day care services, adult; per 15 minutes Ⓐ

☑ **S5101** Day care services, adult; per half day Ⓐ

☑ **S5102** Day care services, adult; per diem Ⓐ

☑ **S5105** Day care services, center-based; services not included in program fee, per diem

☑ **S5108** Home care training to home care client, per 15 minutes

☑ **S5109** Home care training to home care client, per session

☑ **S5110** Home care training, family; per 15 minutes

**S5111** Home care training, family; per session

☑ **S5115** Home care training, nonfamily; per 15 minutes

☑ **S5116** Home care training, nonfamily; per session

☑ **S5120** Chore services; per 15 minutes

☑ **S5121** Chore services; per diem

☑ **S5125** Attendant care services; per 15 minutes

☑ **S5126** Attendant care services; per diem

☑ **S5130** Homemaker service, NOS; per 15 minutes

☑ **S5131** Homemaker service, NOS; per diem

☑ **S5135** Companion care, adult (e.g., IADL/ADL); per 15 minutes Ⓐ

☑ **S5136** Companion care, adult (e.g. IADL/ADL); per diem Ⓐ

☑ **S5140** Foster care, adult; per diem Ⓐ

**S5141** Foster care, adult; per month Ⓐ

**S5145** Foster care, therapeutic, child; per diem Ⓐ

**S5146** Foster care, therapeutic, child; per month Ⓐ

☑ **S5150** Unskilled respite care, not hospice; per 15 minutes

**S5151** Unskilled respite care, not hospice; per diem

**S5160** Emergency response system; installation and testing

**S5161** Emergency response system; service fee, per month (excludes installation and testing)

**S5162** Emergency response system; purchase only

**S5165** Home modifications; per service

**S5170** Home delivered meals, including preparation; per meal

**S5175** Laundry service, external, professional; per order

**S5180** Home health respiratory therapy, initial evaluation

**S5181** Home health respiratory therapy, NOS, per diem

**S5185** Medication reminder service, non-face-to-face; per month

**S5190** Wellness assessment, performed by non-physician

**S5199** Personal care item, NOS, each

**S5497** Home infusion therapy, catheter care/maintenance, not otherwise classified; includes administrative services, professional pharmacy services, care coordination, and all necessary supplies and equipment (drugs and nursing visits coded separately), per diem

░░ Special Coverage Instructions　　░░ Noncovered by Medicare　　░░ Carrier Discretion　　☑ Quantity Alert　　● New Code　　○ Recycled/Reinstated　　▲ Revised Code

**140 — S Codes**　　Ⓐ Age Edit　　Ⓜ Maternity Edit　　♀ Female Only　　♂ Male Only　　Ⓐ-Ⓨ OPPS Status Indicators　　**2008 HCPCS**

S5498    Home infusion therapy, catheter care/maintenance, simple (single lumen), includes administrative services, professional pharmacy services, care coordination and all necessary supplies and equipment, (drugs and nursing visits coded separately), per diem

S5501    Home infusion therapy, catheter care/maintenance, complex (more than one lumen), includes administrative services, professional pharmacy services, care coordination, and all necessary supplies and equipment (drugs and nursing visits coded separately), per diem

S5502    Home infusion therapy, catheter care/maintenance, implanted access device, includes administrative services, professional pharmacy services, care coordination and all necessary supplies and equipment, (drugs and nursing visits coded separately), per diem (use this code for interim maintenance of vascular access not currently in use)

S5517    Home infusion therapy, all supplies necessary for restoration of catheter patency or declotting

S5518    Home infusion therapy, all supplies necessary for catheter repair

S5520    Home infusion therapy, all supplies (including catheter) necessary for a peripherally inserted central venous catheter (PICC) line insertion

S5521    Home infusion therapy, all supplies (including catheter) necessary for a midline catheter insertion

S5522    Home infusion therapy, insertion of peripherally inserted central venous catheter (PICC), nursing services only (no supplies or catheter included)

S5523    Home infusion therapy, insertion of midline venous catheter, nursing services only (no supplies or catheter included)

☑ S5550    Insulin, rapid onset, 5 units

☑ S5551    Insulin, most rapid onset (Lispro or Aspart); 5 units

☑ S5552    Insulin, intermediate acting (NPH or LENTE); 5 units

☑ S5553    Insulin, long acting; 5 units

☑ S5560    Insulin delivery device, reusable pen; 1.5 ml size

☑ S5561    Insulin delivery device, reusable pen; 3 ml size

☑ S5565    Insulin cartridge for use in insulin delivery device other than pump; 150 units

☑ S5566    Insulin cartridge for use in insulin delivery device other than pump; 300 units

☑ S5570    Insulin delivery device, disposable pen (including insulin); 1.5 ml size

☑ S5571    Insulin delivery device, disposable pen (including insulin); 3 ml size

S8030    Scleral application of tantalum ring(s) for localization of lesions for proton beam therapy

S8035    Magnetic source imaging

S8037    Magnetic resonance cholangiopancreatography (MRCP)

S8040    Topographic brain mapping

S8042    Magnetic resonance imaging (MRI), low-field

S8049    Intraoperative radiation therapy (single administration)

S8055    Ultrasound guidance for multifetal pregnancy reduction(s), technical component (only to be used when the physician doing the reduction procedure does not perform the ultrasound. Guidance is included in the CPT code for multifetal pregnancy reduction — 59866)    Ⓜ♀

S8080    Scintimammography (radioimmunoscintigraphy of the breast), unilateral, including supply of radiopharmaceutical

S8085    Fluorine-18 fluorodeoxyglucose (F-18 FDG) imaging using dual-head coincidence detection system (nondedicated PET scan)

S8092    Electron beam computed tomography (also known as ultrafast CT, cine CT)

S8096    Portable peak flow meter

☑ S8097    Asthma kit (including but not limited to portable peak expiratory flow meter, instructional video, brochure, and/or spacer)

S8100    Holding chamber or spacer for use with an inhaler or nebulizer; without mask

S8101    Holding chamber or spacer for use with an inhaler or nebulizer; with mask

S8110    Peak expiratory flow rate (physician services)

☑ S8120    Oxygen contents, gaseous, 1 unit equals 1 cubic foot

☑ S8121    Oxygen contents, liquid, 1 unit equals 1 pound

S8185    Flutter device

S8186    Swivel adaptor

S8189    Tracheostomy supply, not otherwise classified

S8190    Electronic spirometer (or microspirometer)

S8210    Mucus trap

S8262    Mandibular orthopedic repositioning device, each

S8265    Haberman feeder for cleft lip/palate

S8270    Enuresis alarm, using auditory buzzer and/or vibration device

S8301    Infection control supplies, not otherwise specified

S8415    Supplies for home delivery of infant    Ⓜ♀

S8420    Gradient pressure aid (sleeve and glove combination), custom made

S8421    Gradient pressure aid (sleeve and glove combination), ready made

S8422    Gradient pressure aid (sleeve), custom made, medium weight

S8423    Gradient pressure aid (sleeve), custom made, heavy weight

S8424    Gradient pressure aid (sleeve), ready made

S8425    Gradient pressure aid (glove), custom made, medium weight

S8426    Gradient pressure aid (glove), custom made, heavy weight

S8427    Gradient pressure aid (glove), ready made

S8428    Gradient pressure aid (gauntlet), ready made

S8429    Gradient pressure exterior wrap

☑ S8430    Padding for compression bandage, roll

☑ S8431    Compression bandage, roll

Special Coverage Instructions    Noncovered by Medicare    Carrier Discretion    ☑ Quantity Alert    ● New Code    ○ Recycled/Reinstated    ▲ Revised Code

2008 HCPCS    A2-Z3 ASC Payment Indicators    MED: Pub 100/NCD References    ♿ DMEPOS Paid    ⊘ SNF Excluded    PQRI PQRI    S Codes — 141

Temporary National Codes (Non-Medicare)    S5498 — S8431

**Temporary National Codes (Non-Medicare)**

**S8450 — S9214**

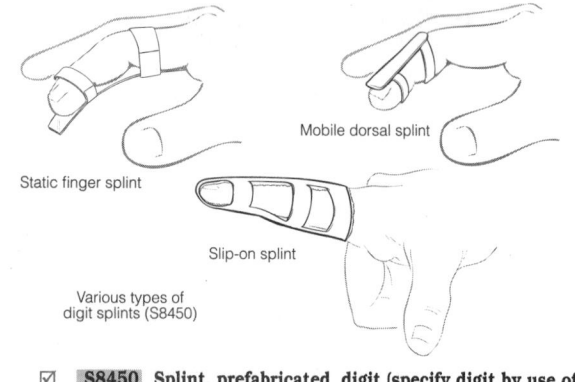

Static finger splint

Mobile dorsal splint

Slip-on splint

Various types of digit splints (S8450)

☑ **S8450** Splint, prefabricated, digit (specify digit by use of modifier)

☑ **S8451** Splint, prefabricated, wrist or ankle

☑ **S8452** Splint, prefabricated, elbow

**S8460** Camisole, post-mastectomy

☑ **S8490** Insulin syringes (100 syringes, any size)

**S8940** Equestrian/hippotherapy, per session

☑ **S8948** Application of a modality (requiring constant provider attendance) to one or more areas; low-level laser; each 15 minutes

☑ **S8950** Complex lymphedema therapy, each 15 minutes

**S8990** Physical or manipulative therapy performed for maintenance rather than restoration

**S8999** Resuscitation bag (for use by patient on artificial respiration during power failure or other catastrophic event)

**S9001** Home uterine monitor with or without associated nursing services  Ⓜ ♀

**S9007** Ultrafiltration monitor

**S9015** Automated EEG monitoring

**S9024** Paranasal sinus ultrasound

**S9025** Omnicardiogram/cardiointegram

▲ **S9034** Extracorporeal shockwave lithotripsy for gall stones (if performed with ERCP, use 43265)

**S9055** Procuren or other growth factor preparation to promote wound healing

**S9056** Coma stimulation per diem

**S9061** Home administration of aerosolized drug therapy (e.g., Pentamidine); administrative services, professional pharmacy services, care coordination, all necessary supplies and equipment (drugs and nursing visits coded separately), per diem

**S9075** Smoking cessation treatment

**S9083** Global fee urgent care centers

**S9088** Services provided in an urgent care center (list in addition to code for service)

☑ **S9090** Vertebral axial decompression, per session

☑ **S9092** Canolith repositioning, per visit

**S9097** Home visit for wound care

**S9098** Home visit, phototherapy services (e.g., Bili-lite), including equipment rental, nursing services, blood draw, supplies, and other services, per diem

**S9109** Congestive heart failure telemonitoring, equipment rental, including telescale, computer system and software, telephone connections, and maintenance, per month

☑ **S9117** Back school, per visit

☑ **S9122** Home health aide or certified nurse assistant, providing care in the home; per hour

☑ **S9123** Nursing care, in the home; by registered nurse, per hour (use for general nursing care only, not to be used when CPT codes 99500-99602 can be used)

☑ **S9124** Nursing care, in the home; by licensed practical nurse, per hour

☑ **S9125** Respite care, in the home, per diem

☑ **S9126** Hospice care, in the home, per diem

☑ **S9127** Social work visit, in the home, per diem

☑ **S9128** Speech therapy, in the home, per diem

☑ **S9129** Occupational therapy, in the home, per diem

☑ **S9131** Physical therapy; in the home, per diem

☑ **S9140** Diabetic management program, follow-up visit to non-MD provider

☑ **S9141** Diabetic management program, follow-up visit to MD provider

**S9145** Insulin pump initiation, instruction in initial use of pump (pump not included)

**S9150** Evaluation by ocularist

● **S9152** Speech therapy, re-evaluation

**S9208** Home management of preterm labor, including administrative services, professional pharmacy services, care coordination, and all necessary supplies or equipment (drugs and nursing visits coded separately), per diem (do not use this code with any home infusion per diem code)  Ⓜ ♀

**S9209** Home management of preterm premature rupture of membranes (PPROM), including administrative services, professional pharmacy services, care coordination, and all necessary supplies or equipment (drugs and nursing visits coded separately), per diem (do not use this code with any home infusion per diem code)  Ⓜ ♀

**S9211** Home management of gestational hypertension, includes administrative services, professional pharmacy services, care coordination and all necessary supplies and equipment (drugs and nursing visits coded separately); per diem (do not use this code with any home infusion per diem code)  Ⓜ ♀

**S9212** Home management of postpartum hypertension, includes administrative services, professional pharmacy services, care coordination, and all necessary supplies and equipment (drugs and nursing visits coded separately), per diem (do not use this code with any home infusion per diem code)  ♀

**S9213** Home management of preeclampsia, includes administrative services, professional pharmacy services, care coordination, and all necessary supplies and equipment (drugs and nursing services coded separately); per diem (do not use this code with any home infusion per diem code)  Ⓜ ♀

**S9214** Home management of gestational diabetes, includes administrative services, professional pharmacy services, care coordination, and all necessary supplies and equipment (drugs and nursing visits coded separately); per diem (do not use this code with any home infusion per diem code)  Ⓜ ♀

Special Coverage Instructions    Noncovered by Medicare    Carrier Discretion    ☑ Quantity Alert    ● New Code    ○ Recycled/Reinstated    ▲ Revised Code

**142 — S Codes**    Ⓐ Age Edit    Ⓜ Maternity Edit    ♀ Female Only    ♂ Male Only    Ⓐ-Ⓨ OPPS Status Indicators    **2008 HCPCS**

**S9325** Home infusion therapy, pain management infusion; administrative services, professional pharmacy services, care coordination, and all necessary supplies and equipment, (drugs and nursing visits coded separately), per diem (do not use this code with S9326, S9327 or S9328)

**S9326** Home infusion therapy, continuous (24 hours or more) pain management infusion; administrative services, professional pharmacy services, care coordination and all necessary supplies and equipment (drugs and nursing visits coded separately), per diem

**S9327** Home infusion therapy, intermittent (less than 24 hours) pain management infusion; administrative services, professional pharmacy services, care coordination, and all necessary supplies and equipment (drugs and nursing visits coded separately), per diem

**S9328** Home infusion therapy, implanted pump pain management infusion; administrative services, professional pharmacy services, care coordination, and all necessary supplies and equipment (drugs and nursing visits coded separately), per diem

**S9329** Home infusion therapy, chemotherapy infusion; administrative services, professional pharmacy services, care coordination, and all necessary supplies and equipment (drugs and nursing visits coded separately), per diem (do not use this code with S9330 or S9331)

**S9330** Home infusion therapy, continuous (24 hours or more) chemotherapy infusion; administrative services, professional pharmacy services, care coordination, and all necessary supplies and equipment (drugs and nursing visits coded separately), per diem

**S9331** Home infusion therapy, intermittent (less than 24 hours) chemotherapy infusion; administrative services, professional pharmacy services, care coordination, and all necessary supplies and equipment (drugs and nursing visits coded separately), per diem

☑ **S9335** Home therapy, hemodialysis; administrative services, professional pharmacy services, care coordination, and all necessary supplies and equipment (drugs and nursing services coded separately), per diem

**S9336** Home infusion therapy, continuous anticoagulant infusion therapy (e.g., Heparin), administrative services, professional pharmacy services, care coordination and all necessary supplies and equipment (drugs and nursing visits coded separately), per diem

**S9338** Home infusion therapy, immunotherapy, administrative services, professional pharmacy services, care coordination, and all necessary supplies and equipment (drugs and nursing visits coded separately), per diem

**S9339** Home therapy; peritoneal dialysis, administrative services, professional pharmacy services, care coordination and all necessary supplies and equipment (drugs and nursing visits coded separately), per diem

**S9340** Home therapy; enteral nutrition; administrative services, professional pharmacy services, care coordination, and all necessary supplies and equipment (enteral formula and nursing visits coded separately), per diem

**S9341** Home therapy; enteral nutrition via gravity; administrative services, professional pharmacy services, care coordination, and all necessary supplies and equipment (enteral formula and nursing visits coded separately), per diem

**S9342** Home therapy; enteral nutrition via pump; administrative services, professional pharmacy services, care coordination, and all necessary supplies and equipment (enteral formula and nursing visits coded separately), per diem

**S9343** Home therapy; enteral nutrition via bolus; administrative services, professional pharmacy services, care coordination, and all necessary supplies and equipment (enteral formula and nursing visits coded separately), per diem

**S9345** Home infusion therapy, anti-hemophilic agent infusion therapy (e.g., factor VIII); administrative services, professional pharmacy services, care coordination, and all necessary supplies and equipment (drugs and nursing visits coded separately), per diem

**S9346** Home infusion therapy, alpha-1-proteinase inhibitor (e.g., Prolastin); administrative services, professional pharmacy services, care coordination, and all necessary supplies and equipment (drugs and nursing visits coded separately), per diem

**S9347** Home infusion therapy, uninterrupted, long-term, controlled rate Intravenous or subcutaneous infusion therapy (e.g. epoprostenol); administrative services, professional pharmacy services, care coordination, and all necessary supplies and equipment (drugs and nursing visits coded separately), per diem

**S9348** Home infusion therapy, sympathomimetic/inotropic agent infusion therapy (e.g., Dobutamine); administrative services, professional pharmacy services, care coordination, all necessary supplies and equipment (drugs and nursing visits coded separately), per diem

**S9349** Home infusion therapy, tocolytic infusion therapy; administrative services, professional pharmacy services, care coordination, and all necessary supplies and equipment (drugs and nursing visits coded separately), per diem  Ⓜ♀

**S9351** Home infusion therapy, continuous or intermittent anti-emetic infusion therapy; administrative services, professional pharmacy services, care coordination, and all necessary supplies and equipment (drugs and visits coded separately), per diem

**S9353** Home infusion therapy, continuous insulin infusion therapy; administrative services, professional pharmacy services, care coordination, and all necessary supplies and equipment (drugs and nursing visits coded separately), per diem

**S9355** Home infusion therapy, chelation therapy; administrative services, professional pharmacy services, care coordination, and all necessary supplies and equipment (drugs and nursing visits coded separately), per diem

**S9357** Home infusion therapy, enzyme replacement intravenous therapy; (e.g., Imiglucerase); administrative services, professional pharmacy services, care coordination, and all necessary supplies and equipment (drugs and nursing visits coded separately), per diem

**S9359** Home infusion therapy, antitumor necrosis factor intravenous therapy; (e.g., Infliximab); administrative services, professional pharmacy services, care coordination, and all necessary supplies and equipment (drugs and nursing visits coded separately), per diem

**S9361** Home infusion therapy, diuretic intravenous therapy; administrative services, professional pharmacy services, care coordination, and all necessary supplies and equipment (drugs and nursing visits coded separately), per diem

---

Special Coverage Instructions    Noncovered by Medicare    Carrier Discretion    ☑ Quantity Alert    ● New Code    ○ Recycled/Reinstated    ▲ Revised Code

**2008 HCPCS**    Ⓐ-Ⓩ ASC Payment Indicators    **MED:** Pub 100/NCD References    DMEPOS Paid    Ⓢ SNF Excluded    ⓅQRI    **S Codes — 143**

**S9363** Home infusion therapy, anti-spasmotic therapy; administrative services, professional pharmacy services, care coordination, and all necessary supplies and equipment (drugs and nursing visits coded separately), per diem

**S9364** Home infusion therapy, total parenteral nutrition (TPN); administrative services, professional pharmacy services, care coordination, and all necessary supplies and equipment including standard TPN formula (lipids, specialty amino acid formulas, drugs other than in standard formula and nursing visits coded separately), per diem (do not use with home infusion codes S9365–S9368 using daily volume scales)

**S9365** Home infusion therapy, total parenteral nutrition (TPN); 1 liter per day, administrative services, professional pharmacy services, care coordination, and all necessary supplies and equipment including standard TPN formula (lipids, specialty amino acid formulas, drugs other than in standard formula and nursing visits coded separately), per diem

**S9366** Home infusion therapy, total parenteral nutrition (TPN); more than 1 liter but no more than 2 liters per day, administrative services, professional pharmacy services, care coordination, and all necessary supplies and equipment including standard TPN formula (lipids, specialty amino acid formulas, drugs other than in standard formula and nursing visits coded separately), per diem

**S9367** Home infusion therapy, total parenteral nutrition (TPN); more than 2 liters but no more than 3 liters per day, administrative services, professional pharmacy services, care coordination, and all necessary supplies and equipment including standard TPN formula (lipids, specialty amino acid formulas, drugs other than in standard formula and nursing visits coded separately), per diem

**S9368** Home infusion therapy, total parenteral nutrition (TPN); more than 3 liters per day, administrative services, professional pharmacy services, care coordination, and all necessary supplies and equipment including standard TPN formula (lipids, specialty amino acid formulas, drugs other than in standard formula and nursing visits coded separately), per diem

**S9370** Home therapy, intermittent anti-emetic injection therapy; administrative services, professional pharmacy services, care coordination, and all necessary supplies and equipment (drugs and nursing visits coded separately), per diem

**S9372** Home therapy; intermittent anticoagulant injection therapy (e.g., Heparin); administrative services, professional pharmacy services, care coordination, and all necessary supplies and equipment (drugs and nursing visits coded separately), per diem (do not use this code for flushing of infusion devices with Heparin to maintain patency)

**S9373** Home infusion therapy, hydration therapy; administrative services, professional pharmacy services, care coordination, and all necessary supplies and equipment (drugs and nursing visits coded separately), per diem (do not use with hydration therapy codes S9374–S9377 using daily volume scales)

**S9374** Home infusion therapy, hydration therapy; one liter per day, administrative services, professional pharmacy services, care coordination, and all necessary supplies and equipment (drugs and nursing visits coded separately), per diem

**S9375** Home infusion therapy, hydration therapy; more than one liter but no more than two liters per day, administrative services, professional pharmacy services, care coordination, and all necessary supplies and equipment (drugs and nursing visits coded separately), per diem

**S9376** Home infusion therapy, hydration therapy; more than two liters but no more than three liters per day, administrative services, professional pharmacy services, care coordination, and all necessary supplies and equipment (drugs and nursing visits coded separately), per diem

**S9377** Home infusion therapy, hydration therapy; more than three liters per day, administrative services, professional pharmacy services, care coordination, and all necessary supplies (drugs and nursing visits coded separately), per diem

**S9379** Home infusion therapy, infusion therapy, not otherwise classified; administrative services, professional pharmacy services, care coordination, and all necessary supplies and equipment (drugs and nursing visits coded separately), per diem

**S9381** Delivery or service to high risk areas requiring escort or extra protection, per visit

**S9401** Anticoagulation clinic, inclusive of all services except laboratory tests, per session

**S9430** Pharmacy compounding and dispensing services

**S9434** Modified solid food supplements for inborn errors of metabolism

**S9435** Medical foods for inborn errors of metabolism

☑ **S9436** Childbirth preparation/Lamaze classes, nonphysician provider, per session　Ⓜ ♀

**S9437** Childbirth refresher classes, nonphysician provider, per session　Ⓜ ♀

☑ **S9438** Cesarean birth classes, nonphysician provider, per session　Ⓜ ♀

☑ **S9439** VBAC (vaginal birth after cesarean) classes, nonphysician provider, per session　Ⓜ ♀

☑ **S9441** Asthma education, non-physician provider, per session

☑ **S9442** Birthing classes, non-physician provider, per session　Ⓜ ♀

☑ **S9443** Lactation classes, non-physician provider, per session　Ⓜ ♀

☑ **S9444** Parenting classes, nonphysician provider, per session

☑ **S9445** Patient education, not otherwise classified, non-physician provider, individual, per session

☑ **S9446** Patient education, not otherwise classified, non-physician provider, group, per session

☑ **S9447** Infant safety (including CPR) classes, nonphysician provider, per session

☑ **S9449** Weight management classes, nonphysician provider, per session

**S9451** Exercise classes, nonphysician provider, per session

**S9452** Nutrition classes, nonphysician provider, per session

**S9453** Smoking cessation classes, nonphysician provider, per session

**S9454** Stress management classes, nonphysician provider, per session

**S9455** Diabetic management program, group session

---

▨ Special Coverage Instructions　　▨ Noncovered by Medicare　　▨ Carrier Discretion　　☑ Quantity Alert　　● New Code　　○ Recycled/Reinstated　　▲ Revised Code

**144 — S Codes**　　Ⓐ Age Edit　　Ⓜ Maternity Edit　　♀ Female Only　　♂ Male Only　　Ⓐ-Ⓨ OPPS Status Indicators　　**2008 HCPCS**

**S9460** Diabetic management program, nurse visit

**S9465** Diabetic management program, dietitian visit

**S9470** Nutritional counseling, dietitian visit

**S9472** Cardiac rehabilitation program, non-physician provider, per diem

**S9473** Pulmonary rehabilitation program, non-physician provider, per diem

**S9474** Enterostomal therapy by a registered nurse certified in enterostomal therapy, per diem

**S9475** Ambulatory setting substance abuse treatment or detoxification services, per diem

☑ **S9476** Vestibular rehabilitation program, nonphysician provider, per diem

**S9480** Intensive outpatient psychiatric services, per diem

☑ **S9482** Family stabilization services, per 15 minutes

☑ **S9484** Crisis intervention mental health services, per hour

**S9485** Crisis intervention mental health services, per diem

**S9490** Home infusion therapy, corticosteroid infusion; administrative services, professional pharmacy services, care coordination, and all necessary supplies and equipment (drugs and nursing visits coded separately), per diem

**S9494** Home infusion therapy, antibiotic, antiviral, or antifungal therapy; administrative services, professional pharmacy services, care coordination, and all necessary supplies and equipment (drugs and nursing visits coded separately, per diem) (do not use this code with home infusion codes for hourly dosing schedules S9497–S9504)

**S9497** Home infusion therapy, antibiotic, antiviral, or antifungal therapy; once every three hours; administrative services, professional pharmacy services, care coordination, and all necessary supplies and equipment (drugs and nursing visits coded separately), per diem

**S9500** Home infusion therapy, antibiotic, antiviral, or antifungal therapy; once every 24 hours; administrative services, professional pharmacy services, care coordination, and all necessary supplies and equipment (drugs and nursing visits coded separately), per diem

**S9501** Home infusion therapy, antibiotic, antiviral, or antifungal therapy; once every 12 hours; administrative services, professional pharmacy services, care coordination, and all necessary supplies and equipment (drugs and nursing visits coded separately), per diem

**S9502** Home infusion therapy, antibiotic, antiviral, or antifungal therapy; once every eight hours, administrative services, professional pharmacy services, care coordination, and all necessary supplies and equipment (drugs and nursing visits coded separately), per diem

**S9503** Home infusion therapy, antibiotic, antiviral, or antifungal; once every six hours; administrative services, professional pharmacy services, care coordination, and all necessary supplies and equipment (drugs and nursing visits coded separately), per diem

**S9504** Home infusion therapy, antibiotic, antiviral, or antifungal; once every four hours; administrative services, professional pharmacy services, care coordination, and all necessary supplies and equipment (drugs and nursing visits coded separately), per diem

**S9529** Routine venipuncture for collection of specimen(s), single home bound, nursing home, or skilled nursing facility patient

**S9537** Home therapy; hematopoietic hormone injection therapy (e.g., erythropoietin, G-CSF, GM-CSF); administrative services, professional pharmacy services, care coordination, and all necessary supplies and equipment (drugs and nursing visits coded separately), per diem

**S9538** Home transfusion of blood product(s); administrative services, professional pharmacy services, care coordination and all necessary supplies and equipment (blood products, drugs, and nursing visits coded separately), per diem

**S9542** Home injectable therapy, not otherwise classified, including administrative services, professional pharmacy services, care coordination, and all necessary supplies and equipment (drugs and nursing visits coded separately), per diem

**S9558** Home injectable therapy; growth hormone, including administrative services, professional pharmacy services, care coordination, and all necessary supplies and equipment (drugs and nursing visits coded separately), per diem

**S9559** Home injectable therapy, interferon, including administrative services, professional pharmacy services, care coordination, and all necessary supplies and equipment (drugs and nursing visits coded separately), per diem

**S9560** Home injectable therapy; hormonal therapy (e.g.; leuprolide, goserelin), including administrative services, professional pharmacy services, care coordination, and all necessary supplies and equipment (drugs and nursing visits coded separately), per diem

**S9562** Home injectable therapy, palivizumab, including administrative services, professional pharmacy services, care coordination, and all necessary supplies and equipment (drugs and nursing visits coded separately), per diem

**S9590** Home therapy, irrigation therapy (e.g., sterile irrigation of an organ or anatomical cavity); including administrative services, professional pharmacy services, care coordination, and all necessary supplies and equipment (drugs and nursing visits coded separately), per diem

**S9810** Home therapy; professional pharmacy services for provision of infusion, specialty drug administration, and/or disease state management, not otherwise classified, per hour (do not use this code with any per diem code)

**S9900** Services by authorized Christian Science practitioner for the process of healing, per diem; not to be used for rest or study; excludes in-patient services

**S9970** Health club membership, annual

☑ **S9975** Transplant related lodging, meals and transportation, per diem

☑ **S9976** Lodging, per diem, not otherwise classified

☑ **S9977** Meals, per diem, NOS

☑ **S9981** Medical records copying fee, administrative

☑ **S9982** Medical records copying fee, per page

**S9986** Not medically necessary service (patient is aware that service not medically necessary)

**S9988** Services provided as part of a Phase 1 clinical trial

**S9989** Services provided outside of the United States of America (list in addition to code(s) for services(s))

**S9990** Services provided as part of a Phase II clinical trial

**S9991** Services provided as part of a Phase III clinical trial

---

Special Coverage Instructions    Noncovered by Medicare    Carrier Discretion    ☑ Quantity Alert    ● New Code    ○ Recycled/Reinstated    ▲ Revised Code

Temporary National Codes (Non-Medicare)

S9992 — S9999

S9992    Transportation costs to and from trial location and local transportation costs (e.g., fares for taxicab or bus) for clinical trial participant and one caregiver/companion

S9994    Lodging costs (e.g., hotel charges) for clinical trial participant and one caregiver/companion

S9996    Meals for clinical trial participant and one caregiver/companion

S9999    Sales tax

☑ Quantity Alert

Special Coverage Instructions    Noncovered by Medicare    Carrier Discretion    ☑ Quantity Alert    ● New Code    ○ Recycled/Reinstated    ▲ Revised Code

**146 — S Codes**    Ⓐ Age Edit    Ⓜ Maternity Edit    ♀ Female Only    ♂ Male Only    Ⓐ-Ⓨ OPPS Status Indicators    **2008 HCPCS**

## NATIONAL T CODES ESTABLISHED FOR STATE MEDICAID AGENCIES T1000-T9999

The T codes are designed for use by Medicaid state agencies to establish codes for items for which there are no permanent national codes but for which codes are necessary to administer the Medicaid program (T codes are not accepted by Medicare but can be used by private insurers). This range of codes describes nursing and home health-related services, substance abuse treatment, and certain training-related procedures.

☑ **T1000** Private duty/independent nursing service(s) — licensed, up to 15 minutes

**T1001** Nursing assessment/evaluation

☑ **T1002** RN services, up to 15 minutes

☑ **T1003** LPN/LVN services, up to 15 minutes

☑ **T1004** Services of a qualified nursing aide, up to 15 minutes

☑ **T1005** Respite care services, up to 15 minutes

**T1006** Alcohol and/or substance abuse services, family/couple counseling

**T1007** Alcohol and/or substance abuse services, treatment plan development and/or modification

**T1009** Child sitting services for children of the individual receiving alcohol and/or substance abuse services

**T1010** Meals for individuals receiving alcohol and/or substance abuse services (when meals not included in the program)

**T1012** Alcohol and/or substance abuse services, skills development

☑ **T1013** Sign language or oral interpretive services, per 15 minutes

**T1014** Telehealth transmission, per minute, professional services bill separately

**T1015** Clinic visit/encounter, all-inclusive

☑ **T1016** Case management, each 15 minutes

☑ **T1017** Targeted case management, each 15 minutes

**T1018** School-based individualized education program (IEP) services, bundled

**T1019** Personal care services, per 15 minutes, not for an inpatient or resident of a hospital, nursing facility, ICF/MR or IMD, part of the individualized plan of treatment (code may not be used to identify services provided by home health aide or certified nurse assistant)

**T1020** Personal care services, per diem, not for an inpatient or resident of a hospital, nursing facility, ICF/MR or IMD, part of the individualized plan of treatment (code may not be used to identify services provided by home health aide or certified nurse assistant)

**T1021** Home health aide or certified nurse assistant, per visit

**T1022** Contracted home health agency services, all services provided under contract, per day

**T1023** Screening to determine the appropriateness of consideration of an individual for participation in a specified program, project or treatment protocol, per encounter

**T1024** Evaluation and treatment by an integrated, specialty team contracted to provide coordinated care to multiple or severely handicapped children, per encounter Ⓐ

**T1025** Intensive, extended multidisciplinary services provided in a clinic setting to children with complex medical, physical, mental and psychosocial impairments, per diem Ⓐ

**T1026** Intensive, extended multidisciplinary services provided in a clinic setting to children with complex medical, physical, medical and psychosocial impairments, per hour Ⓐ

☑ **T1027** Family training and counseling for child development, per 15 minutes

**T1028** Assessment of home, physical and family environment, to determine suitability to meet patient's medical needs

**T1029** Comprehensive environmental lead investigation, not including laboratory analysis, per dwelling

☑ **T1030** Nursing care, in the home, by registered nurse, per diem

☑ **T1031** Nursing care, in the home, by licensed practical nurse, per diem

☑ **T1502** Administration of oral, intramuscular and/or subcutaneous medication by health care agency/professional, per visit

● ☑ **T1503** Administration of medication, other than oral and/or injectable, by a health care agency/professional, per visit

**T1999** Miscellaneous therapeutic items and supplies, retail purchases, NOC; identify product in "remarks"

**T2001** Nonemergency transportation; patient attendant/escort

**T2002** Nonemergency transportation; per diem

**T2003** Nonemergency transportation; encounter/trip

**T2004** Nonemergency transport; commercial carrier, multipass

**T2005** Nonemergency transportation; stretcher van

☑ **T2007** Transportation waiting time, air ambulance and non-emergency vehicle, one-half (1/2) hour increments

☑ **T2010** Preadmission screening and resident review (PASRR) level I identification screening, per screen

**T2011** Preadmission screening and resident review (PASRR) level II evaluation, per evaluation

☑ **T2012** Habilitation, educational; waiver, per diem

☑ **T2013** Habilitation, educational, waiver; per hour

☑ **T2014** Habilitation, prevocational, waiver; per diem

☑ **T2015** Habilitation, prevocational, waiver; per hour

☑ **T2016** Habilitation, residential, waiver; per diem

☑ **T2017** Habilitation, residential, waiver; 15 minutes

☑ **T2018** Habilitation, supported employment, waiver; per diem

☑ **T2019** Habilitation, supported employment, waiver; per 15 minutes

☑ **T2020** Day habilitation, waiver; per diem

☑ **T2021** Day habilitation, waiver; per 15 minutes

☑ **T2022** Case management, per month

☑ **T2023** Targeted case management; per month

**T2024** Service assessment/plan of care development, waiver

**T2025** Waiver services; not otherwise specified (NOS)

☑ **T2026** Specialized childcare, waiver; per diem

Special Coverage Instructions    Noncovered by Medicare    Carrier Discretion    ☑ Quantity Alert    ● New Code    ○ Recycled/Reinstated    ▲ Revised Code

**2008 HCPCS**    A2 A3 ASC Payment Indicators    **MED:** Pub 100/NCD References    ⅋ DMEPOS Paid    ⊘ SNF Excluded    PQ PQRI    **T Codes — 147**

National T Codes

T2027 — T5999

☑ **T2027** Specialized childcare, waiver; per 15 minutes

**T2028** Specialized supply, not otherwise specified, waiver

**T2029** Specialized medical equipment, not otherwise specified, waiver

☑ **T2030** Assisted living, waiver; per month

☑ **T2031** Assisted living; waiver, per diem

☑ **T2032** Residential care, not otherwise specified (NOS), waiver; per month

☑ **T2033** Residential care, not otherwise specified (NOS), waiver; per diem

☑ **T2034** Crisis intervention, waiver; per diem

**T2035** Utility services to support medical equipment and assistive technology/devices, waiver

☑ **T2036** Therapeutic camping, overnight, waiver; each session

☑ **T2037** Therapeutic camping, day, waiver; each session

☑ **T2038** Community transition, waiver; per service

☑ **T2039** Vehicle modifications, waiver; per service

☑ **T2040** Financial management, self-directed, waiver; per 15 minutes

☑ **T2041** Supports brokerage, self-directed, waiver; per 15 minutes

☑ **T2042** Hospice routine home care; per diem

☑ **T2043** Hospice continuous home care; per hour

☑ **T2044** Hospice inpatient respite care; per diem

☑ **T2045** Hospice general inpatient care; per diem

☑ **T2046** Hospice long term care, room and board only; per diem

☑ **T2048** Behavioral health; long-term care residential (nonacute care in a residential treatment program where stay is typically longer than 30 days), with room and board, per diem

☑ **T2049** Nonemergency transportation; stretcher van, mileage; per mile

**T2101** Human breast milk processing, storage and distribution only                                    ♀

☑ **T4521** Adult sized disposable incontinence product, brief/diaper, small, each
MED: 100-3,230.10

☑ **T4522** Adult sized disposable incontinence product, brief/diaper, medium, each
MED: 100-3,230.10

☑ **T4523** Adult sized disposable incontinence product, brief/diaper, large, each
MED: 100-3,230.10

☑ **T4524** Adult sized disposable incontinence product, brief/diaper, extra large, each
MED: 100-3,230.10

☑ **T4525** Adult sized disposable incontinence product, protective underwear/pull-on, small size, each
MED: 100-3,230.10

☑ **T4526** Adult sized disposable incontinence product, protective underwear/pull-on, medium size, each
MED: 100-3,230.10

☑ **T4527** Adult sized disposable incontinence product, protective underwear/pull-on, large size, each
MED: 100-3,230.10

☑ **T4528** Adult sized disposable incontinence product, protective underwear/pull-on, extra large size, each
MED: 100-3,230.10

☑ **T4529** Pediatric sized disposable incontinence product, brief/diaper, small/medium size, each
MED: 100-3,230.10

☑ **T4530** Pediatric sized disposable incontinence product, brief/diaper, large size, each
MED: 100-3,230.10

☑ **T4531** Pediatric sized disposable incontinence product, protective underwear/pull-on, small/medium size, each
MED: 100-3,230.10

☑ **T4532** Pediatric sized disposable incontinence product, protective underwear/pull-on, large size, each
MED: 100-3,230.10

☑ **T4533** Youth sized disposable incontinence product, brief/diaper, each
MED: 100-3,230.10

☑ **T4534** Youth sized disposable incontinence product, protective underwear/pull-on, each
MED: 100-3,230.10

☑ **T4535** Disposable liner/shield/guard/pad/undergarment, for incontinence, each
MED: 100-3,230.10

☑ **T4536** Incontinence product, protective underwear/pull-on, reusable, any size, each
MED: 100-3,230.10

☑ **T4537** Incontinence product, protective underpad, reusable, bed size, each
MED: 100-3,230.10

☑ **T4538** Diaper service, reusable diaper, each diaper
MED: 100-3,230.10

☑ **T4539** Incontinence product, diaper/brief, reusable, any size, each
MED: 100-3,230.10

☑ **T4540** Incontinence product, protective underpad, reusable, chair size, each
MED: 100-3,230.10

☑ **T4541** Incontinence product, disposable underpad, large, each

☑ **T4542** Incontinence product, disposable underpad, small size, each

☑ **T4543** Disposable incontinence product, brief/diaper, bariatric, each

**T5001** Positioning seat for persons with special orthopedic needs

**T5999** Supply, not otherwise specified

Special Coverage Instructions     Noncovered by Medicare     Carrier Discretion     ☑ Quantity Alert     ● New Code     ○ Recycled/Reinstated     ▲ Revised Code

**148 — T Codes**     Ⓐ Age Edit     Ⓜ Maternity Edit     ♀ Female Only     ♂ Male Only     Ⓐ-Ⓨ OPPS Status Indicators     **2008 HCPCS**

## VISION SERVICES V0000-V2999

These V codes include vision-related supplies, including spectacles, lenses, contact lenses, prostheses, intraocular lenses, and miscellaneous lenses.

## FRAMES

[A] **V2020** Frames, purchases
MED: 100-2,15,120; 100-4,3,10.4

[E] **V2025** Deluxe frame
MED: 100-4,1,30.3.5

## SPECTACLE LENSES

See S0500-S0592 for temporary vision codes.

## SINGLE VISION, GLASS, OR PLASTIC

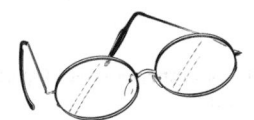

Monofocal spectacles (V2100-V2114)

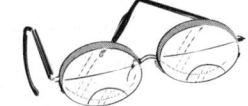

Trifocal spectacles (V2300-V2314)

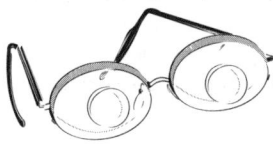

Low vision aids mounted to spectacles (V2610)

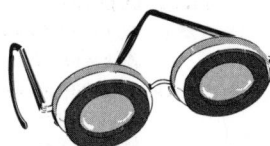

Telescopic or other compound lens fitted on spectacles as a low vision aid (V2615)

[A] ☑ **V2100** Sphere, single vision, plano to plus or minus 4.00, per lens ♿

[A] ☑ **V2101** Sphere, single vision, plus or minus 4.12 to plus or minus 7.00d, per lens ♿

[A] ☑ **V2102** Sphere, single vision, plus or minus 7.12 to plus or minus 20.00d, per lens ♿

[A] ☑ **V2103** Spherocylinder, single vision, plano to plus or minus 4.00d sphere, 0.12 to 2.00d cylinder, per lens ♿

[A] ☑ **V2104** Spherocylinder, single vision, plano to plus or minus 4.00d sphere, 2.12 to 4.00d cylinder, per lens ♿

[A] ☑ **V2105** Spherocylinder, single vision, plano to plus or minus 4.00d sphere, 4.25 to 6.00d cylinder, per lens ♿

[A] ☑ **V2106** Spherocylinder, single vision, plano to plus or minus 4.00d sphere, over 6.00d cylinder, per lens ♿

[A] ☑ **V2107** Spherocylinder, single vision, plus or minus 4.25 to plus or minus 7.00 sphere, 0.12 to 2.00d cylinder, per lens ♿

[A] ☑ **V2108** Spherocylinder, single vision, plus or minus 4.25d to plus or minus 7.00d sphere, 2.12 to 4.00d cylinder, per lens ♿

[A] ☑ **V2109** Spherocylinder, single vision, plus or minus 4.25 to plus or minus 7.00d sphere, 4.25 to 6.00d cylinder, per lens ♿

[A] ☑ **V2110** Spherocylinder, single vision, plus or minus 4.25 to 7.00d sphere, over 6.00d cylinder, per lens ♿

[A] ☑ **V2111** Spherocylinder, single vision, plus or minus 7.25 to plus or minus 12.00d sphere, 0.25 to 2.25d cylinder, per lens ♿

[A] ☑ **V2112** Spherocylinder, single vision, plus or minus 7.25 to plus or minus 12.00d sphere, 2.25d to 4.00d cylinder, per lens ♿

[A] ☑ **V2113** Spherocylinder, single vision, plus or minus 7.25 to plus or minus 12.00d sphere, 4.25 to 6.00d cylinder, per lens ♿

[A] ☑ **V2114** Spherocylinder, single vision, sphere over plus or minus 12.00d, per lens ♿

[A] ☑ **V2115** Lenticular (myodisc), per lens, single vision ♿

[A] **V2118** Aniseikonic lens, single vision ♿

[A] ☑ **V2121** Lenticular lens, per lens, single ♿
MED: 100-2,15,120; 100-4,3,10.4

[A] **V2199** Not otherwise classified, single vision lens

## BIFOCAL, GLASS, OR PLASTIC

[A] ☑ **V2200** Sphere, bifocal, plano to plus or minus 4.00d, per lens ♿

[A] ☑ **V2201** Sphere, bifocal, plus or minus 4.12 to plus or minus 7.00d, per lens ♿

[A] ☑ **V2202** Sphere, bifocal, plus or minus 7.12 to plus or minus 20.00d, per lens ♿

[A] ☑ **V2203** Spherocylinder, bifocal, plano to plus or minus 4.00d sphere, 0.12 to 2.00d cylinder, per lens ♿

[A] ☑ **V2204** Spherocylinder, bifocal, plano to plus or minus 4.00d sphere, 2.12 to 4.00d cylinder, per lens ♿

[A] ☑ **V2205** Spherocylinder, bifocal, plano to plus or minus 4.00d sphere, 4.25 to 6.00d cylinder, per lens ♿

[A] ☑ **V2206** Spherocylinder, bifocal, plano to plus or minus 4.00d sphere, over 6.00d cylinder, per lens ♿

[A] ☑ **V2207** Spherocylinder, bifocal, plus or minus 4.25 to plus or minus 7.00d sphere, 0.12 to 2.00d cylinder, per lens ♿

[A] ☑ **V2208** Spherocylinder, bifocal, plus or minus 4.25 to plus or minus 7.00d sphere, 2.12 to 4.00d cylinder, per lens ♿

[A] ☑ **V2209** Spherocylinder, bifocal, plus or minus 4.25 to plus or minus 7.00d sphere, 4.25 to 6.00d cylinder, per lens ♿

[A] ☑ **V2210** Spherocylinder, bifocal, plus or minus 4.25 to plus or minus 7.00d sphere, over 6.00d cylinder, per lens ♿

[A] ☑ **V2211** Spherocylinder, bifocal, plus or minus 7.25 to plus or minus 12.00d sphere, 0.25 to 2.25d cylinder, per lens ♿

[A] ☑ **V2212** Spherocylinder, bifocal, plus or minus 7.25 to plus or minus 12.00d sphere, 2.25 to 4.00d cylinder, per lens ♿

[A] ☑ **V2213** Spherocylinder, bifocal, plus or minus 7.25 to plus or minus 12.00d sphere, 4.25 to 6.00d cylinder, per lens ♿

[A] ☑ **V2214** Spherocylinder, bifocal, sphere over plus or minus 12.00d, per lens ♿

[A] ☑ **V2215** Lenticular (myodisc), per lens, bifocal ♿

[A] ☑ **V2218** Aniseikonic, per lens, bifocal ♿

[A] ☑ **V2219** Bifocal seg width over 28mm ♿

[A] ☑ **V2220** Bifocal add over 3.25d ♿

[A] **V2221** Lenticular lens, per lens, bifocal ♿
MED: 100-2,15,120; 100-4,3,10.4

[A] **V2299** Specialty bifocal (by report)
Pertinent documentation to evaluate medical appropriateness should be included when this code is reported.

▨ Special Coverage Instructions  ▨ Noncovered by Medicare  ▨ Carrier Discretion  ☑ Quantity Alert  ● New Code  ○ Recycled/Reinstated  ▲ Revised Code

**2008 HCPCS**  [A2]-[Z6] ASC Payment Indicators  **MED:** Pub 100/NCD References  ♿ DMEPOS Paid  ⊘ SNF Excluded  [PQ] PQRI  **V Codes — 149**

**V2020 — V2299**

**Vision Services**

**V2300 — V2615**

## TRIFOCAL, GLASS, OR PLASTIC

Ⓐ ☑ **V2300** Sphere, trifocal, plano to plus or minus 4.00d, per lens ♿

Ⓐ ☑ **V2301** Sphere, trifocal, plus or minus 4.12 to plus or minus 7.00d per lens ♿

Ⓐ ☑ **V2302** Sphere, trifocal, plus or minus 7.12 to plus or minus 20.00, per lens ♿

Ⓐ ☑ **V2303** Spherocylinder, trifocal, plano to plus or minus 4.00d sphere, 0.12 to 2.00d cylinder, per lens ♿

Ⓐ ☑ **V2304** Spherocylinder, trifocal, plano to plus or minus 4.00d sphere, 2.25 to 4.00d cylinder, per lens ♿

Ⓐ ☑ **V2305** Spherocylinder, trifocal, plano to plus or minus 4.00d sphere, 4.25 to 6.00 cylinder, per lens ♿

Ⓐ ☑ **V2306** Spherocylinder, trifocal, plano to plus or minus 4.00d sphere, over 6.00d cylinder, per lens ♿

Ⓐ ☑ **V2307** Spherocylinder, trifocal, plus or minus 4.25 to plus or minus 7.00d sphere, 0.12 to 2.00d cylinder, per lens ♿

Ⓐ ☑ **V2308** Spherocylinder, trifocal, plus or minus 4.25 to plus or minus 7.00d sphere, 2.12 to 4.00d cylinder, per lens ♿

Ⓐ ☑ **V2309** Spherocylinder, trifocal, plus or minus 4.25 to plus or minus 7.00d sphere, 4.25 to 6.00d cylinder, per lens ♿

Ⓐ ☑ **V2310** Spherocylinder, trifocal, plus or minus 4.25 to plus or minus 7.00d sphere, over 6.00d cylinder, per lens ♿

Ⓐ ☑ **V2311** Spherocylinder, trifocal, plus or minus 7.25 to plus or minus 12.00d sphere, 0.25 to 2.25d cylinder, per lens ♿

Ⓐ ☑ **V2312** Spherocylinder, trifocal, plus or minus 7.25 to plus or minus 12.00d sphere, 2.25 to 4.00d cylinder, per lens ♿

Ⓐ ☑ **V2313** Spherocylinder, trifocal, plus or minus 7.25 to plus or minus 12.00d sphere, 4.25 to 6.00d cylinder, per lens ♿

Ⓐ ☑ **V2314** Spherocylinder, trifocal, sphere over plus or minus 12.00d, per lens ♿

Ⓐ ☑ **V2315** Lenticular (myodisc), per lens, trifocal ♿

Ⓐ **V2318** Aniseikonic lens, trifocal ♿

Ⓐ ☑ **V2319** Trifocal seg width over 28 mm ♿

Ⓐ ☑ **V2320** Trifocal add over 3.25d ♿

Ⓐ **V2321** Lenticular lens, per lens, trifocal ♿
MED: 100-2,15,120; 100-4,3,10.4

Ⓐ **V2399** Specialty trifocal (by report)
Pertinent documentation to evaluate medical appropriateness should be included when this code is reported.

## VARIABLE ASPHERICITY LENS, GLASS, OR PLASTIC

Ⓐ ☑ **V2410** Variable asphericity lens, single vision, full field, glass or plastic, per lens ♿

Ⓐ ☑ **V2430** Variable asphericity lens, bifocal, full field, glass or plastic, per lens ♿

Ⓐ **V2499** Variable sphericity lens, other type

## CONTACT LENS

If procedure code 92391 or 92396 is reported, recode with specific lens type listed below (per lens).

Ⓐ ☑ **V2500** Contact lens, PMMA, spherical, per lens ♿

Ⓐ ☑ **V2501** Contact lens, PMMA, toric or prism ballast, per lens ♿

Ⓐ ☑ **V2502** Contact lens, PMMA, bifocal, per lens ♿

Ⓐ ☑ **V2503** Contact lens, PMMA, color vision deficiency, per lens ♿

Ⓐ ☑ **V2510** Contact lens, gas permeable, spherical, per lens ♿

Ⓐ ☑ **V2511** Contact lens, gas permeable, toric, prism ballast, per lens ♿

Ⓐ ☑ **V2512** Contact lens, gas permeable, bifocal, per lens ♿

Ⓐ ☑ **V2513** Contact lens, gas permeable, extended wear, per lens ♿

Ⓐ ☑ **V2520** Contact lens, hydrophilic, spherical, per lens ♿
Hydrophilic contact lenses are covered by Medicare only for aphakic patients. Local contractor if incident to physician services.
MED: 100-3,80.1; 100-3,80.4

Ⓐ ☑ **V2521** Contact lens, hydrophilic, toric, or prism ballast, per lens ♿
Hydrophilic contact lenses are covered by Medicare only for aphakic patients. Local contractor if incident to physician services.
MED: 100-3,80.1; 100-3,80.4

Ⓐ ☑ **V2522** Contact lens, hydrophilic, bifocal, per lens ♿
Hydrophilic contact lenses are covered by Medicare only for aphakic patients. Local contractor if incident to physician services.
MED: 100-3,80.1; 100-3,80.4

Ⓐ ☑ **V2523** Contact lens, hydrophilic, extended wear, per lens ♿
Hydrophilic contact lenses are covered by Medicare only for aphakic patients.
MED: 100-3,80.1; 100-3,80.4

Ⓐ ☑ **V2530** Contact lens, scleral, gas impermeable, per lens (for contact lens modification, see 92325) ♿

Ⓐ ☑ **V2531** Contact lens, scleral, gas permeable, per lens (for contact lens modification, see 92325) ♿
MED: 100-3,80.5

Ⓐ **V2599** Contact lens, other type
Local contractor if incident to physician services.

## VISION AIDS

If procedure code 92392 is reported, recode with specific systems below.

Ⓐ **V2600** Hand held low vision aids and other nonspectacle mounted aids

Ⓐ **V2610** Single lens spectacle mounted low vision aids

Ⓐ **V2615** Telescopic and other compound lens system, including distance vision telescopic, near vision telescopes and compound microscopic lens system

## PROSTHETIC EYE

⬛ Special Coverage Instructions   ⬛ Noncovered by Medicare   ⬛ Carrier Discretion   ☑ Quantity Alert   ● New Code   ○ Recycled/Reinstated   ▲ Revised Code

**150 — V Codes**   Ⓐ Age Edit   Ⓜ Maternity Edit   ♀ Female Only   ♂ Male Only   Ⓐ-Ⓨ OPPS Status Indicators   **2008 HCPCS**

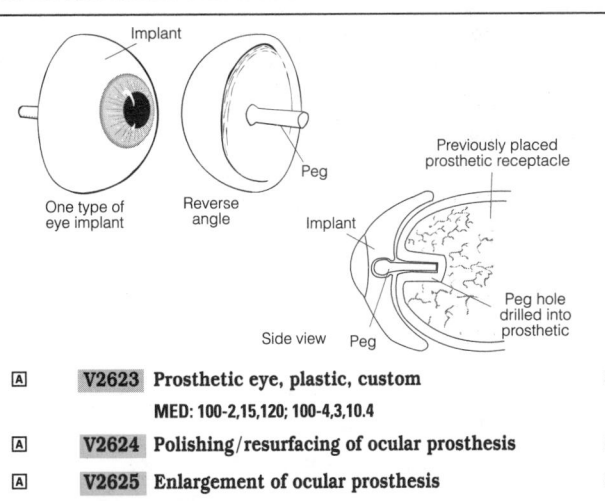

One type of eye implant

Reverse angle

Implant

Peg

Previously placed prosthetic receptacle

Peg hole drilled into prosthetic

Side view

Peg

| | | | | |
|---|---|---|---|---|
| A | | **V2623** | Prosthetic eye, plastic, custom | �2 |

MED: 100-2,15,120; 100-4,3,10.4

| | | | | |
|---|---|---|---|---|
| A | | **V2624** | Polishing/resurfacing of ocular prosthesis | �2 |
| A | | **V2625** | Enlargement of ocular prosthesis | �2 |
| A | | **V2626** | Reduction of ocular prosthesis | �2 |
| A | | **V2627** | Scleral cover shell | �2 |

A scleral shell covers the cornea and the anterior sclera. Medicare covers a scleral shell when it is prescribed as an artificial support to a shrunken and sightless eye or as a barrier in the treatment of severe dry eye.

MED: 100-3,80.5

| | | | | |
|---|---|---|---|---|
| A | | **V2628** | Fabrication and fitting of ocular conformer | �2 |
| A | | **V2629** | Prosthetic eye, other type | |

## INTRAOCULAR LENSES

| | | | | |
|---|---|---|---|---|
| N | | **V2630** | Anterior chamber intraocular lens | N1 |

The IOL must be FDA-approved for reimbursement. Medicare payment for an IOL is included in the payment for ASC facility services. Medicare jurisdiction: local contractor.

MED: 100-2,15,120; 100-4,3,10.4

| | | | | |
|---|---|---|---|---|
| N | | **V2631** | Iris supported intraocular lens | N1 |

The IOL must be FDA-approved for reimbursement. Medicare payment for an IOL is included in the payment for ASC facility services. Medicare jurisdiction: local contractor.

MED: 100-2,15,120; 100-4,3,10.4

| | | | | |
|---|---|---|---|---|
| N | | **V2632** | Posterior chamber intraocular lens | N1 |

The IOL must be FDA-approved for reimbursement. Medicare payment for an IOL is included in the payment for ASC facility services. Medicare jurisdiction: local contractor.

MED: 100-2,15,120; 100-4,3,10.4

## MISCELLANEOUS

| | | | | |
|---|---|---|---|---|
| A | ☑ | **V2700** | Balance lens, per lens | �2 |
| E | | **V2702** | Deluxe lens feature | |

MED: 100-2,15,120; 100-4,3,10.4

| | | | | |
|---|---|---|---|---|
| A | ☑ | **V2710** | Slab off prism, glass or plastic, per lens | �2 |
| A | ☑ | **V2715** | Prism, per lens | �2 |
| A | ☑ | **V2718** | Press-on lens, Fresnel prism, per lens | �2 |
| A | ☑ | **V2730** | Special base curve, glass or plastic, per lens | �2 |
| A | ☑ | **V2744** | Tint, photochromatic, per lens | �2 |

MED: 100-2,15,120; 100-4,3,10.4

| | | | | |
|---|---|---|---|---|
| A | ☑ | **V2745** | Addition to lens; tint, any color, solid, gradient or equal, excludes photochromatic, any lens material, per lens | �2 |

MED: 100-2,15,120; 100-4,3,10.4

| | | | | |
|---|---|---|---|---|
| A | ☑ | **V2750** | Antireflective coating, per lens | �2 |

MED: 100-2,15,120; 100-4,3,10.4

| | | | | |
|---|---|---|---|---|
| A | ☑ | **V2755** | U-V lens, per lens | �2 |

MED: 100-2,15,120; 100-4,3,10.4

| | | | | |
|---|---|---|---|---|
| E | | **V2756** | Eye glass case | |
| A | ☑ | **V2760** | Scratch resistant coating, per lens | �2 |
| B | ☑ | **V2761** | Mirror coating, any type, solid, gradient or equal, any lens material, per lens | |

MED: 100-2,15,120; 100-4,3,10.4

| | | | | |
|---|---|---|---|---|
| A | ☑ | **V2762** | Polarization, any lens material, per lens | �2 |

MED: 100-2,15,120; 100-4,3,10.4

| | | | | |
|---|---|---|---|---|
| A | ☑ | **V2770** | Occluder lens, per lens | �2 |
| A | ☑ | **V2780** | Oversize lens, per lens | �2 |
| B | ☑ | **V2781** | Progressive lens, per lens | |
| A | ☑ | **V2782** | Lens, index 1.54 to 1.65 plastic or 1.60 to 1.79 glass, excludes polycarbonate, per lens | |

MED: 100-2,15,120; 100-4,3,10.4

| | | | | |
|---|---|---|---|---|
| A | ☑ | **V2783** | Lens, index greater than or equal to 1.66 plastic or greater than or equal to 1.80 glass, excludes polycarbonate, per lens | �2 |

MED: 100-2,15,120; 100-4,3,10.4

| | | | | |
|---|---|---|---|---|
| A | ☑ | **V2784** | Lens, polycarbonate or equal, any index, per lens | �2 |

MED: 100-2,15,120; 100-4,3,10.4

| | | | | |
|---|---|---|---|---|
| F | | **V2785** | Processing, preserving and transporting corneal tissue | F4 |

Medicare jurisdiction: local contractor.

| | | | | |
|---|---|---|---|---|
| A | ☑ | **V2786** | Specialty occupational multifocal lens, per lens | �2 |

MED: 100-2,15,120; 100-4,3,10.4

| | | | | |
|---|---|---|---|---|
| ● | E | **V2787** | Astigmatism correcting function of intraocular lens | |
| | E | **V2788** | Presbyopia correcting function of intraocular lens | |
| | N | **V2790** | Amniotic membrane for surgical reconstruction, per procedure | N1 |

Medicare jurisdiction: local contractor.

| | | | |
|---|---|---|---|
| A | **V2797** | Vision supply, accessory and/or service component of another HCPCS vision code | |
| A | **V2799** | Vision service, miscellaneous | |

Determine if an alternative HCPCS Level II or a CPT code better describes the service being reported. This code should be used only if a more specific code is unavailable.

## HEARING SERVICES V5000-V5999

This range of codes describes hearing tests and related supplies and equipment, speech-language pathology screenings, and repair of augmentative communicative system.

| | | | |
|---|---|---|---|
| E | **V5008** | Hearing screening | |

MED: 100-2,16,90

| | | | |
|---|---|---|---|
| E | **V5010** | Assessment for hearing aid | |
| E | **V5011** | Fitting/orientation/checking of hearing aid | |
| E | **V5014** | Repair/modification of a hearing aid | |
| E | **V5020** | Conformity evaluation | |
| E | **V5030** | Hearing aid, monaural, body worn, air conduction | |
| E | **V5040** | Hearing aid, monaural, body worn, bone conduction | |
| E | **V5050** | Hearing aid, monaural, in the ear | |
| E | **V5060** | Hearing aid, monaural, behind the ear | |
| E | **V5070** | Glasses, air conduction | |

---

Special Coverage Instructions    Noncovered by Medicare    Carrier Discretion    ☑ Quantity Alert    ● New Code    ○ Recycled/Reinstated    ▲ Revised Code

**Hearing Services**

**V5080 — V5364**

| | | | |
|---|---|---|---|
| E | | V5080 | Glasses, bone conduction |
| E | | V5090 | Dispensing fee, unspecified hearing aid |
| E | | V5095 | Semi-implantable middle ear hearing prosthesis |

Use this code for Vibrant Soundbridge Implantable Middle Ear Prosthesis.

| | | | |
|---|---|---|---|
| E | | V5100 | Hearing aid, bilateral, body worn |
| E | | V5110 | Dispensing fee, bilateral |
| E | | V5120 | Binaural, body |
| E | | V5130 | Binaural, in the ear |
| E | | V5140 | Binaural, behind the ear |
| E | | V5150 | Binaural, glasses |
| E | | V5160 | Dispensing fee, binaural |
| E | | V5170 | Hearing aid, CROS, in the ear |
| E | | V5180 | Hearing aid, CROS, behind the ear |
| E | | V5190 | Hearing aid, CROS, glasses |
| E | | V5200 | Dispensing fee, CROS |
| E | | V5210 | Hearing aid, BICROS, in the ear |
| E | | V5220 | Hearing aid, BICROS, behind the ear |
| E | | V5230 | Hearing aid, BICROS, glasses |
| E | | V5240 | Dispensing fee, BICROS |
| E | | V5241 | Dispensing fee, monaural hearing aid, any type |
| E | | V5242 | Hearing aid, analog, monaural, CIC (completely in the ear canal) |
| E | | V5243 | Hearing aid, analog, monaural, ITC (in the canal) |
| E | | V5244 | Hearing aid, digitally programmable analog, monaural, CIC |
| E | | V5245 | Hearing aid, digitally programmable, analog, monaural, ITC |
| E | | V5246 | Hearing aid, digitally programmable analog, monaural, ITE (in the ear) |
| E | | V5247 | Hearing aid, digitally programmable analog, monaural, BTE (behind the ear) |
| E | | V5248 | Hearing aid, analog, binaural, CIC |
| E | | V5249 | Hearing aid, analog, binaural, ITC |
| E | | V5250 | Hearing aid, digitally programmable analog, binaural, CIC |
| E | | V5251 | Hearing aid, digitally programmable analog, binaural, ITC |
| E | | V5252 | Hearing aid, digitally programmable, binaural, ITE |
| E | | V5253 | Hearing aid, digitally programmable, binaural, BTE |
| E | | V5254 | Hearing aid, digital, monaural, CIC |
| E | | V5255 | Hearing aid, digital, monaural, ITC |
| E | | V5256 | Hearing aid, digital, monaural, ITE |
| E | | V5257 | Hearing aid, digital, monaural, BTE |
| E | | V5258 | Hearing aid, digital, binaural, CIC |
| E | | V5259 | Hearing aid, digital, binaural, ITC |
| E | | V5260 | Hearing aid, digital, binaural, ITE |
| E | | V5261 | Hearing aid, digital, binaural, BTE |
| E | | V5262 | Hearing aid, disposable, any type, monaural |
| E | ☑ | V5263 | Hearing aid, disposable, any type, binaural |
| E | ☑ | V5264 | Ear mold/insert, not disposable, any type |
| E | ☑ | V5265 | Ear mold/insert, disposable, any type |
| E | ☑ | V5266 | Battery for use in hearing device |

| | | | |
|---|---|---|---|
| E | ☑ | V5267 | Hearing aid supplies/accessories |
| E | ☑ | V5268 | Assistive listening device, telephone amplifier, any type |
| E | | V5269 | Assistive listening device, alerting, any type |
| E | | V5270 | Assistive listening device, television amplifier, any type |
| E | | V5271 | Assistive listening device, television caption decoder |
| E | | V5272 | Assistive listening device, TDD |
| E | | V5273 | Assistive listening device, for use with cochlear implant |
| E | | V5274 | Assistive listening device, not otherwise specified |
| E | ☑ | V5275 | Ear impression, each |
| E | | V5298 | Hearing aid, not otherwise classified |
| B | | V5299 | Hearing service, miscellaneous ⊘ |

Determine if an alternative HCPCS Level II or a CPT code better describes the service being reported. This code should be used only if a more specific code is unavailable.

**MED: 100-2,16,90**

## SPEECH-LANGUAGE PATHOLOGY SERVICES

| | | |
|---|---|---|
| E | V5336 | Repair/modification of augmentative communicative system or device (excludes adaptive hearing aid) |

Medicare jurisdiction: DME regional contractor.

| | | |
|---|---|---|
| E | V5362 | Speech screening |
| E | V5363 | Language screening |
| E | V5364 | Dysphagia screening |

---

Special Coverage Instructions | Noncovered by Medicare | Carrier Discretion | ☑ Quantity Alert | ● New Code | ○ Recycled/Reinstated | ▲ Revised Code

152 — V Codes | A Age Edit | M Maternity Edit | ♀ Female Only | ♂ Male Only | A-Y OPPS Status Indicators | 2008 HCPCS

## APPENDIX 1 — TABLE OF DRUGS

### Introduction and Directions

The HCPCS 2008 Table of Drugs is designed to quickly and easily direct the user to drug names and their corresponding codes. Both generic and brand or trade names are alphabetically listed in the "Drug Name" column of the table. The associated A, C, J, K, Q, or S code is given only for the generic name of the drug.

The "Unit Per" column lists the stated amount for the referenced generic drug as provided by CMS. "Up to" listings are inclusive of all quantities up to and including the listed amount. All other listings are for the amount of the drug as listed. The editors recognize that the availability of some drugs in the quantities listed is dependent on many variables beyond the control of the clinical ordering clerk. The availability in your area of regularly used drugs in the most cost-effective quantities should be relayed to your third-party payers.

The "Route of Administration" column addresses the most common methods of delivering the referenced generic drug as described in current pharmaceutical literature. The official definitions for Level II drug codes generally describe administration other than by oral method. Therefore, with a handful of exceptions, oral-delivered options for most drugs are omitted from the Route of Administration column.

Intravenous administration includes all methods, such as gravity infusion, injections, and timed pushes. When several routes of administration are listed, the first listing is simply the first, or most common, method as described in current reference literature. The "VAR" posting denotes various routes of administration and is used for drugs that are commonly administered into joints, cavities, tissues, or topical applications, in addition to other parenteral administrations. Listings posted with "OTH" alert the user to other administration methods, such as suppositories or catheter injections.

Please be reminded that the Table of Drugs, as well as all HCPCS Level II national definitions and listings, constitutes a post-treatment medical reference for billing purposes only. Although the editors have exercised all normal precautions to ensure the accuracy of the table and related material, the use of any of this information to select medical treatment is entirely inappropriate. Do not code directly from the table of drugs. Refer to the tabular section for complete information.

See Appendix 3 for abbreviations.

| Drug Name | Unit Per: | Route | Code |
|---|---|---|---|
| 10% LMD | 500 ML | IV | J7100 |
| 5% DEXTROSE/NORMAL SALINE | 5% | VAR | J7042 |
| 5% DEXTROSE/WATER | 500 ML | IV | J7060 |
| A-HYDROCORT | 100 MG | IV, IM, SC | J1720 |
| A-METHAPRED | 125 MG | IM, IV | J2930 |
| A-METHAPRED | 40 MG | IM, IV | J2920 |
| ABARELIX | 10 MG | IM | J0128 |
| ABATACEPT | 10 MG | IV | J0129 |
| ABBOKINASE | 250,000 IU | IV | J3365 |
| ABBOKINASE | 5,000 IU | IV | J3364 |
| ABCIXIMAB | 10 MG | IV | J0130 |
| ABELCET | 50 MG | IV | J0285 |
| ABILIFY | 0.25 MG | IM | J0400 ● |
| ABRAXANE | 1 MG | IV | J9264 |
| ACCUNEB NONCOMPOUNDED, CONCENTRATED | 1 MG | INH | J7611 |
| ACCUNEB NONCOMPOUNDED, UNIT DOSE | 1 MG | INH | J7613 |
| ACETADOTE | 1 G | INH | J7608 |
| ACETADOTE | 100 MG | IV | J0132 |
| ACETAZOLAMIDE SODIUM | 500 MG | IM, IV | J1120 |
| ACETYLCYSTEINE NONCOMPOUNDED | 1 G | INH | J7608 |
| ACETYLCYSTEINE COMPOUNDED | PER G | INH | J7604 ● |
| ACTHREL | 1 MCG | IV | J0795 |
| ACTIMMUNE | 0.25 MG | SC | J1830 |
| ACTIMMUNE | 3 MU | SC | J9216 |
| ACTIVASE | 1 MG | IV | J2997 |

| Drug Name | Unit Per: | Route | Code |
|---|---|---|---|
| ACUTECT | DOSE | IV | A9504 |
| ACYCLOVIR | 5 MG | IV | J0133 |
| ADAGEN | 25 IU | IM | J2504 |
| ADALIMUMAB | 20 MG | SC | J0135 |
| ADBEON | 4 MG | IM, IV | J0704 |
| ADENOCARD | 6 MG | IV | J0150 |
| ADENOSCAN | 30 MG | IV | J0152 |
| ADENOSINE | 30 MG | IV | J0152 |
| ADENOSINE | 6 MG | IV | J0150 |
| ADRENALIN | 1 MG | IM, IV, SC | J0170 |
| ADRENALIN CHLORIDE | 1 MG | IM, IV, SC | J0170 |
| ADRENOCORT | 1 MG | IM, IV, OTH | J1100 |
| ADRIAMYCIN | 10 MG | IV | J9000 |
| ADRUCIL | 500 MG | IV | J9190 |
| AEROBID | 1 MG | INH | J7641 |
| AGALSIDASE BETA | 1 MG | IV | J0180 |
| AGGRASTAT | 12.5 MG | IM, IV | J3246 |
| ALATROFLOXACIN MESYLATE | 100 MG | IV | J0200 |
| ALBUTEROL AND IPRATROPIUM BROMIDE NONCOMPOUNDED | 2.5MG/0.5 MG | INH | J7620 |
| ALBUTEROL COMPOUNDED, CONCENTRATED | 1 MG | INH | J7610 |
| ALBUTEROL COMPOUNDED, UNIT DOSE | 1 MG | INH | J7609 |
| ALBUTEROL NONCOMPOUNDED, CONCENETRATED FORM | 1 MG | INH | J7611 |
| ALBUTEROL NONCOMPOUNDED, CONCENETRATED FORM | 1MG | INH | Q4093 |
| ALBUTEROL NONCOMPOUNDED, UNIT DOSE | PER 1 MG | INH | J7603 |
| ALBUTEROL NONCOMPOUNDED, UNIT DOSE FORM | 1MG | INH‡ | Q4094 |
| ALBUTEROL, NONCOMPOUNDED, CONCENTRATED FORM | PER 1 MG | INH | J7602 ● |
| ALDESLEUKIN | 1 VIAL | IV | J9015 |
| ALDURAZYME | 0.1 MG | IV | J1931 |
| ALEFACEPT | 0.5 MG | IV, IM | J0215 |
| ALEMTUZUMAB | 10 MG | IV | J9010 |
| ALFERON N | 250,000 IU | IM | J9215 |
| ALGLUCERASE | 10 U | IV | J0205 |
| ALGLUCOSIDASE ALFA | 10 MG | IV | J0220 |
| ALIMTA | 10 MG | IV | J9305 |
| ALKERAN | 2 MG | ORAL | J8600 |
| ALKERAN | 50 MG | IV | J9245 |
| ALOXI | 25 MCG | IV | J2469 |
| ALPHA 1 - PROTEINASE INHIBITOR — HUMAN | 10 MG | IV | J0256 |
| ALPHANATE | 1 IU | IV | J7190 |
| ALPHANINE SD | 1 IU | IV | J7194 |
| ALPROSTADIL | 1.25 MCG | VAR | J0270 |
| ALPROSTADIL | EA | OTH | J0275 |
| ALTEPLASE RECOMBINANT | 1 MG | IV | J2997 |
| ALUPENT, NONCOMPOUNDED, CONCENTRATED | 10 MG | INH | J7668 |
| ALUPENT, NONCOMPOUNDED, UNIT DOSE | 10 MG | INH | J7669 |
| AMANTADINE HYDROCHLORIDE (BRAND NAME) | 100 MG | ORAL | G9033 |

| Drug Name | Unit Per: | Route | Code | Drug Name | Unit Per: | Route | Code |
|---|---|---|---|---|---|---|---|
| AMANTADINE HYDROCHLORIDE (GENERIC) | 100 MG | ORAL | G9017 | ANZEMET | 50 MG | ORAL | S0174 |
| AMBISOME | 10 MG | IV | J0289 | APLIGRAF | SQ CM | OTH | J7340 |
| AMCORT | 5 MG | IM | J3302 | APOKYN | 1 MG | SC | J0364 |
| AMERGAN | 12.5 MG | ORAL | Q0169 | APOKYN | 1 MG | SC | S0167 |
| AMEVIVE | 0.5 MG | IV, IM | J0215 | APOMORPHINE HYDROCHLORIDE | 1 MG | SC | J0364 |
| AMICAR | 5 G | IV | S0017 | APOMORPHINE HYDROCHLORIDE | 1 MG | SC | S0167 |
| AMIFOSTINE | 500 MG | IV | J0207 | APREPITANT, ORAL, 5 MG | 5 MG | ORAL | J8501 |
| AMIKACIN SULFATE | 100 MG | IM, IV | J0278 | APROTININ | 10,000 KIU | IV | J0365 |
| AMIKIN | 100 MG | IM, IV | S0072 | AQUAMEPHYTON | 1 MG | IM, SC, IV | J3430 |
| AMINOCAPRIOC ACID | 5 G | IV | S0017 | ARA-C | 100 MG | SC, IV | J9100 |
| AMINOPHYLLINE | 250 MG | IV | J0280 | ARAMINE | 10 MG | IV, IM, SC | J0380 |
| AMIODARONE HCL | 30 MG | IV | J0282 | ARANESP, ESRD USE | 1 MCG | SC, IV | J0882 |
| AMITRIPTYLINE HCL | 20 MG | IM | J1320 | ARANESP, NON-ESRD USE | 1 MCG | SC, IV | J0881 |
| AMMONIA N-13 | DOSE | IV | A9526 | ARBUTAMINE HCL | 1 MG | IV | J0395 |
| AMOBARBITAL | 125 MG | IM, IV | J0300 | AREDIA | 30 MG | IV | J2430 |
| AMPHOCIN | 50 MG | IV | J0285 | ARFORMOTEROL | 15 MCG | INH | J7605 ● |
| AMPHOTEC | 10 MG | IV | J0287 | ~~ARGATROBAN~~ | ~~5 MG~~ | ~~IV~~ | ~~C9121~~ |
| AMPHOTERICIN B | 50 MG | IV | J0285 | ARIMIDEX | 1 MG | ORAL | S0170 |
| AMPHOTERICIN B CHOLESTERYL SULFATE COMPLEX | 10 MG | IV | J0288 | ARIPIPRAZOLE | 0.25 MG | IM | J0400 ● |
| AMPHOTERICIN B LIPID COMPLEX | 10 MG | IV | J0287 | ARISTOCORT | 5 MG | IM | J3302 |
| AMPHOTERICIN B LIPOSOME | 10 MG | IV | J0289 | ARISTOCORTE FORTE | 5 MG | IM | J3302 |
| AMPICILLIN SODIUM | 500 MG | IM, IV | J0290 | ARISTOCORTE INTRALESIONAL | 5 MG | OTH | J3302 |
| AMPICILLIN SODIUM/SULBACTAM SODIUM | 1.5 G | IM, IV | J0295 | ARISTOSPAN | 5 MG | VAR | J3303 |
| AMYTAL | 125 MG | IM, IV | J0300 | ARIXTRA | 0.5 MG | SC | J1652 |
| ~~ANABOLIN LA 100~~ | ~~100 MG~~ | ~~IM~~ | ~~J2321~~ | AROMASIN | 25 MG | ORAL | S0156 |
| ANASTROZOLE | 1 MG | ORAL | S0170 | ARRANON | 50 MG | IV | J9261 |
| ANCEF | 500 MG | IV, IM | J0690 | ARRESTIN | 200 MG | IM | J3250 |
| ~~ANDRO LA 200~~ | ~~200 MG~~ | ~~IM~~ | ~~J3130~~ | ARSENIC TRIOXIDE | 1 MG | IV | J9017 |
| ~~ANDROLONE-D 100~~ | ~~100 MG~~ | ~~IM~~ | ~~J2321~~ | ASPARAGINASE | 10,000 U | VAR | J9020 |
| ~~ANDRONAQ 50~~ | ~~50 MG~~ | ~~IM~~ | ~~J3140~~ | ASTRAMORPH PF | 10 MG | IM, IV, SC | J2275 |
| ~~ANDROPOSITORY 100~~ | ~~100 MG~~ | ~~IM~~ | ~~J3120~~ | ATGAM | 250 MG | OTH | J7504 |
| ANECTINE | 20 MG | IM, IV | J0330 | ATIVAN | 2 MG | IM, IV | J2060 |
| ~~ANERGAN 25~~ | ~~50 MG~~ | ~~IM, IV~~ | ~~J2550~~ | ATOPICLAIR | ANY SIZE | OTH | A6250 |
| ~~ANERGAN 50~~ | ~~50 MG~~ | ~~IM, IV~~ | ~~J2550~~ | ATROPEN | 0.3 MG | IV, IM, SC | J0460 |
| AN-DTPA DIAGNOSTIC | UP TO 25 MCI | IV | A9539 ● | ATROPINE SULFATE | 0.3 MG | IV, IM, SC | J0460 |
| AN-DTPA THERAPEUTIC | UP TO 25 MCI | IV | A9567 ● | ATROPINE, COMPOUNDED, CONCENTRATED | I MG | INH | J7635 |
| ANGIOMAX | 1 MG | IV | J0583 | ATROPINE, COMPOUNDED, UNIT DOSE | 1 MG | INH | J7636 |
| ANIDULAFUNGIN | 1 MG | IV | J0348 | ATROVENT, NONCOMPOUNDED, UNIT DOSE | 1 MG | INH | J7644 |
| ANISTREPLASE | 30 U | IV | J0350 | AUROTHIOGLUCOSE | 50 MG | IM | J2910 |
| ANTAGON | 250 MCG | SC | S0132 | AUTOPLEX T | 1 IU | IV | J7198 |
| ANTI-INHIBITOR | 1 IU | IV | J7198 | AVASTIN | 10 MG | IV | J9035 |
| ANTI-THYMOCYTE GLOBULIN, EQUINE | 250 MG | OTH | J7504 | AVELOX | 100 MG | IV | J2280 |
| ~~ANTIFLEX~~ | ~~60 MG~~ | ~~IV, IM~~ | ~~J2360~~ | AVONEX | 11 MCG | IM | Q3025 |
| ANTIHEMOPHILIC FACTOR HUMAN METHOD M MONOCLONAL PURIFIED | 1 IU | IV | J7192 | AVONEX | 33 MCG | IM | J1825 |
| ANTIHEMOPHILIC FACTOR PORCINE | 1 IU | IV | J7191 | AZACITIDINE | 1 MG | SC | J9025 |
| ~~ANTINAUS~~ | ~~50 MG~~ | ~~IM, IV~~ | ~~J2550~~ | AZACTAM | 500 MG | IV | S0073 |
| ANTITHROMBIN III | 1 IU | IV | J7195 | AZASAN | 50 MG | ORAL | J7500 |
| ANTIZOL | 15 MG | IV | J1451 | AZATHIOPRINE | 100 MG | OTH | J7501 |
| ANZEMET | 10 MG | IV | J1260 | AZATHIOPRINE | 50 MG | ORAL | J7500 |
| ANZEMET | 100 MG | ORAL | Q0180 | ~~AZATHIOPRINE SODIUM~~ | ~~100 MG~~ | ~~OTH~~ | ~~J7501~~ |
| | | | | AZITHROMYCIN | 500 MG | IV | J0456 |
| | | | | AZMACORT | PER MG | INH | J7684 |

# APPENDIX 1 — TABLE OF DRUGS

| Drug Name | Unit Per: | Route | Code | Drug Name | Unit Per: | Route | Code |
|---|---|---|---|---|---|---|---|
| AZMACORT CONCENTRATED | PER MG | INH | J7683 | BITOLTEROL MESYLATE, COMPOUNDED CONCENTRATED | PER MG | INH | J7628 |
| AZTREONAM | 500 MG | IV | S0073 | BITOLTEROL MESYLATE, COMPOUNDED UNIT DOSE | PER MG | INH | J7629 |
| AZTREONAM | PER MG | INH | S0143 | BIVALIRUDIN | 1 MG | IV | J0583 |
| BACLOFEN | 10 MG | IT | J0475 | BLENOXANE | 15 U | IM, IV, SC | J9040 |
| BACLOFEN | 50 MCG | OTH | J0476 | BLEOMYCIN LYOPHILLIZED | 15 U | IM, IV, SC | J9040 |
| BACTERIOSTATIC WATER | 5% | VAR | J7051 | BLEOMYCIN SULFATE | 15 U | IM, IV, SC | J9040 |
| BACTOCILL | 250 MG | IM, IV | J2700 | BONIVA | 1 MG | IV | J1740 |
| BACTRIM IV | 10 ML | IV | S0039 | BORTEZOMIB | 0.1 MG | IV | J9041 |
| BAL | 100 MG | IM | J0470 | BOTOX | 1 U | IM | J0585 |
| BANFLEX | 60 MG | IV, IM | J2360 | BOTULINUM TOXIN TYPE A | 1 U | OTH | J0585 |
| BASILIXIMAB | 20 MG | IV | J0480 | BOTULINUM TOXIN TYPE B | 100 U | OTH | J0587 |
| BAYGAM | 1 CC | IM | J1460 | BRAVELLE | 75 IU | SC, IM | J3355 |
| BAYRHO-D | 300 MCG | IM | J2790 | BRETHINE | 1 MG | SC, IV | J3105 |
| BAYTET | 250 U | IM | J1670 | BRETHINE | PER MG | INH | J7681 |
| BCG VACCINE LIVE | VIAL | IV | J9031 | BRETHINE CONCENTRATED | PER MG | INH | J7680 |
| BEBULIN VH | 1 IU | IV | J7194 | BRICANYL | PER MG | INH | J7681 |
| BECAPLERMIN GEL 0.01% | 0.5 G | OTH | S0157 | BRICANYL CONCENTRATED | PER MG | INH | J7680 |
| BECLOMETHASONE COMPOUNDED | 1 MG | INH | J7622 | BRICANYL SUBCUTANEOUS | 1 MG | SC | J3105 |
| BECLOVENT COMPOUNDED | 1 MG | INH | J7622 | BROM-A-COT | 10 MG | IM, SC, IV | J0945 |
| BECONASE COMPOUNDED | 1 MG | INH | J7622 | BROMPHENIRAMINE MALEATE | 10 MG | IM, SC, IV | J0945 |
| BENA-D 10 | 50 MG | IV, IM | J1200 | BRONCHO SALINE | 5 CC | VAR | J7051 |
| BENA-D 50 | 50 MG | IV, IM | J1200 | BUDESONIDE COMPOUNDED, CONCETRATED | 0.25 MG | INH | J7634 |
| BENADRYL | 50 MG | IV, IM | J1200 | BUDESONIDE, COMPOUNDED, UNIT DOSE | 0.5 MG | INH | J7627 • |
| BENAHIST 10 | 50 MG | IV, IM | J1200 | BUDESONIDE, NONCOMPOUNDED, UNIT DOSE | 0.5 MG | INH | J7626 |
| BENAHIST 50 | 50 MG | IV, IM | J1200 | BUDESONIDE, NONCOMPOUNDED, CONCENTRATED | 0.25 MG | INH | J7633 |
| BENEFIX | 1 IU | IV | J7195 | BUMETANIDE | 0.5 MG | IM, IV | S0171 |
| BENOJECT-10 | 50 MG | IV, IM | J1200 | BUPIVACAINE HCL | 30 ML | OTH | S0020 |
| BENOJECT-50 | 50 MG | IV, IM | J1200 | BUPRENEX | 0.1 MG | IM, IV | J0592 |
| BENTYL | 20 MG | IM | J0500 | BUPRENORPHINE HCL | 0.1 MG | IM, IV | J0592 |
| BENZTROPINE MESYLATE | 1 MG | IM, IV | J0515 | BUPROPION HCL | 150 MG | ORAL. | S0106 |
| BERUBIGEN | 1,000 MCG | SC, IM | J3420 | BUSULFAN | 1 MG | IV | J0594 |
| BETA-2 | 1 MG | INH | J7648 | BUSULFAN | 2 MG | OTH | J8510 |
| BETALIN 12 | 1,000 MCG | SC, IM | J3420 | BUSULFEX | 1 MG | IV | J0594 |
| BETAMETHASONE ACETATE AND BETAMETHASONE SODIUM PHOSPHATE | 3 MG, OF EACH | IM | J0702 | BUSULFEX | 2 MG | ORAL | J8510 |
| BETAMETHASONE SODIUM PHOSPHATE | 4 MG | IM, IV | J0704 | BUTORPHANOL TARTRATE | 2 MG | IM, IV | J0595 |
| BETAMETHASONE COMPOUNDED, UNIT DOSE | 1 MG | INH | J7624 | BUTORPHANOL TARTRATE | 25 MG | OTH | S0012 |
| BETASERON | 0.25 MG | SC | J1830 | CABERGOLINE | 0.25 MG | ORAL | J8515 |
| BETHANECHOL CHLORIDE, MYOTONACHOL OR URECHOLINE | 5 MG | SC | J0520 | CAFCIT | 5 MG | IV | J0706 |
| BEVACIZUMAB | 10 MG | IV | J9035 | CAFFEINE CITRATE | 5 MG | IV | J0706 |
| BEXXAR THERAPEUTIC | TX DOSE | IV | A9545 | CALCIJEX | 0.1 MCG | IM | J0636 |
| BICILLIN CR | 1,200,000 U | IM | J0540 | CALCIMAR | UP TO 400 U | SC, IM | J0630 |
| BICILLIN CR | 600,000 U | IM | J0530 | CALCITONIN SALMON | 400 U | SC, IM | J0630 |
| BICILLIN CR 900/300 | 1,200,000 U | IM, IV | J0540 | CALCITRIOL | 0.1 MCG | IM | J0636 |
| BICILLIN CR 900/300 | 2,400,000 U | IM, IV | J0550 | CALCITROL | 0.25 MG | IM | S0161 |
| BICILLIN LA | 1,200,000 U | IM | J0570 | CALCIUM DISODIUM VERSENATE | 1,000 MG | IV, SC, IM | J0600 |
| BICILLIN LA | 2,400,000 U | INJ | J0580 | CALCIUM GLUCONATE | 10 ML | IV | J0610 |
| BICILLIN LA | 600,000 U | IM | J0560 | CALCIUM GLYCEROPHOSPHATE AND CALCIUM LACTATE | 10 ML | IM, SC | J0620 |
| BICNU | 100 MG | IV | J9050 | CAMPATH | 10 MG | IV | J9010 |
| BIOCLATE | 1 IU | IV | J7192 | CAMPTOSAR | 20 MG | IV | J9206 |
| BIOTROPIN | 1 MG | SC | J2941 | CANCIDAS | 5 MG | IV | J0637 |

| Drug Name | Unit Per: | Route | Code |
|---|---|---|---|
| CAPECITABINE | 150 MG | ORAL | J8520 |
| CAPROMAB PENDETIDE | DOSE | IV | A9507 |
| ~~CARBACOT~~ | ~~10 ML~~ | ~~IV, IM~~ | ~~J2800~~ |
| CARBOCAINE | 10 ML | VAR | J0670 |
| CARBOPLATIN | 50 MG | IV | J9045 |
| CARDIOGEN 82 | 60 MCI | IV | A9555 |
| CARDIOLITE | DOSE | IV | A9500 |
| CARIMUNE | 500 MG | IV | J1566 |
| CARMUSTINE | 100 MG | IV | J9050 |
| CARNITOR | 1 G | IV | J1955 |
| CARTICEL | | OTH | J7330 |
| CASPOFUNGIN ACETATE | 5 MG | IV | J0637 |
| CATAPRES | 1 MG | OTH | J0735 |
| CATHFLO | 1 MG | IV | J2997 |
| CAVERJECT | 1.25 MCG | VAR | J0270 |
| CEA SCAN | UP TO 45 MCI | IV | A9568 ● |
| CEENU | 10 MG | ORAL | S0178 |
| CEFEPIME HCL | 500 MG | IV | J0692 |
| CEFIZOX | 500 MG | IV, IM | J0715 |
| CEFOBID | 1 G | IV | S0021 |
| CEFOPERAZONE SODIUM | 1 G | IV | S0021 |
| CEFOTAN | 500 MG | IM, IV | S0074 |
| CEFOTAXIME SODIUM | 1 GM | IV, IM | J0698 |
| CEFOTETAN DISODIUM | 500 MG | IM. IV | S0074 |
| CEFOXITIN | 1 GM | IV, IM | J0694 |
| CEFOXITIN SODIUM | 1 GM | IV, IM | J0694 |
| CEFTAZIDIME | 500 MG | IM, IV | J0713 |
| CEFTIZOXIME SODIUM | 500 MG | IV, IM | J0715 |
| CEFTRIAXONE | 250 MG | IV, IM | J0696 |
| CEFTRIAXONE SODIUM | 250 MG | IV, IM | J0696 |
| CEFUROXIME | 750 MG | IM, IV | J0697 |
| CEFUROXIME SODIUM STERILE | 750 MG | IM, IV | J0697 |
| CELESTONE SOLUSPAN | 3 MG | IM | J0702 |
| CELLCEPT | 250 MG | ORAL | J7517 |
| CENACORT A-40 | 10 MG | IM | J3301 |
| CENACORT FORTE | 5 MG | IM | J3302 |
| ~~CEPHALOTHIN SODIUM~~ | ~~1 G~~ | ~~IM, IV~~ | ~~J1890~~ |
| CEPTAZ | 500 MG | IM, IV | J0713 |
| CEREBRYX | 50 MG | IM, IV | Q2009 |
| CEREBRYX | 750 MG | IM, IV | S0078 |
| CEREDASE | 10 U | IV | J0205 |
| CERETEC | DOSE | IV | A9521 |
| CERETEC | PER STUDY DOSE | IV | A9569 ● |
| CEREZYME | 1 U | IV | J1785 |
| CERUBIDINE | 10 MG | IV | J9150 |
| CESAMET | 1 MG | ORAL | J8650 |
| CETUXIMAB | 10 MG | IV | J9055 |
| CHEALAMIDE | 150 MG | IV | J3520 |
| CHLORAMBUCIL | 2 MG | ORAL | S0172 |
| CHLORAMPHENICOL SODIUM SUCCINATE | 1 G | IV | J0720 |
| CHLORDIAZEPOXIDE HCL | 100 MG | IM, IV | J1990 |
| CHLOROMYCETIN | 1 G | IV | J0720 |
| CHLOROPROCAINE HCL | 30 ML | VAR | J2400 |

| Drug Name | Unit Per: | Route | Code |
|---|---|---|---|
| CHLOROTHIAZIDE SODIUM | 500 MG | IV | J1205 |
| CHLORPROMAZINE HCL | 10 MG | ORAL | Q0171 |
| CHLORPROMAZINE HCL | 25 MG | ORAL | Q0172 |
| CHLORPROMAZINE HCL | 50 MG | IM, IV | J3230 |
| CHOLETEC | UP TO 35 MCI | IV | A9537 ● |
| CHORIONIC GONADOTROPIN | 1,000 USP U | IM | J0725 |
| CHROMIC PHOSPHATE P32 | 1 MCI | IV | A9564 |
| CHROMITOPE SODIUM | 250 UCI | IV | A9553 |
| CHROMIUM CR-51 SODIUM IOTHALAMATE, DIAGNOSTIC | 10 UCI | IV | A9553 |
| CIDOFOVIR | 375 MG | IV | J0740 |
| CILASTATIN SODIUM | 250 MG | IV, IM | J0743 |
| CIMETIDINE HCL | 300 MG | IM, IV | S0023 |
| CIPRO | 200 MG | IV | J0744 |
| CIPROFLOXACIN FOR INTRAVENOUS INFUSION | 200 MG | IV | J0744 |
| CIS-MDP | 30 MCI | IV | A9503 ● |
| CISPLATIN | 10 MG | IV | J9060 |
| CIS-PYRO | UP TO 25 MCI | IV | A9538 ● |
| CLADRIBINE | 1 MG | IV | J9065 |
| CLAFORAN | 1 GM | IV, IM | J0698 |
| CLEOCIN PHOSPHATE | 300 MG | IV | S0077 |
| CLINAGEN LA | UP TO 40 MG | IM | J0970 |
| CLINDAMYCIN PHOSPHATE | 300 MG | IV | S0077 |
| CLOFARABINE | 1 MG | IV | J9027 |
| CLOLAR | 1 MG | IV | J9027 |
| CLONIDINE HCL | 1 MG | OTH | J0735 |
| CLOSTRIDIUM BOTULINUM TOXIN | 1 U | OTH | J0585 |
| CLOZAPINE | 25 MG | ORAL | S0136 |
| CLOZARIL | 25 MG | ORAL | S0136 |
| COBAL | 1,000 MCG | IM, SC | J3420 |
| COBALT CO-57 CYNOCOBALAMIN, DIAGNOSTIC | 1 UCI | ORAL | A9559 |
| COBATOPE 57 | 1 UCI | ORAL | A9559 |
| COBEX | 1,000 MCG | SC, IM | J3420 |
| CODEINE PHOSPHATE | 30 MG | IM, IV, SC | J0745 |
| COGENTIN | 1 MG | IM, IV | J0515 |
| COGNEX | 10 MG | ORAL | S0014 |
| COLCHICINE | 1 MG | IV | J0760 |
| COLHIST | 10 MG | IM, SC, IV | J0945 |
| COLISTIMETHATE SODIUM | 150 MG | IM, IV | J0770 |
| COLISTIMETHATE SODIUM | PER MG | INH | S0142 |
| COLLAGEN, MICROPOROUS NONHUMAN | SQ CM | OTH | C9351 |
| COLLAGEN-GLYCOSAMINOGLYCAN SKIN SUBSTITUTE | SQ CM | OTH | J7343 |
| COLY-MYCIN M | 150 MG | IM, IV | J0770 |
| COMPAZINE | 10 MG | IM, IV | J0780 |
| COMPAZINE | 10 MG | ORAL | Q0165 |
| COMPAZINE | 5 MG | ORAL | Q0164 |
| COMPAZINE | 5 MG | ORAL | S0183 |
| CONTRACEPTIVE SUPPLY, HORMONE CONTAINING PATCH | EACH | OTH | J7304 |
| COPAXONE | 20 MG | SC | J1595 |
| COPPER T MODEL TCU380A IUD COPPER WIRE/COPPER COLLAR | EA | OTH | J7300 |
| CORDARONE | 30 MG | IV | J0282 |

# APPENDIX 1 — TABLE OF DRUGS

| Drug Name | Unit Per: | Route | Code |
|---|---|---|---|
| CORTASTAT | 1 MG | IM, IV, OTH | J1100 |
| CORTASTAT LA | 1 MG | IM | J1094 |
| CORTICORELIN OVINE TRIFLUTATE | 1 MCG | IV | J0795 |
| CORTICOTROPIN | 40 U | IV, IM, SC | J0800 |
| CORTIMED | 80 MG | IM | J1040 |
| CORTROSYN | 0.25 MG | IM, IV | J0835 |
| CORVERT | 1 MG | IV | J1742 |
| COSMEGEN | 0.5 MG | IV | J9120 |
| COSYNTROPIN | 0.25 MG | IM, IV | J0835 |
| ~~COTOLONE~~ | ~~1 ML~~ | ~~IM~~ | ~~J2650~~ |
| COTOLONE | 5 MG | ORAL | J7510 |
| CROMOLYN SODIUM NONCOMPOUNDED | 10 MG | INH | J7631 |
| CROMOLYN SODIUM COMPOUNDED | PER 10 MG | INH | J7632 ● |
| CRYSTAL B12 | 1,000 MCG | IM, SC | J3420 |
| CRYSTICILLIN 300 A.S. | 600,000 UNITS | IM, IV | J2510 |
| CRYSTICILLIN 600 A.S. | 600,000 UNITS | IM, IV | J2510 |
| CUBICIN | 1 MG | IV | J0878 |
| CYANO | 1,000 MCG | IM, SC | J3420 |
| CYANOCOBALAMIN | 1,000 MCG | IM, SC | J3420 |
| CYANOCOBALAMIN COBALT 58/57 | 1 UCI | IV | A9546 |
| CYANOCOBALAMIN COBALT CO-57 | 1 UCI | ORAL | A9559 |
| CYCLOPHOSPHAMIDE | 1 G | IV | J9091 |
| CYCLOPHOSPHAMIDE | 100 MG | IV | J9070 |
| CYCLOPHOSPHAMIDE | 2 G | IV | J9092 |
| CYCLOPHOSPHAMIDE | 200 MG | IV | J9080 |
| CYCLOPHOSPHAMIDE | 25 MG | ORAL | J8530 |
| CYCLOPHOSPHAMIDE | 500 MG | IV | J9090 |
| CYCLOPHOSPHAMIDE LYOPHILIZED | 1 G | IV | J9096 |
| CYCLOPHOSPHAMIDE LYOPHILIZED | 100 MG | IV | J9093 |
| CYCLOPHOSPHAMIDE LYOPHILIZED | 2 G | IV | J9097 |
| CYCLOPHOSPHAMIDE LYOPHILIZED | 200 MG | IV | J9094 |
| CYCLOPHOSPHAMIDE LYOPHILIZED | 500 MG | IV | J9095 |
| CYCLOSPORINE | 100 MG | ORAL | J7502 |
| CYCLOSPORINE | 25 MG | ORAL | J7515 |
| CYCLOSPORINE | 250 MG | OTH | J7516 |
| CYTARABINE | 100 MG | SC, IV | J9100 |
| CYTARABINE | 500 MG | SC, IV | J9110 |
| CYTARABINE LIPOSOME | 10 MG | IT | J9098 |
| CYTOGAM | VIAL | IV | J0850 |
| CYTOMEGALOVIRUS IMMUNE GLOB | VIAL | IV | J0850 |
| CYTOSAR-U | 100 MG | SC, IV | J9100 |
| CYTOSAR-U | 500 MG | SC, IV | J9110 |
| CYTOTEC | 200 MCG | ORAL | S0191 |
| CYTOVENE | 500 MG | IV | J1570 |
| CYTOXAN | 1 G | IV | J9091 |
| CYTOXAN | 100 MG | IV | J9070 |
| CYTOXAN | 2 G | IV | J9092 |
| CYTOXAN | 200 MG | IV | J9080 |
| CYTOXAN | 25 MG | ORAL | J8530 |
| CYTOXAN | 500 MG | IV | J9090 |
| CYTOXAN LYOPHILIZED | 1 G | IV | J9096 |
| CYTOXAN LYOPHILIZED | 100 MG | IV | J9093 |

| Drug Name | Unit Per: | Route | Code |
|---|---|---|---|
| CYTOXAN LYOPHILIZED | 2 G | IV | J9097 |
| CYTOXAN LYOPHILIZED | 200 MG | IV | J9094 |
| CYTOXAN LYOPHILIZED | 500 MG | IV | J9095 |
| D.H.E. 45 | 1 MG | IM, IV | J1110 |
| DACARBAZINE | 100 MG | IV | J9130 |
| DACARBAZINE | 200 MG | IV | J9140 |
| DACLIZUMAB | 25 MG | OTH | J7513 |
| DACOGEN | 1 MG | IV | J0894 |
| DACTINOMYCIN | 0.5 MG | IV | J9120 |
| DALALONE | 1 MG | IM, IV, OTH | J1100 |
| DALALONE LA | 1 MG | IM | J1094 |
| DALTEPARIN SODIUM | 2,500 IU | SC | J1645 |
| DAPTOMYCIN | 1 MG | IV | J0878 |
| DARBEPOETIN ALFA, ESRD USE | 1 MCG | SC, IV | J0882 |
| DARBEPOETIN ALFA, NON-ESRD USE | 1 MCG | SC, IV | J0881 |
| DAUNORUBICIN CITRATE | 10 MG | IV | J9151 |
| DAUNORUBICIN HCL | 10 MG | IV | J9150 |
| DAUNOXOME | 10 MG | IV | J9151 |
| DDAVP | 1 MCG | IV, SC | J2597 |
| ~~DECA-DURABOLIN~~ | ~~100 MG~~ | ~~IM~~ | ~~J2321~~ |
| ~~DECA-DURABOLIN~~ | ~~200 MG~~ | ~~IM~~ | ~~J2322~~ |
| ~~DECA-DURABOLIN~~ | ~~50 MG~~ | ~~IM~~ | ~~J2320~~ |
| DECADRON | 0.25 MG | ORAL | J8540 |
| DECAJECT | 1 MG | IM, IV, OTH | J1100 |
| DECITABINE | 1 MG | IV | J0894 |
| ~~DECOLONE-100~~ | ~~100 MG~~ | ~~IM~~ | ~~J2321~~ |
| DECOLONE-50 | 50 MG | IM | J2320 |
| DEFEROXAMINE MESYLATE | 500 MG | IM, SC, IV | J0895 |
| ~~DELATEST~~ | ~~100 MG~~ | ~~IM~~ | ~~J3120~~ |
| DELATESTRYL | 100 MG | IM | J3120 |
| DELATESTRYL | 200 MG | IM | J3130 |
| DELESTROGEN | 10 MG | IM | J1380 |
| DELESTROGEN | 20 MG | IM | J1390 |
| DELESTROGEN | UP TO 40 MG | IM | J0970 |
| DELTA-CORTEF | 5 MG | ORAL | J7510 |
| DELTASONE | 5 MG | ORAL | J7506 |
| DELTASONE | 5 MG | OTH | J7506 |
| DEMADEX | 10 MG | IV | J3265 |
| DEMEROL | 100 MG | IM, IV, SC | J2175 |
| DENILEUKIN DIFTITOX | 300 MCG | IV | J9160 |
| DEPANDRATE | 1 CC, 200 MG | IM | J1080 |
| DEPANDROGYN | 1 ML | IM | J1060 |
| DEPGYNOGEN | UP TO 5 MG | IM | J1000 |
| DEPHENACEN-50 | 50 MG | IM, IV | J1200 |
| DEPMEDALONE | 40 MG | IM | J1030 |
| DEPMEDALONE | 80 MG | IM | J1040 |
| DEPODUR | UP TO 10 MG | IV | J2270 ● |
| DEPODUR | UP TO 10 MG | IV | J2271 ● |
| DEPO-ESTRADIOL CYPIONATE | UP TO 5 MG | IM | J1000 |
| DEPO-MEDROL | 20 MG | IM | J1020 |
| DEPO-MEDROL | 40 MG | IM | J1030 |
| DEPO-MEDROL | 80 MG | IM | J1040 |
| DEPO-PROVERA | 150 MG | IM | J1055 |
| DEPO-PROVERA | 50 MG | IM | J1051 |

| Drug Name | Unit Per: | Route | Code | Drug Name | Unit Per: | Route | Code |
|---|---|---|---|---|---|---|---|
| DEPO-TESTADIOL | 1 ML | IM | J1060 | DEXTROAMPHETAMINE SULFATE | 5 MG | ORAL | S0160 |
| DEPO-TESTOSTERONE | 1 CC, 200 MG | IM | J1080 | DEXTROSE | 500 ML | IV | J7060 |
| DEPO-TESTOSTERONE | UP TO 100 MG | IM | J1070 | DEXTROSE, STERILE WATER, AND/OR DEXTROSE DILUENT/FLUSH | 10 ML | VAR | A46216 |
| DEPO-TESTOSTERONE CYPIONATE | UP TO 100 MG | IM | J1070 | DEXTROSE/SODIUM CHLORIDE | 5% | VAR | J7042 |
| DEPOCYT | 10 MG | IT | J9098 | DEXTROSE/THEOPHYLLINE | 40 MG | IV | J2810 |
| DEPOGEN | UP TO 5 MG | IM | J1000 | DEXTROSTAT | 5 MG | ORAL | S0160 |
| DEPTESTROGEN | UP TO 100 MG | IM | J1070 | DIALYSIS/STRESS VITAMINS | 100 CAPS | ORAL | S0194 |
| DERMAGRAFT | SQ CM | OTH | J7342 | DIAMOX | 500 MG | IM, IV | J1120 |
| DERMAL AND EPIDERMAL, TISSUE OF NONHUMAN ORIGIN, WITH OR WITHOUT OTHER BIOENGINEERED OR PROCESSED ELEMENTS, WITHOUT METABOLICALLY ACTIVE ELEMENTS | SQ CM | OTH | J7343 ▲ | DIASTAT | 5 MG | IV, IM | J3360 |
| | | | | DIAZEPAM | 5 MG | IV, IM | J3360 |
| | | | | DIAZOXIDE | 300 MG | IV | J1730 |
| | | | | DICYCLOMINE HCL | 20 MG | IM | J0500 |
| DERMAL (SUBSTITUTE) TISSUE OF NONHUMAN ORIGIN, WITH OR WITHOUT OTHER BIOENGINEERED OR PROCESSED ELEMENTS, WITHOUT METABOLICALLY ACTIVE ELEMENTS (INTEGRA MATRIX) | UNIT PER SQ CM | OTH | J7347 ● | DIDANOSINE (DDI) | 25 MG | ORAL | S0137 |
| | | | | DIDRONEL | 300 MG | IV | J1436 |
| | | | | DIETHYLSTILBESTROL DIPHSPHATE | 250 MG | INJ | J9165 |
| | | | | DIFLUCAN | 200 MG | IV | J1450 |
| | | | | DIGIBIND | VIAL | IV | J1162 |
| DERMAL (SUBSTITUTE) TISSUE OF NONHUMAN ORIGIN, WITH OR WITHOUT OTHER BIOENGINEERED OR PROCESSED ELEMENTS, WITHOUT METABOLICALLY ACTIVE ELEMENTS (PRIMATRIX) | SQ CM | OTH | J7349 ● | DIGIFAB | VIAL | IV | J1162 |
| | | | | DIGOXIN | 0.5 MG | IM, IV | J1160 |
| | | | | DIGOXIN IMMUNE FAB | VIAL | IV | J1162 |
| | | | | DIHYDROERGOTAMINE MESYLATE | 1 MG | IM, IV | J1110 |
| DERMAL (SUBSTITUTE) TISSUE OF NONHUMAN ORIGIN, WITH OR WITHOUT OTHER BIOENGINEERED OR PROCESSED ELEMENTS, WITHOUT METABOLICALLY ACTIVE ELEMENTS (TISSUEMEND) | SQ CM | OTH | J7348 ● | DILANTIN | 50 MG | IM, IV | J1165 |
| | | | | DILAUDID | 250 MG | OTH | S0092 |
| | | | | DILAUDID | 4 MG | SC, IM, IV | J1170 |
| | | | | ~~DILOR~~ | ~~UP TO 500 MG~~ | ~~IM~~ | ~~J1180~~ |
| DERMAL TISSUE, OF HUMAN ORIGIN, WITH OR WITHOUT OTHER BIOENGINEERED OR PROCESSED ELEMENTS, WITH METABOLICALLY ACTIVE ELEMENTS | SQ CM | OTH | J7342 ▲ | DIMENHYDRINATE | 50 MG | IM, IV | J1240 |
| | | | | DIMERCAPROL | 100 MG | IM | J0470 |
| | | | | DIMINE | 50 MG | IV, IM | J1200 |
| | | | | DINATE | 50 MG | IM, IV | J1240 |
| DERMAL TISSUE, OF HUMAN ORIGIN, WITH OR WITHOUT OTHER BIOENGINEERED OR PROCESSED ELEMENTS, WITHOUT METABOLICALLY ACTIVE ELEMENTS | SQ CM | OTH | J7344 ▲ | DIOVAL | 10 MG | IM | J1380 |
| | | | | DIOVAL | 20 MG | IM | J1390 |
| | | | | DIOVAL 40 | 10 MG | IM | J1380 |
| | | | | DIOVAL 40 | 20 MG | IM | J1390 |
| DESFERAL | 500 MG | IM, SC, IV | J0895 | DIOVAL XX | 10 MG | IM | J1380 |
| DESMOPRESSIN ACETATE | 1 MCG | IV, SC | J2597 | DIOVAL XX | 20 MG | IM | J1390 |
| DEXAMETHASONE | 0.25 MG | ORAL | J8540 | DIPHENHYDRAMINE HCL | 50 MG | IV, IM | J1200 |
| DEXAMETHASONE ACETATE | 1 MG | IM | J1094 | DIPHENHYDRAMINE HCL | 50 MG | ORAL | Q0163 |
| DEXAMETHASONE ACETATE ANHYDROUS | 1 MG | IM | J1094 | DIPYRIDAMOLE | 10 MG | IV | J1245 |
| DEXAMETHASONE SODIUM PHOSPHATE | 1 MG | IM, IV, OTH | J1100 | DISOTATE | 150 MG | IV | J3520 |
| DEXAMETHASONE, COMPOUNDED, CONCENTRATED | PER MG | INH | J7637 | DIURIL | 500 MG | IV | J1205 |
| DEXAMETHASONE, COMPOUNDED, UNIT DOSE | PER MG | INH | J7638 | DIURIL SODIUM | 500 MG | IV | J1205 |
| | | | | DIZAC | 5 MG | IV, IM | J3360 |
| DEXASONE | 1 MG | IM, IV, OTH | J1100 | DMSA | VIAL | IV | C1201 |
| DEXEDRINE | 5 MG | ORAL | S0160 | DMSA KIT | VIAL | IV | C1201 |
| DEXFERRUM | 50 MG | IM, IV | J1752 | DMSO, DIMETHYL SULFOXIDE | 50%, 50 ML | OTH | J1212 |
| DEXIM | 1 MG | IM, IV, OTH | J1100 | DOBUTAMINE HCL | 250 MG | IV | J1250 |
| DEXONE | 0.25 MG | ORAL | J8540 | ~~DOBUTREX~~ | ~~PER 250 MG~~ | ~~IV~~ | ~~J1250~~ |
| DEXONE | 1 MG | IM, IV, OTH | J1100 | DOCETAXEL | 20 MG | IV | J9170 |
| DEXONE LA | 1 MG | IM | J1094 | DOLASETRON MESYLATE | 10 MG | IV | J1260 |
| DEXRAZOXANE | 250 MG | IV | J1190 | DOLASETRON MESYLATE | 100 MG | ORAL | Q0180 |
| DEXRAZOXANE HYDROCHLORIDE | 250 MG | IV | J1190 | DOLASETRON MESYLATE | 50 MG | ORAL | S0174 |
| DEXTRAN 40 | 500 ML | IV | J7100 | DOLOPHINE | 5 MG | ORAL | S0109 |
| | | | | DOLOPHINE HCL | 10 MG | IM, SC | J1230 |

# APPENDIX 1 — TABLE OF DRUGS

| Drug Name | Unit Per: | Route | Code | Drug Name | Unit Per: | Route | Code |
|---|---|---|---|---|---|---|---|
| DOMMANATE | 50 MG | IM, IV | J1240 | ELLIOTTS B SOLUTION | 1 ML | IV, IT | J9175 |
| DOPAMINE HCL | 40 MG | IV | J1265 | ELOXATIN | 0.5 MG | IV | J9263 |
| DORNASE ALPHA | PER MG | INH | J7639 | ELSPAR | 10,000 U | VAR | J9020 |
| DOSTINEX | 0.25 MG | ORAL | J8515 | EMEND | 5 MG | ORAL | J8501 |
| DOXERCALCIFEROL | 1 MG | IV | J1270 | EMINASE | 30 U | IV | J0350 |
| DOXIL | 10 MG | IV | J9001 | ENBREL | 25 MG | IM, IV | J1438 |
| DOXORUBICIN HCL | 10 MG | IV | J9000 | ENDOXAN-ASTA | 1 G | IV | J9091 |
| DRAMAMINE | 50 MG | IM, IV | J1240 | ENDOXAN-ASTA | 100 MG | IV | J9070 |
| DRAMILIN | 50 MG | IM, IV | J1240 | ENDOXAN-ASTA | 200 MG | IV | J9080 |
| DRAMOCEN | 50 MG | IM, IV | J1240 | ENDOXAN-ASTA | 500 MG | IV | J9090 |
| DRAMOJECT | 50 MG | IM, IV | J1240 | ENDRATE | 150 MG | IV | J3520 |
| DRAXIMAGE MDP-10 | 30 MCI | IV | A9503 ● | ENFUVIRTIDE | 1 MG | SC | J1324 |
| DRAXIMAGE MDP-25 | 30 MCI | IV | A9503 ● | ~~ENOVIL~~ | ~~20 MG~~ | ~~IM~~ | ~~J1320~~ |
| DRONABINAL | 2.5 MG | ORAL | Q0167 | ENOXAPARIN SODIUM | 10 MG | SC | J1650 |
| DRONABINAL | 5 MG | ORAL | Q0168 | EPINEPHRINE | 1 MG | IM, IV, SC, VAR | J0170 |
| DROPERIDOL | 5 MG | IM, IV | J1790 | EPIPEN | 0.3 MG | IM | J0170 |
| DROPERIDOL AND FENTANYL CITRATE | 2 ML | IM, IV | J1810 | EPIRUBICIN HCL | 2 MG | IV | J9178 |
| DROXIA | 500 MG | ORAL | S0176 | EPOETIN ALFA, ESRD USE | 1,000 U | SC, IV | J0886 |
| DTIC-DOME | 100 MG | IV | J9130 | EPOETIN ALFA, NON-ESRD USE | 1,000 U | SC, IV | J0885 |
| DTIC-DOME | 200 MG | IV | J9140 | EPOGEN/ESRD | 1,000 U | SC, IV | J0886 ▲ |
| DTPA | UP TO 25 MCI | IV | A9539 ● | EPOGEN/NON-ESRD | 1,000 U | SC, IV | J0885 ▲ |
| DTPA | UP TO 25 MCI | INH | A9567 ● | EPOPROSTENOL | 0.5 MG | IV | J1325 |
| DUO-SPAN | 1 ML | IM | J1060 | EPOPROSTENOL STERILE DILUTANT | 50 ML | IV | S0155 |
| DUO-SPAN II | 1 ML | IM | J1060 | EPTIFIBATIDE | 5 MG | IM, IV | J1327 |
| DURACILLIN A.S. | 600,000 UNITS | IM, IV | J2510 | ERAXIS | 1 MG | IV | J0348 |
| | | | | ERBITUX | 10 MG | IV | J9055 |
| DURACLON | 1 MG | OTH | J0735 | ERGAMISOL | 50 MG | ORAL | S0177 |
| DURAGEN-10 | 10 MG | IM | J1380 | ERGONOVINE MALEATE | 0.2 MG | IM, IV | J1330 |
| DURAGEN-10 | 20 MG | IM | J1390 | ERTAPENEM SODIUM | 500 MG | IM, IV | J1335 |
| DURAGEN-20 | 10 MG | IM | J1380 | ERYTHROCIN LACTOBIONATE | 500 MG | IV | J1364 |
| DURAGEN-20 | 20 MG | IM | J1390 | ESTONE AQUEOUS | 1 MG | IM, IV | J1435 |
| DURAGEN-40 | 10 MG | IM | J1380 | ESTRA-L 20 | 10 MG | IM | J1380 |
| DURAGEN-40 | 20 MG | IM | J1390 | ESTRA-L 20 | 20 MG | IM | J1390 |
| DURAMORPH | 10 MG | IM, IV, SC | J2275 | ESTRA-L 40 | 10 MG | IM | J1380 |
| DURAMORPH | 500 MG | OTH | S0093 | ESTRA-L 40 | 20 MG | IM | J1390 |
| ~~DURATHATE-200~~ | ~~100 MG~~ | ~~IM~~ | ~~J3130~~ | ESTRADIOL CYPIONATE | UP TO 5 MG | IM | J1000 |
| DURO CORT | 80 MG | IM | J1040 | ESTRADIOL L.A. | 10 MG | IM | J1380 |
| DYMENATE | 50 MG | IM, IV | J1240 | ESTRADIOL L.A. | 20 MG | IM | J1390 |
| DYPHYLLINE | 500 MG | IM | J1180 | ESTRADIOL L.A. 20 | 10 MG | IM | J1380 |
| ECHOCARDIOGRAM IMAGE ENHANCER | 1 ML | IV | Q9955 | ESTRADIOL L.A. 20 | 20 MG | IM | J1390 |
| ECHOCARDIOGRAM IMAGE ENHANCER | 1 ML | INJ | Q9956 | ESTRADIOL L.A. 40 | 10 MG | IM | J1380 |
| | | | | ESTRADIOL L.A. 40 | 20 MG | IM | J1390 |
| ECULIZUMAB | 10 MG | IV | J1300 | ESTRADIOL VALERATE | 10 MG | IM | J1380 |
| EDETATE CALCIUM DISODIUM | 1,000 MG | IV, SC, IM | J0600 | ESTRADIOL VALERATE | 20 MG | IM | J1390 |
| EDETATE DISODIUM | 150 MG | IV | J3520 | ESTRADIOL VALERATE | UP TO 40 MG | IM | J0970 |
| EDEX | 1.25 MCG | VAR | J0270 | ESTRAGYN | 1 MG | IV, IM | J1435 |
| E.D.T.A | 150 MG | IV | J3520 | ESTRO-A | 1 MG | IV, IM | J1435 |
| EFALIZUMAB | 125 MG | SC | S0162 | ESTROGEN CONJUGATED | 25 MG | IV, IM | J1410 |
| ELAPRASE | 1 MG | IV | C9232 | ESTRONE | 1 MG | IV, IM | J1435 |
| ELAVIL | 20 MG | IM | J1320 | ESTRONOL | 1 MG | IM, IV | J1435 |
| ELIGARD | 7.5 MG | IM | J9217 | ETANERCEPT | 25 MG | IM, IV | J1438 |
| ELIGARD | PER 3.75 MG | SC | J1950 ● | ETHAMOLIN | 100 MG | IV | J1430 |
| ELITEK | 50 MCG | IM | J2783 | ETHANOLAMINE OLEATE | 100 MG | IV | J1430 |
| ELLENCE | 2 MG | IV | J9178 | ETHYOL | 500 MG | IV | J0207 |

| Drug Name | Unit Per: | Route | Code |
|---|---|---|---|
| ETIDRONATE DISODIUM | 300 MG | IV | J1436 |
| ETONOGESTREL | PER IMPLANT | OTH | J7307 ● |
| ETOPOSIDE | 10 MG | IV | J9181 |
| ETOPOSIDE | 100 MG | IV | J9182 |
| ETOPOSIDE | 50 MG | ORAL | J8560 |
| EUFLEXXA | PER DOSE | OTH | J7323 ● |
| EULEXIN | 125 MG | ORAL | S0175 |
| EVERONE | 100 MG | IM | J3120 |
| EVERONE | 100 MG | IM | J3130 |
| EXMESTANE | 25 MG | ORAL | S0156 |
| EXAMETAZIME LABELED AUTOLOGOUS WHITE BLOOD CELLS, TECHNETIUM TC-99M | PER STUDY DOSE | IV | A9569 ● |
| FABRAZYME | 1 MG | IV | J0180 |
| FACTOR IX NON-RECOMBINANT | 1 IU | IV | J7193 |
| FACTOR IX RECOMBINANT | 1 IU | IV | J7195 |
| FACTOR IX+ COMPLEX | 1 IU | IV | J7194 |
| FACTOR VIIA RECOMBINANT | 1 MCG | IV | J7189 |
| FACTOR VIII PORCINE | 1 IU | IV | J7191 |
| FACTOR VIII RECOMBINANT | 1 IU | IV | J7192 |
| FACTOR VIII, HUMAN | 1 IU | IV | J7190 |
| FACTREL | 100 MCG | SC, IV | J1620 |
| FAMOTIDINE | 20 MG | IV | S0028 |
| FASLODEX | 25 MG | IM | J9395 |
| FDG | STUDY DOSE | | A9552 |
| FEIBA-VH AICC | 1 IU | IV | J7198 |
| FENTANYL CITRATE | 0.1 MG | IM, IV | J3010 |
| FERIDEX IV | 1 ML | IV | Q9953 |
| FERRLECIT | 12.5 MG | IV | J2916 |
| FERTINEX | 75 IU | SC | J3355 |
| FILGRASTIM | 300 MCG | SC, IV | J1440 |
| FILGRASTIM | 480 MCG | SC, IV | J1441 |
| FINASTERIDE | 5 MG | ORAL | S0138 |
| FLAGYL | 500 MG | IV | S0030 |
| FLEBOGAMMA | 500 MG | IV | Q4091 |
| FLEXOJECT | 60 MG | IV, IM | J2360 |
| FLEXON | 60 MG | IV, IM | J2360 |
| FLOLAN | 0.5 MG | IV | J1325 |
| FLOXIN IV | 400 MG | IV | S0034 |
| FLOXURIDINE | 500 MG | IV | J9200 |
| FLUCONAZOLE | 200 MG | IV | J1450 |
| FLUDARA | 50 MG | IV | J9185 |
| FLUDARABINE PHOSPHATE | 50 MG | IV | J9185 |
| FLUDEOXYGLUCOSE F18 | STUDY DOSE | IV | A9552 |
| FLUNISOLIDE, COMPOUNDED, UNIT DOSE | 1 MG | INH | J7641 |
| FLUOCINOLONE ACETONIDE INTRAVITREAL | IMPLANT | OTH | J7311 |
| FLUORODEOXYGLUCOSE F-18 FDG, DIAGNOSTIC | 45 MCI | IV | A9552 |
| FLUOROURACIL | 500 MG | IV | J9190 |
| FLUPHENAZINE DECANOATE | 25 MG | SC, IM | J2680 |
| FLUTAMIDE | 125 MG | ORAL | S0175 |
| FOLEX | 5 MG | IV, IM, IT, IA | J9250 |
| FOLEX | 50 MG | IV, IM, IT, IA | J9260 |

| Drug Name | Unit Per: | Route | Code |
|---|---|---|---|
| FOLEX PFS | 5 MG | IV, IM, IT, IA | J9250 |
| FOLEX PFS | 50 MG | IV, IM, IT, IA | J9260 |
| FOLLISTIM | 75 IU | SC, IM | S0128 |
| FOLLITROPIN ALFA | 75 IU | SC | S0126 |
| FOLLITROPIN BETA | 75 IU | SC, IM | S0128 |
| FOMEPIZOLE | 15 MG | IV | J1451 |
| FOMIVIRSEN SODIUM | 1.65 MG | OTH | J1452 |
| FONDAPARINUX SODIUM | 0.5 MG | SC | J1652 |
| FORMOTEROL, COMPOUNDED, UNIT DOSE | 12 MCG | INH | J7640 |
| FORTAZ | 500 MG | IM, IV | J0713 |
| FORTEO | 10 MCG | SC | J3110 |
| FORTOVASE | 200 MG | ORAL | S0140 |
| FOSCARNET SODIUM | 1,000 MG | IV | J1455 |
| FOSCAVIR | 1,000 MG | IV | J1455 |
| FOSPHENYTOIN | 50 MG | IM, IV | Q2009 |
| FOSPHENYTOIN SODIUM | 750 MG | IM, IV | S0078 |
| FRAGMIN | 2,500 IU | SC | J1645 |
| FUDR | 500 MG | IV | J9200 |
| FULVESTRANT | 25 MG | IM | J9395 |
| FUNGIZONE | 50 MG | IV | J0285 |
| FUROCOT | 20 MG | IM, IV | J1940 |
| FUROMIDE M.D. | 20 MG | IM, IV | J1940 |
| FUROSEMIDE | 20 MG | IM, IV | J1940 |
| FUZEON | 1 MG | SC | J1324 |
| GADOBENATE DIMEGLUMINE (MULTIHANCE MULTIPACK) | PER ML | IV | A9577 |
| GADOLINIUM-BASED MAGNETIC RESONANCE CONTRAST AGENT | 1 ML | IV | Q9952 |
| GADOTERIDOL (PROHANCE MULTIPACK) | PER ML | IV | A9576 |
| GALLIUM GA-67 | 1 MCI | IV | A9556 |
| GALLIUM NITRATE | 1 MG | IV | J1457 |
| GALSULFASE | 1 MG | IV | J1458 |
| GAMASTAN | 1 CC | IM | J1460 |
| GAMASTAN | 2 CC | IM | J1470 |
| GAMASTAN | 3 CC | IM | J1480 |
| GAMASTAN | 4 CC | IM | J1490 |
| GAMASTAN | 5 CC | IM | J1500 |
| GAMASTAN | 6 CC | IM | J1510 |
| GAMASTAN | 7 CC | IM | J1520 |
| GAMASTAN | 8 CC | IM | J1530 |
| GAMASTAN | 9 CC | IM | J1540 |
| GAMASTAN | 10 CC | IM | J1550 |
| GAMASTAN | OVER 10 CC | IM | J1560 |
| GAMIMMUNE N | 500 MG | IV | J1567 |
| GAMMA GLOBULIN | 1 CC | IM | J1460 |
| GAMMA GLOBULIN | 2 CC | IM | J1470 |
| GAMMA GLOBULIN | 3 CC | IM | J1480 |
| GAMMA GLOBULIN | 4 CC | IM | J1490 |
| GAMMA GLOBULIN | 5 CC | IM | J1500 |
| GAMMA GLOBULIN | 6 CC | IM | J1510 |
| GAMMA GLOBULIN | 7 CC | IM | J1520 |
| GAMMA GLOBULIN | 8 CC | IM | J1530 |
| GAMMA GLOBULIN | 9 CC | IM | J1540 |
| GAMMA GLOBULIN | 10 CC | IM | J1550 |

# APPENDIX 1 — TABLE OF DRUGS

| Drug Name | Unit Per: | Route | Code |
|---|---|---|---|
| GAMMA GLOBULIN | OVER 10 CC | IM | J1560 |
| GAMMAGARD | 500 MG | IV | J1569 |
| GAMMAGARD S/D | 500 MG | IV | J1566 |
| GAMMAR | 1 CC | IM | J1460 |
| GAMMAR | 2 CC | IM | J1470 |
| GAMMAR | 3 CC | IM | J1480 |
| GAMMAR | 4 CC | IM | J1490 |
| GAMMAR | 5 CC | IM | J1500 |
| GAMMAR | 6 CC | IM | J1510 |
| GAMMAR | 7 CC | IM | J1520 |
| GAMMAR | 8 CC | IM | J1530 |
| GAMMAR | 9 CC | IM | J1540 |
| GAMMAR | 10 CC | IM | J1550 |
| GAMMAR | OVER 10 CC | IM | J1560 |
| GAMMAR P | 500 MG | IV | J1566 |
| GAMULIN RH | 300 MCG | IM | J2790 |
| GAMUNEX | 500 MG | IV | J1567 |
| GAMUNEX | 500 MG | IV | J1561 |
| GANCICLOVIR | 4.5 MG | OTH | J7310 |
| GANCICLOVIR SODIUM | 500 MG | IV | J1570 |
| GANIRELIX ACETATE | 250 MCG | SC | S0132 |
| GANITE | 1 MG | IV | J1457 |
| GANITE | PER MCI | IV | A9556 ● |
| GARAMYCIN | 80 MG | IM, IV | J1580 |
| GASTROCROM | 10 MG | INH | J7631 |
| GASTROMARK | 1 ML | ORAL | Q9954 |
| GATIFLOXACIN | 10 MG | IV | J1590 |
| GEFITINIB | 250 MG | ORAL | J8565 |
| GEMCITABINE HCL | 200 MG | IV | J9201 |
| GEMTUZUMAB | 5 MG | IV | J9300 |
| GEMZAR | 200 MG | IV | J9201 |
| GENARC | 1 IU | IV | J7192 |
| GENGRAF | 100 MG | ORAL | J7502 |
| GENGRAF | 25 MG | ORAL | J7515 |
| GENOTROPIN | 1 MG | SC | J2941 |
| GENOTROPIN MINIQUICK | 1 MG | SC | J2941 |
| GENOTROPIN NUTROPIN | 1 MG | SC | J2941 |
| GENTAMICIN | 80 MG | IM, IV | J1580 |
| GENTRAN | 500 ML | IV | J7100 |
| GENTRAN 75 | 500 ML | IV | J7110 |
| GEODON | 10 MG | IM | J3486 |
| GEREF | 1MCG | SC | Q0515 |
| ~~GESTERONE~~ | ~~50 MG~~ | ~~IM~~ | ~~J2675~~ |
| ~~GESTRIN~~ | ~~50 MG~~ | ~~IM~~ | ~~J2675~~ |
| GLATIRAMER ACETATE | 20 MG | SC | J1595 |
| GLEEVEC | 100 MG | ORAL | S0088 |
| GLOFIL-125 | 10 UCI | IV | A9554 |
| GLUCAGEN | 1 MG | SC, IM, IV | J1610 |
| GLUCAGON | 1 MG | SC, IM, IV | J1610 |
| GLUCOTOPE | STUDY DOSE | IV | A9552 |
| GLYCOPYRROLATE, COMPOUNDED CONCENTRATED | PER MG | INH | J7642 |
| GLYCOPYRROLATE, COMPOUNDED, UNIT DOSE | 1 MG | INH | J7643 |
| GOLD SODIUM THIOMALATE | 50 MG | IM | J1600 |

| Drug Name | Unit Per: | Route | Code |
|---|---|---|---|
| GONADORELIN HCL | 100 MCG | SC, IV | J1620 |
| GONAL-F | 75 IU | SC | S0126 |
| GOSERELIN ACETATE | 3.6 MG | SC | J9202 |
| GRAFTJACKET REGULAR MATRIX | PER 16 SQ CM | OTH | C9221 |
| GRAFTJACKET SOFT TISSUE MATRIX | 1 CC | OTH | C9222 |
| GRANISETRON HCL | 1 MG | ORAL | Q0166 |
| GRANISETRON HCL | 1 MG | IV | S0091 |
| GRANISETRON HCL | 100 MCG | IV | J1626 |
| GYNOGEN L.A. 10 | 10 MG | IM | J1380 |
| GYNOGEN L.A. 10 | 20 MG | IM | J1390 |
| GYNOGEN L.A. 20 | 10 MG | IM | J1380 |
| GYNOGEN L.A. 20 | 20 MG | IM | J1390 |
| GYNOGEN L.A. 40 | 10 MG | IM | J1380 |
| GYNOGEN L.A. 40 | 20 MG | IM | J1390 |
| GYNOGEN LA | 20 MG | IM | J1390 |
| H.P. ACTHAR GEL | UP TO 40 UNITS | OTH | J0800 ▲ |
| HALDOL | 5 MG | IM, IV | J1630 |
| HALDOL DECANOATE | 50 MG | IM | J1631 |
| HALOPERIDOL | 5 MG | IM, IV | J1630 |
| HAVID | 0.375 MG | ORAL | S0141 |
| HECTOROL | 1 MG | IV | J1270 |
| HELIXATE | 1 IU | IV | J7192 |
| HEMIN | 1 MG | IV | J1640 |
| HEMOFIL-M | 1 IU | IV | J7190 |
| HEP LOCK | 10 U | IV | J1642 |
| HEP-PAK | 10 UNITS | IV | J1642 |
| HEPAGAM | 0.5 ML | IM | Q4090 |
| HEPARIN SODIUM | 1,000 U | IV, SC | J1644 |
| HEPARIN SODIUM | 10 U | IV | J1642 |
| HEPATOLITE | UP TO 15 MCI | IV | A9510 ● |
| HERCEPTIN | 10 MG | IV | J9355 |
| HEXABRIX 320 | 1 ML | IV | Q9949 |
| HEXADROL | 0.25 MG | ORAL | J8540 |
| HIGH OSMOLAR CONTRAST MATERIAL, UP TO 149 MG/ML IODINE CONCENTRATION | 1 ML | IV | Q9958 |
| HIGH OSMOLAR CONTRAST MATERIAL, UP TO 150-199 MG/ML IODINE CONCENTRATION | 1 ML | IV | Q9959 |
| HIGH OSMOLAR CONTRAST MATERIAL, UP TO 200-249 MG/ML IODINE CONCENTRATION | 1 ML | IV | Q9960 |
| HIGH OSMOLAR CONTRAST MATERIAL, UP TO 250-299 MG/ML IODINE CONCENTRATION | 1 ML | IV | Q9961 |
| HIGH OSMOLAR CONTRAST MATERIAL, UP TO 300-349 MG/ML IODINE CONCENTRATION | 1 ML | IV | Q9962 |
| HIGH OSMOLAR CONTRAST MATERIAL, UP TO 350-399 MG/ML IODINE CONCENTRATION | 1 ML | IV | Q9963 |
| HIGH OSMOLAR CONTRAST MATERIAL, UP TO 400 OR GREATER MG/ML IODINE CONCENTRATION | 1 ML | IV | Q9964 |
| ~~HISTERONE 100~~ | ~~50 MG~~ | ~~IM~~ | ~~J3140~~ |
| ~~HISTERONE 50~~ | ~~50 MG~~ | ~~IM~~ | ~~J3140~~ |
| HISTRELIN ACETATE | 10 MG | INJ | J1675 |

| Drug Name | Unit Per: | Route | Code |
|---|---|---|---|
| HISTERLIN IMPLANT | 50 MG | OTH | J9225 ● |
| HUMALOG | 5 U | SC | J1815 |
| HUMALOG | 5 U | SC | S5551 |
| HUMALOG | 50 U | SC | J1817 |
| HUMATE-P | 1 IU | IV | J7187 |
| HUMATROPE | 1 MG | SC | J2941 |
| HUMIRA | 20 MG | SC | J0135 |
| HUMULIN | 5 U | SC | J1815 |
| HUMULIN | 50 U | SC | J1817 |
| HUMULIN R | 5 U | SC | J1815 |
| HUMULIN R U-500 | 5 U | SC | J1815 |
| HYALGAN | PER DOSE | OTH | J7321 |
| HYALURONAN, EUFLEXXA | PER DOSE | OTH | J7323 ● |
| HYALURONAN, HYALGAN OR SUPARTZ | PER DOSE | OTH | J7321 ● |
| HYALURONAN, ORTHOVISC | PER DOSE | OTH | J7324 ● |
| HYALURONAN, SYNVISC | PER DOSE | OTH | J7322 ● |
| HYALURONIDASE | 150 UNITS | VAR | J3470 |
| HYALURONIDASE RECOMBINANT | 1 USP UNIT | SC | J3473 |
| HYALURONIDASE, OVINE, PRESERVATIVE FREE | 1 USP | OTH | J3471 |
| HYALURONIDASE, OVINE, PRESERVATIVE FREE | 1000 USP | OTH | J3472 |
| HYATE C | 1 IU | IV | J7191 |
| ~~HYBOLIN DECANOATE~~ | ~~100 MG~~ | ~~IM~~ | ~~J2321~~ |
| ~~HYBOLIN DECANOATE~~ | ~~50 MG~~ | ~~IM~~ | ~~J2320~~ |
| HYCAMTIN | 4 MG | IV | J9350 |
| HYDRALAZINE HCL | 20 MG | IV, IM | J0360 |
| HYDRATE | 50 MG | IM, IV | J1240 |
| HYDREA | 500 MG | ORAL | S0176 |
| HYDROCORTISONE ACETATE | 25 MG | IV, IM, SC | J1700 |
| HYDROCORTISONE SODIUM PHOSPHATE | 50 MG | IV, IM, SC | J1710 |
| HYDROCORTISONE SODIUM SUCCINATE | 100 MG | IV, IM, SC | J1720 |
| HYDROCORTONE PHOSPHATE | 50 MG | SC, IM, IV | J1710 |
| HYDROMORPHONE HCL | 4 MG | SC, IM, IV | J1170 |
| HYDROMORPHONE HYDROCHLORIDE | 250 MG | OTH | S0092 |
| HYDROXOCOBALAMIN | 1,000 MCG | IM, SC | J3420 |
| HYDROXYCOBAL | 1,000 MCG | IM, SC | J3420 |
| HYDROXYUREA | 500 MG | ORAL | S0176 |
| HYDROXYZINE HCL | 25 MG | IM | J3410 |
| HYDROXYZINE PAMOATE | 25 MG | ORAL | Q0177 |
| HYDROXYZINE PAMOATE | 50 MG | ORAL | Q0178 |
| ~~HYLENEX~~ | ~~1 USP UNIT~~ | ~~SC~~ | ~~J3473~~ |
| HYOSCYAMINE SULFATE | 0.25 MG | SC, IM, IV | J1980 |
| ~~HYPERSTAT~~ | ~~300 MG~~ | ~~IV~~ | ~~J1730~~ |
| HYPRHO-D | 300 MCG | IM | J2790 |
| ~~HYPRHO-D~~ | ~~50 MCG~~ | ~~IM~~ | ~~J2788~~ |
| HYREXIN | 50 MG | IV, IM | J1200 |
| HYZINE | 25 MG | IM | J3410 |
| HYZINE-50 | 25 MG | IM | J3410 |
| I-131 TOSITUMOMAB DIAGNOSTIC | DOSE | IV | A9544 |
| I-131 TOSITUMOMAB THERAPEUTIC | DOSE | IV | A9545 |
| IBANDRONATE SODIUM | 1 MG | IV | J1740 |

| Drug Name | Unit Per: | Route | Code |
|---|---|---|---|
| IBRITUMOMAB TUXETAN | 5 MCI | IV | A9542 |
| IBUTILIDE FUMARATE | 1 MG | IV | J1742 |
| IDAMYCIN | 5 MG | IV | J9211 |
| IDAMYCIN PFS | 5 MG | IV | J9211 |
| IDARUBICIN HCL | 5 MG | IV | J9211 |
| IDURSULFASE | 1 MG | IV | C9232 |
| IFEX | 1 G | IV | J9208 |
| IFOSFAMIDE | 1 G | IV | J9208 |
| IL-2 | 1 VIAL | IV | J9015 |
| ILETIN | 5 UNITS | SC | J1815 |
| ILETIN II NPH PORK | 50 U | SC | J1817 |
| ILETIN II REGULAR PORK | 5 U | SC | J1815 |
| ILOPROST INHALATION SOLUTION | 20 UCI | INH | Q4080 |
| IMAGENT | 1 ML | IV | Q9955 |
| IMATINIB | 100 MG | ORAL | S0088 |
| IMIGLUCERASE | 1 U | IV | J1785 |
| IMITREX | 6 MG | SC | J3030 |
| IMMUNE GLOBULIN (GAMMAGARD LIQUID) | 500 MG | IV | J1569 ● |
| IMMUNE GLOBULIN (GAMUNEX) | 500 MG | IV | J1561 ● |
| IMMUNE GLOBULIN (OCTAGAM) | 500 MG | IV | J1568 ● |
| IMMUNE GLOBULIN (RHOPHYLAC) | 10 IU | IV | J2791 ● |
| IMMUNE GLOBULIN LYOPHILIZED | 500 MG | IV | J1566 |
| ~~IMMUNE GLOBULIN NONLYOPHILIZED~~ | ~~500 MG~~ | ~~IV~~ | ~~J1567~~ |
| IMMUNE GLOBULIN SUBCUTANEOUS | 100 MG | SC | J1562 |
| IMPLANON | PER IMPLANT | OTH | J7307 ● |
| IMURAN | 50 MG | ORAL | J7500 |
| IN-111 SATUMOMAB PENDETIDE | DOSE | IV | A4642 |
| INAPSINE | 5 MG | IM, IV | J1790 |
| INDERAL | 1 MG | IV | J1800 |
| INDIUM IN-111 LABELED AUTOLOGOUS PLATELETS | PER STUDY DOSAGE | IV | A9571 ● |
| INDIUM IN-111 LABELED AUTOLOGOUS WHITE BLOOD CELLS | PER STUDY DOSE | IV | A9570 ● |
| INDIUM IN-111PENTETREOTIDE | PER STUDY DOSE | IV | A9572 ● |
| INDIUM IN-111 IBRITUMOMAB TIUXETAN, DIAGNOSTIC | 5 MCI | IV | A9542 |
| INDIUM IN-111 OXYQUINOLINE | 0.5 MCI | IV | A9547 |
| INDIUM IN-111 PENTETREOTIDE | 1 MCI | IV | A9565 |
| INDURSALFASE | 1 MG | IV | J1743 ● |
| INFED | 50 MG | IM, IV | J1751 |
| INFERGEN | 1 MCG | SC | J9212 |
| INFLIXIMAB | 100 MG | IV | J1745 |
| INFUMORPH | 10 MG | IM, IV, SC | J2270 |
| INFUMORPH | 10 MG | OTH | J2275 |
| INFUMORPH PRESERVATIVE FREE | 100 MG | IM, IV, SC | J2271 |
| INNOHEP | 1,000 IU | SC | J1655 |
| ~~INNOVAR~~ | ~~2 ML~~ | ~~IM, IV~~ | ~~J1810~~ |
| INSULIN | 5 U | SC | J1815 |
| INSULIN | 50 U | SC | J1817 |
| INSULIN LISPRO | 5 U | SC | J1815 |
| INSULIN LISPRO | 5 U | SC | S5551 |
| INSULIN PURIFIED REGULAR PORK | 5 U | SC | J1815 |

# APPENDIX 1 — TABLE OF DRUGS

| Drug Name | Unit Per: | Route | Code |
|---|---|---|---|
| INTAL | 10 MG | INH | J7631 |
| INTEGRA MATRIX | PER SQ. CM. | OTH | J7347 ● |
| INTEGRILIN | 5 MG | IM, IV | J1327 |
| INTERFERON ALFA-2A | 3,000,000 U | SC, IM | J9213 |
| INTERFERON ALFA-2B | 1,000,000 U | SC, IM | J9214 |
| INTERFERON ALFA-N3 | 250,000 IU | IM | J9215 |
| INTERFERON ALFACON-1 | 1 MCG | SC | J9212 |
| INTERFERON BETA-1A | 11 MCG | IM | Q3025 |
| INTERFERON BETA-1A | 11 MCG | SC | Q3026 |
| INTERFERON BETA-1A | 33 MCG | IM | J1825 |
| INTERFERON BETA-1B | 0.25 MG | SC | J1830 |
| INTERFERON, ALFA-2A, RECOMBINANT | 3,000,000 U | SC, IM | J9213 |
| INTERFERON, ALFA-2B, RECOMBINANT | 1,000,000 U | SC, IM | J9214 |
| INTERFERON, ALFA-N3, (HUMAN LEUKOCYTE DERIVED) | 250,000 IU | IM | J9215 |
| INTERFERON, GAMMA 1-B | 3 MU | SC | J9216 |
| INTERLUEKIN | 1 VIAL | IV | J9015 |
| INTRON A | 1,000,000 U | SC, IM | J9214 |
| ~~INTROPIN~~ | ~~40 MG~~ | ~~IV~~ | ~~J1265~~ |
| INVANZ | 500 MG | IM, IV | J1335 |
| INVIRASE | 200 MG | ORAL | S0140 |
| IOBENGUANE SULFATE I-131 | 0.5 MCI | IV | A9508 |
| IODINE I-123 SODIUM IODIDE CAPSULE(S), DIAGNOSTIC | 100 UCI | ORAL | A9516 |
| IODINE I-123 SODIUM IODIDE | PER MCI | IV | A9509 ● |
| IODINE I-125 SERUM ALBUMIN, DIAGNOSTIC | 10 UCI | IV | A9554 |
| IODINE I-125 SODIUM IOTHALAMATE, DIAGNOSTIC | 10 UCI | IV | A9554 |
| IODINE I-125, SODIUM IODIDE SOLUTION, THERAPEUTIC | 1 UCI | ORAL | A9527 |
| IODINE I-131 IODINATED SERIUM ALBUMIN, DIAGNOSTIC | PER 5 UCI | ORAL | A9524 |
| IODINE I-131 SERUM ALBUMIN, DIAGNOSTIC | 5 UCI | IV | A9532 |
| IODINE I-131 SODIUM IODIDE CAPSULE(S), DIAGNOSTIC | 1 MCI | ORAL | A9528 |
| IODINE I-131 SODIUM IODIDE CAPSULE(S), THERAPEUTIC | 1 MCI | ORAL | A9517 |
| IODINE I-131 SODIUM IODIDE SOLUTION, DIAGNOSTIC | 1 MCI | ORAL | A9529 |
| IODINE I-131 SODIUM IODIDE SOLUTION, THERAPEUTIC | 1 MCI | ORAL | A9530 |
| IODINE I-131 SODIUM IODIDE, DIAGNOSTIC | 100 UCI | IV | A9531 |
| IODINE I-131 TOSITUMOMAB, DIAGNOSTIC | STUDY DOSE | IV | A9544 |
| IODINE I-131 TOSITUMOMAB, THERAPEUTIC | STUDY DOSE | IV | A9545 |
| IODOTOPE THERAPEUTIC CAPSULE(S) | 1 MCI | ORAL | A9517 |
| IODOTOPE THERAPEUTIC SOLUTION | 1 MCI | ORAL | A9530 |
| ION-BASED MAGNETIC RESONANCE CONTRAST AGENT | 1 ML | IV | Q9953 |
| IOTHALAMATE SODIUM I-125 | STUDY DOSE | IV | A9554 |
| IPLEX | 1 MG | SC | J2170 ● |
| IPRATROPIUM BROMIDE, NONCOMPOUNDED, UNIT DOSE | 1 MG | INH | J7644 |

| Drug Name | Unit Per: | Route | Code |
|---|---|---|---|
| IPTRATROPIUM BROMIDE COMPOUNDED, UNIT DOSE | 1 MG | INH | J7645 |
| IRESSA | 250 MG | ORAL | J8565 |
| IRINOTECAN | 20 MG | IV | J9206 |
| IRON DEXTRAN 165 | 50 MG | IM, IV | J1751 |
| IRON DEXTRAN 237 | 50 MG | IM, IV | J1752 |
| IRON SUCROSE | 1 MG | IV | J1756 |
| ISOCAINE | 10 ML | VAR | J0670 |
| ISOETHARINE HCL COMPOUNDED, CONCENTRATED | 1 MG | INH | J7647 |
| ISOETHARINE HCL NONCOMPOUNDED, CONCENTRATED | 1 MG | INH | J7650 |
| ISOETHARINE HCL, NONCOMPOUNDED CONCENTRATED | PER MG | INH | J7648 |
| ISOETHARINE HCL, NONCOMPOUNDED, UNIT DOSE | 1 MG | INH | J7649 |
| ISOJEX | 5 MCI | IV | A9532 |
| ISOPROTERENOL HCL COMPOUNDED, CONCENTRATED | 1 MG | INH | J7657 |
| ISOPROTERENOL HCL COMPOUNDED, UNIT DOSE | 1 MG | INH | J7660 |
| ISOPROTERENOL HCL, NONCOMPOUNDED CONCENTRATED | 1 MG | INH | J7658 |
| ISOPROTERNOL HCL, NONCOMPOUNDED, UNIT DOSE | PER MG | INH | J7659 |
| ITRACONAZOLE | 50 MG | IV | J1835 |
| IVEEGAM | 500 MG | IV | J1566 |
| ~~K-FLEX~~ | ~~60 MG~~ | ~~IV, IM~~ | ~~J2360~~ |
| ~~KABIKINASE~~ | ~~250,000 IU~~ | ~~IV~~ | ~~J2995~~ |
| KANAMYCIN | 500 MG | IM, IV | J1840 |
| KANTREX | 500 MG | IM, IV | J1840 |
| KANTREX | 75 MG | IM, IV | J1850 |
| KEFZOL | 500 MG | IV, IM | J0690 |
| KENAJECT-40 | 10 MG | IM | J3301 |
| KENALOG-10 | 10 MG | IM | J3301 |
| KENALOG-40 | 10 MG | IM | J3301 |
| KEPIVANCE | 50 MCG | IV | J2425 |
| KEPIVANCE | 60 MCG | IV | J2425 ● |
| KESTRONE | 1 MG | IV, IM | J1435 |
| KETOROLAC TROMETHAMINE | 15 MG | IM, IV | J1885 |
| ~~KEY-PRED 25~~ | ~~1 ML~~ | ~~IM~~ | ~~J2650~~ |
| ~~KEY-PRED 50~~ | ~~1 ML~~ | ~~IM~~ | ~~J2650~~ |
| KINEVAC | 5 MCG | IV | J2805 |
| KOATE-DVI | 1 IU | IV | J7190 |
| KOGENATE | 1 IU | IV | J7190 |
| KOGENATE | 1 IU | IV | J7192 |
| KONAKION | 1 MG | SC, IM, IV | J3430 |
| KONYNE 80 | 1 IU | IV | J7194 |
| KYTRIL | 1 MG | ORAL | Q0166 |
| KYTRIL | 1 MG | IV | S0091 |
| KYTRIL | 100 MCG | IV | J1626 |
| ~~L-CARNITINE~~ | ~~1 G~~ | ~~IV~~ | ~~J1955~~ |
| L-PHENYLALANINE MUSTARD | 50 MG | IV | J9245 |
| L.A.E. 20 | 10 MG | IM | J1380 |
| L.A.E. 20 | 20 MG | IM | J1390 |
| LANOXIN | 0.5 MG | IM, IV | J1160 |
| LANTUS | 50 U | SC | J1817 |

| Drug Name | Unit Per: | Route | Code |
|---|---|---|---|
| LARONIDASE | 0.1 MG | IV | J1931 |
| LASIX | 20 MG | IM, IV | J1940 |
| LENTE ILETIN I | 5 U | SC | J1815 |
| LEPIRUDIN | 50 MG | IV | J1945 |
| LEUCOVORIN CALCIUM | 50 MG | IM, IV | J0640 |
| LEUKERAN | 2 MG | ORAL | S0172 |
| LEUKINE | 50 MCG | IV | J2820 |
| LEUPROLIDE ACETATE | 1 MG | IM | J9218 |
| LEUPROLIDE ACETATE | 7.5 MG | IM | J9217 |
| LEUPROLIDE ACETATE (FOR DEPOT SUSPENSION) | 3.75 MG | IM | J1950 |
| LEUPROLIDE ACETATE DEPOT | 7.5 MG | IM | J9217 |
| LEUPROLIDE ACETATE IMPLANT | 65 MG | OTH | J9219 |
| LEUSTATIN | 1 MG | IV | J9065 |
| LEVABUTEROL COMPOUNDED, UNIT DOSE | 1 MG | INH | J7615 |
| LEVABUTEROL, COMPOUNDED, CONCENTRATED | 0.5 MG | INH | J7607 |
| ~~LEVALBUTEROL NONCOMPOUNDED, CONCENTRATED FORM~~ | ~~0.5 MG~~ | ~~INH~~ | ~~J7612~~ |
| LEVALBUTEROL NONCOMPOUNDED, CONCENTRATED FORM | 0.5 MG | INH | J7612 |
| LEVALBUTEROL, NONCOMPOUNDED, CONCENTRATED FORM | PER 0.5 MG | INH | J7602 ● |
| ~~LEVALBUTEROL, NONCOMPOUNED UNIT DOSE~~ | ~~0.5 MG~~ | ~~INH~~ | ~~J7614~~ |
| ~~LEVALBUTEROL, NONCOMPOUNED UNIT DOSE~~ | ~~0.5 MG~~ | ~~INH~~ | ~~Q4095~~ |
| LEVALBUTEROL, NONCOMPOUNDED, UNIT DOSE | PER 0.5 MG | INH | J7603 |
| LEVAMISOLE HCL | 50 MG | ORAL | S0177 |
| LEVAQUIN | 1 G | IV | J1956 |
| LEVOCARNITINE | 1 G | IV | J1955 |
| LEVOFLOXACIN | 1 G | IV | J1956 |
| LEVONORGESTREL | 52 MG | OTH | J7302 |
| LEVORPHANOL TARTRATE | 2 MG | SC, IV, IM | J1960 |
| LEVOXYL | 5 MG | ORAL | J7506 |
| LEVSIN | 0.25 MG | SC, IM, IV | J1980 |
| LEVULAN KERASTICK | SINGLE UNIT DOSE (354 MG) | OTH | J7308 |
| LIBRIUM | 100 MG | IM, IV | J1990 |
| LIDOCAINE HCL | 10 MG | IV | J2001 |
| LINCOCIN HCL | 300 MG | IV | J2010 |
| LINCOMYCIN HCL | 300 MG | IM, IV | J2010 |
| LINEZOLID | 200 MG | IV | J2020 |
| LIORESAL | 10 MG | IT | J0475 |
| LIORESAL INTRATHECAL REFILL | 50 MCG | IT | J0476 |
| LIQUAEMIN SODIUM | 1,000 UNITS | SC, IV | J1644 |
| LIQUID PRED SYRUP | 5 MG | OTH | J7506 |
| LISPRO-PFC | 50 U | SC | J1817 |
| LOK-PAK | 10 UNITS | IV | J1642 |
| LOMUSTINE | 10 MG | ORAL | S0178 |
| LONITEN | 10 MG | ORAL | S0139 |
| LORAZEPAM | 2 MG | IM, IV | J2060 |
| LOVENOX | 10 MG | SC | J1650 |

| Drug Name | Unit Per: | Route | Code |
|---|---|---|---|
| LOW OSMOLAR CONTRAST MATERIAL, 400 OR GREATER MG/ML IODINE CONCENTRATION | 1 ML | IV | Q9951 |
| ~~LOW OSMOLAR CONTRAST MATERIAL, UP TO 150-199 MG/ML IODINE CONCENTRATION~~ | ~~1 ML~~ | ~~IV~~ | ~~Q9946~~ |
| LOW OSMOLAR CONTRAST MATERIAL, 100-199 MG/ML IODINE CONCENTRATIONS | PER ML | IV | Q9965 ● |
| ~~LOW OSMOLAR CONTRAST MATERIAL, UP TO 200-249 MG/ML IODINE CONCENTRATION~~ | ~~1 ML~~ | ~~IV~~ | ~~Q9947~~ |
| ~~LOW OSMOLAR CONTRAST MATERIAL, UP TO 250-299 MG/ML IODINE CONCENTRATION~~ | ~~1 ML~~ | ~~IV~~ | ~~Q9948~~ |
| LOW OSMOLAR CONTRAST MATERIAL, 200-299 MG/ML IODINE CONCENTRATION | PER ML | IV | Q9966 ● |
| ~~LOW OSMOLAR CONTRAST MATERIAL, UP TO 300-349 MG/ML IODINE CONCENTRATION~~ | ~~1 ML~~ | ~~IV~~ | ~~Q9949~~ |
| ~~LOW OSMOLAR CONTRAST MATERIAL, UP TO 350-399 MG/ML IODINE CONCENTRATION~~ | ~~1 ML~~ | ~~IV~~ | ~~Q9950~~ |
| LOW OSMOLAR CONTRAST MATERIAL, 300-399 MG/ML IODINE CONCENTRATION | PER ML | IV | Q9967 ● |
| LUCENTIS | 0.1 MG | IV | J2778 ● |
| ~~LUFYLLIN~~ | ~~500 MG~~ | ~~IM~~ | ~~J1180~~ |
| ~~LUMINAL SODIUM~~ | ~~120 MG~~ | ~~IM, IV~~ | ~~J2560~~ |
| LUNELLE | 5 MG/25 MG | IM | J1056 |
| LUPRON | 1 MG | IM | J9218 |
| LUPRON | 7.5 MG | IM | J9217 |
| LUPRON | PER 3.75 MG | SC | J1950 ● |
| LUPRON-3 | PER 3.75 MG | SC | J1950 ● |
| LUPRON-4 | PER 3.75 MG | SC | J1950 ● |
| LUPRON DEPOT | 3.75 MG | IM | J1950 |
| LUPRON DEPOT | 7.5 MG | IM | J9217 |
| LUPRON IMPLANT | 65 MG | OTH | J9219 |
| LUTREPULSE | 100 MCG | SC, IV | J1620 |
| LYMPHOCYTE IMMUNE GLOBULIN, ANTITHYMOCYTE GLOBULIN, EQUINE | 250 MG | OTH | J7504 |
| LYMPHOCYTE IMMUNE GLOBULIN, ANTITHYMOCYTE GLOBULIN, RABBIT | 25 MG | OTH | J7511 |
| MACUGEN | 0.3 MG | OTH | J2503 |
| MAGNESIUM SULFATE | 10 MG | IV | J3475 |
| MAGNETIC RESONANCE CONTRAST AGENT | 1 ML | ORAL | Q9954 |
| MAGNAVIST | UP TO 25 MCI | IV | A9539 ● |
| MAGNAVIST | UP TO 25 MCI | INH | A9567 ● |
| MAGROTEC | 10 MCI | IV | A9540 |
| MANNITOL | 25% IN 50 ML | IV | J2150 |
| MARCAINE HCL | 30 ML | VAR | S0020 |
| MARINOL | 2.5 MG | ORAL | Q0167 |
| MARINOL | 5 MG | ORAL | Q0168 |
| MARMINE | 50 MG | IM, IV | J1240 |
| MATULANE | 50 MG | ORAL | S0182 |
| MAXIPIME | 500 MG | IV | J0692 |
| MDP-BRACCO | 30 MCI | IV | A9503 ● |
| MECASERMIN | 1 MG | SC | J2170 |

# APPENDIX 1 — TABLE OF DRUGS

| Drug Name | Unit Per: | Route | Code |
|---|---|---|---|
| MECHLORETHAMINE HYDROCHLORIDE | 10 MG | IV | J9230 |
| MEDIDEX | 1 MG | IM, IV, OTH | J1100 |
| MEDROL | 4 MG | ORAL | J7509 |
| MEDROXYPROGESTERONE ACETATE | 150 MG | IM | J1055 |
| MEDROXYPROGESTERONE ACETATE | 50 MG | IM | J1051 |
| MEDROXYPROGESTERONE ACETATE/ESTRADIOL CYPIONATE | 5 MG/25 MG | IM | J1056 |
| MEFOXIN | 1 G | IV | J0694 |
| MEGACE | 20 MG | ORAL | S0179 |
| MEGESTROL ACETATE | 20 MG | ORAL | S0179 |
| MELPHALAN HCL | 2 MG | ORAL | J8600 |
| MELPHALAN HCL | 50 MG | IV | J9245 |
| MENADIONE | 1 MG | IM, SC, IV | J3430 |
| MENOTROPINS | 75 IU | SC, IM, IV | S0122 |
| MEPERGAN | 50 MG | IM, IV | J2180 |
| MEPERIDINE AND PROMETHAZINE HCL | 50 MG | IM, IV | J2180 |
| MEPERIDINE HCL | 100 MG | IM, IV, SC | J2175 |
| MEPIVACAINE HCL | 10 ML | VAR | J0670 |
| MERCAPTOPURINE | 50 MG | ORAL | S0108 |
| MERITATE | 150 MG | IV | J3520 |
| MEROPENEM | 100 MG | IV | J2185 |
| MERREM | 100 MG | IV | J2185 |
| MESNA | 200 MG | IV | J9209 |
| MESNEX | 200 MG | IV | J9209 |
| METAPROTERENOL SULFATE COMPOUNDED, UNIT DOSE | 10 MG | INH | J7670 |
| METAPROTERENOL SULFATE, NONCOMPOUNDED, UNIT DOSE | 10 MG | INH | J7669 |
| METAPROTERENOL SULFATE, NONCOMPOUNDED, CONCENTRATED | 10 MG | INH | J7668 |
| METARAMINOL BITARTRATE | 10 MG | IV, IM, SC | J0380 |
| METASTRON STRONTIUM 89 CHLORIDE | 1 MCI | IV | A9600 |
| METATRACE | STUDY DOSE | IV | A9552 |
| METHACHOLINE CHLORIDE | 1 MG | INH | J7674 |
| METHADONE | 5 MG | ORAL | S0109 |
| METHADONE HCL | 10 MG | IM, SC | J1230 |
| METHAPREL, COMPOUNDED, UNIT DOSE | 10 MG | INH | J7670 |
| METHAPREL, NONCOMPOUNDED, CONCENTRATED | 10 MG | INH | J7668 |
| METHAPREL, NONCOMPOUNDED, UNIT DOSE | 10 MG | INH | J7669 |
| METHERGINE | 0.2 MG | IM, IV | J2210 |
| METHOCARBAMOL RELAXIN | 10 ML | IV, IM | J2800 |
| METHOTREXATE | 5 MG | IV, IM, IT, IA | J9250 |
| METHOTREXATE | 50 MG | IV, IM, IT, IA | J9260 |
| METHOTREXATE LPF | 5 MG | IV, IM, IT, IA | J9250 |
| METHOTREXATE LPF | 50 MG | IV, IM, IT, IA | J9260 |
| METHOTREXATE SODIUM | 2.5 MG | ORAL | J8610 |
| METHOTREXATE SODIUM | 5 MG | IV, IM, IT, IA | J9250 |
| METHOTREXATE SODIUM | 50 MG | IV, IM, IT, IA | J9260 |
| METHYLCOTOLONE | 80 MG | IM | J1040 |
| METHYLDOPA HCL | 250 MG | IV | J0210 |
| METHYLDOPATE HCL | 5 MG | IV | J0210 |

| Drug Name | Unit Per: | Route | Code |
|---|---|---|---|
| METHYLENE BLUE | 1 ML | IV | A9535 |
| METHYLERGONOVINE MALEATE | 0.2 MG | IM, IV | J2210 |
| METHYLPRED | 4 MG | ORAL | J7509 |
| METHYLPREDNISOLONE | 125 MG | IM, IV | J2930 |
| METHYLPREDNISOLONE | 4 MG | ORAL | J7509 |
| METHYLPREDNISOLONE | UP TO 40 MG | IM, IV | J2920 |
| METHYLPREDNISOLONE ACETATE | 20 MG | IM | J1020 |
| METHYLPREDNISOLONE ACETATE | 40 MG | IM | J1030 |
| METHYLPREDNISOLONE ACETATE | 80 MG | IM | J1040 |
| METOCLOPRAMIDE | 10 MG | IV | J2765 |
| METRONIDAZOLE | 500 MG | IV | S0030 |
| MIACALCIN | 400 U | SC, IM | J0630 |
| MIBG | 0.5 MCI | IV | A9508 |
| MICAFUNGIN SODIUM | 1 MG | IV | J2248 |
| MIDAZOLAM HCI | 1 MG | IM, IV | J2250 |
| MILRINONE LACTATE | 5 MG | IV | J2260 |
| MINOXIDIL | 10 MG | ORAL | S0139 |
| MIO REL | 60 MG | IV, IM | J2360 |
| MIRENA | 52 MG | OTH | J7302 |
| MISOPROSTOL | 200 MG | ORAL | S0191 |
| MITHRACIN | 2,500 MCG | IV | J9270 |
| MITOMYCIN | 20 MG | IV | J9290 |
| MITOMYCIN | 40 MG | IV | J9291 |
| MITOMYCIN | 5 MG | IV | J9280 |
| MITOXANA | 1 G | IV | J9208 |
| MITOXANTRONE HYDROCHLORIDE | 5 MG | IV | J9293 |
| MONARC-M | 1 IU | IV | J7190 |
| MONOCLATE-P | 1 IU | IV | J7190 |
| MONONINE | 1 IU | IV | J7193 |
| MONOPUR | 75 IU | SC, IM | S0122 |
| MORPHINE SULFATE | 10 MG | IM, IV, SC | J2270 |
| MORPHINE SULFATE | 100 MG | IM, IV, SC | J2271 |
| MORPHINE SULFATE | 500 MG | OTH | S0093 |
| MORPHINE SULFATE, PRESERVATIVE FREE, STERILE SOLUTION | 10 MG | IM, IV, SC | J2275 |
| MOXIFLOXACIN | 100 MG | IV | J2280 |
| MPI INDIUM DTPA | 0.5 MCI | IV | A9548 |
| MS CONTIN | 500 MG | OTH | S0093 |
| MUCOMYST | 1 G | INH | J7608 |
| MUCOSIL | 1 G | INH | J7608 |
| MULTIHANCE | 1 ML | IV | Q9952 |
| MULTIHANCE (GADOBENATE DIMEGLUMINE) | PER ML | IV | A9577 |
| MUROMONAB-CD3 | 5 MG | OTH | J7505 |
| MUSE | EA | OTH | J0275 |
| MUSTARGEN | 10 MG | IV | J9230 |
| MUTAMYCIN | 20 MG | IV | J9290 |
| MUTAMYCIN | 40 MG | IV | J9291 |
| MUTAMYCIN | 5 MG | IV | J9280 |
| MYCAMINE | 1 MG | IV | J2248 |
| MYCOPHENOLATE MOFETIL | 250 MG | ORAL | J7517 |
| MYCOPHENOLIC ACID | 180 MG | ORAL | J7518 |
| MYFORTIC DELAYED RELEASE | 180 MG | ORAL | J7518 |
| MYLERAN | 2 MG | ORAL | J8510 |

**Appendix 1 — Table of Drugs**

| Drug Name | Unit Per: | Route | Code |
|---|---|---|---|
| MYLOCEL | 500 MG | ORAL | S0176 |
| MYLOTARG | 5 MG | IV | J9300 |
| MYOBLOC | 100 U | IM | J0587 |
| MYOCHRYSINE | 50 MG | IM | J1600 |
| ~~MYOLIN~~ | ~~60 MG~~ | ~~IV, IM~~ | ~~J2360~~ |
| ~~MYOPHEN~~ | ~~60 MG~~ | ~~IV, IM~~ | ~~J2360~~ |
| MYOVIEW | DOSE | IV | A9502 |
| ~~MYOZYME~~ | ~~10 MG~~ | ~~IV~~ | ~~C9234~~ |
| ~~MYOZYME~~ | ~~20 MG~~ | ~~IV~~ | ~~S0147~~ |
| NABILONE | 1 MG | ORAL | J8650 |
| NAFCILLIN SODIUM | 2 GM | IM, IV | S0032 |
| NAGLAZYME | 1 MG | IV | J1458 |
| NALBUPHINE HCL | 10 MG | IM, IV, SC | J2300 |
| NALLPEN | 2 GM | IM, IV | S0032 |
| NALOXONE HCL | 1 MG | IM, IV, SC | J2310 |
| NALTREXONE, DEPOT FORM | 1 MG | IM | J2315 |
| ~~NANDROBOLIC L.A.~~ | ~~100 MG~~ | ~~IM~~ | ~~J2321~~ |
| NANDROLONE DECANOATE | 100 MG | IM | J2321 |
| NANDROLONE DECANOATE | 200 MG | IM | J2322 |
| NANDROLONE DECANOATE | 50 MG | IM | J2320 |
| NARCAN | 1 MG | IM, IV, SC | J2310 |
| NAROPIN | 1 MG | VAR | J2795 |
| NASAHIST B | 10 MG | IM | J0945 |
| NASALCROM | 10 MG | INH | J7631 |
| NATALIZUMAB | 1 MG | IV | J2323 |
| NATRECOR | 0.1 MG | IV | J2325 |
| NATURAL ESTROGENIC SUBSTANCE | 1 MG | IM, IV | J1410 |
| NAVELBINE | 10 MG | IV | J9390 |
| ND-STAT | 10 MG | IM, SC, IV | J0945 |
| NEBCIN | 80 MG | IM, IV | J3260 |
| NEBUPENT | 300 MG | INH | J2545 |
| NEBUPENT | 300 MG | IM, IV | S0080 |
| NELARABINE | 50 MG | IV | J9261 |
| ~~NEMBUTAL SODIUM~~ | ~~120 MG~~ | ~~IM, IV~~ | ~~J2560~~ |
| NEMBUTAL SODIUM | 50 MG | IM, IV, OTH | J2515 |
| ~~NEO SYNEPHRINE HCL~~ | ~~1 ML~~ | ~~SC, IM, IV~~ | ~~J2370~~ |
| ~~NEO-DURABOLIC~~ | ~~100 MG~~ | ~~IM~~ | ~~J2321~~ |
| ~~NEO-DURABOLIC~~ | ~~200 MG~~ | ~~IM~~ | ~~J2322~~ |
| ~~NEO-DURABOLIC~~ | ~~50 MG~~ | ~~IM~~ | ~~J2320~~ |
| ~~NEOCYTEN~~ | ~~60 MG~~ | ~~IV, IM~~ | ~~J2360~~ |
| NEORAL | 25 MG | ORAL | J7515 |
| NEORAL | 250 MG | ORAL | J7516 |
| NEOSAR | 1 G | IV | J9091 |
| NEOSAR | 100 MG | IV | J9070 |
| NEOSAR | 2 G | IV | J9092 |
| NEOSAR | 200 MG | IV | J9080 |
| NEOSAR | 500 MG | IV | J9090 |
| NEOSCAN | 1 MCI | IV | A9556 |
| NEOSTIGMINE METHYLSULFATE | 250 MG | IM, IV | J2710 |
| NEOTECT | STUDY DOSE | IV | A9536 |
| NESACAINE | 30 ML | VAR | J2400 |
| NESACAINE-MPF | 30 ML | VAR | J2400 |
| NESIRITIDE | 0.1 MG | IV | J2325 |
| NEULASTA | 6 MG | SC, SQ | J2505 |

| Drug Name | Unit Per: | Route | Code |
|---|---|---|---|
| NEUMEGA | 5 MG | SC | J2355 |
| NEUPOGEN | 300 MCG | SC, IV | J1440 |
| NEUPOGEN | 480 MCG | SC, IV | J1441 |
| NEUROLITE | 25 MCI | IV | A9557 |
| NEUTREXIN | 25 MG | IV | J3305 |
| NEUTROSPEC | 25 MCI | IV | A9566 |
| NIPENT | 10 MG | IV | J9268 |
| NITROGEN N-13 AMMONIA, DIAGNOSTIC | STUDY DOSE, UP TO 40 MCI | INJ | A9526 |
| NOC DRUGS, INHALATION SOLUTION ADMINISTERED THROUGH DME | 1 EA | | J7699 |
| NOLVADEX | 10 MG | ORAL | S0187 |
| NOLVADEX | 10 MG | ORAL | S0187 |
| NORDITROPIN | 1 MG | SC | J2941 |
| NORDYL | 50 MG | IV, IM | J1200 |
| NORFLEX | 60 MG | IV, IM | J2360 |
| ~~NORMAL SALINE~~ | ~~2 ML~~ | ~~IV~~ | ~~J2912~~ |
| NORPLANT II | PER IMPLANT | OTH | J7306 ▲ |
| ~~NORZINE~~ | ~~10 MG~~ | ~~IM~~ | ~~J3280~~ |
| NOT OTHERWISE CLASSIFIED, ANTINEOPLASTIC DRUGS | | | J9999 |
| NOV-ONXOL | 30 MG | IV | J9265 |
| NOVANTRONE | 5 MG | IV | J9293 |
| NOVAREL | 1,000 USP U | IM | J0725 |
| NOVASTAN | 5 MG | IV | C9121 |
| NOVO NORDISK | 5 UNITS | SC | J1815 |
| NOVOLIN | 50 U | SC | J1817 |
| NOVOLIN R | 5 U | SC | J1815 |
| NOVOLOG | 50 U | SC | J1817 |
| NOVOSEVEN | 1 MCG | IV | J7189 |
| NPH | 5 UNITS | SC | J1815 |
| NUBAIN | 10 MG | IM, IV, SC | J2300 |
| NUMORPHAN | 1 MG | IV, SC, IM | J2410 |
| ~~NUMORPHAN H.P.~~ | ~~1 MG~~ | ~~IV, SC, IM~~ | ~~J2410~~ |
| NUTRI-TWELVE | 1,000 MCG | IM, SC | J3420 |
| NUTROPIN | 1 MG | SC | J2941 |
| NUTROPIN A.Q. | 1 MG | SC | J2941 |
| NUVARING VAGINAL RING | EA | OTH | J7303 |
| ~~O-FLEX~~ | ~~60 MG~~ | ~~IV, IM~~ | ~~J2360~~ |
| ~~OCATMIDE PFS~~ | ~~10 MG~~ | ~~IV~~ | ~~J2765~~ |
| OCTAFLUOROPROPANE UCISPHERES | 1 ML | IV | Q9956 |
| OCTAGAM | 500 MG | IV | J1568 ● |
| OCTAGAM IMMUNE GLOBULIN | 1 GM | IV | J1563 |
| ~~OCTOGAM IMMUNE GLOBULIN~~ | ~~500 MG~~ | ~~IV~~ | ~~Q4087~~ |
| OCTREOSCAN | 1 MCI | IV | A9565 |
| OCTREOTIDE ACETATE DEPOT | 1 MG | IM | J2353 |
| OCTREOTIDE, NON-DEPOT FORM | 25 MCG | SC, IV | J2354 |
| OFLOXACIN | 400 MG | IV | S0034 |
| OLANZAPINE | 2.5 MG | IM | S0166 |
| OMALIZUMAB | 5 MG | SC | J2357 |
| OMNIPAQUE 140 | PER ML | IV | Q9965 ▲ |
| OMNIPAQUE 180 | PER ML | IV | Q9965 ▲ |
| OMNIPAQUE 240 | PER ML | IV | Q9966 ▲ |

| Drug Name | Unit Per: | Route | Code | Drug Name | Unit Per: | Route | Code |
|---|---|---|---|---|---|---|---|
| OMNIPAQUE 300 | PER ML | IV | Q9966 ▲ | PARICALCITOL | 1 MCG | IV, IM | J2501 |
| OMNIPAQUE 350 | PER ML | IV | Q9967 ▲ | PEDIAPRED | 5 MG | ORAL | J7510 |
| OMNISCAN | PER ML | IV | A9579 ▲ | PEG-INTRON | 10 MCG | SC | S0146 |
| ONCASPAR | VIAL | IM, IV | J9266 | PEG-INTRON | 180 MCG | SC | S0145 |
| ONCOSCINT | DOSE | IV | A4642 | PEGADEMASE BOVINE | 25 IU | IM | J2504 |
| ONDANSETRON HCL | 4 MG | ORAL | S0181 | PEGAPTANIB SODIUM | 0.3 MG | OTH | J2503 |
| ONDANSETRON HCL | 8 MG | ORAL | Q0179 | PEGASPARGASE | VIAL | IM, IV | J9266 |
| ONDANSETRON HYDROCHLORIDE | 1 MG | IV | J2405 | PEGASYS | 10 MCG | SC | S0146 |
| ONTAK | 300 MCG | IV | J9160 | PEGFILGRASTIM | 6 MG | SC | J2505 |
| ONXOL | 30 MG | IV | J9265 | PEGINTERFERON ALFA-2A | 180 MCG | SC | S0145 |
| OPRELVEKIN | 5 MG | SC | J2355 | PEGYLATED INTERFERON ALFA-2A | 180 MCG | SC | S0145 |
| ~~OPTIMARK~~ | ~~1 ML~~ | ~~IV~~ | ~~Q9952~~ | PEGYLATED INTERFERON ALFA-2B | 10 MCG | SC | S0146 |
| OPTIRAY | PER ML | IV | Q9967 ▲ | PEMETREXED | 10 MG | IV | J9305 |
| OPTIRAY 160 | PER ML | IV | Q9965 ▲ | PEN G BENZ/PEN G PROCAINE | 600,000 U | IM | J0530 |
| OPTIRAY 240 | PER ML | IV | Q9966 ▲ | PENICILLIN G BENZATHINE | 1,200,000 U | IM | J0570 |
| OPTIRAY 300 | PER ML | IV | Q9967 ▲ | PENICILLIN G BENZATHINE | 2,400,000 U | IM | J0580 |
| OPTIRAY 320 | PER ML | IV | Q9967 ▲ | PENICILLIN G BENZATHINE | 600,000 U | IM | J0560 |
| OPTISON | 1 ML | IV | Q9957 | PENICILLIN G BENZATHINE AND PENICILLIN G PROCAINE | 1,200,000 U | IM | J0540 |
| ORAL MAGNETIC RESONANCE CONTRAST AGENT, PER 100 ML | 100 ML | ORAL | Q9954 | PENICILLIN G POTASSIUM | 600,000 U | IM, IV | J2540 |
| ORCEL | SQ CM | OTH | J7340 | PENICILLIN G PROCAINE | 600,000 U | IM, IV | J2510 |
| ORENCIA | 10 MG | IV | J0129 | PENTACARINAT | 300 MG | INH | S0080 |
| ORPHENADRINE CITRATE | 60 MG | IV, IM | J2360 | PENTAM | 300 MG | IM, IV | J2545 |
| ~~ORPHENATE~~ | ~~60 MG~~ | ~~IV, IM~~ | ~~J2360~~ | PENTAM 300 | 300 MG | IM, IV | S0080 |
| ORTHOCLONE OKT3 | 5 MG | OTH | J7505 | PENTAMIDINE ISETHIONATE NONCOMPOUNDED | 300 MG | INH | J2545 |
| ORTHOVISC | PER DOSE | OTH | J7324 ▲ | PENTAMIDINE ISETHIONATE | 300 MG | IM, IV | S0080 |
| OSELTAMIVIR PHOSPHATE (BRAND NAME) | 75 MG | ORAL | G9035 | PENTAMIDINE ISETHIONATE COMPOUNDED | PER 300 MG | INH | J7676 ● |
| OSELTAMIVIR PHOSPHATE (GENERIC) | 75 MG | ORAL | G9019 | PENTASPAN | 100 ML | IV | J2513 |
| OSMITROL | 25% IN 50 ML | IV | J2150 | PENTASTARCH 10% SOLUTION | 100 ML | IV | J2513 |
| OSTREOSCAN | UP TO 6 MCI | IV | A9572 ● | PENTATE CALCIUM TRISODIUM | UP TO 25 MCI | IV | A9539 ● |
| OXACILLIN SODIUM | 250 MG | IM, IV | J2700 | PENTATE CALCIUM TRISODIUM | UP TO 25 MCI | INH | A9567 ● |
| OXALIPLATIN | 0.5 MG | IV | J9263 | PENTATE ZINC TRISODIUM | UP TO 25 MCI | IV | A9539 ● |
| OXILAN 300 | PER ML | IV | Q9967 | PENTATE ZINC TRISODIUM | UP TO 25 MCI | INH | A9567 ● |
| OXILAN 350 | PER ML | IV | Q9967 | PENTAZOCINE | 30 MG | IM, SC, IV | J3070 |
| OXYMORPHONE HCL | 1 MG | IV, SC, IM | J2410 | PENTOBARBITAL SODIUM | 50 MG | IM, IV, OTH | J2515 |
| OXYTETRACYCLINE HCL | 50 MG | IM | J2460 | PENTOSTATIN | 10 MG | IV | J9268 |
| OXYTOCIN | 10 U | IV, IM | J2590 | PEPCID | 20 MG | IV | S0028 |
| PACIS BCG | VIAL | OTH | J9031 | PERFLEXANE LIPID UCISPHERE | 1 ML | IV | Q9955 |
| PACLITAXEL | 30 MG | IV | J9265 | PERFLUTREN LIPID UCISPHERE | 1 ML | IV | Q9957 |
| PACLITAXEL PROTEIN-BOUND PARTICLES | 1 MG | IV | J9264 | PERMAPEN | 600,000 | IM | J0560 |
| PALIFERMIN | 50 MCG | IV | J2425 | PERMAPEN | > 2,400,000 U | IM | J0580 |
| PALIVIZUMAB-RSV-IGM | 50 MG | IM | C9003 | PERMAPEN | >1,200,000 U | IM | J0570 |
| PALONOSETRON HCL | 25 MCG | IV | J2469 | PERPHENAZINE | 4 MG | ORAL | Q0175 |
| PAMIDRONATE DISODIUM | 30 MG | IV | J2430 | PERPHENAZINE | 5 MG | IM, IV | J3310 |
| PANGLOBULIN | 1 G | IV | J1563 | PERSANTINE | 10 MG | IV | J1245 |
| PANHEMATIN | 1 MG | IV | J1640 | PFIZERPEN A.S. | 600,000 UNITS | IM, IV | J2510 |
| PANITUMUMAB | 10 MG | IV | J9303 ▲ | ~~PHENAZINE 25~~ | ~~50 MG~~ | ~~IM, IV~~ | ~~J2550~~ |
| PANTOPRAZOLE SODIUM | 40 MG | IV | S0164 | ~~PHENAZINE 50~~ | ~~50 MG~~ | ~~IM, IV~~ | ~~J2550~~ |
| PANTOPRAZOLE SODIUM | VIAL | IV | C9113 | PHENERGAN | 12.5 MG | ORAL | Q0169 |
| PAPAVERINE HCL | 60 MG | IV, IM | J2440 | PHENERGAN | 50 MG | IM, IV | J2550 |
| PARAGARD T380A | EA | OTH | J7300 | PHENOBARBITAL SODIUM | 120 MG | IM, IV | J2560 |
| PARAPLANTIN | 50 MG | IV | J9045 | PHENTOLAMINE MESYLATE | 5 MG | IM, IV | J2760 |
| | | | | PHENYLEPHRINE HCL | 1 ML | SC, IM, IV | J2370 |

| Drug Name | Unit Per: | Route | Code | Drug Name | Unit Per: | Route | Code |
|-----------|-----------|-------|------|-----------|-----------|-------|------|
| PHENYTOIN SODIUM | 50 MG | IM, IV | J1165 | PROCRIT, NON-ESRD USE | 1,000 U | SC, IV | J0885 |
| PHOSPHOCOL | 1 MCI | IV | A9563 | PROFILNINE HEAT-TREATED | 1 IU | IV | J7194 |
| PHOSPHOTEC | 25 MCI | IV | A9538 | PROFILNINE SD | 1 IU | IV | J7194 |
| PHOTOFRIN | 75 MG | IV | J9600 | PROFONIX | VIAL | INJ | C9113 |
| PHYTONADIONE | 1 MG | IM, SC, IV | J3430 | PROGESTERONE | 50 MG | IM | J2675 |
| PIPERACILLIN SODIUM | 500 MG | IM, IV | S0081 | PROGRAF | 1 MG | ORAL | J7507 |
| PIPERACILLIN SODIUM/TAZOBACTAM SODIUM | 1 G/1.125 GM | IV | J2543 | PROGRAF | 5 MG | OTH | J7525 |
| | | | | PROHANCE | 1 ML | IV | Q9952 |
| PITOCIN | 10 U | IV, IM | J2590 | PROHANCE MULTIPACK (GADOTERIDOL) | PER ML | IV | A9576 |
| PLATINOL AQ | 10 MG | IV | J9060 | PROKINE | 50 MCG | IV | J2820 |
| PLATINOL AQ | 50 MG | IV | J9062 | PROLASTIN | 10 MG | IV | J0256 |
| PLENAXIS | 10 MG | IM | J0128 | PROLEUKIN | 1 VIAL | VAR | J9015 |
| PLICAMYCIN | 2,500 MCG | IV | J9270 | PROLIXIN DECANOATE | 25 MG | SC, IM | J2680 |
| PNEUMOCOCCAL CONJUGATE | EA | IM | S0195 | PROMAZINE HCL | 25 MG | IM | J2950 |
| PNEUMOVAX II | EA | IM | S0195 | PROMETHAZINE HCL | 12.5 MG | ORAL | Q0169 |
| POLOCAINE | 10 ML | VAR | J0670 | PROMETHAZINE HCL | 50 MG | IM, IV | J2550 |
| POLY-L-LACTIC ACID | 1 ML | SC | S0196 | PRONESTYL | 1 G | IM, IV | J2690 |
| POLYGAM | 500 MG | IV | J1566 | PROPECIA | 5 MG | ORAL | S0138 |
| POLYGAM S/D | 500 MG | IV | J1566 | PROPLEX SX-T | 1 IU | IV | J7194 |
| PORFIMER SODIUM | 75 MG | IV | J9600 | PROPLEX T | 1 IU | IV | J7194 |
| PORK INSULIN | 5 UNITS | SC | J1815 | PROPRANOLOL HCL | 1 MG | IV | J1800 |
| POTASSIUM CHLORIDE | 2 MEQ | IV | J3480 | PROREX | 50 MG | IM, IV | J2550 |
| PRALIDOXIME CHLORIDE | 1 MG | IV, IM, SC | J2730 | PROSCAR | 5 MG | ORAL | S0138 |
| PREDACORT | 1 ML | IM | J2650 | PROSTAPHLIN | 250 MG | IM, IV | J2700 |
| PREDALONE-50 | 1 ML | IM | J2650 | PROSTASCINT | DOSE | IV | A9507 |
| PREDCOR-25 | 1 ML | IM | J2650 | PROSTIGMIN | 0.5 MG | IM, IV | J2710 |
| PREDCOR-50 | 1 ML | IM | J2650 | PROSTIN VR | 1.25 MCG | INJ | J0270 |
| PREDICORT-50 | 1 ML | IM | J2650 | PROTAMINE SULFATE | 10 MG | IV | J2720 |
| PREDNICOT | 5 ML | ORAL | J7506 | PROTEIN C CONCENTRATE | 10 IU | IV | J2724 ● |
| PREDNISOLONE | 5 MG | ORAL | J7510 | PROTEINASE INHIBITOR (HUMAN) | 10 MG | IV | J0256 |
| PREDNISOLONE ACETATE | 1 ML | IM | J2650 | PROTHAZINE | 50 MG | IM, IV | J2550 |
| PREDNISONE | 5 MG | ORAL | J7506 | PROTIRELIN | 250 MCG | IV | J2725 |
| PREDNORAL | 5 MG | ORAL | J7510 | PROTONIX IV | 40 MG | IV | S0164 |
| PREDOJECT-50 | 1 ML | IM | J2650 | PROTONIX IV | VIAL | IV | C9113 |
| PREDONE | 5 MG | ORAL | J7506 | PROTOPAM CHLORIDE | 1 G | SC, IM, IV | J2730 |
| PREGNYL | 1,000 USP U | IM | J0725 | PROTROPIN | 1 MG | SC, IM | J2940 |
| PRELONE | 5 MG | ORAL | J7510 | PROVENTIL NONCOMPOUNDED, CONCENTRATED | 1 MG | INH | J7611 |
| PREMARIN | 25 MG | IV, IM | J1410 | | | | |
| PRENATAL VITAMINS | 30 TABS | ORAL | S0197 | PROVENTIL NONCOMPOUNDED, UNIT DOSE | 1 MG | INH | J7613 |
| PRI-ANDRIOL LA | 50 MG | IM | J2320 | PROVOCHOLINE POWDER | 1 MG | INH | J7674 |
| PRIALT | 1 MCG | OTH | J2278 | PROZINE-50 | 25 MG | IM | J2950 |
| PRIMACOR | 5 MG | IV | J2260 | PULMICORT | 0.25 MG | INH | J7633 |
| PRIMATRIX | PER SQ. CM. | OTH | J7349 ● | PULMICORT RESPULES | 0.5 MG | INH | J7627 |
| PRIMAXIN | 250 MG | IV, IM | J0743 | PULMICORT RESPULES NONCOMPOUNDED, CONCETRATED | 0.25 MG | INH | J7626 |
| PRIMESTRIN AQUEOUS | 1 MG | IM, IV | J1410 | | | | |
| PRIMETHASONE | 1 MG | IM, IV, OTH | J1100 | PULMOZYME | 1 MG | INH | J7639 |
| PRI-METHYLATE | 80 MG | IM | J1040 | PURINETHOL | 50 MG | ORAL | S0108 |
| PRISCOLINE HCL | 25 MG | IV | J2670 | PYRIDOXINE HCL | 100 MG | INJ | J3415 |
| PROCAINAMIDE HCL | 1 G | IM, IV | J2690 | QUADRAMET | 50 MCI | IV | A9605 |
| PROCARBAZINE HCL | 50 MG | ORAL | S0182 | QUELICIN | 20 MG | IM, IV | J0330 |
| PROCHLOPERAZINE MALEATE | 5 MG | ORAL | S0183 | QUINUPRISTIN/DALFOPRISTIN | 500 MG | IV | J2770 |
| PROCHLORPERAZINE | 10 MG | IM, IV | J0780 | RANIBIZUMAB | 0.5 MG | OTH | C9233 |
| PROCHLORPERAZINE MALEATE | 10 MG | ORAL | Q0165 | RANITIDINE HCL | 25 MG | INJ | J2780 |
| PROCHLORPERAZINE MALEATE | 5 MG | ORAL | Q0164 | RAPAMUNE | 1 MG | ORAL | J7520 |
| PROCRIT, ESRD USE | 1,000 U | SC, IV | J0886 | | | | |

Appendix 1 — Table of Drugs

# APPENDIX 1 — TABLE OF DRUGS

| Drug Name | Unit Per: | Route | Code |
|---|---|---|---|
| RAPTIVA | 125 MG | SC | S0162 |
| RASBURICASE | 50 MCG | IM | J2783 |
| REBETRON KIT | 1,000,000 UNITS | SC, IM | J9214 |
| REBIF | 11 MCG | SC | Q3026 |
| REBIF | 33 MCG | SC | J1825 |
| RECLAST | 1 MG | IV | J3488 ▲ |
| RECOMBINATE | 1 IU | IV | J7192 |
| REDISOL | 1,000 MCG | SC. IM | J3420 |
| REFACTO | 1 IU | IV | J7192 |
| REFLUDAN | 50 MG | IM, IV | J1945 |
| REGITINE | 5 MG | IM, IV | J2760 |
| REGLAN | 10 MG | IV | J2765 |
| REGRANEX GEL | 0.5 G | OTH | J0157 |
| REGRANEX GEL | 0.5 G | OTH | S0157 |
| REGULAR INSULIN | 5 UNITS | SC | J1815 |
| RELAXIN | 10 ML | IV, IM | J2800 |
| RELION | 5 U | SC | J1815 |
| RELION NOVOLIN | 50 U | SC | J1817 |
| REMICADE | 10 MG | IV | J1745 |
| REMODULIN | 1 MG | SC | J3285 |
| REODULIN | 1 MG | SC | J3285 |
| REOPRO | 10 MG | IV | J0130 |
| REPRONEX | 75 IU | SC, IM, IV | S0122 |
| RESP SYNCYTIAL VIR IMMUNE GLOB | 50 MG | IV | J1565 |
| RESPIGAM | 50 MG | IV | J1565 |
| RESPIROL NONCOMPOUNDED, CONCENTRATED | 1 MG | INH | J7611 |
| RESPIROL NONCOMPOUNDED, UNIT DOSE | 1 MG | INH | J7613 |
| RETAVASE | 18.1 MG | IV | J2993 |
| RETEPLASE | 18.1 MG | IV | J2993 |
| RETISERT | IMPLANT | OTH | J7311 |
| RETROVIR | 10 MG | IV | J3485 |
| RETROVIR | 100 MG | ORAL | S0104 |
| RHEOMACRODEX | 500 ML | IV | J7100 |
| RHEUMATREX DOSE PACK | 2.5 MG | ORAL | J8610 |
| RHO D IMMUNE GLOBULIN | 100 IU | IV | J2792 |
| RHO D IMMUNE GLOBULIN | 50 MCG | IM | J2788 |
| RHOGAM | 300 MCG | IM | J2790 |
| RHOGAM | 50 MCG | IM | J2788 |
| RHOPHYLAC | 100 IU | IM, IV | J2791 ▲ |
| RIMANTADINE HYDROCHLORIDE | 100 MG | ORAL | G9036 |
| RIMANTADINE HYDROCHLORIDE (GENERIC) | 100 MG | ORAL | G9020 |
| RIMSO 50 | 50 ML | IV | J1212 ▲ |
| RINGERS LACTATE INFUSION | 1,000 ML | VAR | J7120 |
| RISPERDAL COSTA LONG ACTING | 0.5 MG | IM | J2794 |
| RISPERIDONE, LONG ACTING | 0.5 MG | IM | J2794 |
| RITUXAN | 100 MG | IV | J9310 |
| RITUXIMAB | 100 MG | IV | J9310 |
| ROBAXIN | 10 ML | IV, IM | J2800 |
| ROBINUL | 1 MG | INH | J7643 |
| ROCEPHIN | 250 MG | IV, IM | J0696 |
| ROFERON-A | 3,000,000 U | SC, IM | J9213 |

| Drug Name | Unit Per: | Route | Code |
|---|---|---|---|
| ROPIVACAINE HYDROCHLORIDE | 1 MG | VAR | J2795 |
| RUBEX | 10 MG | IV | J9000 |
| RUBIDIUM RB-82 | 60 MCI | IV | A9555 |
| RUBRAMIN PC | 1,000 MCG | SC, IM | J3420 |
| RUBRATOPE 57 | 1 MCI | ORAL | A9559 |
| SAIZEN | 1 MG | SC | J2941 |
| SAIZEN SOMATROPIN RDNA ORIGIN | 1 MG | SC | J2941 |
| SALINE OR STERILE WATER, METERED DOSE DISPENSER | 10 ML | INH | A4218 |
| SALINE, STERILE WATER, AND/OR DEXTROSE DILUENT/FLUSH | 10 ML | VAR | A4216 |
| SALINE/STERILE WATER | 500 ML | VAR | A4217 |
| SAMARIUM LEXIDRONAMM | 50 MCI | IV | A9605 |
| SANDIMMUNE | 100 MG | ORAL | J7502 |
| SANDIMMUNE | 25 MG | ORAL | J7515 |
| SANDIMMUNE | 250 MG | OTH | J7516 |
| SANDOGLOBULIN | 1 G | IV | J1563 |
| SCANDONEST | PER 10 ML | IV | J0670 ● |
| SANDOSTATIN | 25 MCG | SC, IV | J2354 |
| SANDOSTATIN LAR | 1 MG | IM | J2353 |
| SANGCYA | 100 MG | ORAL | J7502 |
| SANO-DROL | 40 MG | IM | J1030 |
| SANO-DROL | 80 MG | IM | J1040 |
| SAQUINAVIR | 200 MG | ORAL | S0140 |
| SARGRAMOSTIM (GM-CSF) | 50 MCG | IV | J2820 |
| SECREFLO | 1 MCG | IV | J2850 |
| SECRETIN, SYNTHETIC, HUMAN | 1 MCG | IV | J2850 |
| SENSORCAINE | 30 ML | VAR | S0200 |
| SEPTRA IV | 10 ML | IV | S0039 |
| SERMORELIN ACETATE | 1 MCG | IV | Q0515 |
| SEROSTIM | 1 MG | SC | J2941 |
| SEROSTIM RDNA ORIGIN | 1 MG | SC | J2941 |
| SILDENAFIL CITRATE | 25 MG | ORAL | S0090 |
| SIMULECT | 20 MG | IV | J0480 |
| SINCALIDE | 5 MCG | IV | J2805 |
| SIROLIMUS | 1 MG | ORAL | J7520 |
| SMZ-TMP | 10 ML | IV | S0039 |
| SODIUM FERRIC GLUCONATE COMPLEX IN SUCROSE | 12.5 MG | IV | J2916 |
| SODIUM HYALURONATE | 1 MG | OTH | J7318 |
| SODIUM HYALURONATE | INJ | OTH | J7319 |
| SODIUM IODIDE I-131 CAPSULE DIAGNOSTIC | 1 MCI | ORAL | A9528 |
| SODIUM IODIDE I-131 CAPSULE THERAPEUTIC | 1 MCI | ORAL | A9517 |
| SODIUM IODIDE I-131 SOLUTION THERAPEUTIC | 1 MCI | ORAL | A9530 |
| SODIUM PHOSPHATE P32 | 1 MCI | IV | A9563 |
| SOLGANAL | 50 MG | IM | J2910 |
| SOLIRIS | 10 MG | IV | J1300 ▲ |
| SOLUREX | 1 MG | IM, IV, OTH | J1100 |
| SOLTAMOX | 10 MG | ORAL | S0187 |
| SOLU-CORTEF | 100 MG | IV, IM, SC | J1720 |
| SOLU-MEDROL | 125 MG | IM, IV | J2930 |
| SOLU-MEDROL | 40 MG | IM, IV | J2920 |
| SOMATREM | 1 MG | SC, IM | J2940 |

**Appendix 1 — Table of Drugs**

| Drug Name | Unit Per: | Route | Code |
|---|---|---|---|
| SOMATROPIN | 1 MG | SC | J2941 |
| SPARINE | 25 MG | IM | J2950 |
| SPECTINOMYCIN DIHYDROCHLORIDE | 2 G | IM | J3320 |
| SPECTRO-DEX | 1 MG | IM, IV, OTH | J1100 |
| SPORANOX | 50 MG | IV | J1835 |
| STADOL | 1 MG | IM, IV | J0595 |
| STADOL NS | 25 MG | OTH | S0012 |
| STERAPRED | 5 MG | ORAL | J7506 |
| STERILE WATER OR SALINE, METERED DOSE DISPENSER | 10 ML | INH | A4218 |
| STERILE WATER, SALINE, AND/OR DEXTROSE DILUENT/FLUSH | 10 ML | VAR | A4216 |
| STERILE WATER/SALINE | 500 ML | VAR | A4217 |
| STREPTASE | 250,000 IU | IV | J2995 |
| STREPTOKINASE | 250,000 IU | IV | J2995 |
| STREPTOMYCIN | 1 G | IM | J3000 |
| STREPTOZOCIN | 1 GM | IV | J9320 |
| STRONTIUM 89 CHLORIDE | 1 MCI | IV | A9600 |
| SUBLIMAZE | 0.1 MG | IM, IV | J3010 |
| SUCCINYLCHOLINE CHLORIDE | 20 MG | IM, IV | J0330 |
| SULFAMETHOXAZOLE AND TRIMETHOPRIM | 10 ML | IV | S0039 |
| SULFUTRIM | 10 ML | IV | S0039 |
| SUMATRIPTAN SUCCINATE | 6 MG | SC | J3030 |
| SUPARTZ | PER DOSE | OTH | J7321 ▲ |
| SUPPRELIN LA | 10 MCG | OTH | J1675 ● |
| SUS-PHRINE | UP TO 1 ML | VAR | J0170 |
| SYNAGIS | 50 MG | IM | C9003 |
| SYNERCID | 500 MG | IV | J2770 |
| SYNTOCINON | 10 UNITS | IV | J2590 |
| SYNVISC | PER DOSE | OTH | J7322 ▲ |
| SYTOBEX | 1,000 MCG | SC, IM | J3420 |
| T-GEN | 250 MG | ORAL | Q0173 |
| TACRINE HCL | 10 MG | ORAL | S0014 |
| TACROLIMUS | 1 MG | ORAL | J7507 |
| TACROLIMUS | 5 MG | OTH | J7525 |
| TAGAMET HCL | 300 MG | IM, IV | S0023 |
| TALWIN | 30 MG | IM, SC, IV | J3070 |
| TAMOXIFEN CITRATE | 10 MG | ORAL | S0187 |
| TAXOL | 30 MG | IV | J9265 |
| TAXOTERE | 20 MG | IV | J9170 |
| TAZICEF | 500 MG | IM, IV | J0713 |
| TEBAMIDE | 250 MG | ORAL | Q0173 |
| TEBOROXIME, TECHNETIUM TC-99 M | PER STUDY DOSE | IV | A9501 ● |
| TECHNEPLEX | 25 MCI | IV | A9539 |
| TECHNESCAN | UP TO 30 MCI | IV | A9561 ▲ |
| TECHNESCAN FANOLESOMAB | STUDY DOSE | IV | A9566 |
| TECHNESCAN MAA | 10 MCI | IV | A9540 |
| TECHNESCAN MAG3 | STUDY DOSE | IV | A9562 |
| TECHNESCAN PYP | 25 MCI | IV | A9538 |
| TECHNESCAN PYP KIT | UP TO 25 MCI | IV | A9538 ● |
| TECHNETIUM SESTAMBI | 40 MCI | IV | A9500 |
| TECHNETIUM TC 99M ACRITUMOMAB | 25 MCI | IV | A9549 |

| Drug Name | Unit Per: | Route | Code |
|---|---|---|---|
| TECHNETIUM TC 99M APCITIDE | 20 MCI | IV | A9504 |
| TECHNETIUM TC 99M ARCITUMOMAB, DIAGNOSTIC | 45 MCI | IV | A9568 |
| TECHNETIUM TC 99M BICISATE | 25 MCI | IV | A9557 |
| TECHNETIUM TC 99M DEPREOTIDE | 35 MCI | IV | A9536 |
| TECHNETIUM TC 99M EXAMETAZIME | 25 MCI | IV | A9521 |
| TECHNETIUM TC-99M EXAMETAZIME LABELED AUTOLOGOUS WHITE BLOOD CELLS | PER STUDY DOSE | IV | A9596 |
| TECHNETIUM TC 99M FANOLESOMAB | 25 MCI | IV | A9566 |
| TECHNETIUM TC 99M LABELED RED BLOOD CELLS | 30 MCI | IV | A9560 |
| TECHNETIUM TC 99M MACROAGGREGATED ALBUMIN | 10 MCI | IV | A9540 |
| TECHNETIUM TC 99M MDI-MDP | 30 MCI | IV | A9503 ● |
| TECHNETIUM TC 99M MEBROFENIN | 15 MCI | IV | A9537 |
| TECHNETIUM TC 99M MEDRONATE | 30 MCI | IV | A9503 ● |
| TECHNETIUM TC 99M MERTIATIDE | 15 MCI | IV | A9562 |
| TECHNETIUM TC 99M OXIDRONATE | 30 MCI | IV | A9561 |
| TECHNETIUM TC 99M PENTETATE | 25 MCI | IV | A9539 |
| TECHNETIUM TC 99M PENTETATE | 75 MCI | INH | A9539 |
| TECHNETIUM TC 99M PYROPHOSPHATE | 25 MCI | IV | A9538 |
| TECHNETIUM TC 99M SODIUM GLUCEPATATE | 25 MCI | IV | A9550 |
| TECHNETIUM TC 99M SUCCIMER | 10 MCI | IV | A9551 |
| TECHNETIUM TC 99M SULFUR COLLOID | 20 MCI | IV | A9541 |
| TECHNETIUM TC-99M TEBOROXIME | PER STUDY DOSE | IV | A9501 ● |
| TECHNETIUM TC 99M TETROFOSMIN | 40 MCI | IV | A9502 |
| TECHNILITE | PER MCI | IV | A9512 ● |
| TEMODAR | 100 MG | ORAL | J8700 |
| TEMOZOLOMIDE | 100 MG | ORAL | J8700 |
| TENECTEPLASE | 50 MG | IV | J3100 |
| TENIPOSIDE | 50 MG | IV | Q2017 |
| TEQUIN | 10 MG | IV | J1590 |
| TERBUTALINE SULFATE | 1 MG | SC, IV | J3105 |
| TERBUTALINE SULFATE, COMPOUNDED, CONCENTRATED | 1 MG | INH | J7680 |
| TERBUTALINE SULFATE, COMPOUNDED, UNIT DOSE | 1 MG | INH | J7681 |
| TERIPARATIDE | 10 MCG | SC | J3110 |
| TERRAMYCIN | 50 MG | IM | J2460 |
| TESTAQUA | 50 MG | IM | J3140 |
| TESTERONE | 50 MG | IM | J3140 |
| TESTEX | 50 MG | IM | J3150 |
| TESTOJECT-50 | 50 MG | IM | J3140 |
| TESTONE LA 100 | 100 MG | IM | J3120 |
| TESTONE LA 200 | 100 MG | IM | J3130 |
| TESTOSTERONE AQUEOUS | 50 MG | IM | J3140 |
| TESTOSTERONE CYPIONATE | 1 CC, 200 MG | IM | J1080 |
| TESTOSTERONE CYPIONATE | UP TO 100 MG | IM | J1070 |
| TESTOSTERONE CYPIONATE & ESTRADIOL CYPIONATE | 1 ML | IM | J1060 |
| TESTOSTERONE ENANTHATE | 100 MG | IM | J3120 |

# APPENDIX 1 — TABLE OF DRUGS

| Drug Name | Unit Per: | Route | Code |
|-----------|-----------|-------|------|
| TESTOSTERONE ENANTHATE | 200 MG | IM | J3130 |
| TESTOSTERONE ENANTHATE & ESTRADIOL VALERATE | UP TO 1 CC | IM | J0900 |
| TESTOSTERONE PELLET | 75 MG | OTH | S0189 |
| TESTOSTERONE PROPIONATE | 100 MG | IM | J3150 |
| TESTOSTERONE SUSPENSION | 50 MG | IM | J3140 |
| ~~TESTRIIN PA~~ | ~~100 MG~~ | ~~IM~~ | ~~J3130~~ |
| TESTRO AQ | 50 MG | IM | J3140 |
| TETANUS IMMUNE GLOBULIN | 250 U | IM | J1670 |
| TETRACYCLINE HCL | 250 MG | IV | J0120 |
| THALLOUS CHLORIDE | 1 MCI | IV | A9505 |
| THALLOUS CHLORIDE TL-201 | 1 MCI | IV | A9505 |
| THALLOUS CHLORIDE USP | 1 MCI | IV | A9505 |
| THEELIN AQUEOUS | 1 MG | IM, IV | J1435 |
| THEOPHYLLINE | 40 MG | IV | J2810 |
| THERACYS | VIAL | IV | J9031 |
| THIAMINE HCL | 100 MG | INJ | J3411 |
| THIETHYLPERAZINE MALEATE | 10 MG | IM | J3280 |
| THIETHYLPERAZINE MALEATE | 10 MG | ORAL | Q0174 |
| THIMAZIDE | 250 MG | ORAL | Q0173 |
| THIOTEPA | 15 MG | IV | J9340 |
| THORAZINE | 10 MG | ORAL | Q0171 |
| THORAZINE | 25 MG | ORAL | Q0172 |
| THORAZINE | 50 MG | IM, IV | J3230 |
| THROMBATE III | 1 IU | IV | J7197 |
| THYMOGLOBULIN | 25 MG | OTH | J7511 |
| THYROGEN | 0.9 MG | IM, SC | J3240 |
| THYROTROPIN ALPHA | 0.9 MG | IM, SC | J3240 |
| ~~THYTROPAR~~ | ~~0.9 MG~~ | ~~SC, IM~~ | ~~J3240~~ |
| TICARCILLIN DISODIUM AND CLAVULANATE | 3.1 G | IV | S0040 |
| TICE BCG | VIAL | OTH | J9031 |
| TICON | 250 MG | IM | Q0173 ▲ |
| TIGAN | 200 MG | IM | J3250 |
| TIGECYCLINE | 1 MG | IV | J3243 |
| TIJECT-20 | 200 MG | IM | J3250 |
| TIMENTIN | 3.1 G | IV | S0040 |
| TINZAPARIN | 1,000 IU | SC | J1655 |
| TIROFIBAN HCL | 0.25 MG | IM, IV | J3246 |
| ~~TIROFIBAN HYDROCHLORIDE~~ | ~~12.5 MG~~ | ~~IM, IV~~ | ~~J3246~~ |
| TISSUEMEND | PER SQ. CM. | OTH | J7348 ● |
| TNKASE | 50 MG | IV | J3100 |
| TOBI | 300 MG | INH | J7682 |
| TOBRAMYCIN COMPOUNDED, UNIT DOSE | 300 MG | INH | J7685 |
| TOBRAMYCIN SULFATE | 80 MG | IM, IV | J3260 |
| TOBRAMYCIN, NONCOMPOUNDED, UNIT DOSE | 300 MG | INH | J7682 |
| TOLAZOLINE HCL | 25 MG | IV | J2670 |
| TOPOSAR | 10 MG | IV | J9181 |
| TOPOSAR | 100 MG | IV | J9182 |
| TOPOTECAN | 4 MG | IV | J9350 |
| ~~TORADOL IV/IM~~ | ~~15 MG~~ | ~~IM, IV~~ | ~~J1885~~ |
| TORECAN | 10 MG | ORAL | Q0174 ▲ |
| TORNALATE | PER MG | INH | J7629 |
| TORNALATE CONCENTRATE | PER MG | INH | J7628 |

| Drug Name | Unit Per: | Route | Code |
|-----------|-----------|-------|------|
| TORSEMIDE | 10 MG | IV | J3265 |
| TOSITUMOMAB DIAGNOSTIC | DOSE | IV | A9544 |
| TOSITUMOMAB THERAPEUTIC | DOSE | IV | A9545 |
| TOTECT | PER 250 MG | IV | J1190 ● |
| TRANSCYTE | PER 247 SQ CM | OTH | J7340 |
| TRASTUZUMAB | 10 MG | IV | J9355 |
| TRASYLOL | 10,000 KIU | IV | J0365 |
| TRELSTAR DEPOT | 3.75 MG | IM | J3315 |
| TRELSTAR DEPOT PLUS DEBIOCLIP KIT | 3.75 MG | IM | J3315 |
| TRELSTAR LA | 3.75 MG | IM | J3315 |
| TREPROSTINIL | 1 MG | SC | J3285 |
| TRETINOIN | 5 G | OTH | S0117 |
| TRI-KORT | 10 MG | IM | J3301 |
| TRIAM-A | 10 MG | IM | J3301 |
| TRIAMCINOLONE ACETONIDE | 10 MG | IM | J3301 |
| TRIAMCINOLONE DIACETATE | 5 MG | IM | J3302 |
| TRIAMCINOLONE HEXACETONIDE | 5 MG | VAR | J3303 |
| TRIAMCINOLONE, COMPOUNDED, CONCENTRATED | 1 MG | INH | J7683 |
| TRIAMCINOLONE, COMPOUNDED, UNIT DOSE | 1 MG | INH | J7684 |
| TRIBAN | 250 MG | ORAL | Q0173 |
| TRILIFON | 4 MG | ORAL | Q0175 |
| TRILOG | 10 MG | IM | J3301 |
| TRILONE | 5 MG | IM | J3302 |
| TRIMETHOBENZAMIDE HCL | 200 MG | IM | J3250 |
| TRIMETHOBENZAMIDE HCL | 250 MG | ORAL | Q0173 |
| TRIMETREXATE GLUCURONATE | 25 MG | IV | J3305 |
| TRIPTORELIN PAMOATE | 3.75 MG | IM | J3315 |
| TRISENOX | 1 MG | IV | J9017 |
| TROBICIN | 2 G | IM | J3320 |
| TRUXADRYL | 50 MG | IV, IM | J1200 |
| ~~TRYPTANOL~~ | ~~20 MG~~ | ~~IM~~ | ~~J1320~~ |
| TYGACIL | 1 MG | IV | J3243 |
| TYPE A BOTOX | 1 U | OTH | J0585 |
| TYSABRI | 1 MG | IV | J2323 ● |
| ULTRALENTE | 5 UNITS | SC | J1815 |
| ULTRA-TECHNEKOW | PER MCI | IV | A9512 ● |
| ULTRATAG | 30 MCI | IV | A9560 |
| ULTRAVIST | 1 ML | IV | Q9949 |
| ULTRAVIST 150 | 1 ML | IV | Q9946 |
| ULTRAVIST 240 | 1 ML | IV | Q9947 |
| ULTRAVIST 370 | 1 ML | IV | Q9950 |
| UNASYN | 1.5 G | IM, IV | J0295 |
| UNCLASSIFIED BIOLOGICS | | | J3590 |
| UREA | 40 G | IV | J3350 |
| ~~UREAPHIL~~ | ~~40 G~~ | ~~IV~~ | ~~J3350~~ |
| UROFOLLITROPIN | 75 IU | SC, IM | J3355 |
| UROKINASE | 250,000 IU | IV | J3365 |
| UROKINASE | 5,000 IU | IV | J3364 |
| ~~V-GAN 25~~ | ~~50 MG~~ | ~~IM, IV~~ | ~~J2550~~ |
| ~~V-GAN 50~~ | ~~50 MG~~ | ~~IM, IV~~ | ~~J2550~~ |
| VALERGEN | 10 MG | IM | J1380 |
| VALERGEN | 20 MG | IM | J1390 |

| Drug Name | Unit Per: | Route | Code |
|---|---|---|---|
| VALIUM | 5 MG | IV, IM | J3360 |
| VALRUBICIN | 200 MG | OTH | J9357 |
| VALSTAR | 200 MG | OTH | J9357 |
| VANCOCIN | 500 MG | IM, IV | J3370 |
| VANCOMYCIN HCL | 500 MG | IV, IM | J3370 |
| VANTAS | 50 MG | OTH | J9225 |
| VECTIBIX | 10 MG | IV | C9235 |
| VECTIBIX | 10 MG | IV | J9303 ● |
| VELCADE | 0.1 MG | IV | J9041 |
| VELOSULIN | 5 UNITS | SC | J1815 |
| VELOSULIN BR | 5 U | SC | J1815 |
| VENOFER | 1 MG | IV | J1756 |
| VENOGLOBULIN-S | 1 G | IV | J1563 |
| VENTOLIN NONCOMPOUNDED, CONCENTRATED | 1 MG | INH | J7611 |
| VENTOLIN NONCOMPOUNDED, UNIT DOSE | 1 MG | INH | J7613 |
| VEPESID | 10 MG | IV | J9181 |
| VEPESID | 100 MG | IV | J9182 |
| VEPESID | 50 MG | ORAL | J8560 |
| VERSED | 1 MG | IM, IV | J2250 |
| VERTEPORFIN | 0.1 MG | IV | J3396 |
| VFEND | 200 MG | IV | J3465 |
| VIAGRA | 25 MG | ORAL | S0090 |
| VIDAZA | 1 MG | SC | J9025 |
| VIDEX | 25 MG | ORAL | S0137 |
| VINBLASTINE SULFATE | 1 MG | IV | J9360 |
| VINCRISTINE SULFATE | 1 MG | IV | J9370 |
| VINCRISTINE SULFATE | 2 MG | IV | J9375 |
| VINORELBINE TARTRATE | 10 MG | IV | J9390 |
| VIRILON | 1 CC, 200 MG | IM | J1080 |
| VISIPAQUE 270 | 1 ML | IV | Q9948 |
| VISIPAQUE 320 | 1 ML | IV | Q9949 |
| VISTAJECT-25 | 25 MG | IM | J3410 |
| VISTARIL | 25 MG | IM | J3410 |
| VISTARIL | 25 MG | ORAL | Q0177 |
| VISTIDE | 375 MG | IV | J0740 |
| VISUDYNE | 0.1 MG | IV | J3396 |
| VITAMIN B-12 CYANOCOBALAMIN | 1,000 MCG | IM, SC | J3420 |
| VITRASE | 1 USP | OTH | J3471 |
| VITRASE | 1,000 USP | OTH | J3472 |
| VITRASERT | 4.5 MG | OTH | J7310 |
| VITRAVENE | 1.65 MG | OTH | J1452 |
| VIVITROL | 1 MG | IM | J2315 |
| VON WILLEBRAND FACTOR COMPLEX, RISTOCETIN COFACTOR | IU | IV | J7187 |
| VORICONAZOLE | 200 MG | IV | J3465 |
| VUMON | 50 MG | IV | Q2017 |
| WEHAMINE | 50 MG | IM, IV | J1240 |
| WEHDRYL | 50 MG | IM, IV | J1200 |
| WELBUTRIN SR | 150 MG | ORAL | S0106 |
| WINRHO SDF | 100 IU | IV | J2792 |
| WYCILLIN | 600,000 U | IM, IV | J2510 |
| ~~WYDASE~~ | ~~150 UNITS~~ | ~~VAR~~ | ~~J3470~~ |
| XELODA | 150 MG | ORAL | J8520 |

| Drug Name | Unit Per: | Route | Code |
|---|---|---|---|
| XELODA | 500 MG | ORAL | J8521 |
| XENON XE-133 | 10 MCI | OTH | A9558 |
| XOLAIR | 5 MG | SC | J2357 |
| ~~XOPENENEX HFA NONCOMPOUNDED, CONCENTRATED~~ | ~~0.5 MG~~ | ~~INH~~ | ~~J7612~~ |
| ~~XOPENEX NONCOMPOUNDED, UNIT DOSE~~ | ~~0.5 MG~~ | ~~INH~~ | ~~J7614~~ |
| XYLOCAINE | 10 MG | IV | J2001 |
| YTTRIUM 90 IBRITUMOMAB TIUXETAN | TX DOSE | IV | A9543 |
| ZALCITABINE (DDC) | 0.375 MG | ORAL | S0141 |
| ZANAMIVIR (BRAND NAME) | 10 MG | INH | G9034 |
| ZANAMIVIR (GENERIC) | 10 MG | INH | G9018 |
| ZANOSAR | 1 GM | IV | J9320 |
| ZANTAC | 25 MG | INJ | J2780 |
| ZEMAIRA | 10 MG | IV | J0256 |
| ZEMPLAR | 1 MCG | IV, IM | J2501 |
| ZENAPAX | 25 MG | OTH | J7513 |
| ~~ZETRAN~~ | ~~5 MG~~ | ~~IM, IV~~ | ~~J3360~~ |
| ZEVALIN | UP TO 5 MCI | IV | A9542 ● |
| ZEVALIN DIAGNOSTIC | TX DOSE | IV | A9542 |
| ZEVALIN THERAPEUTIC | TX DOSE | IV | A9543 |
| ZICONOTIDE | 1 MCG | IT | J2278 |
| ZIDOVUDINE | 10 MG | IV | J3485 |
| ZIDOVUDINE | 100 MG | ORAL | S0104 |
| ZINACEFT | PER 750 MG | IM, IV | J0697 ● |
| ZINECARD | 250 MG | IV | J1190 |
| ZIPRASIDONE MESYLATE | 10 MG | IM | J3486 |
| ZITHROMAX | 1 G | ORAL | Q0144 |
| ZITHROMAX | 500 MG | IV | J0456 |
| ZOFRAN | 1 MG | IV | J2405 |
| ZOFRAN | 4 MG | ORAL | S0181 |
| ZOFRAN | 8 MG | ORAL | Q0179 |
| ZOLADEX | 3.6 MG | SC | J9202 |
| ZOLEDRONIC ACID | 1 MG | IV | J3487 |
| ZOLEDRONIC ACID FOR PAGET'S DISEASE | 1 MG | IV | Q4095 |
| ZOLEDRONIC ACID (RECLAST) | 1 MG | IV | J3488 ● |
| ZOMETA | 1 MG | IV | J3487 |
| ZORBTIVE | 1 MG | SC | J2941 |
| ZOSYN | 1 G/1.125 GM | IV | J2543 |
| ZOVIRAX | 5 MG | IV | J0133 |
| ZOVIRAX | 50 MG | IV | S0071 |
| ZYPREXA | 2.5 MG | IM | S0166 |
| ZYVOX | 200 MG | IV | J2020 |

## NOT OTHERWISE CLASSIFIED DRUGS

| Drug Name | Unit Per: | Route | Code |
|---|---|---|---|
| ALGUCOSIDE ALFA | 1 MG | IV | J3490 |
| ALLOPURINOL SODIUM | 500 MG | IV | J3490 |
| AMINOCAPROIC ACID | 250 MG | IV | J3490 |
| ARFORMOTEROL TATRATE | 15 MCG | INH | J3490 |
| ARGININE HYDROCHLORIDE | 300 ML | IV | J3490 |
| ASCORBIC ACID | 250 MG | IV | J3490 |

# APPENDIX 1 — TABLE OF DRUGS

| Drug Name | Unit Per: | Route | Code |
|---|---|---|---|
| ATROPINE SULFATE/EDROPHONIUM CHLORIDE | 10 MG | IV | J3490 |
| AZTREONAM | 500 MG | IV | J3490 |
| BUMETANIDE | 0.25 MG | IM, IV | J3490 |
| BUPIVACAINE, 0.25% | 1 ML | OTH | J3490 |
| BUPIVACAINE, 0.50% | 1 ML | OTH | J3490 |
| BUPIVACAINE, 0.75% | 1 ML | OTH | J3490 |
| CALCIUM CHLORIDE | 100 MG | IV | J3490 |
| CIMETIDINE HCL | 150 MG | IM, IV | J3490 |
| CLAVULANTE POTASSIUM/TICARCILLIN DISODIUM | 0.1-3 GM | IV | J3490 |
| CLINDAMYCIN PHOSPHATE | 150 MG | IV | J3490 |
| COPPER SULFATE | 0.4 MG | INJ | J3490 |
| DEXTROSE 50% | 50 ML | IV | J3490 |
| DILTIAZEM HCL | 5 MG | IV | J3490 |
| DOXYCYCLINE HYCLATE | 100 MG | INJ | J3490 |
| ECULIZUMAB | 1 MG | IV | J3490 |
| EDROPHONIUM CHLORIDE | 10 MG | IM, IV | J3490 |
| ENALAPRILAT | 1.25 MG | IV | J3490 |
| ESMOLOL HCL | 10 MG | IV | J3490 |
| ESOMEPRAZOLE SODIUM | 20 MG | IV | J3490 |
| ETOMIDATE | 2 MG | IV | J3490 |
| FAMOTIDINE | 10 MG | IV | J3490 |
| FLUMAZENIL | 0.1 MG | IV | J3490 |
| FOLIC ACID | 5 MG | SC, IM, IV | J3490 |
| GLYCOPYRROLATE | 0.2 MG | IM, IV | J3490 |
| HEPAGAMB INTRAVENOUS | 0.5 ML | IV | J3490 |
| IDURSULFASE | 1 MG | IV | J3490 |
| KETAMINE HCL | 10 MG | IM, IV | J3490 |

| Drug Name | Unit Per: | Route | Code |
|---|---|---|---|
| LABETALOL HCL | 5 MG | INJ | J3490 |
| LIDOCAINE | 1 ML | VAR | J3490 |
| METOPROLOL TARTRATE | 1 MG | IV | J3490 |
| METRONIDAZOLE INJ | 500 MG | IV | J3490 |
| MORRHUATE SODIUM | 50 MG | OTH | J3490 |
| NAFCILLIN SODIUM | 1 GM | IM, IV | J3490 |
| NITROGLYCERIN | 5 MG | IV | J3490 |
| OLANZAPINE | 0.5 MG | IM | J3490 |
| PANITUMUMAB | 1 MG | IV | J3490 |
| PANITUMUMAB | 1MG | IV | J3490 |
| PEGASYS | 180 MCG | SC | J3490 |
| PEGINTERFERON ALFA-2A | 180 MCG | SC | J3490 |
| POTASSIUM ACETATE | 2 MEQ | IV | J3490 |
| POTASSIUM POSPHATE | 3 MMOL | IV | J3490 |
| PROPOFOL | 10 MG | IV | J3490 |
| PROTONIX | 40 MG | IV | J3490 |
| RANIBIZUMAB INJ | 0.5 MG | OTH | J3490 |
| RIFAMPIN | 600 MG | IV | J3490 |
| SARRACENIA PURPURA | 1 ML | INJ | J3490 |
| SODIUM ACETATE | 2 MEQ | | J3490 |
| SODIUM BICARBONATE, 8.4% | 50 ML | IV | J3490 |
| SODIUM CHLORIDE, HYPERTONIC | 250 CC | IV | J3490 |
| SODIUM THIOSULFATE | 100 MG | IV | J3490 |
| VALPROATE SODIUM | 100 MG | IV | J3490 |
| VASOPRESSIN | 20 UNITS | SC, IM | J3490 |
| VECURONIUM BROMIDE | 1 MG | IV | J3490 |
| VERAPAMIL HCL | 2.5 MG | IV | J3490 |

# APPENDIX 2 — MODIFIERS

| | |
|---|---|
| A1 | Dressing for one wound |
| A2 | Dressing for two wounds |
| A3 | Dressing for three wounds |
| A4 | Dressing for four wounds |
| A5 | Dressing for five wounds |
| A6 | Dressing for six wounds |
| A7 | Dressing for seven wounds |
| A8 | Dressing for eight wounds |
| A9 | Dressing for nine or more wounds |
| AA | Anesthesia services performed personally by anesthesiologist |
| AD | Medical supervision by a physician: more than four concurrent anesthesia procedures |
| AE | Registered dietician |
| AF | Specialty physician |
| AG | Primary physician |
| AH | Clinical psychologist |
| AJ | Clinical social worker |
| AK | Nonparticipating physician |
| AM | Physician, team member service |
| AP | Determination of refractive state was not performed in the course of diagnostic ophthalmological examination |
| AQ | Physician provider service in a physician scarcity area |
| AR | Physician assistant |
| AS | PA, nurse practitioner, or clinical nurse specialist services for assistant at surgery |
| AT | Acute treatment (this modifier should be used when reporting service 98940, 98941, 98942) |
| AU | Item furnished in conjunction with a urological, ostomy, or tracheostomy supply |
| AV | Item furnished in conjunction with a prosthetic device, prosthetic or orthotic |
| AW | Item furnished in conjunction with a surgical dressing |
| AX | Item furnished in conjunction with dialysis services |
| BA | Item furnished in conjunction with parenteral enteral nutrition (PEN) services |
| BL | Special acquisition of blood and blood products |
| BO | Orally administered nutrition, not by feeding tube |
| BP | The beneficiary has been informed of the purchase and rental options and has elected to purchase the item |
| BR | The beneficiary has been informed of the purchase and rental options and has elected to rent the item |
| BU | The beneficiary has been informed of the purchase and rental options and after 30 days has not informed the supplier of his/her decision |
| CA | Procedure payable only in the inpatient setting when performed emergently on an outpatient who expires prior to admission |
| CB | Service ordered by a renal dialysis facility (RDF) physician as part of the ESRD beneficiary's dialysis benefit, is not part of the composite rate, and is separately reimbursable |
| CC | Procedure code change (use CC when the procedure code submitted was changed either for administrative reasons or because an incorrect code was filed) |
| CD | AMCC test has been ordered by an ESRD facility or MCP physician that is a part of the composite rate and is not separately billable |
| CE | AMCC test has been ordered by an ESRD facility or MCP physician that is a composite rate test but is beyond the normal frequency covered under the rate and is separately reimbursable based on medically necessary |
| CF | AMCC test has been ordered by an ESRD facility or MCP physician that is not part of the composite rate and is separately billable |

| | |
|---|---|
| CR | Catastrophe/Disaster related |
| E1 | Upper left, eyelid |
| E2 | Lower left, eyelid |
| E3 | Upper right, eyelid |
| E4 | Lower right, eyelid |
| EA | Erythropoetic stimulating agent (ESA) administered to treat anemia due to anticancer chemotherapy |
| EB | Erythropoetic stimulating agent (ESA) administered to treat anemia due to anticancer radiotherapy |
| EC | Erythropoetic stimulating agent (ESA) administered to treat anemia due to anticancer radiotherapy or anticancer chemotherapy |
| ED | Hematocrit level has exceeded 39% (or hemoglobin level has exceeded 13.0 G/DL) for three or more consecutive billing cycles immediately prior to and including the current cycle |
| EE | Hematocrit level has not exceeded 39% (or hemoglobin level has not exceeded 13.0 G/DL) for three or more consecutive billing cycles immediately prior to and including the current cycle |
| EJ | Subsequent claims for a defined course of therapy, e.g., EPO, sodium hyaluronate, infliximab |
| EM | Emergency reserve supply (for ESRD benefit only) |
| EP | Service provided as part of Medicaid early periodic screening diagnosis and treatment (EPSDT) program |
| ET | Emergency services |
| EY | No physician or other licensed health care provider order for this item or service |
| F1 | Left hand, second digit |
| F2 | Left hand, third digit |
| F3 | Left hand, fourth digit |
| F4 | Left hand, fifth digit |
| F5 | Right hand, thumb |
| F6 | Right hand, second digit |
| F7 | Right hand, third digit |
| F8 | Right hand, fourth digit |
| F9 | Right hand, fifth digit |
| FA | Left hand, thumb |
| FB | Item provided without cost to provider, supplier or practitioner, or full credit received for replaced device (examples, but not limited to, covered under warranty, replaced due to defect, free samples) |
| FC | Partial credit received for replaced device |
| FP | Service provided as part of family planning program |
| G1 | Most recent URR reading of less than 60 |
| G2 | Most recent URR reading of 60 to 64.9 |
| G3 | Most recent URR reading of 65 to 69.9 |
| G4 | Most recent URR reading of 70 to 74.9 |
| G5 | Most recent URR reading of 75 or greater |
| G6 | ESRD patient for whom less than six dialysis sessions have been provided in a month |
| G7 | Pregnancy resulted from rape or incest or pregnancy certified by physician as life threatening |
| G8 | Monitored anesthesia care (MAC) for deep complex, complicated, or markedly invasive surgical procedure |
| G9 | Monitored anesthesia care (MAC) for patient who has history of severe cardiopulmonary condition |
| GA | Waiver of liability statement on file |
| GB | Claim being resubmitted for payment because it is no longer covered under a global payment demonstration |
| GC | This service has been performed in part by a resident under the direction of a teaching physician |
| GD | Units of service exceeds medically unlikely edit value and represents reasonable and necessary services |

# APPENDIX 2 — MODIFIERS

| | |
|---|---|
| GE | This service has been performed by a resident without the presence of a teaching physician under the primary care exception |
| GF | Nonphysician (e.g., nurse practitioner (NP), certified registered nurse anesthetist (CRNA), certified registered nurse (CRN), clinical nurse specialist (CNS), physician assistant (PA)) services in a critical access hospital |
| GG | Performance and payment of a screening mammogram and diagnostic mammogram on the same patient, same day |
| GH | Diagnostic mammogram converted from screening mammogram on same day |
| GJ | Opt out physician or practitioner emergency or urgent service |
| GK | Reasonable and necessary item/service associated with GA or GZ modifier |
| GL | Medically unnecessary upgrade provided instead of nonupgraded item, no charge, no advance beneficiary notice (ABN) |
| GM | Multiple patients on one ambulance trip |
| GN | Service delivered under an outpatient speech-language pathology plan of care |
| GO | Service delivered under an outpatient occupational therapy plan of care |
| GP | Service delivered under an outpatient physical therapy plan of care |
| GQ | Via asynchronous telecommunications system |
| GR | This service was performed in whole or in part by a resident in a department of veterans affairs medical center or clinic, supervised in accordance with VA policy |
| GS | Dosage of EPO or darbepoetin alfa has been reduced and maintained in response to hematocrit or hemoglobulin level |
| GT | Via interactive audio and video telecommunication systems |
| GV | Attending physician not employed or paid under arrangement by the patient's hospice provider |
| GW | Service not related to the hospice patient's terminal condition |
| GY | Item or service statutorily excluded, does not meet the definition of any Medicare benefit or, for non-Medicare insurers, is not a contract benefit |
| GZ | Item or service expected to be denied as not reasonable and necessary |
| H9 | Court-ordered |
| HA | Child/adolescent program |
| HB | Adult program, nongeriatric |
| HC | Adult program, geriatric |
| HD | Pregnant/parenting womens' program |
| HE | Mental health program |
| HF | Substance abuse program |
| HG | Opioid addiction treatment program |
| HH | Integrated mental health substance abuse program |
| HI | Integrated mental health and mental retardation/developmental disabilities program |
| HJ | Employee assistance program |
| HK | Specialized mental health programs for high-risk populations |
| HL | Intern |
| HM | Less than bachelor degree level |
| HN | Bachelors degree level |
| HO | Masters degree level |
| HP | Doctoral level |
| HQ | Group setting |
| HR | Family/couple with client present |
| HS | Family/couple without client present |
| HT | Multi-disciplinary team |
| HU | Funded by child welfare agency |
| HV | Funded state addictions agency |

| | |
|---|---|
| HW | Funded by state mental health agency |
| HX | Funded by county/local agency |
| HY | Funded by juvenile justice agency |
| HZ | Funded by criminal justice agency |
| J1 | Competitive acquisition program (CAP) no-pay submission for a prescription number |
| J2 | Competitive acquisition program (CAP), restocking of emergency drugs after emergency administration |
| J3 | Competitive acquisition program (CAP), drug not available through CAP as written, reimbursed under average sales price methodology |
| JA | Administered intravenously |
| JB | Administered subcutaneously |
| JW | Drug amount discarded/not administered to any patient |
| K0 | Lower extremity prosthesis functional level 0-does not have the ability or potential to ambulate or transfer safely with or without assistance and a prosthesis does not enhance their quality of life or mobility |
| K1 | Lower extremity prosthesis functional level 1-does have the ability or potential to use a prosthesis for transfer or ambulation on level surfaces at fixed cadence, typical of the limited and unlimited household ambulator. |
| K2 | Lower extremity prosthesis functional level 2-has the ability or potential for ambulation with the ability to traverse low level environmental barriers such as curbs, stairs, or uneven surfaces, typical of limited community ambulator |
| K3 | Lower extremity prosthesis functional level 3-has the ability or potential for ambulation with variable cadence, typical of the community ambulator who has the ability to traverse most environmental barriers and may have vocational, therapeutic, or exercise activity that demands prosthetic utilization beyond simple locomotion |
| K4 | Lower extremity prosthesis functional level 4-has the ability or potential for prosthetic ambulation that exceeds basic ambulation skills, exhibiting high impact, stress, or energy levels, typical of the prosthetic demands of the child, active adult, or athlete |
| KA | Add-on option/accessory for wheelchair |
| KB | Beneficiary requested upgrade for ABN, more than four modifiers identified on claim |
| KC | Replacement of special power wheelchair interface |
| KD | Drug or biological infused through DME |
| KF | Item designated by FDA as class III device |
| KG | DMEPOS item subject to DMEPOS competitive bidding program number 1 |
| KH | DMEPOS item, initial claim, purchase or first month rental |
| KI | DMEPOS item, second or third month rental |
| KJ | DMEPOS item, parenteral enteral nutrition (PEN) pump or capped rental, months four to 15 |
| KK | DMEPOS item subject to DMEPOS competitive bidding program number 2 |
| KL | DMEPOS item delivered via mail |
| KM | Replacement of facial prosthesis including new impression/moulage |
| KN | Replacement of facial prosthesis using previous master model |
| KO | Single drug unit dose formulation |
| KP | First drug of a multiple drug unit dose formulation |
| KQ | Second or subsequent drug of a multiple drug unit dose formulation |
| KR | Rental item, billing for partial month |
| KS | Glucose monitor supply for diabetic beneficiary not treated with insulin |
| KT | Beneficiary resides in a competitive bidding area and travels to a non-competitive area and receives item from a non-contract supplier |
| KU | DMEPOS item subject to DMEPOS competitive bidding program number 3 |

| | |
|---|---|
| **KV** | DMEPOS item subject to DMEPOS competitive bidding program that is furnished as part of a professional service |
| **KW** | DMEPOS item subject to DMEPOS competitive bidding program number 4 |
| **KX** | Requirements specified in the medical policy have been met |
| **KY** | DMEPOS item subject to DMEPOS competitive bidding program number 5 |
| **KZ** | New coverage not implemented by managed care |
| **LC** | Left circumflex coronary artery |
| **LD** | Left anterior descending coronary artery |
| **LL** | Lease/rental (use the LL modifier when DME equipment rental is to be applied against the purchase price) |
| **LR** | Laboratory round trip |
| **LS** | FDA-monitored intraocular lens implant |
| **LT** | Left side (used to identify procedures performed on the left side of the body) |
| **M2** | Medicare secondary payer (MSP) |
| **MS** | Six month maintenance and servicing fee for reasonable and necessary parts and labor which are not covered under any manufacturer or supplier warranty |
| **NR** | New when rented (use the NR modifier when DME which was new at the time of rental is subsequently purchased) |
| **NU** | New equipment |
| **P1** | Anesthesia physical status-Normal, healthy patient |
| **P2** | Anesthesia physical status-Patient with mild, systemic disease |
| **P3** | Anesthesia physical status-Patient with severe, systemic disease |
| **P4** | Anesthesia physical status-Patient with severe, systemic disease that is a constant threat to life |
| **P5** | Anesthesia physical status-Moribund patient who is not expected to survive without the operation |
| **P6** | Anesthesia physical status-Declared brain-dead patient whose organs are being removed for donor purposes |
| **PL** | Progressive addition lenses |
| **Q0** | Investigational clinical service provided in a clinical research study |
| **Q1** | Routine clinical service provided in a clinical research study that is in an approved clinical research study |
| **Q2** | HCFA/ORD demonstration project procedure/service |
| **Q3** | Live kidney donor surgery and related services |
| **Q4** | Service for ordering/referring physician qualifies as a service exemption |
| **Q5** | Service furnished by a substitute physician under a reciprocal billing arrangement |
| **Q6** | Service furnished by a locum tenens physician |
| **Q7** | One Class A finding |
| **Q8** | Two Class B findings |
| **Q9** | One Class B and two Class C findings |
| **QA** | FDA investigational device exemption |
| **QB** | Physician providing service in a rural HPSA |
| **QC** | Single channel monitoring |
| **QD** | Recording and storage in solid state memory by a digital recorder |
| **QE** | Prescribed amount of oxygen is less than one liter per minute (LPM) |
| **QF** | Prescribed amount of oxygen exceeds four LPM and portable oxygen is prescribed |
| **QG** | Prescribed amount of oxygen is greater than four liters per minute (LPM) |
| **QH** | Oxygen conserving device is being used with an oxygen delivery system |
| **QJ** | Services/items provided to a prisoner or patient in state or local custody. However, the state or local government, as applicable, meets the requirements in 42 CFR 411.4(B) |
| **QK** | Medical direction of two, three or four concurrent anesthesia procedures involving qualified individuals |
| **QL** | Patient pronounced dead after ambulance called |
| **QM** | Ambulance service provided under arrangement by a provider of services |
| **QN** | Ambulance service furnished directly by a provider of services |
| **QP** | Documentation is on file showing that the laboratory test(s) was ordered individually or ordered as a CPT-recognized panel other than automated profile codes 80002-80019, G0058, G0059, and G0060 |
| **QQ** | Claim submitted with a written statement of intent |
| **QR** | Item or service provided in a Medicare specified study |
| **QS** | Monitored anesthesia care service |
| **QT** | Recording and storage on tape by an analog tape recorder |
| **QU** | Physician providing service in an urban HPSA |
| **QV** | Item or service provided as routine care in a Medicare qualifying clinical trial |
| **QW** | CLIA waived test |
| **QX** | CRNA service: with medical direction by a physician |
| **QY** | Medical direction of one certified registered nurse anesthetist (CRNA) by an anesthesiologist |
| **QZ** | CRNA service: without medical direction by a physician |
| **RC** | Right coronary artery |
| **RD** | Drug provided to beneficiary, but not administered incident to |
| **RP** | Replacement and repair -RP may be used to indicate replacement of DME, orthotic and prosthetic devices which have been in use for sometime. The claim shows the code for the part, followed by the 'RP' modifier and the charge for the part. |
| **RR** | Rental (use the RR modifier when DME is to be rented) |
| **RT** | Right side (used to identify procedures performed on the right side of the body) |
| **SA** | Nurse practitioner rendering service in collaboration with a physician |
| **SB** | Nurse midwife |
| **SC** | Medically necessary service or supply |
| **SD** | Services provided by registered nurse with specialized, highly technical home infusion training |
| **SE** | State and/or federally-funded programs/services |
| **SF** | Second opinion ordered by a professional review organization (PRO) per section 9401, p.l. 99-272 (100% reimbursement - no Medicare deductible or coinsurance) |
| **SG** | Ambulatory surgical center (ASC) facility service |
| **SH** | Second concurrently administered infusion therapy |
| **SJ** | Third or more concurrently administered infusion therapy |
| **SK** | Member of high risk population (use only with codes for immunization) |
| **SL** | State supplied vaccine |
| **SM** | Second surgical opinion |
| **SN** | Third surgical opinion |
| **SQ** | Item ordered by home health |
| **SS** | Home infusion services provided in the infusion suite of the IV therapy provider |
| **ST** | Related to trauma or injury |
| **SU** | Procedure performed in physician's office (to denote use of facility and equipment) |
| **SV** | Pharmaceuticals delivered to patient's home but not utilized |
| **SW** | Services provided by a certified diabetic educator |
| **SY** | Persons who are in close contact with member of high-risk population (use only with codes for immunization) |
| **T1** | Left foot, second digit |
| **T2** | Left foot, third digit |

| | |
|---|---|
| T3 | Left foot, fourth digit |
| T4 | Left foot, fifth digit |
| T5 | Right foot, great toe |
| T6 | Right foot, second digit |
| T7 | Right foot, third digit |
| T8 | Right foot, fourth digit |
| T9 | Right foot, fifth digit |
| TA | Left foot, great toe |
| TC | Technical component. Under certain circumstances, a charge may be made for the technical component alone. Under those circumstances the technical component charge is identified by adding modifier 'TC' to the usual procedure number. Technical component charges are institutional charges and not billed separately by physicians. However, portable x-ray suppliers only bill for technical component and should utilize modifier TC. The charge data from portable x-ray suppliers will then be used to build customary and prevailing profiles. |
| TD | RN |
| TE | LPN/LVN |
| TF | Intermediate level of care |
| TG | Complex/high tech level of care |
| TH | Obstetrical treatment/services, prenatal or postpartum |
| TJ | Program group, child and/or adolescent |
| TK | Extra patient or passenger, nonambulance |
| TL | Early intervention/individualized family service plan (IFSP) |
| TM | Individualized education program (IEP) |
| TN | Rural/outside providers' customary service area |
| TP | Medical transport, unloaded vehicle |
| TQ | Basic life support by volunteer ambulance provider |
| TR | School-based individualized education program (IEP) services provided outside the public school district responsible for the student |
| TS | Follow-up service |
| TT | Individualized service provided to more than one patient in same setting |
| TU | Special payment rate, overtime |
| TV | Special payment rates, holidays/weekends |
| TW | Back-up equipment |
| U1 | Medicaid level of care 1, as defined by each state |
| U2 | Medicaid level of care 2, as defined by each state |
| U3 | Medicaid level of care 3, as defined by each state |
| U4 | Medicaid level of care 4, as defined by each state |
| U5 | Medicaid level of care 5, as defined by each state |
| U6 | Medicaid level of care 6, as defined by each state |
| U7 | Medicaid level of care 7, as defined by each state |
| U8 | Medicaid level of care 8, as defined by each state |
| U9 | Medicaid level of care 9, as defined by each state |
| UA | Medicaid level of care 10, as defined by each state |
| UB | Medicaid level of care 11, as defined by each state |

| | |
|---|---|
| UC | Medicaid level of care 12, as defined by each state |
| UD | Medicaid level of care 13, as defined by each state |
| UE | Used durable medical equipment |
| UF | Services provided in the morning |
| UG | Services provided in the afternoon |
| UH | Services provided in the evening |
| UJ | Services provided at night |
| UK | Services provided on behalf of the client to someone other than the client (collateral relationship) |
| UN | Two patients served |
| UP | Three patients served |
| UQ | Four patients served |
| UR | Five patients served |
| US | Six or more patients served |
| VP | Aphakic patient |

# APPENDIX 3 — ABBREVIATIONS AND ACRONYMS

## HCPCS Abbreviations and Acronyms

The following abbreviations and acronyms are used in the HCPCS descriptions:

| | |
|---|---|
| / | or |
| < | less than |
| <= | less than equal to |
| > | greater than |
| >= | greater than equal to |
| AC | alternating current |
| AFO | ankle-foot orthosis |
| AICC | anti-inhibitor coagulant complex |
| AK | above the knee |
| AKA | above knee amputation |
| ALS | advanced life support |
| AMP | ampule |
| ART | artery |
| ART | Arterial |
| ASC | ambulatory surgery center |
| ATT | attached |
| A-V | Arteriovenous |
| AVF | arteriovenous fistula |
| BICROS | bilateral routing of signals |
| BK | below the knee |
| BLS | basic life support |
| BP | blood pressure |
| BTE | behind the ear (hearing aid) |
| CAPD | continuous ambulatory peritoneal dialysis |
| Carb | carbohydrate |
| CBC | complete blood count |
| cc | cubic centimeter |
| CCPD | continuous cycling peritoneal analysis |
| CHF | congestive heart failure |
| CIC | completely in the canal (hearing aid) |
| CIM | Coverage Issue Manual |
| Clsd | closed |
| cm | centimeter |
| CMN | certificate of medical necessity |
| CMS | Centers for Medicare and Medicaid Services |
| CMV | Cytomegalovirus |
| Conc | concentrate |
| Conc | concentrated |
| Cont | continuous |
| CP | clinical psychologist |
| CPAP | continuous positive airway pressure |
| CPT | Current Procedural Terminology |
| CRF | chronic renal failure |
| CRNA | certified registered nurse anesthetist |
| CROS | contralateral routing of signals |
| CSW | clinical social worker |
| CT | computed tomography |
| CTLSO | cervical-thoracic-lumbar-sacral orthosis |
| cu | cubic |
| DC | direct current |
| DI | diurnal rhythm |
| Dx | diagnosis |
| DLI | donor leukocyte infusion |
| DME | durable medical equipment |
| DME MAC | durable medical equipment Medicare administrative contractor |
| DMEPOS | Durable Medical Equipment, Prosthestics, Orthotics and Other Supplies |
| DMERC | durable medical equipment regional carrier |
| DR | diagnostic radiology |
| DX | diagnostic |
| e.g. | for example |
| Ea | each |
| ECF | extended care facility |
| EEG | electroencephalogram |
| EKG | electrocardiogram |
| EMG | electromyography |
| EO | elbow orthosis |
| EP | electrophysiologic |
| EPO | epoetin alfa |
| EPSDT | early periodic screening, diagnosis and treatment |
| ESRD | end-stage renal disease |
| Ex | extended |
| Exper | experimental |
| Ext | external |
| F | french |
| FDA | Food and Drug Administration |
| FDG-PET | Positron emission with tomography with 18 fluorodeoxyglucose |
| Fem | female |
| FO | finger orthosis |
| FPD | fixed partial denture |
| Fr | french |
| ft | foot |
| G-CSF | filgrastim (granulocyte colony-stimulating factor) |
| gm | gram (g) |
| H2O | water |
| HCl | hydrochloric acid, hydrochloride |
| HCPCS | Healthcare Common Procedural Coding System |
| HCT | hematocrit |
| HFO | hand-finger orthosis |
| HHA | home health agency |
| HI | high |
| HI-LO | high-low |
| HIT | home infusion therapy |
| HKAFO | hip-knee-ankle foot orthosis |
| HLA | human leukocyte antigen |
| HMES | heat and moisture exchange system |
| HNPCC | hereditary non-polyposis colorectal cancer |
| HO | hip orthosis |
| HPSA | health professional shortage area |
| IA | intra-arterial administration |
| ip | interphalangeal |
| I-131 | Iodine 131 |
| ICF | intermediate care facility |
| ICU | intensive care facility |
| IM | intramuscular |
| in | inch |
| INF | infusion |
| INH | inhalation solution |
| INJ | injection |
| IOL | intraocular lens |
| IPD | intermittent peritoneal dialysis |
| IPPB | intermittent positive pressure breathing |
| IT | intrathecal administration |
| ITC | in the canal (hearing aid) |
| ITE | in the ear (hearing aid) |
| IU | international units |
| IV | intravenous |

| | | | | |
|---|---|---|---|---|
| IVF | in vitro fertilization | | PI | paramedic intercept |
| KAFO | knee-ankle-foot orthosis | | PICC | peripherally inserted central venous catheter |
| KO | knee orthosis | | PKR | photorefractive keratotomy |
| KOH | potassium hydroxide | | Pow | powder |
| L | left | | PRK | photoreactive keratectomy |
| LASIK | laser in situ keratomileusis | | PRO | peer review organization |
| LAUP | laser assisted uvulopalatoplasty | | PSA | prostate specific antigen |
| lbs | pounds | | PTB | patellar tendon bearing |
| LDL | low density lipoprotein | | PTK | phototherapeutic keratectomy |
| Lo | low | | PVC | polyvinyl chloride |
| LPM | liters per minute | | R | right |
| LPN/LVN | Licensed Practical Nurse/Licensed Vocational Nurse | | Repl | replace |
| LSO | lumbar-sacral orthosis | | RN | registered nurse |
| MAC | Medicare administrative contractor | | RP | retrograde pyelogram |
| mp | metacarpophalangeal | | Rx | prescription |
| mcg | microgram | | SACH | solid ankle, cushion heel |
| mCi | millicurie | | SC | subcutaneous |
| MCM | Medicare Carriers Manual | | SCT | specialty care transport |
| MCP | metacarparpophalangeal joint | | SEO | shoulder-elbow orthosis |
| MCP | monthly capitation payment | | SEWHO | shoulder-elbow-wrist-hand orthosis |
| mEq | milliequivalent | | SEXA | single energy x-ray absorptiometry |
| MESA | microsurgical epididymal sperm aspiration | | SGD | speech generating device |
| mg | milligram | | SGD | sinus rhythm |
| mgs | milligrams | | SM | samarium |
| MHT | megahertz | | SNCT | sensory nerve conduction test |
| ml | milliliter | | SNF | skilled nursing facility |
| mm | millimeter | | SO | sacroilliac othrosis |
| mmHg | millimeters of Mercury | | SO | shoulder orthosis |
| MRA | magnetic resonance angiography | | Sol | solution |
| MRI | magnetic resonance imaging | | SQ | square |
| NA | sodium | | SR | screen |
| NCI | National Cancer Institute | | ST | standard |
| NEC | not elsewhere classified | | ST | sustained release |
| NG | nasogastric | | Syr | syrup |
| NH | nursing home | | TABS | tablets |
| NMES | neuromuscular electrical stimulation | | Tc | Technetium |
| NOC | not otherwise classified | | Tc 99m | technetium isotope |
| NOS | not otherwise specified | | TENS | transcutaneous electrical nerve stimulator |
| O2 | oxygen | | THKAO | thoracic-hip-knee-ankle orthosis |
| OBRA | Omnibus Budget Reconciliation Act | | TLSO | thoracic-lumbar-sacral-orthosis |
| OMT | osteopathic manipulation therapy | | TM | temporomandibular |
| OPPS | outpatient prospective payment system | | TMJ | temporomandibular joint |
| ORAL | oral administration | | TPN | total parenteral nutrition |
| OSA | obstructive sleep apnea | | U | unit |
| Ost | ostomy | | uCi | microcurie |
| OTH | other routes of administration | | VAR | various routes of administration |
| oz | ounce | | w | with |
| PA | physician's assistant | | w/ | with |
| PAR | parenteral | | w/o | with or without |
| PCA | patient controlled analgesia | | WAK | wearable artificial kidney |
| PCH | pouch | | wc | wheelchair |
| PEN | parenteral and enteral nutrition | | WHFO | wrist-hand-finger orthotic |
| PENS | percutaneous electrical nerve stimulation | | Wk | week |
| PET | positron emission tomography | | w/o | without |
| PHP | pre-paid health plan | | Xe | xenon (isotope mass of xenon 133) |
| PHP | physician hospital plan | | | |

# APPENDIX 4 — PUB 100 REFERENCES

The Centers for Medicare and Medicaid Services restructured its paper-based manual system as a web-based system on October 1, 2003. Called the online CMS manual system, it combines all of the various program instructions into internet-only manuals (IOMs), which are used by all CMS programs and contractors. Complete versions of all of the manuals can be found at http://www.cms.hhs.gov/manuals.

Effective September 30, 2003, the former method of publishing program memoranda (PMs) to communicate program instructions was replaced by the following four templates:

- One-time notification
- Manual revisions
- Business requirements
- Confidential requirements

The web-based system has been organized by functional area (e.g., eligibility, entitlement, claims processing, benefit policy, program integrity) in an effort to eliminate redundancy within the manuals, simplify updating, and make CMS program instructions available more quickly. The web-based system contains the functional areas included below:

Pub. 100        Introduction
Pub. 100-1      Medicare General Information, Eligibility, and Entitlement Manual
Pub. 100-2      Medicare Benefit Policy Manual
Pub. 100-3      Medicare National Coverage Determinations Manual
Pub. 100-4      Medicare Claims Processing Manual
Pub. 100-5      Medicare Secondary Payer Manual
Pub. 100-6      Medicare Financial Management Manual
Pub. 100-7      State Operations Manual
Pub. 100-8      Medicare Program Integrity Manual
Pub. 100-9      Medicare Contractor Beneficiary and Provider Communications Manual
Pub. 100-10     Quality Improvement Organization Manual
Pub. 100-11     Reserved
Pub. 100-12     State Medicaid Manual (under development)
Pub. 100-13     Medicaid State Children's Health Insurance Program (under development)
Pub. 100-14     Medicare ESRD Network Organizations Manual
Pub. 100-15     State Buy-In Manual
Pub. 100-16     Medicare Managed Care Manual
Pub. 100-17     CMS/Business Partners Systems Security Manual
Pub. 100-18     Reserved
Pub. 100-19     Demonstrations
Pub. 100-20     One-Time Notification
Pub. 100-21     Recurring Update Notification

A brief description of the Medicare manuals primarily used for *CPC Expert* follows:

The **National Coverage Determinations Manual** (NCD), is organized according to categories such as diagnostic services, supplies, and medical procedures. The table of contents lists each category and subject within that category. Revision transmittals identify any new or background material, recap the changes, and provide an effective date for the change.

When complete, the manual will contain two chapters. Chapter 1 currently includes a description of CMS's national coverage determinations. When available, chapter 2 will contain a list of HCPCS codes related to each coverage determination. The manual is organized in accordance with CPT category sequences.

The **Medicare Benefit Policy Manual** contains Medicare general coverage instructions that are not national coverage determinations. As a general rule, in the past these instructions have been found in chapter II of the **Medicare Carriers Manual**, the **Medicare Intermediary Manual**, other provider manuals, and program memoranda.

The **Medicare Claims Processing Manual** contains instructions for processing claims for contractors and providers.

The **Medicare Program Integrity Manual** communicates the priorities and standards for the Medicare integrity programs.

## 100-1,1,10.1

### Hospital Insurance (Part A) for Inpatient Hospital, Hospice, HomeHealth and Skilled Nursing Facility (SNF) Services - A Brief Description

Hospital insurance is designed to help patients defray the expenses incurred by hospitalization and related care. In addition to inpatient hospital benefits, hospital insurance covers post hospital extended care in SNFs and post hospital care furnished by a home health agency in the patient's home. Blood clotting factors, for hemophilia patients competent to use such factors to control bleeding without medical or other supervision, and items related to the administration of such factors, are also a Part A benefit for beneficiaries in a covered Part A stay. The purpose of these additional benefits is to provide continued treatment after hospitalization and to encourage the appropriate use of more economical alternatives to inpatient hospital care. Program payments for services rendered to beneficiaries by providers (i.e., hospitals, SNFs, and home health agencies) are generally made to the provider. In each benefit period, payment may be made for up to 90 inpatient hospital days, and 100 days of post hospital extended care services .Hospices also provide Part A hospital insurance services such as short-term inpatient care. In order to be eligible to elect hospice care under Medicare, an individual must be entitled to Part A of Medicare and be certified as being terminally ill. An individual is considered to be terminally ill if the individual has a medical prognosis that his or her life expectancy is 6 months or less if the illness runs its normal course.

## 100-1,3,20.5

### Blood Deductibles (Part A and Part B)

Program payment may not be made for the first 3 pints of whole blood or equivalent units of packed red cells received under Part A and Part B combined in a calendar year. However, blood processing (e.g., administration, storage) is not subject to the deductible.

The blood deductibles are in addition to any other applicable deductible and coinsurance amounts for which the patient is responsible.

The deductible applies only to the first 3 pints of blood furnished in a calendar year, even if more than one provider furnished blood.

## 100-1,3,20.5.2

### Part B Blood Deductible

Blood is furnished on an outpatient basis or is subject to the Part B blood deductible and is counted toward the combined limit. It should be noted that payment for blood may be made to the hospital under Part B only for blood furnished in an outpatient setting. Blood is not covered for inpatient Part B services.

## 100-1,3,20.5.3

### Items Subject to Blood Deductibles

The blood deductibles apply only to whole blood and packed red cells. The term whole blood means human blood from which none of the liquid or cellular components have been removed. Where packed red cells are furnished, a unit of packed red cells is considered equivalent to a pint of whole blood. Other components of blood such as platelets, fibrinogen, plasma, gamma globulin, and serum albumin are not subject to the blood deductible. However, these components of blood are covered as biologicals.

Refer to Pub. 100-04, Medicare Claims Processing Manual, chapter 4, §231 regarding billing for blood and blood products under the Hospital Outpatient Prospective Payment System (OPPS).

## 100-1,5,90.2

### Laboratory Defined

Laboratory means a facility for the biological, microbiological, serological, chemical, immuno-hematological, hematological, biophysical, cytological, pathological, or other examination of materials derived from the human body for the purpose of providing information for the diagnosis, prevention, or treatment of any disease or impairment of, or the assessment of the health of, human beings. These examinations also include procedures to determine, measure, or otherwise describe the presence or absence of various substances or organisms in the body. Facilities only collecting or preparing specimens (or both) or only serving as a mailing service and not performing testing are not considered laboratories.

## 100-2,1,10

### Covered Inpatient Hospital Services Covered Under Part A

A3-3101, HO-210

Patients covered under hospital insurance are entitled to have payment made on their behalf for inpatient hospital services. (Inpatient hospital services do not include extended care services provided by hospitals pursuant to swing bed approvals. See Pub. 100-1, Chapter 8, §10.1, "Hospital Providers of Extended Care Services."). However, both inpatient hospital and inpatient SNF benefits are provided under Part A - Hospital Insurance Benefits for the Aged and Disabled, of Title XVIII).

Additional information concerning the following topics can be found in the following manual chapters:

- Benefit periods is found in Chapter 3, "Duration of Covered Inpatient Services";
- Copayment days is found in Chapter 2, "Duration of Covered Inpatient Services";
- Lifetime reserve days is found in Chapter 5, "Lifetime Reserve Days";
- Related payment information is housed in the Provider Reimbursement Manual.

Blood must be furnished on a day which counts as a day of inpatient hospital services to be covered as a Part A service and to count toward the blood deductible. Thus, blood is not covered under Part A and does not count toward the Part A blood deductible when furnished to an inpatient after the inpatient has exhausted all benefit days in a benefit period, or where the individual has elected not to use lifetime reserve days. However, where the patient is discharged on their first day of entitlement or on the hospital's first day of participation, the hospital is permitted to submit a billing form with no accommodation charge, but with ancillary charges including blood.

The records for all Medicare hospital inpatient discharges are maintained in CMS for statistical analysis and use in determining future PPS DRG classifications and rates.

Non-PPS hospitals do not pay for noncovered services generally excluded from coverage in the Medicare Program. This may result in denial of a part of the billed charges or in denial of the entire admission, depending upon circumstance. In PPS hospitals, the following are also possible:

1. In appropriately admitted cases where a noncovered procedure was performed, denied services may result in payment of a different DRG (i.e., one which excludes payment for the noncovered procedure); or
2. In appropriately admitted cases that become cost outlier cases, denied services may lead to denial of some or all of an outlier payment.

The following examples illustrate this principle. If care is noncovered because a patient does not need to be hospitalized, the intermediary denies the admission and makes no Part A (i.e., PPS) payment unless paid under limitation on liability. Under limitation on liability, Medicare payment may be made when the provider and the beneficiary were not aware the services were not necessary and could not reasonably be expected to know that he services were not necessary. For detailed instructions, see the Medicare Claims Processing Manual, Chapter 30,"Limitation on Liability." If a patient is appropriately hospitalized but receives (beyond routine services) only noncovered care, the admission is denied.

NOTE: The intermediary does not deny an admission that includes covered care, even if noncovered care was also rendered. Under PPS, Medicare assumes that it is paying for only the covered care rendered whenever covered services needed to treat and/or diagnose the illness were in fact provided.

If a noncovered procedure is provided along with covered nonroutine care, a DRG change rather than an admission denial might occur. If noncovered procedures are elevating costs into the cost outlier category, outlier payment is denied in whole or in part.

When the hospital is included in PPS, most of the subsequent discussion regarding coverage of inpatient hospital services is relevant only in the context of determining the appropriateness of admissions, which DRG, if any, to pay, and the appropriateness of payment for any outlier cases.

If a patient receives items or services in excess of, or more expensive than, those for which payment can be made, payment is made only for the covered items or services or for only the appropriate prospective payment amount. This provision applies not only to inpatient services, but also to all hospital services under Parts A and B of the program. If the items or services were requested by the patient, the hospital may charge him the difference between the amount customarily charged for the services requested and the amount customarily charged for covered services.

An inpatient is a person who has been admitted to a hospital for bed occupancy for purposes of receiving inpatient hospital services. Generally, a patient is considered an inpatient if formally admitted as inpatient with the expectation that he or she will remain at least overnight and occupy a bed even though it later develops that the patient can be discharged or transferred to another hospital and not actually use a hospital bed overnight.

The physician or other practitioner responsible for a patient's care at the hospital is also responsible for deciding whether the patient should be admitted as an inpatient. Physicians should use a 24-hour period as a benchmark, i.e., they should order admission for patients who are expected to need hospital care for 24 hours or more, and treat other patients on an outpatient basis. However, the decision to admit a patient is a complex medical judgment which can be made only after the physician has considered a number of factors, including the patient's medical history and current medical needs, the types of facilities available to inpatients and to outpatients, the hospital's by-laws and admissions policies, and the relative appropriateness of treatment in each setting. Factors to be considered when making the decision to admit include such things as: The severity of the signs and symptoms exhibited by the patient;

The medical predictability of something adverse happening to the patient;

The need for diagnostic studies that appropriately are outpatient services (i.e., their performance does not ordinarily require the patient to remain at the hospital for 24 hours or more) to assist in assessing whether the patient should be admitted; and

The availability of diagnostic procedures at the time when and at the location where the patient presents.

Admissions of particular patients are not covered or noncovered solely on the basis of the length of time the patient actually spends in the hospital. In certain specific situations coverage of services on an inpatient or outpatient basis is determined by the following rules:

Minor Surgery or Other Treatment - When patients with known diagnoses enter a hospital for a specific minor surgical procedure or other treatment that is expected to keep them in the hospital for only a few hours (less than 24), they are considered outpatients for coverage purposes regardless of: the hour they came to the hospital, whether they used a bed, and whether they remained in the hospital past midnight.

Renal Dialysis - Renal dialysis treatments are usually covered only as outpatient services but may under certain circumstances be covered as inpatient services depending on the patient's condition. Patients staying at home, who are ambulatory, whose conditions are stable and who come to the hospital for routine chronic dialysis treatments, and not for a diagnostic workup or a change in therapy, are considered outpatients. On the other hand, patients undergoing short-term dialysis until their kidneys recover from an acute illness (acute dialysis), or persons with borderline renal failure who develop acute renal failure every time they have an illness and require dialysis (episodic dialysis) are usually inpatients. A patient may begin dialysis as an inpatient and then progress to an outpatient status.

Under original Medicare, the Quality Improvement Organization (QIO), for each hospital is responsible for deciding, during review of inpatient admissions on a case-by-case basis, whether the admission was medically necessary. Medicare law authorizes the QIO to make these judgments, and the judgments are binding for purposes of Medicare coverage. In making these judgments, however, QIOs consider only the medical evidence which was available to the physician at the time an admission decision had to be made. They do not take into account other information (e.g., test results) which became available only after admission, except in cases where considering the post-admission information would support a finding that an admission was medically necessary.

Refer to Parts 4 and 7 of the QIO Manual with regard to initial determinations for these services. The QIO will review the swing bed services in these PPS hospitals as well.

NOTE: When patients requiring extended care services are admitted to beds in a hospital, they are considered inpatients of the hospital. In such cases, the services furnished in the hospital will not be considered extended care services, and payment may not be made under the program for such services unless the services are extended care services furnished pursuant to a swing bed agreement granted to the hospital by the Secretary of Health and Human Services.

### 100-2,1,10.1.4

#### Charges for Deluxe Private Room
A3-3101.1.D, HO-210.1.D

Beneficiaries found to need a private room (either because they need isolation for medical reasons or because they need immediate admission when no other accommodations are available) may be assigned to any of the provider's private rooms. They do not have the right to insist on the private room of their choice, but their preferences should be given the same consideration as if they were paying all provider charges themselves. The program does not, under any circumstances, pay for personal comfort items. Thus, the program does not pay for deluxe accommodations and/or services. These would include a suite, or a room substantially more spacious than is required for treatment, or specially equipped or decorated, or serviced for the comfort and convenience of persons willing to pay a differential for such amenities. If the beneficiary (or representative) requests such deluxe accommodations, the provider should advise that there will be a charge, not covered by Medicare, of a specified amount per day (not exceeding the differential defined in the next sentence); and may charge the beneficiary that amount for each day he/she occupies the deluxe accommodations. The maximum amount the provider may charge the beneficiary for such accommodations is the differential between the most prevalent private room rate at the time of admission and the customary charge for the room occupied. Beneficiaries may not be charged this differential if they (or their representative) do not request the deluxe accommodations.

The beneficiary may not be charged such a differential in private room rates if that differential is based on factors other than personal comfort items. Such factors might include differences between older and newer wings, proximity to lounge, elevators or nursing stations, desirable view, etc. Such rooms are standard 1-bed units and not deluxe rooms for purposes of these instructions, even though the provider may call them deluxe and have a higher customary charge for them. No additional charge may be imposed upon the beneficiary who is assigned to a room that may be somewhat more desirable because of these factors.

## 100-2,1,40

### Supplies, Appliances, and Equipment

Supplies, appliances, and equipment, which are ordinarily furnished by the hospital for the care and treatment of the beneficiary solely during the inpatient hospital stay, are covered inpatient hospital services.

Under certain circumstances, supplies, appliances, and equipment used during the beneficiary's inpatient stay are covered under Part A even though the supplies, appliances and equipment leave the hospital with the patient upon discharge. These are circumstances in which it would be unreasonable or impossible from a medical standpoint to limit the patient's use of the item to the periods during which the individual is an inpatient. Examples of items covered under this rule are:

- Items permanently installed in or attached to the patient's body while an inpatient, such as cardiac valves, cardiac pacemakers, and artificial limbs; and

- Items which are temporarily installed in or attached to the patient's body while an inpatient, and which are also necessary to permit or facilitate the patient's release from the hospital, such as tracheotomy or drainage tubes.

Hospital "admission packs" containing primarily toilet articles, such as soap, toothbrushes, toothpaste, and combs, are covered under Part A if routinely furnished by the hospital to all its inpatients. If not routinely furnished to all patients, the packs are not covered. In that situation, the hospital may charge beneficiaries for the pack, but only if they request it with knowledge of what they are requesting and what the charge to them will be.

Supplies, appliances, and equipment furnished to an inpatient for use only outside the hospital are not, in general, covered as inpatient hospital services. However, a temporary or disposable item, which is medically necessary to permit or facilitate the patient's departure from the hospital and is required until the patient can obtain a continuing supply, is covered as an inpatient hospital service.

Oxygen furnished to hospital inpatients is covered under Part A as an inpatient supply.

## 100-2,10,20

### Coverage Guidelines for Ambulance Service Claims
B3-2125

Payment may be made for expenses incurred by a patient for ambulance service provided conditions I, 2, and 3 in the left-hand column have been met. The right-hand column indicates the documentation needed to establish that the condition has been met.

| Conditions | Review Action |
|---|---|
| 1. Patient was transported by an approved supplier of ambulance services. | 1. Ambulance supplier is listed in the table of approved ambulance companies (§10.1.3) |
| 2. The patient was suffering from an illness or injury, which contraindicated transportation by other means. (§10.2) | 2. (a) The contractor presumes the requirement was met if the submitted documentation indicates that the patient: <br>• Was transported in an emergency situation, e.g., as a result of an accident, injury or acute illness, or<br>• Needed to be restrained to prevent injury to the beneficiary or others; or<br>• Was unconscious or in shock; or<br>• Required oxygen or other emergency treatment during transport to the nearest appropriate facility; or<br>• Exhibits signs and symptoms of acute respiratory distress or cardiac distress such as shortness of breath or chest pain; or<br>• Exhibits signs and symptoms that indicate the possibility of acute stroke; or<br>• Had to remain immobile because of a fracture that had not been set or the possibility of a fracture; or<br>• Was experiencing severe hemorrhage; or |

| Conditions | Review Action |
|---|---|
| | • Could be moved only by stretcher; or<br>• Was bed-confined before and after the ambulance trip. |
| | (b) In the absence of any of the conditions listed in (a) above additional documentation should be obtained to establish medical need where the evidence indicates the existence of the circumstances listed below: |
| | (i) Patient's condition would not ordinarily require movement by stretcher, or |
| | (ii) The individual was not admitted as a hospital inpatient (except in accident cases), or |
| | (iii) The ambulance was used solely because other means of transportation were unavailable, or |
| | (iv) The individual merely needed assistance in getting from his room or home to a vehicle. |
| | (c) Where the information indicates a situation not listed in 2(a) or 2(b) above, refer the case to your supervisor. |
| 3. The patient was transported from and to points listed below. | 3. Claims should show the ZIP code of the point of pickup |
| (a) From patient's residence (or other place where need arose) to hospital or skilled nursing facility. | (a)<br>i. Condition met if trip began within the institution's service area as shown in the carrier's locality guide<br>ii. Condition met where the trip began outside the institution's service area if the institution was the nearest one with appropriate facilities. |

NOTE: A patient's residence is the place where he or she makes his/her home and dwells permanently, or for an extended period of time. A skilled nursing facility is one, which is listed in the Directory of Medical Facilities as a participating SNF or as an institution which meets §1861(j)(1) of the Act.

NOTE: A claim for ambulance service to a participating hospital or skilled nursing facility should not be denied on the grounds that there is a nearer nonparticipating institution having appropriate facilities.

| Conditions | Review Action |
|---|---|
| (b) Skilled nursing facility to a hospital or hospital to a skilled nursing facility. | (b)<br>(i) Condition met if the ZIP code of the pickup point is within the service area of the destination as shown in the carrier's locality guide.<br>(ii) Condition met where the ZIP code of the pickup point is outside the service area of the destination if the destination institution was the nearest appropriate facility. |
| (c) Hospital to hospital or skilled nursing facility to skilled nursing facility. | (c) Condition met if the discharging institution was not an appropriate facility and the admitting institution was the nearest appropriate facility. |
| (d) From a hospital or skilled nursing facility to patient's residence. | (d)<br>(i) Condition met if patient's residence is within the institution's service area as shown in the carrier's locality guide.<br>(ii) Condition met where the patient's residence is outside the institution's service area if the institution was the nearest appropriate facility. |
| (e) Round trip for hospital or participating skilled nursing facility inpatients to the nearest hospital or nonhospital treatment facility. | (e) Condition met if the reasonable and necessary diagnostic or therapeutic service required by patient's condition is not available at the institution where the beneficiary is an inpatient. |

NOTE: Ambulance service to a physician's office or a physician-directed clinic is not covered. See §10.3.7 above, where a stop is made at a physician's office en route to a hospital and §10.3.3 for additional exceptions.)

| Conditions | Review Action |
|---|---|
| 4. Ambulance services involving hospital admissions in Canada or Mexico are covered (Medicare Claims Processing Manual, Chapter 1, "General Billing Requirements, " §§10.1.3.) if the following conditions are met: | (a) The foreign hospitalization has been determined to be covered; and<br><br>(b) The ambulance service meets the coverage requirements set forth in §§10-10.3. If the foreign hospitalization has been determined to be covered on the basis of emergency services (See the Medicare Claims Processing Manual, Chapter 1, "General Billing Requirements," §10.1.3), the necessity requirement (§10.2 ) and the destination requirement (§10.3 ) are considered met. |
| 5. The carrier will make partial payment for otherwise covered ambulance service, which exceeded limits defined in item | (a) From the pickup point to the nearest appropriate facility, or<br><br>(b) From the nearest appropriate facility to the beneficiary's residence where he or she is being returned home from a distant institution. |
| 6. The carrier will base the payment on the amount payable had the patient been transported: | |

## 100-2,11,130

### Inpatient Hospital Dialysis
A3-3173, A3-3173.1, A3-3173.2

Dialysis services provided by any participating Medicare hospital are covered if the inpatient stay is medically necessary and the primary reason for the admission is not maintenance dialysis. Reimbursement for the maintenance dialysis is included in the PPS reimbursement for the DRG that represents care for the actual reason for admission. In many cases, ESRD patients who require inpatient care are experiencing complications that affect the nature of the dialysis services. Payment for medically necessary inpatient dialysis is not subject to the composite rate.

A hospital may decide not to provide dialysis services directly to an inpatient. In this situation, the hospital must make arrangements with a certified ESRD facility to provide the dialysis services.

Inpatient dialysis services are also covered if an ESRD emergency occurs. However, when the emergency is over, outpatient maintenance dialysis must be performed in an ESRD certified facility or coverage will be denied. The intermediary should examine all claims for inpatient dialysis services, from hospitals that are not certified under the ESRD conditions for coverage, to ensure that one or more of these special situations exist.

## 100-2,11,130.1

### Inpatient Dialysis in Nonparticipating Hospitals
A3-3173.3

Emergency inpatient dialysis services provided by a nonparticipating U.S. hospital are covered if the requirements in §130 above are met.

## 100-2,15,100

### Surgical Dressings, Splints, Casts, and Other Devices Used for Reductions of Fractures and Dislocations
B3-2079, A3-3110.3, HO-228.3

Surgical dressings are limited to primary and secondary dressings required for the treatment of a wound caused by, or treated by, a surgical procedure that has been performed by a physician or other health care professional to the extent permissible under State law. In addition, surgical dressings required after debridement of a wound are also covered, irrespective of the type of debridement, as long as the debridement was reasonable and necessary and was performed by a health care professional acting within the scope of his/her legal authority when performing this function. Surgical dressings are covered for as long as they are medically necessary. Primary dressings are therapeutic or protective coverings applied directly to wounds or lesions either on the skin or caused by an opening to the skin. Secondary dressing materials that serve a therapeutic or protective function and that are needed to secure a primary dressing are also covered. Items such as adhesive tape, roll gauze, bandages, and disposable compression material are examples of secondary dressings. Elastic stockings, support hose, foot coverings, leotards, knee supports, surgical leggings, gauntlets, and pressure garments for the arms and hands are examples of items that are not ordinarily covered as surgical dressings. Some items, such as transparent film, may be used as a primary or secondary dressing. If a physician, certified nurse midwife, physician assistant, nurse practitioner, or clinical nurse specialist applies surgical dressings as part of a professional service that is billed to Medicare, the surgical dressings are considered incident to the professional services of the health care practitioner. (See §§60.1, 180, 190, 200, and 210.) When surgical dressings are not covered incident to the services of a health care practitioner and are obtained by the patient from a supplier (e.g., a drugstore, physician, or other health care practitioner that qualifies as a supplier) on an order from a physician or other health care professional authorized under State law or regulation to make such an order, the surgical dressings are covered separately under Part B. Splints and casts, and other devices used for reductions of fractures and dislocations are covered under Part B of Medicare. This includes dental splints.

## 100-2,15,110

### Durable Medical Equipment - General
B3-2100, A3-3113, HO-235, HHA-220

Expenses incurred by a beneficiary for the rental or purchases of durable medical equipment (DME) are reimbursable if the following three requirements are met:

- The equipment meets the definition of DME (§110.1);•The equipment is necessary and reasonable for the treatment of the patient's illness or injury or to improve the functioning of his or her malformed body member (§110.1); and

- The equipment is used in the patient's home. The decision whether to rent or purchase an item of equipment generally resides with the beneficiary, but the decision on how to pay rests with CMS. For some DME, program payment policy calls for lump sum payments and in others for periodic payment. Where covered DME is furnished to a beneficiary by a supplier of services other than a provider of services, the DMERC makes the reimbursement. If a provider of services furnishes the equipment, the intermediary makes the reimbursement. The payment method is identified in the annual fee schedule update furnished by CMS. The CMS issues quarterly updates to a fee schedule file that contains rates by HCPCS code and also identifies the classification of the HCPCS code within the following categories. Category Code Definition IN Inexpensive and Other Routinely Purchased Items FS Frequently Serviced Items CR Capped Rental Items OX Oxygen and Oxygen Equipment OS Ostomy, Tracheostomy & Urological Items SD Surgical Dressings PO Prosthetics & Orthotics SU Supplies TE Transcutaneous Electrical Nerve Stimulators The DMERCs, carriers, and intermediaries, where appropriate, use the CMS files to determine payment rules. See the Medicare Claims Processing Manual, Chapter 20, "Durable Medical Equipment, Surgical Dressings and Casts, Orthotics and Artificial Limbs, and Prosthetic Devices," for a detailed description of payment rules for each classification. Payment may also be made for repairs, maintenance, and delivery of equipment and for expendable and nonreusable items essential to the effective use of the equipment subject to the conditions in §110.2. See the Medicare Benefit Policy Manual, Chapter 11, "End Stage Renal Disease," for hemodialysis equipment and supplies.

## 100-2,15,110.1

### Definition of Durable Medical Equipment
B3-2100.1, A3-3113.1, HO-235.1, HHA-220.1, B3-2100.2, A3-3113.2, HO-235.2, HHA-220.2

Durable medical equipment is equipment which:

- Can withstand repeated use;

- Is primarily and customarily used to serve a medical purpose;

- Generally is not useful to a person in the absence of an illness or injury; and

- Is appropriate for use in the home.

All requirements of the definition must be met before an item can be considered to be durable medical equipment. The following describes the underlying policies for determining whether an item meets the definition of DME and may be covered.

#### A. Durability
An item is considered durable if it can withstand repeated use, i.e., the type of item that could normally be rented. Medical supplies of an expendable nature, such as incontinent pads, lambs wool pads, catheters, ace bandages, elastic stockings, surgical facemasks, irrigating kits, sheets, and bags are not considered "durable" within the meaning of the definition. There are other items that, although durable in nature, may fall into other coverage categories such as supplies, braces, prosthetic devices, artificial arms, legs, and eyes.

#### B. Medical Equipment
Medical equipment is equipment primarily and customarily used for medical purposes and is not generally useful in the absence of illness or injury. In most instances, no development will be needed to determine whether a specific item of equipment is medical in nature. However, some cases will require development to determine whether the item constitutes medical equipment. This development would include the advice of local medical organizations (hospitals, medical schools, medical societies) and specialists in the field of physical medicine and rehabilitation. If the equipment is new on the market, it may be necessary, prior to seeking professional advice, to obtain information from the supplier or manufacturer explaining the design, purpose, effectiveness and method of using the equipment in the home as well as the results of any tests or clinical studies that have been conducted.

1. Equipment Presumptively Medical
   Items such as hospital beds, wheelchairs, hemodialysis equipment, iron lungs, respirators, intermittent positive pressure breathing machines, medical regulators,

oxygen tents, crutches, canes, trapeze bars, walkers, inhalators, nebulizers, commodes, suction machines, and traction equipment presumptively constitute medical equipment. (Although hemodialysis equipment is covered as a prosthetic device (§120), it also meets the definition of DME, and reimbursement for the rental or purchase of such equipment for use in the beneficiary's home will be made only under the provisions for payment applicable to DME. See the Medicare Benefit Policy Manual, Chapter 11, "End Stage Renal Disease," §30.1, for coverage of home use of hemodialysis.) NOTE: There is a wide variety in types of respirators and suction machines. The DMERC's medical staff should determine whether the apparatus specified in the claim is appropriate for home use.

2. Equipment Presumptively Nonmedical

Equipment which is primarily and customarily used for a nonmedical purpose may not be considered "medical" equipment for which payment can be made under the medical insurance program. This is true even though the item has some remote medically related use. For example, in the case of a cardiac patient, an air conditioner might possibly be used to lower room temperature to reduce fluid loss in the patient and to restore an environment conducive to maintenance of the proper fluid balance. Nevertheless, because the primary and customary use of an air conditioner is a nonmedical one, the air conditioner cannot be deemed to be medical equipment for which payment can be made. Other devices and equipment used for environmental control or to enhance the environmental setting in which the beneficiary is placed are not considered covered DME. These include, for example, room heaters, humidifiers, dehumidifiers, and electric air cleaners. Equipment which basically serves comfort or convenience functions or is primarily for the convenience of a person caring for the patient, such as elevators, stairway elevators, and posture chairs, do not constitute medical equipment. Similarly, physical fitness equipment (such as an exercycle), first-aid or precautionary-type equipment (such as preset portable oxygen units), self-help devices (such as safety grab bars), and training equipment (such as Braille training texts) are considered nonmedical in nature.

3. Special Exception Items

Specified items of equipment may be covered under certain conditions even though they do not meet the definition of DME because they are not primarily and customarily used to serve a medical purpose and/or are generally useful in the absence of illness or injury. These items would be covered when it is clearly established that they serve a therapeutic purpose in an individual case and would include:

a. Gel pads and pressure and water mattresses (which generally serve a preventive purpose) when prescribed for a patient who had bed sores or there is medical evidence indicating that they are highly susceptible to such ulceration; and

b. Heat lamps for a medical rather than a soothing or cosmetic purpose, e.g., where the need for heat therapy has been established.

In establishing medical necessity for the above items, the evidence must show that the item is included in the physician's course of treatment and a physician is supervising its use.

NOTE: The above items represent special exceptions and no extension of coverage to other items should be inferred

## C. Necessary and Reasonable

Although an item may be classified as DME, it may not be covered in every instance. Coverage in a particular case is subject to the requirement that the equipment be necessary and reasonable for treatment of an illness or injury, or to improve the functioning of a malformed body member. These considerations will bar payment for equipment which cannot reasonably be expected to perform a therapeutic function in an individual case or will permit only partial therapeutic function in an individual case or will permit only partial payment when the type of equipment furnished substantially exceeds that required for the treatment of the illness or injury involved. See the Medicare Claims Processing Manual, Chapter 1, "General Billing Requirements;" §60, regarding the rules for providing advance beneficiary notices (ABNs) that advise beneficiaries, before items or services actually are furnished, when Medicare is likely to deny payment for them. ABNs allow beneficiaries to make an informed consumer decision about receiving items or services for which they may have to pay out-of-pocket and to be more active participants in their own health care treatment decisions.

1. Necessity for the Equipment

Equipment is necessary when it can be expected to make a meaningful contribution to the treatment of the patient's illness or injury or to the improvement of his or her malformed body member. In most cases the physician's prescription for the equipment and other medical information available to the DMERC will be sufficient to establish that the equipment serves this purpose.

2. Reasonableness of the Equipment

Even though an item of DME may serve a useful medical purpose, the DMERC or intermediary must also consider to what extent, if any, it would be reasonable for the Medicare program to pay for the item prescribed. The following considerations should enter into the determination of reasonableness:

1. Would the expense of the item to the program be clearly disproportionate to the therapeutic benefits which could ordinarily be derived from use of the equipment?

2. Is the item substantially more costly than a medically appropriate and realistically feasible alternative pattern of care?

3. Does the item serve essentially the same purpose as equipment already available to the beneficiary?

3. Payment Consistent With What is Necessary and Reasonable

Where a claim is filed for equipment containing features of an aesthetic nature or features of a medical nature which are not required by the patient's condition or where there exists a reasonably feasible and medically appropriate alternative pattern of care which is less costly than the equipment furnished, the amount payable is based on the rate for the equipment or alternative treatment which meets the patient's medical needs. The acceptance of an assignment binds the supplier-assignee to accept the payment for the medically required equipment or service as the full charge and the supplier-assignee cannot charge the beneficiary the differential attributable to the equipment actually furnished.

4. Establishing the Period of Medical Necessity

Generally, the period of time an item of durable medical equipment will be considered to be medically necessary is based on the physician's estimate of the time that his or her patient will need the equipment. See the Medicare Program Integrity Manual, Chapters 5 and 6, for medical review guidelines.

## D. Definition of a Beneficiary's Home

For purposes of rental and purchase of DME a beneficiary's home may be his/her own dwelling, an apartment, a relative's home, a home for the aged, or some other type of institution. However, an institution may not be considered a beneficiary's home if it:

- Meets at least the basic requirement in the definition of a hospital, i.e., it is primarily engaged in providing by or under the supervision of physicians, to inpatients, diagnostic and therapeutic services for medical diagnosis, treatment, and care of injured, disabled, and sick persons, or rehabilitation services for the rehabilitation of injured, disabled, or sick persons; or

- Meets at least the basic requirement in the definition of a skilled nursing facility, i.e., it is primarily engaged in providing to inpatients skilled nursing care and related services for patients who require medical or nursing care, or rehabilitation services for the rehabilitation of injured, disabled, or sick persons.

Thus, if an individual is a patient in an institution or distinct part of an institution which provides the services described in the bullets above, the individual is not entitled to have separate Part B payment made for rental or purchase of DME. This is because such an institution may not be considered the individual's home. The same concept applies even if the patient resides in a bed or portion of the institution not certified for Medicare.

If the patient is at home for part of a month and, for part of the same month is in an institution that cannot qualify as his or her home, or is outside the U.S., monthly payments may be made for the entire month. Similarly, if DME is returned to the provider before the end of a payment month because the beneficiary died in that month or because the equipment became unnecessary in that month, payment may be made for the entire month.

## 100-2,15,110.2

### Repairs, Maintenance, Replacement, and Delivery

Under the circumstances specified below, payment may be made for repair, maintenance, and replacement of medically required DME, including equipment which had been in use before the user enrolled in Part B of the program. However, do not pay for repair, maintenance, or replacement of equipment in the frequent and substantial servicing or oxygen equipment payment categories. In addition, payments for repair and maintenance may not include payment for parts and labor covered under a manufacturer's or supplier's warranty.

### A. Repairs

To repair means to fix or mend and to put the equipment back in good condition after damage or wear. Repairs to equipment which a beneficiary owns are covered when necessary to make the equipment serviceable. However, do not pay for repair of previously denied equipment or equipment in the frequent and substantial servicing or oxygen equipment payment categories. If the expense for repairs exceeds the estimated expense of purchasing or renting another item of equipment for the remaining period of medical need, no payment can be made for the amount of the excess. (See subsection C where claims for repairs suggest malicious damage or culpable neglect.) Since renters of equipment recover from the rental charge the expenses they incur in maintaining in working order the equipment they rent out, separately itemized charges for repair of rented equipment are not covered. This includes items in the frequent and substantial servicing, oxygen equipment, capped rental, and inexpensive or routinely purchased payment categories which are being rented. A new Certificate of Medical Necessity (CMN) and/or physician's order is not needed for repairs. For replacement items, see Subsection C below.

## B. Maintenance

Routine periodic servicing, such as testing, cleaning, regulating, and checking of the beneficiary's equipment, is not covered. The owner is expected to perform such routine maintenance rather than a retailer or some other person who charges the beneficiary. Normally, purchasers of DME are given operating manuals which describe the type of servicing an owner may perform to properly maintain the equipment. It is reasonable to expect that beneficiaries will perform this maintenance. Thus, hiring a third party to do such work is for the convenience of the beneficiary and is not covered. However, more extensive maintenance which, based on the manufacturers' recommendations, is to be performed by authorized technicians, is covered as repairs for medically necessary equipment which a beneficiary owns. This might include, for example, breaking down sealed components and performing tests which require specialized testing equipment not available to the beneficiary. Do not pay for maintenance of purchased items that require frequent and substantial servicing or oxygen equipment. Since renters of equipment recover from the rental charge the expenses they incur in maintaining in working order the equipment they rent out, separately itemized charges for maintenance of rented equipment are generally not covered. Payment may not be made for maintenance of rented equipment other than the maintenance and servicing fee established for capped rental items. For capped rental items which have reached the 15-month rental cap, contractors pay claims for maintenance and servicing fees after 6 months have passed from the end of the final paid rental month or from the end of the period the item is no longer covered under the supplier's or manufacturer's warranty, whichever is later. See the Medicare Claims Processing Manual, Chapter 20, "Durable Medical Equipment, Prosthetics and Orthotics, and Supplies (DMEPOS)," for additional instruction and an example. A new CMN and/or physician's order is not needed for covered maintenance.

## C. Replacement

Replacement refers to the provision of an identical or nearly identical item. Situations involving the provision of a different item because of a change in medical condition are not addressed in this section.

Equipment which the beneficiary owns or is a capped rental item may be replaced in cases of loss or irreparable damage. Irreparable damage refers to a specific accident or to a natural disaster (e.g., fire, flood). A physician's order and/or new Certificate of Medical Necessity (CMN), when required, is needed to reaffirm the medical necessity of the item.

Irreparable wear refers to deterioration sustained from day-to-day usage over time and a specific event cannot be identified. Replacement of equipment due to irreparable wear takes into consideration the reasonable useful lifetime of the equipment. If the item of equipment has been in continuous use by the patient on either a rental or purchase basis for the equipment's useful lifetime, the beneficiary may elect to obtain a new piece of equipment. Replacement may be reimbursed when a new physician order and/or new CMN, when required, is needed to reaffirm the medical necessity of the item.

The reasonable useful lifetime of durable medical equipment is determined through program instructions. In the absence of program instructions, carriers may determine the reasonable useful lifetime of equipment, but in no case can it be less than 5 years. Computation of the useful lifetime is based on when the equipment is delivered to the beneficiary, not the age of the equipment. Replacement due to wear is not covered during the reasonable useful lifetime of the equipment. During the reasonable useful lifetime, Medicare does cover repair up to the cost of replacement (but not actual replacement) for medically necessary equipment owned by the beneficiary. (See subsection A.)

Charges for the replacement of oxygen equipment, items that require frequent and substantial servicing or inexpensive or routinely purchased items which are being rented are not covered. Cases suggesting malicious damage, culpable neglect, or wrongful disposition of equipment should be investigated and denied where the DMERC determines that it is unreasonable to make program payment under the circumstances. DMERCs refer such cases to the program integrity specialist in the RO.

## D. Delivery

Payment for delivery of DME whether rented or purchased is generally included in the fee schedule allowance for the item. See Pub. 100-04, Medicare Claims Processing Manual, Chapter 20, "Durable Medical Equipment, Prosthetics and Orthotics, and Supplies (DMEPOS)," for the rules that apply to making reimbursement for exceptional cases.

## 100-2,15,110.3

### Coverage of Supplies and Accessories

B3-2100.5, A3-3113.4, HO-235.4, HHA-220.5Payment may be made for supplies, e.g., oxygen, that are necessary for the effective use of durable medical equipment. Such supplies include those drugs and biologicals which must be put directly into the equipment in order to achieve the therapeutic benefit of the durable medical equipment or to assure the proper functioning of the equipment, e.g., tumor chemotherapy agents used with an infusion pump or heparin used with a home dialysis system. However, the coverage of such drugs or biologicals does not preclude the need for a determination that the drug or biological itself is reasonable and necessary for treatment of the illness or injury or to improve the functioning of a malformed body member.

In the case of prescription drugs, other than oxygen, used in conjunction with durable medical equipment, prosthetic, orthotics, and supplies (DMEPOS) or prosthetic devices, the entity that dispenses the drug must furnish it directly to the patient for whom a prescription is written. The entity that dispenses the drugs must have a Medicare supplier number, must possess a current license to dispense prescription drugs in the State in which the drug is dispensed, and must bill and receive payment in its own name. A supplier that is not the entity that dispenses the drugs cannot purchase the drugs used in conjunction with DME for resale to the beneficiary. Reimbursement may be made for replacement of essential accessories such as hoses, tubes, mouthpieces, etc., for necessary DME, only if the beneficiary owns or is purchasing the equipment.

## 100-2,15,120

### Prosthetic Devices

B3-2130, A3-3110.4, HO-228.4, A3-3111, HO-229

### A. General

Prosthetic devices (other than dental) which replace all or part of an internal body organ (including contiguous tissue), or replace all or part of the function of a permanently inoperative or malfunctioning internal body organ are covered when furnished on a physician's order. This does not require a determination that there is no possibility that the patient's condition may improve sometime in the future. If the medical record, including the judgment of the attending physician, indicates the condition is of long and indefinite duration, the test of permanence is considered met. (Such a device may also be covered under §60.I as a supply when furnished incident to a physician's service.)

Examples of prosthetic devices include artificial limbs, parenteral and enteral (PEN) nutrition, cardiac pacemakers, prosthetic lenses (see subsection B), breast prostheses (including a surgical brassiere) for postmastectomy patients, maxillofacial devices, and devices which replace all or part of the ear or nose. A urinary collection and retention system with or without a tube is a prosthetic device replacing bladder function in case of permanent urinary incontinence. The foley catheter is also considered a prosthetic device when ordered for a patient with permanent urinary incontinence. However, chucks, diapers, rubber sheets, etc., are supplies that are not covered under this provision. Although hemodialysis equipment is a prosthetic device, payment for the rental or purchase of such equipment in the home is made only for use under the provisions for payment applicable to durable medical equipment.

An exception is that if payment cannot be made on an inpatient's behalf under Part A, hemodialysis equipment, supplies, and services required by such patient could be covered under Part B as a prosthetic device, which replaces the function of a kidney. See the Medicare Benefit Policy Manual, Chapter 11, "End Stage Renal Disease," for payment for hemodialysis equipment used in the home. See the Medicare Benefit Policy Manual, Chapter 1, "Inpatient Hospital Services," §10, for additional instructions on hospitalization for renal dialysis.

NOTE: Medicare does not cover a prosthetic device dispensed to a patient prior to the time at which the patient undergoes the procedure that makes necessary the use of the device. For example, the carrier does not make a separate Part B payment for an intraocular lens (IOL) or pacemaker that a physician, during an office visit prior to the actual surgery, dispenses to the patient for his or her use. Dispensing a prosthetic device in this manner raises health and safety issues. Moreover, the need for the device cannot be clearly established until the procedure that makes its use possible is successfully performed. Therefore, dispensing a prosthetic device in this manner is not considered reasonable and necessary for the treatment of the patient's condition.

Colostomy (and other ostomy) bags and necessary accoutrements required for attachment are covered as prosthetic devices. This coverage also includes irrigation and flushing equipment and other items and supplies directly related to ostomy care, whether the attachment of a bag is required.

Accessories and/or supplies which are used directly with an enteral or parenteral device to achieve the therapeutic benefit of the prosthesis or to assure the proper functioning of the device may also be covered under the prosthetic device benefit subject to the additional guidelines in the Medicare National Coverage Determinations Manual.

Covered items include catheters, filters, extension tubing, infusion bottles, pumps (either food or infusion), intravenous (I.V.) pole, needles, syringes, dressings, tape, Heparin Sodium (parenteral only), volumetric monitors (parenteral only), and parenteral and enteral nutrient solutions. Baby food and other regular grocery products that can be blenderized and used with the enteral system are not covered. Note that some of these items, e.g., a food pump and an I.V. pole, qualify as DME. Although coverage of the enteral and parenteral nutritional therapy systems is provided on the basis of the prosthetic device benefit, the payment rules relating to lump sum or monthly payment for DME apply to such items.

The coverage of prosthetic devices includes replacement of and repairs to such devices as explained in subsection D.

Finally, the Benefits Improvement and Protection Act of 2000 amended §1834(h)(1) of the Act by adding a provision (1834 (h)(1)(G)(i)) that requires Medicare payment to be made for the replacement of prosthetic devices which are artificial limbs, or for the replacement of any part of such devices, without regard to continuous use or useful lifetime restrictions if an ordering physician determines that the replacement device, or replacement part of such a device, is necessary.

Payment may be made for the replacement of a prosthetic device that is an artificial limb, or replacement part of a device if the ordering physician determines that the replacement device or part is necessary because of any of the following:

1. A change in the physiological condition of the patient;

2. An irreparable change in the condition of the device, or in a part of the device; or

3. The condition of the device, or the part of the device, requires repairs and the cost of such repairs would be more than 60 percent of the cost of a replacement device, or, as the case may be, of the part being replaced.

This provision is effective for items replaced on or after April 1, 2001. It supersedes any rule that that provided a 5-year or other replacement rule with regard to prosthetic devices.

### B. Prosthetic Lenses

The term "internal body organ" includes the lens of an eye. Prostheses replacing the lens of an eye include post-surgical lenses customarily used during convalescence from eye surgery in which the lens of the eye was removed. In addition, permanent lenses are also covered when required by an individual lacking the organic lens of the eye because of surgical removal or congenital absence. Prosthetic lenses obtained on or after the beneficiary's date of entitlement to supplementary medical insurance benefits may be covered even though the surgical removal of the crystalline lens occurred before entitlement.

1. Prosthetic Cataract Lenses

   One of the following prosthetic lenses or combinations of prosthetic lenses furnished by a physician (see §30.4 for coverage of prosthetic lenses prescribed by a doctor of optometry) may be covered when determined to be reasonable and necessary to restore essentially the vision provided by the crystalline lens of the eye:

   • Prosthetic bifocal lenses in frames;

   • Prosthetic lenses in frames for far vision, and prosthetic lenses in frames for near vision; or

   • When a prosthetic contact lens(es) for far vision is prescribed (including cases of binocular and monocular aphakia), make payment for the contact lens(es) and prosthetic lenses in frames for near vision to be worn at the same time as the contact lens(es), and prosthetic lenses in frames to be worn when the contacts have been removed.

   Lenses which have ultraviolet absorbing or reflecting properties may be covered, in lieu of payment for regular (untinted) lenses, if it has been determined that such lenses are medically reasonable and necessary for the individual patient.

   Medicare does not cover cataract sunglasses obtained in addition to the regular (untinted) prosthetic lenses since the sunglasses duplicate the restoration of vision function performed by the regular prosthetic lenses.

2. Payment for Intraocular Lenses (IOLs) Furnished in Ambulatory Surgical Centers (ASCs)
   Effective for services furnished on or after March 12, 1990, payment for intraocular lenses (IOLs) inserted during or subsequent to cataract surgery in a Medicare certified ASC is included with the payment for facility services that are furnished in connection with the covered surgery. Refer to the Medicare Claims Processing Manual, Chapter 14, "Ambulatory Surgical Centers," for more information.

3. Limitation on Coverage of Conventional Lenses
   One pair of conventional eyeglasses or conventional contact lenses furnished after each cataract surgery with insertion of an IOL is covered.

### C. Dentures

Dentures are excluded from coverage. However, when a denture or a portion of the denture is an integral part (built-in) of a covered prosthesis (e.g., an obturator to fill an opening in the palate), it is covered as part of that prosthesis.

### D. Supplies, Repairs, Adjustments, and Replacement

Supplies are covered that are necessary for the effective use of a prosthetic device (e.g., the batteries needed to operate an artificial larynx). Adjustment of prosthetic devices required by wear or by a change in the patient's condition is covered when ordered by a physician. General provisions relating to the repair and replacement of durable medical equipment in §110.2 for the repair and replacement of prosthetic devices are applicable. (See the Medicare Benefit Policy Manual, Chapter 16, "General Exclusions from Coverage," §40.4, for payment for devices

replaced under a warranty.) Replacement of conventional eyeglasses or contact lenses furnished in accordance with §120.B.3 is not covered. Necessary supplies, adjustments, repairs, and replacements are covered even when the device had been in use before the user enrolled in Part B of the program, so long as the device continues to be medically required.

### 100-2,15,130

### Leg, Arm, Back, and Neck Braces, Trusses, and Artificial Legs, Arms, and Eyes

B3-2133, A3-3110.5, HO-228.5, AB-01-06 dated 1/18/01

These appliances are covered under Part B when furnished incident to physicians' services or on a physician's order. A brace includes rigid and semi-rigid devices which are used for the purpose of supporting a weak or deformed body member or restricting or eliminating motion in a diseased or injured part of the body. Elastic stockings, garter belts, and similar devices do not come within the scope of the definition of a brace. Back braces include, but are not limited to, special corsets, e.g., sacroiliac, sacrolumbar, dorsolumbar corsets, and belts. A terminal device (e.g., hand or hook) is covered under this provision whether an artificial limb is required by the patient. Stump stockings and harnesses (including replacements) are also covered when these appliances are essential to the effective use of the artificial limb.

Adjustments to an artificial limb or other appliance required by wear or by a change in the patient's condition are covered when ordered by a physician.

Adjustments, repairs and replacements are covered even when the item had been in use before the user enrolled in Part B of the program so long as the device continues to be medically required.

### 100-2,15,140

### Therapeutic Shoes for Individuals with Diabetes

B3-2134Coverage of therapeutic shoes (depth or custom-molded) along with inserts for individuals with diabetes is available as of May 1, 1993. These diabetic shoes are covered if the requirements as specified in this section concerning certification and prescription are fulfilled. In addition, this benefit provides for a pair of diabetic shoes even if only one foot suffers from diabetic foot disease. Each shoe is equally equipped so that the affected limb, as well as the remaining limb, is protected. Claims for therapeutic shoes for diabetics are processed by the Durable Medical Equipment Regional Carriers (DMERCs).

Therapeutic shoes for diabetics are not DME and are not considered DME nor orthotics, but a separate category of coverage under Medicare Part B. (See §1861(s)(12) and §1833(o) of the Act.)

#### A. Definitions

The following items may be covered under the diabetic shoe benefit:

1. Custom-Molded ShoesCustom-molded shoes are shoes that:

   • Are constructed over a positive model of the patient's foot;

   • Are made from leather or other suitable material of equal quality;

   • Have removable inserts that can be altered or replaced as the patient's condition warrants; and

   • Have some form of shoe closure.

2. Depth Shoes
   Depth shoes are shoes that:

   • Have a full length, heel-to-toe filler that, when removed, provides a minimum of 3/16 inch of additional depth used to accommodate custom-molded or customized inserts;

   • Are made from leather or other suitable material of equal quality;

   • Have some form of shoe closure; and

   • Are available in full and half sizes with a minimum of three widths so that the sole is graded to the size and width of the upper portions of the shoes according to the American standard last sizing schedule or its equivalent. (The American standard last sizing schedule is the numerical shoe sizing system used for shoes sold in the United States.)

3. Inserts
   Inserts are total contact, multiple density, removable inlays that are directly molded to the patient's foot or a model of the patient's foot and that are made of a suitable material with regard to the patient's condition.

#### B. Coverage

1. Limitations
   For each individual, coverage of the footwear and inserts is limited to one of the following within one calendar year:

   • No more than one pair of custom-molded shoes (including inserts provided with such shoes) and two additional pairs of inserts; or

- No more than one pair of depth shoes and three pairs of inserts (not including the noncustomized removable inserts provided with such shoes).

2. Coverage of Diabetic Shoes and Brace

Orthopedic shoes, as stated in the Medicare Claims Processing Manual, Chapter 20, "Durable Medical Equipment, Surgical Dressings and Casts, Orthotics and Artificial Limbs, and Prosthetic Devices," generally are not covered. This exclusion does not apply to orthopedic shoes that are an integral part of a leg brace. In situations in which an individual qualifies for both diabetic shoes and a leg brace, these items are covered separately. Thus, the diabetic shoes may be covered if the requirements for this section are met, while the brace may be covered if the requirements of §130 are met.

3. Substitution of Modifications for Inserts

An individual may substitute modification(s) of custom-molded or depth shoes instead of obtaining a pair(s) of inserts in any combination. Payment for the modification(s) may not exceed the limit set for the inserts for which the individual is entitled. The following is a list of the most common shoe modifications available, but it is not meant as an exhaustive list of the modifications available for diabetic shoes:

- Rigid Rocker Bottoms- These are exterior elevations with apex positions for 51 percent to 75 percent distance measured from the back end of the heel. The apex is a narrowed or pointed end of an anatomical structure. The apex must be positioned behind the metatarsal heads and tapered off sharply to the front tip of the sole. Apex height helps to eliminate pressure at the metatarsal heads. Rigidity is ensured by the steel in the shoe. The heel of the shoe tapers off in the back in order to cause the heel to strike in the middle of the heel;

- Roller Bottoms (Sole or Bar)- These are the same as rocker bottoms, but the heel is tapered from the apex to the front tip of the sole;

- Metatarsal Bars- An exterior bar is placed behind the metatarsal heads in order to remove pressure from the metatarsal heads. The bars are of various shapes, heights, and construction depending on the exact purpose;

- Wedges (Posting)- Wedges are either of hind foot, fore foot, or both and may be in the middle or to the side. The function is to shift or transfer weight bearing upon standing or during ambulation to the opposite side for added support, stabilization, equalized weight distribution, or balance; and

- Offset Heels- This is a heel flanged at its base either in the middle, to the side, or a combination, that is then extended upward to the shoe in order to stabilize extreme positions of the hind foot. Other modifications to diabetic shoes include, but are not limited to flared heels, Velcro closures, and inserts for missing toes.

4. Separate Inserts Inserts may be covered and dispensed independently of diabetic shoes if the supplier of the shoes verifies in writing that the patient has appropriate footwear into which the insert can be placed. This footwear must meet the definitions found above for depth shoes and custom-molded shoes.

## C. Certification

The need for diabetic shoes must be certified by a physician who is a doctor of medicine or a doctor of osteopathy and who is responsible for diagnosing and treating the patient's diabetic systemic condition through a comprehensive plan of care. This managing physician must:

- Document in the patient's medical record that the patient has diabetes;

- Certify that the patient is being treated under a comprehensive plan of care for diabetes, and that the patient needs diabetic shoes; and

- Document in the patient's record that the patient has one or more of the following conditions:

  - Peripheral neuropathy with evidence of callus formation;

  - History of pre-ulcerative calluses;

  - History of previous ulceration;

  - Foot deformity;

  - Previous amputation of the foot or part of the foot; or

  - Poor circulation.

## D. Prescription

Following certification by the physician managing the patient's systemic diabetic condition, a podiatrist or other qualified physician who is knowledgeable in the fitting of diabetic shoes and inserts may prescribe the particular type of footwear necessary.

## E. Furnishing

FootwearThe footwear must be fitted and furnished by a podiatrist or other qualified individual such as a pedorthist, an orthotist, or a prosthetist. The certifying physician may not furnish the diabetic shoes unless the certifying physician is the only qualified individual in the area. It is left to the discretion of each carrier to determine the meaning of "in the area."

## 100-2,15,150

### Dental Services

B3-2136

As indicated under the general exclusions from coverage, items and services in connection with the care, treatment, filling, removal, or replacement of teeth or structures directly supporting the teeth are not covered. "Structures directly supporting the teeth" means the periodontium, which includes the gingivae, dentogingival junction, periodontal membrane, cementum of the teeth, and alveolar process.

In addition to the following, see Pub 100-01, the Medicare General Information, Eligibility, and Entitlement Manual, Chapter 5, Definitions and Pub 3, the Medicare National Coverage Determinations Manual for specific services which may be covered when furnished by a dentist. If an otherwise noncovered procedure or service is performed by a dentist as incident to and as an integral part of a covered procedure or service performed by the dentist, the total service performed by the dentist on such an occasion is covered.

EXAMPLE 1:

The reconstruction of a ridge performed primarily to prepare the mouth for dentures is a noncovered procedure. However, when the reconstruction of a ridge is performed as a result of and at the same time as the surgical removal of a tumor (for other than dental purposes), the totality of surgical procedures is a covered service.

EXAMPLE 2:

Medicare makes payment for the wiring of teeth when this is done in connection with the reduction of a jaw fracture.

The extraction of teeth to prepare the jaw for radiation treatment of neoplastic disease is also covered. This is an exception to the requirement that to be covered, a noncovered procedure or service performed by a dentist must be an incident to and an integral part of a covered procedure or service performed by the dentist. Ordinarily, the dentist extracts the patient's teeth, but another physician, e.g., a radiologist, administers the radiation treatments.

When an excluded service is the primary procedure involved, it is not covered, regardless of its complexity or difficulty. For example, the extraction of an impacted tooth is not covered. Similarly, an alveoplasty (the surgical improvement of the shape and condition of the alveolar process) and a frenectomy are excluded from coverage when either of these procedures is performed in connection with an excluded service, e.g., the preparation of the mouth for dentures. In a like manner, the removal of a torus palatinus (a bony protuberance of the hard palate) may be a covered service. However, with rare exception, this surgery is performed in connection with an excluded service, i.e., the preparation of the mouth for dentures. Under such circumstances, Medicare does not pay for this procedure.

Dental splints used to treat a dental condition are excluded from coverage under 1862(a)(12) of the Act. On the other hand, if the treatment is determined to be a covered medical condition (i.e., dislocated upper/lower jaw joints), then the splint can be covered.

Whether such services as the administration of anesthesia, diagnostic x-rays, and other related procedures are covered depends upon whether the primary procedure being performed by the dentist is itself covered. Thus, an x-ray taken in connection with the reduction of a fracture of the jaw or facial bone is covered. However, a single x-ray or x-ray survey taken in connection with the care or treatment of teeth or the periodontium is not covered.

Medicare makes payment for a covered dental procedure no matter where the service is performed. The hospitalization or nonhospitalization of a patient has no direct bearing on the coverage or exclusion of a given dental procedure.

Payment may also be made for services and supplies furnished incident to covered dental services. For example, the services of a dental technician or nurse who is under the direct supervision of the dentist or physician are covered if the services are included in the dentist's or physician's bill.

## 100-2,15,230

### Practice of Physical Therapy, Occupational Therapy, and Speech-Language Pathology

#### A. Group Therapy Services.

Contractors pay for outpatient physical therapy services (which includes outpatient speech-language pathology services) and outpatient occupational therapy services provided simultaneously to two or more individuals by a practitioner as group therapy services (97150). The individuals can be, but need not be performing the same activity. The physician or therapist involved in group therapy services must be in constant attendance, but one-on-one patient contact is not required.

#### B. Therapy Students

1. General

Only the services of the therapist can be billed and paid under Medicare Part B. The services performed by a student are not reimbursed even if provided under "line of sight" supervision of the therapist; however, the presence of the student "in the room" does not make the service unbillable. Pay for the direct (one-to-one) patient contact services of thephysician or therapist provided to Medicare Part B patients. Group therapy services performed by a therapist or physician may be billed when a student is also present "in the room".

EXAMPLES:

Therapists may bill and be paid for the provision of services in the following scenarios:

- The qualified practitioner is present and in the room for the entire session. The student participates in the delivery of services when the qualified practitioner is directing the service, making the skilled judgment, and is responsible for the assessment and treatment.

- The qualified practitioner is present in the room guiding the student in service delivery when the therapy student and the therapy assistant student are participating in the provision of services, and the practitioner is not engaged in treating another patient or doing other tasks at the same time

- The qualified practitioner is responsible for the services and as such, signs all documentation. (A student may, of course, also sign but it is not necessary since the Part B payment is for the clinician's service, not for the student's services).

2. Therapy Assistants as Clinical Instructors
Physical therapist assistants and occupational therapy assistants are not precluded from serving as clinical instructors for therapy students, while providing services within their scope of work and performed under the direction and supervision of a licensed physical or occupational therapist to a Medicare beneficiary.

3. Services Provided Under Part A and Part B"
The payment methodologies for Part A and B therapy services rendered by a student are different. Under the MPFS (Medicare Part B), Medicare pays for services provided by physicians and practitioners that are specifically authorized by statute. Students do not meet the definition of practitioners under Medicare Part B. Under SNF PPS, payments are based upon the case mix or Resource Utilization Group (RUG) category that describes the patient. In the rehabilitation groups, the number of therapy minutes delivered to the patient determines the RUG category. Payment levels for each category are based upon the costs of caring for patients in each group rather than providing pecific payment for each therapy service as is done in Medicare Part B.

## 100-2,15,280.1

### Glaucoma Screening

**A. Conditions of Coverage**
The regulations implementing the Benefits Improvements and Protection Act of 2000, §102, provide for annual coverage for glaucoma screening for beneficiaries in the following high risk categories:

- Individuals with diabetes mellitus;

- Individuals with a family history of glaucoma; or

- African-Americans age 50 and over. In addition, beginning with dates of service on or after January 1, 2006, 42 CFR 410.23(a)(2), revised, the definition of an eligible beneficiary in a high-risk category is expanded to include:

- Hispanic-Americans age 65 and over.

Medicare will pay for glaucoma screening examinations where they are furnished by or under the direct supervision in the office setting of an ophthalmologist or optometrist, who is legally authorized to perform the services under State law. Screening for glaucoma is defined to include:

- A dilated eye examination with an intraocular pressure measurement; and

- A direct ophthalmoscopy examination, or a slit-lamp biomicroscopic examination.

Payment may be made for a glaucoma screening examination that is performed on an eligible beneficiary after at least 11 months have passed following the month in which the last covered glaucoma screening examination was performed.

The following HCPCS codes apply for glaucoma screening:

G0117   Glaucoma screening for high-risk patients furnished by an optometrist or ophthalmologist; and

G0118   Glaucoma screening for high-risk patients furnished under the direct supervision of an optometrist or ophthalmologist.

The type of service for the above G codes is: TOS Q.

For providers who bill intermediaries, applicable types of bill for screening glaucoma services are 13X, 22X, 23X, 71X, 73X, 75X, and 85X. The following revenue codes should be reported when billing for screening glaucoma services:

- Comprehensive outpatient rehabilitation facilities (CORFs), critical access hospitals (CAHs), skilled nursing facilities (SNFs), independent and provider-based RHCs and free standing and provider-based FQHCs bill for this service under revenue code 770. CAHs

electing the optional method of payment for outpatient services report this service under revenue codes 96X, 97X, or 98X.

- Hospital outpatient departments bill for this service under any valid/appropriate revenue code. They are not required to report revenue code 770.

**B. Calculating the Frequency**
Once a beneficiary has received a covered glaucoma screening procedure, the beneficiary may receive another procedure after 11 full months have passed. To determine the 11-month period, start the count beginning with the month after the month in which the previous covered screening procedure was performed.

**C. Diagnosis Coding Requirements**
Providers bill glaucoma screening using screening ("V") code V80.1 (Special Screening for Neurological, Eye, and Ear Diseases, Glaucoma). Claims submitted without a screening diagnosis code may be returned to the provider as unprocessable.

**D. Payment Methodology**

1. Carriers
Contractors pay for glaucoma screening based on the Medicare physician fee schedule. Deductible and coinsurance apply. Claims from physicians or other providers where assignment was not taken are subject to the Medicare limiting charge (refer to the Medicare Claims Processing Manual, Chapter 12, "Physician/Non-physician Practitioners," for more information about the Medicare limiting charge).

2. Intermediaries
Payment is made for the facility expense as follows:

- Independent and provider-based RHC/free standing and provider-based FQHC - payment is made under the all inclusive rate for the screening glaucoma service based on the visit furnished to the RHC/FQHC patient;

- CAH - payment is made on a reasonable cost basis unless the CAH has elected the optional method of payment for outpatient services in which case, procedures outlined in the Medicare Claims Processing Manual, Chapter 3, §30.1.1, should be followed;

- CORF - payment is made under the Medicare physician fee schedule;

- Hospital outpatient department - payment is made under outpatient prospective payment system (OPPS);

- Hospital inpatient Part B - payment is made under OPPS;

- SNF outpatient - payment is made under the Medicare physician fee schedule (MPFS); and

- SNF inpatient Part B - payment is made under MPFS.

Deductible and coinsurance apply.

**E. Special Billing Instructions for RHCs and FQHCs**
Screening glaucoma services are considered RHC/FQHC services. RHCs and FQHCs bill the contractor under bill type 71X or 73X along with revenue code 770 and HCPCS codes G0117 or G0118 and RHC/FQHC revenue code 520 or 521 to report the related visit. Reporting of revenue code 770 and HCPCS codes G0117 and G0118 in addition to revenue code 520 or 521 is required for this service in order for CWF to perform frequency editing.

Payment should not be made for a screening glaucoma service unless the claim also contains a visit code for the service. Therefore, the contractor installs an edit in its system to assure payment is not made for revenue code 770 unless the claim also contains a visit revenue code (520 or 521).

## 100-2,15,290

### Foot Care

**A. Treatment of Subluxation of Foot**
Subluxations of the foot are defined as partial dislocations or displacements of joint surfaces, tendons ligaments, or muscles of the foot. Surgical or nonsurgical treatments undertaken for the sole purpose of correcting a subluxated structure in the foot as an isolated entity are not covered.

However, medical or surgical treatment of subluxation of the ankle joint (talo-crural joint) is covered. In addition, reasonable and necessary medical or surgical services, diagnosis, or treatment for medical conditions that have resulted from or are associated with partial displacement of structures is covered. For example, if a patient has osteoarthritis that has resulted in a partial displacement of joints in the foot, and the primary treatment is for the osteoarthritis, coverage is provided.

**B. Exclusions from Coverage**
The following foot care services are generally excluded from coverage under both Part A and Part B. (See §167;290.F and §167;290.G for instructions on applying foot care exclusions.)

1. Treatment of Flat Foot
The term "flat foot" is defined as a condition in which one or more arches of the foot have

flattened out. Services or devices directed toward the care or correction of such conditions, including the prescription of supportive devices, are not covered.

2. Routine Foot Care
Except as provided above, routine foot care is excluded from coverage. Services that normally are considered routine and not covered by Medicare include the following:

- The cutting or removal of corns and calluses;

- The trimming, cutting, clipping, or debriding of nails; and

- Other hygienic and preventive maintenance care, such as cleaning and soaking the feet, the use of skin creams to maintain skin tone of either ambulatory or bedfast patients, and any other service performed in the absence of localized illness, injury, or symptoms involving the foot.

3. Supportive Devices for Feet
Orthopedic shoes and other supportive devices for the feet generally are not covered. However, this exclusion does not apply to such a shoe if it is an integral part of a leg brace, and its expense is included as part of the cost of the brace. Also, this exclusion does not apply to therapeutic shoes furnished to diabetics.

## C. Exceptions to Routine Foot Care Exclusion

1. Necessary and Integral Part of Otherwise Covered Services
In certain circumstances, services ordinarily considered to be routine may be covered if they are performed as a necessary and integral part of otherwise covered services, such as diagnosis and treatment of ulcers, wounds, or infections.

2. Treatment of Warts on Foot
The treatment of warts (including plantar warts) on the foot is covered to the same extent as services provided for the treatment of warts located elsewhere on the body.

3. Presence of Systemic Condition
The presence of a systemic condition such as metabolic, neurologic, or peripheral vascular disease may require scrupulous foot care by a professional that in the absence of such condition(s) would be considered routine (and, therefore, excluded from coverage). Accordingly, foot care that would otherwise be considered routine may be covered when systemic condition(s) result in severe circulatory embarrassment or areas of diminished sensation in the individual's legs or feet. (See subsection A.)

In these instances, certain foot care procedures that otherwise are considered routine (e.g., cutting or removing corns and calluses, or trimming, cutting, clipping, or debriding nails) may pose a hazard when performed by a nonprofessional person on patients with such systemic conditions. (See §167;290.G for procedural instructions.)

4. Mycotic Nails
In the absence of a systemic condition, treatment of mycotic nails may be covered.

The treatment of mycotic nails for an ambulatory patient is covered only when the physician attending the patient's mycotic condition documents that (1) there is clinical evidence of mycosis of the toenail, and (2) the patient has marked limitation of ambulation, pain, or secondary infection resulting from the thickening and dystrophy of the infected toenail plate.

The treatment of mycotic nails for a nonambulatory patient is covered only when the physician attending the patient's mycotic condition documents that (1) there is clinical evidence of mycosis of the toenail, and (2) the patient suffers from pain or secondary infection resulting from the thickening and dystrophy of the infected toenail plate.

For the purpose of these requirements, documentation means any written information that is required by the carrier in order for services to be covered. Thus, the information submitted with claims must be substantiated by information found in the patient's medical record. Any information, including that contained in a form letter, used for documentation purposes is subject to carrier verification in order to ensure that the information adequately justifies coverage of the treatment of mycotic nails.

## D. Systemic Conditions That Might Justify Coverage
Although not intended as a comprehensive list, the following metabolic, neurologic, and peripheral vascular diseases (with synonyms in parentheses) most commonly represent the underlying conditions that might justify coverage for routine foot care.

- Diabetes mellitus *

- Arteriosclerosis obliterans (A.S.O., arteriosclerosis of the extremities, occlusive peripheral arteriosclerosis)

- Buerger's disease (thromboangiitis obliterans)

- Chronic thrombophlebitis *

- Peripheral neuropathies involving the feet - Associated with malnutrition and vitamin deficiency *

  – Malnutrition (general, pellagra)

  – Alcoholism

  – Malabsorption (celiac disease, tropical sprue)

  – Pernicious anemia

- Associated with carcinoma *

- Associated with diabetes mellitus *

- Associated with drugs and toxins *

- Associated with multiple sclerosis *

- Associated with uremia (chronic renal disease) *

- Associated with traumatic injury

- Associated with leprosy or neurosyphilis

- Associated with hereditary disorders

  – Hereditary sensory radicular neuropathy

  – Angiokeratoma corporis diffusum (Fabry's)

  – Amyloid neuropathy

When the patient's condition is one of those designated by an asterisk (*), routine procedures are covered only if the patient is under the active care of a doctor of medicine or osteopathy who documents the condition.

## E. Supportive Devices for Feet
Orthopedic shoes and other supportive devices for the feet generally are not covered. However, this exclusion does not apply to such a shoe if it is an integral part of a leg brace, and its expense is included as part of the cost of the brace. Also, this exclusion does not apply to therapeutic shoes furnished to diabetics.

## F. Presumption of Coverage
In evaluating whether the routine services can be reimbursed, a presumption of coverage may be made where the evidence available discloses certain physical and/or clinical findings consistent with the diagnosis and indicative of severe peripheral involvement. For purposes of applying this presumption the following findings are pertinent:

Class A Findings
Nontraumatic amputation of foot or integral skeletal portion thereof.

Class B Findings
Absent posterior tibial pulse;

Advanced trophic changes as: hair growth (decrease or absence) nail changes (thickening) pigmentary changes (discoloration) skin texture (thin, shiny) skin color (rubor or redness) (Three required); and

Absent dorsalis pedis pulse.

Class C Findings
Claudication;

Temperature changes (e.g., cold feet);

Edema;

Paresthesias (abnormal spontaneous sensations in the feet); and

Burning.

The presumption of coverage may be applied when the physician rendering the routine foot care has identified:

1. A Class A finding;

2. Two of the Class B findings; or

3. One Class B and two Class C findings.

Cases evidencing findings falling short of these alternatives may involve podiatric treatment that may constitute covered care and should be reviewed by the intermediary's medical staff and developed as necessary.

For purposes of applying the coverage presumption where the routine services have been rendered by a podiatrist, the contractor may deem the active care requirement met if the claim or other evidence available discloses that the patient has seen an M.D. or D.O. for treatment and/or evaluation of the complicating disease process during the 6-month period prior to the rendition of the routine-type services. The intermediary may also accept the podiatrist's statement that the diagnosing and treating M.D. or D.O. also concurs with the podiatrist's findings as to the severity of the peripheral involvement indicated.

Services ordinarily considered routine might also be covered if they are performed as a necessary and integral part of otherwise covered services, such as diagnosis and treatment of diabetic ulcers, wounds, and infections.

### G. Application of Foot Care Exclusions to Physician's Services

The exclusion of foot care is determined by the nature of the service. Thus, payment for an excluded service should be denied whether performed by a podiatrist, osteopath, or a doctor of medicine, and without regard to the difficulty or complexity of the procedure.

When an itemized bill shows both covered services and noncovered services not integrally related to the covered service, the portion of charges attributable to the noncovered services should be denied. (For example, if an itemized bill shows surgery for an ingrown toenail and also removal of calluses not necessary for the performance of toe surgery, any additional charge attributable to removal of the calluses should be denied.)

In reviewing claims involving foot care, the carrier should be alert to the following exceptional situations:

1. Payment may be made for incidental noncovered services performed as a necessary and integral part of, and secondary to, a covered procedure. For example, if trimming of toenails is required for application of a cast to a fractured foot, the carrier need not allocate and deny a portion of the charge for the trimming of the nails. However, a separately itemized charge for such excluded service should be disallowed. When the primary procedure is covered the administration of anesthesia necessary for the performance of such procedure is also covered.

2. Payment may be made for initial diagnostic services performed in connection with a specific symptom or complaint if it seems likely that its treatment would be covered even though the resulting diagnosis may be one requiring only noncovered care.

The name of the M.D. or D.O. who diagnosed the complicating condition must be submitted with the claim. In those cases, where active care is required, the approximate date the beneficiary was last seen by such physician must also be indicated.

NOTE: Section 939 of P.L. 96-499 removed §8220;warts§8221; from the routine foot care exclusion effective July 1, 1981.

Relatively few claims for routine-type care are anticipated considering the severity of conditions contemplated as the basis for this exception. Claims for this type of foot care should not be paid in the absence of convincing evidence that nonprofessional performance of the service would have been hazardous for the beneficiary because of an underlying systemic disease. The mere statement of a diagnosis such as those mentioned in §167;D above does not of itself indicate the severity of the condition. Where development is indicated to verify diagnosis and/or severity the carrier should follow existing claims processing practices which may include review of carrier's history and medical consultation as well as physician contacts.

The rules in §290.F concerning presumption of coverage also apply.

Codes and policies for routine foot care and supportive devices for the feet are not exclusively for the use of podiatrists. These codes must be used to report foot care services regardless of the specialty of the physician who furnishes the services. Carriers must instruct physicians to use the most appropriate code available when billing for routine foot care.

### 100-2,15,50

#### Drugs and Biologicals
B3-2049, A3-3112.4.B, HO-230.4.B

The Medicare program provides limited benefits for outpatient drugs. The program covers drugs that are furnished "incident to" a physician's service provided that the drugs are not usually self-administered by the patients who take them.

Generally, drugs and biologicals are covered only if all of the following requirements are met:

- They meet the definition of drugs or biologicals (see §50.1);
- They are of the type that are not usually self-administered. (see §50.2);
- They meet all the general requirements for coverage of items as incident to a physician's services (see §§50.1 and 50.3);
- They are reasonable and necessary for the diagnosis or treatment of the illness or injury for which they are administered according to accepted standards of medical practice (see §50.4);
- They are not excluded as noncovered immunizations (see §50.4.4.2); and
- They have not been determined by the FDA to be less than effective. (See §§50.4.4).

Medicare Part B does generally not cover drugs that can be self-administered, such as those in pill form, or are used for self-injection. However, the statute provides for the coverage of some self-administered drugs. Examples of self-administered drugs that are covered include blood-clotting factors, drugs used in immunosuppressive therapy, erythropoietin for dialysis patients, osteoporosis drugs for certain homebound patients, and certain oral cancer drugs. (See §110.3 for coverage of drugs, which are necessary to the effective use of Durable Medical Equipment (DME) or prosthetic devices.)

### 100-2,15,50.2

#### Determining Self-Administration of Drug or Biological
AB-02-072, AB-02-139, B3-2049.2The Medicare program provides limited benefits for outpatient prescription drugs. The program covers drugs that are furnished "incident to" a physician's service provided that the drugs are not usually self-administered by the patients who take them. Section 112 of the Benefits, Improvements & Protection Act of 2000 (BIPA) amended sections 1861(s)(2)(A) and 1861(s)(2)(B) of the Act to redefine this exclusion. The prior statutory language referred to those drugs "which cannot be self-administered." Implementation of the BIPA provision requires interpretation of the phrase "not usually self-administered by the patient".

#### A. Policy
Fiscal intermediaries and carriers are instructed to follow the instructions below when applying the exclusion for drugs that are usually self-administered by the patient. Each individual contractor must make its own individual determination on each drug. Contractors must continue to apply the policy that not only the drug is medically reasonable and necessary for any individual claim, but also that the route of administration is medically reasonable and necessary. That is, if a drug is available in both oral and injectable forms, the injectable form of the drug must be medically reasonable and necessary as compared to using the oral form.

For certain injectable drugs, it will be apparent due to the nature of the condition(s) for which they are administered or the usual course of treatment for those conditions, they are, or are not, usually self-administered. For example, an injectable drug used to treat migraine headaches is usually self-administered. On the other hand, an injectable drug, administered at the same time as chemotherapy, used to treat anemia secondary to chemotherapy is not usually self-administered.

#### B. Administered
The term "administered" refers only to the physical process by which the drug enters the patient's body. It does not refer to whether the process is supervised by a medical professional (for example, to observe proper technique or side-effects of the drug). Only injectable (including intravenous) drugs are eligible for inclusion under the "incident to" benefit. Other routes of administration including, but not limited to, oral drugs, suppositories, topical medications are all considered to be usually self-administered by the patient.

#### C. Usually
For the purposes of applying this exclusion, the term "usually" means more than 50 percent of the time for all Medicare beneficiaries who use the drug. Therefore, if a drug is self-administered by more than 50 percent of Medicare beneficiaries, the drug is excluded from coverage and the contractor may not make any Medicare payment for it. In arriving at a single determination as to whether a drug is usually self-administered, contractors should make a separate determination for each indication for a drug as to whether that drug is usually self-administered.

After determining whether a drug is usually self-administered for each indication, contractors should determine the relative contribution of each indication to total use of the drug (i.e., weighted average) in order to make an overall determination as to whether the drug is usually self-administered. For example, if a drug has three indications, is not self-administered for the first indication, but is self administered for the second and third indications, and the first indication makes up 40 percent of total usage, the second indication makes up 30 percent of total usage, and the third indication makes up 30 percent of total usage, then the drug would be considered usually self-administered.

Reliable statistical information on the extent of self-administration by the patient may not always be available. Consequently, CMS offers the following guidance for each contractor's consideration in making this determination in the absence of such data:

1. Absent evidence to the contrary, presume that drugs delivered intravenously are not usually self-administered by the patient.

2. Absent evidence to the contrary, presume that drugs delivered by intramuscular injection are not usually self-administered by the patient. (Avonex, for example, is delivered by intramuscular injection, not usually self-administered by the patient.) The contractor may consider the depth and nature of the particular intramuscular injection in applying this presumption. In applying this presumption, contractors should examine the use of the particular drug and consider the following factors:

3. Absent evidence to the contrary, presume that drugs delivered by subcutaneous injection are self-administered by the patient. However, contractors should examine the use of the particular drug and consider the following factors:

   A. Acute Condition - Is the condition for which the drug is used an acute condition? If so, it is less likely that a patient would self-administer the drug. If the condition were longer term, it would be more likely that the patient would self-administer the drug.

   B. Frequency of Administration - How often is the injection given? For example, if the drug is administered once per month, it is less likely to be self-administered by the patient. However, if it is administered once or more per week, it is likely that the drug is self-administered by the patient.

In some instances, carriers may have provided payment for one or perhaps several doses of a drug that would otherwise not be paid for because the drug is usually self-administered. Carriers may have exercised this discretion for limited coverage, for example, during a brief time when the patient is being trained under the supervision of a physician in the proper technique for self-administration. Medicare will no longer pay for such doses. In addition, contractors may no longer pay for any drug when it is administered on an outpatient emergency basis, if the drug is excluded because it is usually self-administered by the patient.

### D. Definition of Acute Condition

For the purposes of determining whether a drug is usually self-administered, an acute condition means a condition that begins over a short time period, is likely to be of short duration and/or the expected course of treatment is for a short, finite interval. A course of treatment consisting of scheduled injections lasting less than two weeks, regardless of frequency or route of administration, is considered acute. Evidence to support this may include Food and Drug administration (FDA) approval language, package inserts, drug compendia, and other information.

### E. By the Patient

The term "by the patient" means Medicare beneficiaries as a collective whole. The carrier includes only the patients themselves and not other individuals (that is, spouses, friends, or other care-givers are not considered the patient). The determination is based on whether the drug is self-administered by the patient a majority of the time that the drug is used on an outpatient basis by Medicare beneficiaries for medically necessary indications.

The carrier ignores all instances when the drug is administered on an inpatient basis. The carrier makes this determination on a drug-by-drug basis, not on a beneficiary-by-beneficiary basis. In evaluating whether beneficiaries as a collective whole self-administer, individual beneficiaries who do not have the capacity to self-administer any drug due to a condition other than the condition for which they are taking the drug in question are not considered. For example, an individual afflicted with paraplegia or advanced dementia would not have the capacity to self-administer any injectable drug, so such individuals would not be included in the population upon which the determination for self-administration by the patient was based. Note that some individuals afflicted with a less severe stage of an otherwise debilitating condition would be included in the population upon which the determination for "self-administered by the patient" was based; for example, an early onset of dementia.

### F. Evidentiary Criteria

Contractors are only required to consider the following types of evidence: peer reviewed medical literature, standards of medical practice, evidence-based practice guidelines, FDA approved label, and package inserts. Contractors may also consider other evidence submitted by interested individuals or groups subject to their judgment.

Contractors should also use these evidentiary criteria when reviewing requests for making a determination as to whether a drug is usually self-administered, and requests for reconsideration of a pending or published determination.

Please note that prior to the August 1, 2002, one of the principal factors used to determine whether a drug was subject to the self-administered exclusion was whether the FDA label contained instructions for self-administration. However, CMS notes that under the new standard, the fact that the FDA label includes instructions for self-administration is not, by itself, a determining factor that a drug is subject to this exclusion.

### G. Provider Notice of Noncovered Drugs

Contractors must describe on their Web site the process they will use to determine whether a drug is usually self-administered and thus does not meet the "incident to" benefit category. Contractors must publish a list of the injectable drugs that are subject to the self-administered exclusion on their Web site, including the data and rationale that led to the determination. Contractors will report the workload associated with developing new coverage statements in CAFM 21208.

Contractors must provide notice 45 days prior to the date that these drugs will not be covered. During the 45-day time period, contractors will maintain existing medical review and payment procedures. After the 45-day notice, contractors may deny payment for the drugs subject to the notice.

Contractors must not develop local medical review policies (LMRPs) for this purpose because further elaboration to describe drugs that do not meet the 'incident to' and the 'not usually self-administered' provisions of the statute are unnecessary. Current LMRPs based solely on these provisions must be withdrawn. LMRPs that address the self-administered exclusion and other information may be reissued absent the self-administered drug exclusion material. Contractors will report this workload in CAFM 21206. However, contractors may continue to use and write LMRPs to describe reasonable and necessary uses of drugs that are not usually self-administered.

### H. Conferences Between Contractors

Contractors' Medical Directors may meet and discuss whether a drug is usually self-administered without reaching a formal consensus. Each contractor uses its discretion as to whether or not it will participate in such discussions. Each contractor must make its own individual determinations, except that fiscal intermediaries may, at their discretion, follow the determinations of the local carrier with respect to the self-administered exclusion.

### I. Beneficiary Appeals

If a beneficiary's claim for a particular drug is denied because the drug is subject to the "self-administered drug" exclusion, the beneficiary may appeal the denial. Because it is a "benefit category" denial and not a denial based on medical necessity, an Advance Beneficiary Notice (ABN) is not required. A "benefit category" denial (i.e., a denial based on the fact that there is no benefit category under which the drug may be covered) does not trigger the financial liability protection provisions of Limitation On Liability (under §1879 of the Act). Therefore, physicians or providers may charge the beneficiary for an excluded drug.

### J. Provider and Physician Appeals

A physician accepting assignment may appeal a denial under the provisions found in Chapter 29 of the Medicare Claims Processing Manual.

### K. Reasonable and Necessary

Carriers and fiscal intermediaries will make the determination of reasonable and necessary with respect to the medical appropriateness of a drug to treat the patient's condition. Contractors will continue to make the determination of whether the intravenous or injection form of a drug is appropriate as opposed to the oral form. Contractors will also continue to make the determination as to whether a physician's office visit was reasonable and necessary. However, contractors should not make a determination of whether it was reasonable and necessary for the patient to choose to have his or her drug administered in the physician's office or outpatient hospital setting. That is, while a physician's office visit may not be reasonable and necessary in a specific situation, in such a case an injection service would be payable.

### L. Reporting Requirements

Each carrier and intermediary must report to CMS, every September 1 and March 1, its complete list of injectable drugs that the contractor has determined are excluded when furnished incident to a physician's service on the basis that the drug is usually self-administered. The CMS anticipates that contractors will review injectable drugs on a rolling basis and publish their list of excluded drugs as it is developed. For example, contractors should not wait to publish this list until every drug has been reviewed.

Contractors must send their exclusion list to the following e-mail address: drugdata@cms.hhs.gov a template that CMS will provide separately, consisting of the following data elements in order:

1. Carrier Name
2. State
3. Carrier ID#
4. HCPCS
5. Descriptor
6. Effective Date of Exclusion
7. End Date of Exclusion
8. Comments

Any exclusion list not provided in the CMS mandated format will be returned for correction.

To view the presently mandated CMS format for this report, open the file located at: http://cms.hhs.gov/manuals/pm_trans/AB02_139a.zip

## 100-2,15,50.4.2

### Unlabeled Use of Drug

B3-2049.3

An unlabeled use of a drug is a use that is not included as an indication on the drug's label as approved by the FDA. FDA approved drugs used for indications other than what is indicated on the official label may be covered under Medicare if the carrier determines the use to be medically accepted, taking into consideration the major drug compendia, authoritative medical literature and/or accepted standards of medical practice. In the case of drugs used in an anti-cancer chemotherapeutic regimen, unlabeled uses are covered for a medically accepted indication as defined in §50.5. These decisions are made by the contractor on a case-by-case basis.

## 100-2,15,50.5

### Self-Administered Drugs and Biologicals

B3-2049.5

Medicare Part B does not cover drugs that are usually self-administered by the patient unless the statute provides for such coverage. The statute explicitly provides coverage, for blood clotting factors, drugs used in immunosuppressive therapy, erythropoietin for dialysis patients, certain oral anti-cancer drugs and anti-emetics used in certain situations.

## 100-2,15,80.1

### Clinical Laboratory Services
B3-2070.1

Section 1833 and 1861 of the Act provides for payment of clinical laboratory services under Medicare Part B. Clinical laboratory services involve the biological, microbiological, serological, chemical, immunohematological, hematological, biophysical, cytological, pathological, or other examination of materials derived from the human body for the diagnosis, prevention, or treatment of a disease or assessment of a medical condition. Laboratory services must meet all applicable requirements of the Clinical Laboratory Improvement Amendments of 1988 (CLIA), as set forth at 42 CFR part 493. Section 1862(a)(1)(A) of the Act provides that Medicare payment may not be made for services that are not reasonable and necessary. Clinical laboratory services must be ordered and used promptly by the physician who is treating the beneficiary as described in 42 CFR 410.32(a), or by a qualified nonphysician practitioner, as described in 42 CFR 410.32(a)(3). See the Medicare Claims Processing Manual Chapter 16 for related claims processing instructions.

## 100-2,16,10

### General Exclusions From Coverage
A3-3150, HO-260, HHA-232, B3-2300

No payment can be made under either the hospital insurance or supplementary medical insurance program for certain items and services, when the following conditions exist:

- Not reasonable and necessary (§20);
- No legal obligation to pay for or provide (§40);
- Paid for by a governmental entity (§50);
- Not provided within United States (§60);
- Resulting from war (§70);
- Personal comfort (§80);
- Routine services and appliances (§90);
- Custodial care (§110);
- Cosmetic surgery (§120);
- Charges by immediate relatives or members of household (§130);
- Dental services (§140);
- Paid or expected to be paid under workers' compensation (§150);
- Nonphysician services provided to a hospital inpatient that were not provided directly or arranged for by the hospital (§170);
- Services Related to and Required as a Result of Services Which are not Covered Under Medicare (§180);
- Excluded foot care services and supportive devices for feet (§30); or
- Excluded investigational devices (See Chapter 14, §30).

## 100-2,16,20

### Services Not Reasonable and Necessary
A3-3151, HO-260.1, B3-2303, AB-00-52 - 6/00

Items and services which are not reasonable and necessary for the diagnosis or treatment of illness or injury or to improve the functioning of a malformed body member are not covered, e.g., payment cannot be made for the rental of a special hospital bed to be used by the patient in their home unless it was a reasonable and necessary part of the patient's treatment. See also §80.

A health care item or service for the purpose of causing, or assisting to cause, the death of any individual (assisted suicide) is not covered. This prohibition does not apply to the provision of an item or service for the purpose of alleviating pain or discomfort, even if such use may increase the risk of death, so long as the item or service is not furnished for the specific purpose of causing death.

## 100-2,16,90

### Routine Services and Appliances
A3-3157, HO-260.7, B3-2320, R-1797A3 - 5/00

Routine physical checkups; eyeglasses, contact lenses, and eye examinations for the purpose of prescribing, fitting, or changing eyeglasses; eye refractions by whatever practitioner and for whatever purpose performed; hearing aids and examinations for hearing aids; and immunizations are not covered.

The routine physical checkup exclusion applies to (a) examinations performed without relationship to treatment or diagnosis for a specific illness, symptom, complaint, or injury; and (b) examinations required by third parties such as insurance companies business establishments, or Government agencies.

If the claim is for a diagnostic test or examination performed solely for the purpose of establishing a claim under title IV of Public Law 91-173, "Black Lung Benefits," the service is not covered under Medicare and the claimant should be advised to contact their Social Security office regarding the filing of a claim for reimbursement under the "Black Lung" program.

The exclusions apply to eyeglasses or contact lenses, and eye examinations for the purpose of prescribing, fitting, or changing eyeglasses or contact lenses for refractive errors. The exclusions do not apply to physicians' services (and services incident to a physicians' service) performed in conjunction with an eye disease, as for example, glaucoma or cataracts, or to post-surgical prosthetic lenses which are customarily used during convalescence from eye surgery in which the lens of the eye was removed, or to permanent prosthetic lenses required by an individual lacking the organic lens of the eye whether by surgical removal or congenital disease. Such prosthetic lens is a replacement for an internal body organ - the lens of the eye. (See the Medicare Benefit Policy Manual, Chapter 15, "Covered Medical and Other Health Services," §120). Expenses for all refractive procedures, whether performed by an ophthalmologist (or any other physician) or an optometrist and without regard to the reason for performance of the refraction, are excluded from coverage.

### A. Immunizations
Vaccinations or inoculations are excluded as immunizations unless they are either

- Directly related to the treatment of an injury or direct exposure to a disease or condition, such as antirabies treatment, tetanus antitoxin or booster vaccine, botulin antitoxin, antivenin sera, or immune globulin. (In the absence of injury or direct exposure, preventive immunization (vaccination or inoculation) against such diseases as smallpox, polio, diphtheria, etc., is not covered.); or

- Specifically covered by statute, as described in the Medicare Benefit Policy Manual, Chapter 15, "Covered Medical and Other Health Services," §50.

### B. Antigens
Prior to the Omnibus Reconciliation Act of 1980, a physician who prepared an antigen for a patient could not be reimbursed for that service unless the physician also administered the antigen to the patient. Effective January 1, 1981, payment may be made for a reasonable supply of antigens that have been prepared for a particular patient even though they have not been administered to the patient by the same physician who prepared them if:

- The antigens are prepared by a physician who is a doctor of medicine or osteopathy, and

- The physician who prepared the antigens has examined the patient and has determined a plan of treatment and a dosage regimen.

A reasonable supply of antigens is considered to be not more than a 12-week supply of antigens that has been prepared for a particular patient at any one time. The purpose of the reasonable supply limitation is to assure that the antigens retain their potency and effectiveness over the period in which they are to be administered to the patient. (See the Medicare Benefit Policy Manual, Chapter 15, "Covered Medical and Other Health Services," §50.4.4.2)

## 100-2,16,140

### Dental Services Exclusion
A3-3162, HO-260.13, B3-2336

Items and services in connection with the care, treatment, filling, removal, or replacement of teeth, or structures directly supporting the teeth are not covered. Structures directly supporting the teeth mean the periodontium, which includes the gingivae, dentogingival junction, periodontal membrane, cementum, and alveolar process. However, payment may be made for certain other services of a dentist. (See the Medicare Benefit Policy Manual, Chapter 15, "Covered Medical and Other Health Services," §150.)

The hospitalization or nonhospitalization of a patient has no direct bearing on the coverage or exclusion of a given dental procedure.

When an excluded service is the primary procedure involved, it is not covered regardless of its complexity or difficulty. For example, the extraction of an impacted tooth is not covered. Similarly, an alveoplasty (the surgical improvement of the shape and condition of the alveolar process) and a frenectomy are excluded from coverage when either of these procedures is performed in connection with an excluded service, e.g., the preparation of the mouth for dentures. In like manner, the removal of the torus palatinus (a bony protuberance of the hard palate) could be a covered service. However, with rare exception, this surgery is performed in connection with an excluded service, i.e., the preparation of the mouth for dentures. Under such circumstances, reimbursement is not made for this purpose.

The extraction of teeth to prepare the jaw for radiation treatments of neoplastic disease is also covered. This is an exception to the requirement that to be covered, a noncovered procedure or service performed by a dentist must be an incident to and an integral part of a covered procedure or service performed by the dentist. Ordinarily, the dentist extracts the patient's teeth, but another physician, e.g., a radiologist, administers the radiation treatments.

Whether such services as the administration of anesthesia, diagnostic x-rays, and other related procedures are covered depends upon whether the primary procedure being performed by the dentist is covered. Thus, an x-ray taken in connection with the reduction of a fracture of the jaw or facial bone is covered. However, a single x-ray or xray survey taken in connection with the care or treatment of teeth or the periodontium is not covered.

See also the Medicare Benefit Policy Manual, Chapter 1, "Inpatient Hospital Services, §70, and Chapter 15, "Covered Medical and Other Health Services," §150 for additional information on dental services.

## 100-2,6,10

### Medical and Other Health Services Furnished to Inpatients of Participating Hospitals

Payment may be made under Part B for physician services and for the nonphysician medical and other health services listed below when furnished by a participating hospital (either directly or under arrangements) to an inpatient of the hospital, but only if payment for these services cannot be made under Part A.

In PPS hospitals, this means that Part B payment could be made for these services if:

- No Part A prospective payment is made at all for the hospital stay because of patient exhaustion of benefit days before admission;

- The admission was disapproved as not reasonable and necessary (and waiver of liability payment was not made);

- The day or days of the otherwise covered stay during which the services were provided were not reasonable and necessary (and no payment was made under waiver of liability);

- The patient was not otherwise eligible for or entitled to coverage under Part A (See the Medicare Benefit Policy Manual, Chapter 1, §150, for services received as a result of noncovered services); or

- No Part A day outlier payment is made (for discharges before October 1997) for one or more outlier days due to patient exhaustion of benefit days after admission but before the case's arrival at outlier status, or because outlier days are otherwise not covered and waiver of liability payment is not made.

However, if only day outlier payment is denied under Part A (discharges before October 1997), Part B payment may be made for only the services covered under Part B and furnished on the denied outlier days.

In non-PPS hospitals, Part B payment may be made for services on any day for which Part A payment is denied (i.e., benefit days are exhausted; services are not at the hospital level of care; or patient is not otherwise eligible or entitled to payment under Part A).

Services payable are:

- Diagnostic x-ray tests, diagnostic laboratory tests, and other diagnostic tests;

- X-ray, radium, and radioactive isotope therapy, including materials and services of technicians;

- Surgical dressings, and splints, casts, and other devices used for reduction of fractures and dislocations;

- Prosthetic devices (other than dental) which replace all or part of an internal body organ (including contiguous tissue), or all or part of the function of a permanently inoperative or malfunctioning internal body organ, including replacement or repairs of such devices;

- Leg, arm, back, and neck braces, trusses, and artificial legs, arms, and eyes including adjustments, repairs, and replacements required because of breakage, wear, loss, or a change in the patient's physical condition;

- Outpatient physical therapy, outpatient speech-language pathology services, and outpatient occupational therapy (see the Medicare Benefit Policy Manual, Chapter 15, "Covered Medical and Other Health Services," §§220 and 230);

- Screening mammography services;

- Screening pap smears;

- Influenza, pneumococcal pneumonia, and hepatitis B vaccines;

- Colorectal screening;

- Bone mass measurements;

- Diabetes self-management;

- Prostate screening;

- Ambulance services;

- Hemophilia clotting factors for hemophilia patients competent to use these factors without supervision);

- Immunosuppressive drugs;

- Oral anti-cancer drugs;

- Oral drug prescribed for use as an acute anti-emetic used as part of an anti-cancer chemotherapeutic regimen; and

- Epoetin Alfa (EPO).

Coverage rules for these services are described in the Medicare Benefit Policy Manual, Chapters: 11, "End Stage Renal Disease (ESRD);" 14, "Medical Devices;" or 15, "Medical and Other Health Services.

For services to be covered under Part A or Part B, a hospital must furnish nonphysician services to its inpatients directly or under arrangements. A nonphysician service is one which does not meet the criteria defining physicians' services specifically provided for in regulation at 42 CFR 415.102. Services "incident to" physicians' services (except for the services of nurse anesthetists employed by anesthesiologists) are nonphysician services for purposes of this provision. This provision is applicable to all hospitals participating in Medicare, including those paid under alternative arrangements such as State cost control systems, and to emergency hospital services furnished by nonparticipating hospitals.

In all hospitals, every service provided to a hospital inpatient other than those listed in the next paragraph must be treated as an inpatient hospital service to be paid for under Part A, if Part A coverage is available and the beneficiary is entitled to Part A. This is because every hospital must provide directly or arrange for any nonphysician service rendered to its inpatients, and a hospital can be paid under Part B for a service provided in this manner only if Part A coverage does not exist.

These services, when provided to a hospital inpatient, may be covered under Part B, even though the patient has Part A coverage for the hospital stay. This is because these services are covered under Part B and not covered under Part A. They are:

- Physicians' services (including the services of residents and interns in unapproved teaching programs);

- Influenza vaccine;

- Pneumoccocal vaccine and its administration;

- Hepatitis B vaccine and its administration;

- Screening mammography services;

- Screening pap smears and pelvic exams;

- Colorectal screening;

- Bone mass measurements;

- Diabetes self management training services; and

- Prostate screening.

However, note that in order to have any Medicare coverage at all (Part A or Part B), any nonphysician service rendered to a hospital inpatient must be provided directly or arranged for by the hospital.

## 100-2,6,20.5

### Outpatient Observation Services
#### A. Outpatient Observation Services Defined

Observation care is a well-defined set of specific, clinically appropriate services, which include ongoing short term treatment, assessment, and reassessment before a decision can be made regarding whether patients will require further treatment as hospital inpatients or if they are able to be discharged from the hospital. Observation status is commonly assigned to patients who present to the emergency department and who then require a significant period of treatment or monitoring before a decision is made concerning their admission or discharge.

Observation services are covered only when provided by the order of a physician or another individual authorized by State licensure law and hospital staff bylaws to admit patients to the hospital or to order outpatient tests. In the majority of cases, the decision whether to discharge a patient from the hospital following resolution of the reason for the observation care or to admit the patient as an inpatient can be made in less than 48 hours, usually in less than 24 hours. In only rare and exceptional cases do reasonable and necessary outpatient observation services span more than 48 hours.

Hospitals may bill for patients who are "direct admissions" to observation. A "direct admission" occurs when a physician in the community refers a patient to the hospital for observation, bypassing the clinic or emergency department (ED). Effective for services furnished on or after January 1, 2003, hospitals may bill for patients directly admitted for observation services.

See Pub. 100-04, Medicare Claims Processing Manual, Chapter 4, §290, at http://www.cms.hhs.gov/manuals/downloads/clm104c04.pdf for billing and payment instructions for outpatient observation services.

## B. Coverage of Outpatient Observation Services

When a physician orders that a patient be placed under observation, the patient's status is that of an outpatient. The purpose of observation is to determine the need for further treatment or for inpatient admission. Thus, a patient in observation may improve and be released, or be admitted as an inpatient (see Pub. 100-02, Medicare Benefit Policy Manual, Chapter 1, §10 "Covered Inpatient Hospital Services Covered Under Part A" at http://www.cms.hhs.gov/manuals/Downloads/bp102c01.pdf ).

## C. Notification of Beneficiary

All hospital observation services, regardless of the duration of the observation care, that are medically reasonable and necessary are covered by Medicare, and hospitals receive OPPS payments for such observation services. A separate APC payment is made for outpatient observation services involving three specific conditions: chest pain, asthma, and congestive heart failure (see the Medicare Claims Processing Manual, §290.4.2) for additional criteria which must be met. Payments for all other reasonable and necessary observation services are packaged into the payments for other separately payable services provided to the patient on the same day. An ABN should not be issued in the context of reasonable and necessary observation services, whether packaged or paid separately.

If a hospital intends to place or retain a beneficiary in observation for a noncovered service, it must give the beneficiary proper written advance notice of noncoverage under limitation on liability procedures (see Pub. 100-04, Medicare Claims Processing Manual; Chapter 30, "Financial Liability Protections," §20, at http://www.cms.hhs.gov/manuals/downloads/clm104c30.pdf for information regarding Limitation On Liability (LOL) Under §1879 Where Medicare Claims Are Disallowed).

Noncovered," in this context, refers to such services as those listed in paragraph D, below.

## D. Services That Are Not Covered as Outpatient Observation

The following types of services are not covered as outpatient observation services:

- Services that are not reasonable or necessary for the diagnosis or treatment of the patient.

- Services that are provided for the convenience of the patient, the patient's family, or a physician, (e.g., following an uncomplicated treatment or a procedure, physician busy when patient is physically ready for discharge, patient awaiting placement in a long term care facility).

- Services that are covered under Part A, such as a medically appropriate inpatient admission, or services that are part of another Part B service, such as postoperative monitoring during a standard recovery period, (e.g., 4-6 hours), which should be billed as recovery room services. Similarly, in the case of patients who undergo diagnostic testing in a hospital outpatient department, routine preparation services furnished prior to the testing and recovery afterwards are included in the payment for those diagnostic services. Observation should not be billed concurrently with therapeutic services such as chemotherapy.

- Standing orders for observation following outpatient surgery.

Claims for the preceding services are to be denied as not reasonable and necessary, under §1862(a)(1)(A) of the Act.

## 100-4,1,10.1.4.1

## Physician and Ambulance Services Furnished in Connection With Covered Foreign Inpatient Hospital Services

Payment is made for necessary physician and ambulance services that meet the other coverage requirements of the Medicare program, and are furnished in connection with and during a period of covered foreign hospitalization.

## A. Coverage of Physician and Ambulance Services Furnished Outside the U.S.

Where inpatient services in a foreign hospital are covered, payment may also be made for

- Physicians' services furnished to the beneficiary while he/she is an inpatient,

- Physicians' services furnished to the beneficiary outside the hospital on the day of his/her admission as an inpatient, provided the services were for the same condition for which the beneficiary was hospitalized (including the services of a Canadian ship's physician who furnishes emergency services in Canadian waters on the day the patient is admitted to a Canadian hospital for a covered emergency stay and,

- Ambulance services, where necessary, for the trip to the hospital in conjunction with the beneficiary's admission as an inpatient. Return trips from a foreign hospital are not covered.

In cases involving foreign ambulance services, the general requirements in Chapter 15 are also applicable, subject to the following special rules:

- If the foreign hospitalization was determined to be covered on the basis of emergency services, the medical necessity requirements outlined in Chapter 15 are considered met.

- The definition of "physician," for purposes of coverage of services furnished outside the U.S., is expanded to include a foreign practitioner, provided the practitioner is legally licensed to practice in the country in which the services are furnished.

- Only the enrollee can file for Part B benefits; the assignment method may not be used.

- Where the enrollee is deceased, the rules for settling Part B underpayments are applicable. Payment is made to the foreign physician or foreign ambulance company on an unpaid bill provided the physician or ambulance company accepts the payment as the full charge for the service, or payment an be made to a person who has agreed to assume legal liability to pay the physician or supplier. Where the bill is paid, payment may be made in accordance with Medicare regulations. The regular deductible and coinsurance requirements apply to physicians' and ambulance services furnished outside the U.S.

## 100-4,1,30.3.5

## Effect of Assignment Upon Purchase of Cataract Glasses FromParticipating Physician or Supplier on Claims Submitted to Carriers
B3-3045.4

A pair of cataract glasses is comprised of two distinct products: a professional product (the prescribed lenses) and a retail commercial product (the frames). The frames serve not only as a holder of lenses but also as an article of personal apparel. As such, they are usually selected on the basis of personal taste and style. Although Medicare will pay only for standard frames, most patients want deluxe frames. Participating physicians and suppliers cannot profitably furnish such deluxe frames unless they can make an extra (noncovered) charge for the frames even though they accept assignment.

Therefore, a participating physician or supplier (whether an ophthalmologist, optometrist, or optician) who accepts assignment on cataract glasses with deluxe frames may charge the Medicare patient the difference between his/her usual charge to private pay patients for glasses with standard frames and his/her usual charge to such patients for glasses with deluxe frames, in addition to the applicable deductible and coinsurance on glasses with standard frames, if all of the following requirements are met:

A. The participating physician or supplier has standard frames available, offers them for saleto the patient, and issues and ABN to the patient that explains the price and other differences between standard and deluxe frames. Refer to Chapter 30.

B. The participating physician or supplier obtains from the patient (or his/her representative) and keeps on file the following signed and dated statement:

_____

Name of Patient Medicare Claim Number

Having been informed that an extra charge is being made by the physician or supplier for deluxe frames, that this extra charge is not covered by Medicare, and that standard frames are available for purchase from the physician or supplier at no extra charge, I have chosen to purchase deluxe frames. _____

Signature Date

C. The participating physician or supplier itemizes on his/her claim his/her actual charge for the lenses, his/her actual charge for the standard frames, and his/her actual extra charge for the deluxe frames (charge differential). Once the assigned claim for deluxe frames has been processed, the carrier will follow the ABN instructions as described in §60.

## 100-4,11,40.1.3.1
### Care Plan Oversight

Care plan oversight (CPO) exists where there is physician supervision of patients under care of hospices that require complex and multidisciplinary care modalities involving regular physician development and/or revision of care plans. Implicit in the concept of CPO is the expectation that the physician has coordinated an aspect of the patient's care with the hospice during the month for which CPO services were billed.

For a physician or NP employed by or under arrangement with a hospice agency, CPO functions are incorporated and are part of the hospice per diem payment and as such may not be separately billed.

For information on separately billable CPO services by the attending physician or nurse practitioner see Chapter 12, §180 of this manual.

## 100-4,12,180
### Care Plan Oversight Services

The Medicare Benefit Policy Manual, Chapter 15, contains requirements for coverage for medical and other health services including those of physicians and non-physician practitioners.

Care plan oversight (CPO) is the physician supervision of a patient receiving complex and/or multidisciplinary care as part of Medicare-covered services provided by a participating home health agency or Medicare approved hospice.

CPO services require complex or multidisciplinary care modalities involving:

- Regular physician development and/or revision of care plans;

- Review of subsequent reports of patient status;

- Review of related laboratory and other studies;

- Communication with other health professionals not employed in the same practice who are involved in the patient's care;

- Integration of new information into the medical treatment plan; and/or

- Adjustment of medical therapy.

The CPO services require recurrent physician supervision of a patient involving 30 or more minutes of the physician's time per month. Services not countable toward the 30 minutes threshold that must be provided in order to bill for CPO include, but are not limited to:

- Time associated with discussions with the patient, his or her family or friends to adjust medication or treatment;

- Time spent by staff getting or filing charts;

- Travel time; and/or

- Physician's time spent telephoning prescriptions into the pharmacist unless the telephone conversation involves discussions of pharmaceutical therapies.

Implicit in the concept of CPO is the expectation that the physician has coordinated an aspect of the patient's care with the home health agency or hospice during the month for which CPO services were billed. The physician who bills for CPO must be the same physician who signs the plan of care.

Nurse practitioners, physician assistants, and clinical nurse specialists, practicing within the scope of State law, may bill for care plan oversight. These non-physician practitioners must have been providing ongoing care for the beneficiary through evaluation and management services. These non-physician practitioners may not bill for CPO if they have been involved only with the delivery of the Medicare-covered home health or hospice service.

## A. Home Health CPO

Non-physician practitioners can perform CPO only if the physician signing the plan of care provides regular ongoing care under the same plan of care as does the NPP billing for CPO and either:

- The physician and NPP are part of the same group practice; or

- If the NPP is a nurse practitioner or clinical nurse specialist, the physician signing the plan of care also has a collaborative agreement with the NPP; or

- If the NPP is a physician assistant, the physician signing the plan of care is also the physician who provides general supervision of physician assistant services for the practice.

Billing may be made for care plan oversight services furnished by an NPP when:

- The NPP providing the care plan oversight has seen and examined the patient;

- The NPP providing care plan oversight is not functioning as a consultant whose participation is limited to a single medical condition rather than multidisciplinary coordination of care; and

- The NPP providing care plan oversight integrates his or her care with that of the physician who signed the plan of care.

NPPs may not certify the beneficiary for home health care.

## B. Hospice CPO

The attending physician or nurse practitioner (who has been designated as the attending physician) may bill for hospice CPO when they are acting as an "attending physician".

An "attending physician" is one who has been identified by the individual, at the time he/she elects hospice coverage, as having the most significant role in the determination and delivery of their medical care. They are not employed nor paid by the hospice.The care plan oversight services are billed using Form CMS-1500 or electronic equivalent.

For additional information on hospice CPO, see Chapter 11, §40.1.3.1 of this manual.

### 100-4,12,180.1

## Care Plan Oversight Billing Requirements
### A. Codes for Which Separate Payment May Be Made
Effective January 1, 1995, separate payment may be made for CPO oversight services for 30 minutes or more if the requirements specified in the Medicare Benefits Policy Manual, Chapter 15 are met.

Providers billing for CPO must submit the claim with no other services billed on that claim and may bill only after the end of the month in which the CPO services were rendered. CPO services may not be billed across calendar months and should be submitted (and paid) only for one unit of service.

Physicians may bill and be paid separately for CPO services only if all the criteria in the Medicare Benefit Policy Manual, Chapter 15 are met.

### B. Physician Certification and Recertification of Home Health Plans of Care
Effective 2001, two new HCPCS codes for the certification and recertification and development of plans of care for Medicare-covered home health services were created. See the Medicare General Information, Eligibility, and Entitlement Manual, Pub. 100-01, Chapter 4, "Physician Certification and Recertification of Services," §10-60, and the Medicare Benefit Policy Manual, Pub. 100-02, Chapter 7, "Home Health Services", §30.

The home health agency certification code can be billed only when the patient has not received Medicare-covered home health services for at least 60 days. The home health agency recertification code is used after a patient has received services for at least 60 days (or one certification period) when the physician signs the certification after the initial certification period. The home health agency recertification code will be reported only once every 60 days, except in the rare situation when the patient starts a new episode before 60 days elapses and requires a new plan of care to start a new episode.

### C. Provider Number of Home Health Agency (HHA) or Hospice
For claims for CPO submitted on or after January 1, 1997, physicians must enter on the Medicare claim form the 6-character Medicare provider number of the HHA or hospice providing Medicare-covered services to the beneficiary for the period during which CPO services was furnished and for which the physician signed the plan of care. Physicians are responsible for obtaining the HHA or hospice Medicare provider numbers. Additionally, physicians should provide their UPIN to the HHA or hospice furnishing services to their patient.

NOTE:There is currently no place on the HIPAA standard ASC X12N 837 professional format to specifically include the HHA or hospice provider number required for a care plan oversight claim. For this reason, the requirement to include the HHA or hospice provider number on a care plan oversight claim is temporarily waived until a new version of this electronic standard format is adopted under HIPAA and includes a place to provide the HHA and hospice provider numbers for care plan oversight claims.

### 100-4,12,190

## Medicare Payment for Telehealth Services
A3-3497, A3-3660.2, B3-4159, B3-15516

### 100-4,12,210.1

## Application of Limitation
B3-2472 - 2472.5

### A. Status of Patient
The limitation is applicable to expenses incurred in connection with the treatment of an individual who is not an inpatient of a hospital. Thus, the limitation applies to mental health services furnished to a person in a physician's office, in the patient's home, in a skilled nursing facility, as an outpatient, and so forth. The term "hospital" in this context means an institution, which is primarily engaged in providing to inpatients, by or under the supervision of physician(s):

- Diagnostic and therapeutic services for medical diagnosis, treatment and care of injured, disabled, or sick persons;

- Rehabilitation services for injured, disabled, or sick persons; or

- Psychiatric services for the diagnosis and treatment of mentally ill patients.

### B. Disorders Subject to Limitation
The term "mental, psychoneurotic, and personality disorders" is defined as the specificpsychiatric conditions described in the American Psychiatric Association's (APA)Diagnostic and Statistical Manual of Mental Disorders, Third Edition - Revised (DSMIII-R).

When the treatment services rendered are both for a psychiatric condition as defined in the DSM-III-R and one or more nonpsychiatric conditions, separate the expenses for the psychiatric aspects of treatment from the expenses for the nonpsychiatric aspects of treatment. However, in any case in which the psychiatric treatment component is not readily distinguishable from the nonpsychiatric treatment component, all of the expenses are allocated to whichever component constitutes the primary diagnosis.

1. Diagnosis Clearly Meets Definition - If the primary diagnosis reported for a particular service is the same as or equivalent to a condition described in the APA's DSM-III-R, the expense for the service is subject to the limitation except as described in subsection D.

2. Diagnosis Does Not Clearly Meet Definition - When it is not clear whether the primary diagnosis reported meets the definition of mental, psychoneurotic, and personality disorders, it may be necessary to contact the practitioner to clarify the diagnosis. In deciding whether contact is necessary in a given case, give consideration to such factors

as the type of services rendered, the diagnosis, and the individual's previous utilization history.

## C. Services Subject to Limitation

Carriers apply the limitation to claims for professional services that represent mental health treatment furnished to individuals who are not hospital inpatients by physicians, clinical psychologists, clinical social workers, and other allied health professionals. Items and supplies furnished by physicians or other mental health practitioners in connection with treatment are also subject to the limitation. (The limitation also applies to CORF claims processed by intermediaries.)

Carriers apply the limitation only to treatment services. It does not apply to diagnostic services as described in subsection D. Testing services performed to evaluate a patient's progress during treatment are considered part of treatment and are subject to the limitation.

D. Services Not Subject to Limitation

1. Diagnosis of Alzheimer's Disease or Related Disorder - When the primary diagnosis reported for a particular service is Alzheimer's Disease (coded 331.0 in theInternational Classification of Diseases, 9th Revision") or Alzheimer's or other disorders coded 290.XX in the APA's DSM-III-R, carriers look to the nature of the service that has been rendered in determining whether it is subject to the limitation. Typically, treatment provided to a patient with a diagnosis of Alzheimer's Disease or a related disorder represents medical management of the patient's condition (rather than psychiatric treatment) and is not subject to the limitation. However, when the primary treatment rendered to a patient with such a diagnosis is psychotherapy, it is subject to the limitation.

2. Brief Office Visits for Monitoring or Changing Drug Prescriptions - Brief office visits for the sole purpose of monitoring or changing drug prescriptions used in the treatment of mental, psychoneurotic and personality disorders are not subject to the limitation. These visits are reported using HCPCS code M0064 (brief office visit for the sole purpose of monitoring or changing drug prescriptions used in the treatment of mental, psychoneurotic, and personality disorders). Claims where the diagnosis reported is a mental, psychoneurotic, or personality disorder (other than a diagnosis specified in subsection A) are subject to the limitation except for the procedure identified by HCPCS code M0064.

3. Diagnostic Services - Carriers do not apply the limitation to tests and evaluations performed to establish or confirm the patient's diagnosis. Diagnostic services include psychiatric or psychological tests and interpretations, diagnostic consultations, and initial evaluations.

An initial visit to a practitioner for professional services often combines diagnostic evaluation and the start of therapy. Such a visit is neither solely diagnostic nor solely therapeutic. Therefore, carriers deem the initial visit to be diagnostic so that the limitation does not apply. Separating diagnostic and therapeutic components of a visit is not administratively feasible, unless the practitioner already has separately identified them on the bill. Determining the entire visit to be therapeutic is not justifiable since some diagnostic work must be done before even a tentative diagnosis can be made and certainly before therapy can be instituted. Moreover, the patient should not be disadvantaged because therapeutic as well as diagnostic services were provided in the initial visit. In the rare cases where a practitioner's diagnostic services take more than one visit, carriers do not apply the limitation to the additional visits. However, it is expected such cases are few. Therefore, when a practitioner bills for more than one visit for professional diagnostic services, carriers request documentation to justify the reason for more than one diagnostic visit.

4. Partial Hospitalization Services Not Directly Provided by Physician - The limitation does not apply to partial hospitalization services that are not directly provided by a physician. These services are billed by hospitals and community mental health centers (CMHCs) to intermediaries.

## E. Computation of Limitation

Carriers determine the Medicare allowed payment amount for services subject to the limitation. They:

- Multiply this amount by 0.625;
- Subtract any unsatisfied deductible; and,
- Multiply the remainder by 0.8 to obtain the amount of Medicare payment.

The beneficiary is responsible for the difference between the amount paid by Medicare and the full allowed amount.

EXAMPLE A:

A beneficiary is referred to a Medicare participating psychiatrist who performs a diagnostic evaluation that costs $350. Those services are not subject to the limitation, and they satisfy the deductible. The psychiatrist then conducts 10 weekly therapy sessions for which he/she charges $125 each. The Medicare allowed amount is $90 each, for a total of $900.

Apply the limitation by multiplying 0.625 times $900, which equals $562.50.

Apply regular 20 percent coinsurance by multiplying 0.8 times $562.50, which equals $450 (the amount of Medicare payment).

The beneficiary is responsible for $450 (the difference between Medicare payment and the allowed amount).

EXAMPLE B:

A beneficiary was an inpatient of a psychiatric hospital and was discharged on January 1, 1992. During his/her inpatient stay he/she was diagnosed and therapy was begun under a treatment team that included a clinical psychologist. He/she received post-discharge therapy from the psychologist for 12 sessions, at which point the psychologist administered testing that showed the patient had recovered sufficiently to warrant termination of therapy. The allowed amount for the therapy sessions was $80 each, and the amount for the testing was $125, for a total of $1085. All services in 1992 were subject to the limitation, since the diagnosis had been completed in the hospital and the subsequent testing was a part of therapy.

Apply the limitation by multiplying 0.625 times $1085, which gives $678.13.

Since the deductible must be met for 1992, subtract $100 from $678.13, for a remainder of $578.13.

Determine Medicare payment by multiplying the remainder by 0.8, which equals $462.50.

The beneficiary is responsible for $622.50.

## 100-4,12,30.4

## Cardiovascular System (Codes 92950-93799)

### A. Echocardiography Contrast Agents

Effective October 1, 2000, physicians may separately bill for contrast agents used in echocardiography. Physicians should use HCPCS Code A9700 (Supply of Injectable Contrast Material for Use in Echocardiography, per study). The type of service code is 9. This code will be carrier-priced.

### B. Electronic Analyses of Implantable Cardioverter-defibrillators and Pacemakers

The CPT codes 93731, 93734, 93741 and 93743 are used to report electronic analyses of single or dual chamber pacemakers and single or dual chamber implantable cardioverterdefibrillators. In the office, a physician uses a device called a programmer to obtain information about the status and performance of the device and to evaluate the patient's cardiac rhythm and response to the implanted device. Advances in information technology now enable physicians to evaluate patients with implanted cardiac devices without requiring the patient to be present in the physician's office. Using a manufacturer's specific monitor/transmitter, a patient can send complete device data and specific cardiac data to a distant receiving station or secure Internet server. The electronic analysis of cardiac device data that is remotely obtained provides immediate and long-term data on the device and clinical data on the patient's cardiac functioning equivalent to that obtained during an in-office evaluation. Physicians should report the electronic analysis of an implanted cardiac device using remotely obtained data as described above with CPT code 93731, 93734, 93741 or 93743, depending on the type  of cardiac device implanted in the patient.

## 100-4,12,30.6.1.1

## Initial Preventive Physical Examination (HCPCS Codes G0344, G0366, G0367 and G0368)

### A. Definition

The initial preventive physical examination (IPPE), or "Welcome to Medicare Visit", is a preventive evaluation and management service (E/M) that includes: (1) review of the individual's medical and social history with attention to modifiable risk factors for disease detection, (2) review of the individual's potential (risk factors) for depression or other mood disorders, (3) review of the individual's functional ability and level of safety; (4) a physical examination to include measurement of the individual's height, weight, blood pressure, a visual acuity screen, and other factors as deemed appropriate by the examining physician or qualified nonphysician practitioner (NPP), (5) performance and interpretation of an electrocardiogram (EKG); (6) education, counseling, and referral, as deemed appropriate, based on the results of the review and evaluation services described in the previous 5 elements, and (7) education, counseling, and referral including a brief written plan (e.g., a checklist or alternative) provided to the individual for obtaining the appropriate screening and other preventive services, which are separately covered under Medicare Part B benefits. (For billing requirements, refer to Pub. 100-04, Chapter 18, Section 80.)

### B. Who May Perform

The IPPE may be performed by a doctor of medicine or osteopathy as defined in section 1861 (r)(1) of the Social Security Act or by a qualified NPP (nurse practitioner, physician assistant and clinical nurse specialist). The carrier will pay the appropriate physician fee schedule amount based on the rendering UPIN/PIN.

## C. Eligibility

Medicare will pay for one IPPE per beneficiary per lifetime. A beneficiary is eligible when he first enrolls in Medicare Part B on or after January 1, 2005, and receives the IPPE benefit within the first 6 months of the effective date of the initial Part B coverage period.

## D. The EKG Component

If the physician or qualified NPP is not able to perform both the examination and the screening EKG, an arrangement may be made to ensure that another physician or entity performs the screening EKG and reports the EKG separately using the appropriate HCPCS G code. The primary physician or qualified NPP shall document the results of the screening EKG into the beneficiary's medical record to complete and bill for the IPPE benefit. NOTE: Both components of the IPPE (the examination and the screening EKG) must be performed before the claims can be submitted by the physician, qualified NPP and/or entity.

## E. Codes Used to Bill the IPPE

The physician or qualified NPP shall bill HCPCS code G0344 for the physical examination performed face-to-face and HCPCS code G0366 for performing a screening EKG that includes both the interpretation and report. If the primary physician or qualified NPP performs only the examination, he/she shall bill HCPCS code G0344 only.   The physician or entity that performs the screening EKG that includes both the interpretation and report shall bill HCPCS code G0366. The physician or entity that  performs the screening EKG tracing only (without interpretation and report) shall bill HCPCS code G0367. The physician or entity that performs the interpretation and report  only (without the EKG tracing) shall bill HCPCS code G0368. Medicare will pay for a screening EKG only as part of the IPPE. NOTE: For an IPPE performed during the global period of surgery refer to section 30.6.6, chapter 12, Pub 100-04 for reporting instructions.

## F. Documentation

The physician and qualified NPP shall use the appropriate screening tools typically used in routine physician practice. As for all E/M services, the 1995 and 1997 E/M documentation guidelines (http://www.cms.hhs.gov/medlearn/emdoc.asp) should be followed for recording the appropriate clinical information in the beneficiary's medical record. All referrals and a written medical plan must be included in this documentation.

## G. Reporting A Medically Necessary E/M at Same IPPE Visit

When the physician or qualified NPP provide a medically necessary E/M service in addition to the IPPE, CPT codes 99201 – 99215 may be used depending on the clinical appropriateness of the circumstances. CPT Modifier –25 shall be appended to the medically necessary E/M service identifying this service as a separately identifiable service from the IPPE code G0344 reported. NOTE: Some of the components of a medically necessary E/M service (e.g., a portion of history or physical exam portion) may have been part of the IPPE and should not be included when determining the most appropriate level of E/M service to be billed for the medically necessary E/M service.

## 100-4,12,70

### Payment Conditions for Radiology Services
B3-15022

See chapter 13, for claims processing instructions for radiology.

## 100-4,13,140

### Bone Mass Measurements (BMMs)

Sections 1861(s)(15) and (rr)(1) of the Social Security Act (the Act) (as added by §4106 of the Balanced Budget Act (BBA) of 1997) standardize Medicare coverage of medically necessary bone mass measurements by providing for uniform coverage under Medicare Part B. This coverage is effective for claims with dates of service furnished on or after July 1, l998.

Effective for dates of service on and after January 1, 2007, the CY 2007 Physician Fee Schedule final rule expanded the number of beneficiaries qualifying for BMM by reducing the dosage requirement for glucocorticoid (steroid) therapy from 7.5 mg of prednisone per day to 5.0 mg. It also changed the definition of BMM by removing coverage for a single-photon absorptiometry as it is not considered reasonable and necessary under section 1862 (a)(1)(A) of the Act.

Conditions of Coverage for BMMs are located in Pub.100-02, Medicare Benefit Policy Manual, chapter 15.

## 100-4,13,20

### Payment Conditions for Radiology Services
B3-15022

## 100-4,13,40.1.2

### HCPCS Coding Requirements

Providers must report HCPCS codes when submitting claims for MRA of the chest, abdomen, head, neck or peripheral vessels of lower extremities. The following HCPCS codes should be used to report these services:

| | |
|---|---|
| MRA of head | 70544, 70544-26, 70544-TC |
| MRA of head | 70545, 70545-26, 70545-TC |
| MRA of head | 70546, 70546-26, 70546-TC |
| MRA of neck | 70547, 70547-26, 70547-TC |
| MRA of neck | 70548, 70548-26, 70548-TC |
| MRA of neck | 70549, 70549-26, 70549-TC |
| MRA of chest | 71555, 71555-26, 71555-TC |
| MRA of pelvis | 72198, 72198-26, 72198-TC |
| MRA of abdomen (dates of service on or after July 1, 2003) – see below. | 74185, 74185-26, 74185-TC |
| MRA of peripheral vessels of lower extremities | 73725, 73725-26, 73725-TC |

Hospitals subject to OPPS should report the following C codes in place of the above HCPCS codes as follows:

- MRA of chest 71555: C8909 – C8911
- MRA of abdomen 74185: C8900 – C8902
- MRA of peripheral vessels of lower extremities 73725: C8912 – C8914

For claims with dates of service on or after July 1, 2003, coverage under this benefit has been expanded for the use of MRA for diagnosing pathology in the renal or aortoiliac arteries. The following HCPCS code should be used to report this expanded coverage of MRA:

- MRA, pelvis, with or without contrast material(s) 72198, 72198-26, 72198-TC

Hospitals subject to OPPS report the following C codes in place of HCPCS code 72198:

- MRA, pelvis, with or without contrast material(s) 72198: C8918 - C8920

Providers utilizing the UB-92 flat file, use record type 61, HCPCS code (Field No. 6) to report HCPCS/CPT code. Providers utilizing the hard copy UB-92, report the HCPCS/CPT code in FL 44 "HCPCS/Rates." Providers utilizing the Medicare A 837 Health Care Claim version 3051 implementations 3A.01 and 1A.C1, report the HCPCS/CPT in 2-395-SV202-02.

## 100-4,13,60.14

### Billing Requirements for PET Scans for Non-Covered Indications

For services performed on or after January 28, 2005, contractors shall accept claims with the following  HCPCS code for non-covered PET indications:

- G0235: PET imaging, any site not otherwise specified

Short Descriptor: PET not otherwise specified

Type of Service: 4

NOTE:This code is for a non-covered service.

## 100-4,13,60.3

### PET Scan Qualifying Conditions and HCPCS Code Chart
(Rev. 527, Issued: 04-15-05, Effective: 01-28-05, Implementation: 04-18-05)

Below is a summary of all covered PET scan conditions, with effective dates.

NOTE: The G codes below except those a # can be used to bill for PET Scan services through January 27, 2005. Effective for dates of service on or after January 28, 2005, providers must bill for PET Scan services using the appropriate CPT codes. See section 60.3.1. The G codes with a # can continue to be used for billing after January 28, 2005 and these remain non-covered by Medicare. (NOTE: PET Scanners must be FDA-approved.)

| Conditions | Coverage Effective Date | ****HCPCS/CPT |
|---|---|---|
| *Myocardial perfusion imaging (following previous PET G0030-G0047) single study, rest or stress (exercise and/or pharmacologic) | 3/14/95 | G0030 |
| *Myocardial perfusion imaging (following previous PET G0030-G0047) multiple studies, rest or stress (exercise and/or pharmacologic) | 3/14/95 | G0031 |
| *Myocardial perfusion imaging (following rest SPECT, 78464); single study, rest or stress (exercise and/or pharmacologic) | 3/14/95 | G0032 |
| *Myocardial perfusion imaging (following rest SPECT 78464); multiple studies, rest or stress (exercise and/or pharmacologic) | 3/14/95 | G0033 |
| *Myocardial perfusion (following stress SPECT 78465); single study, rest or stress (exercise and/or pharmacologic) | 3/14/95 | G0034 |
| *Myocardial Perfusion Imaging (following stress SPECT 78465); multiple studies, rest or stress (exercise and/or pharmacologic) | 3/14/95 | G0035 |
| *Myocardial Perfusion Imaging (following coronary angiography 93510-93529); single study, rest or stress (exercise and/or pharmacologic) | 3/14/95 | G0036 |
| *Myocardial Perfusion Imaging (following stress planar myocardial perfusion, 78460); multiple studies, rest or stress (exercise and/or pharmacologic) | 3/14/95 | G0039 |
| *Myocardial Perfusion Imaging (following stress echocardiogram 93350; single study, rest or stress (exercise and/or pharmacologic) | 3/14/95 | G0040 |
| *Myocardial Perfusion Imaging (following stress echocardiogram, 93350); multiple studies, rest or stress (exercise and/or pharmacologic) | 3/14/95 | G0041 |
| *Myocardial Perfusion Imaging (following stress nuclear ventriculogram 78481 or 78483); single study, rest or stress (exercise and/or pharmacologic) | 3/14/95 | G0042 |
| *Myocardial Perfusion Imaging (following stress nuclear ventriculogram 78481 or 78483); multiple studies, rest or stress (exercise and/or pharmacologic) | 3/14/95 | G0043 |
| *Myocardial Perfusion Imaging (following stress ECG, 93000); single study, rest or stress (exercise and/or pharmacologic) | 3/14/95 | G0044 |
| *Myocardial perfusion (following stress ECG, 93000), multiple studies; rest or stress (exercise and/or pharmacologic) | 3/14/95 | G0045 |
| *Myocardial perfusion (following stress ECG, 93015), single study; rest or stress (exercise and/or pharmacologic) | 3/14/95 | G0046 |
| *Myocardial perfusion (following stress ECG, 93015); multiple studies, rest or stress (exercise and/or pharmacologic) | 3/14/95 | G0047 |
| PET imaging regional or whole body; single pulmonary nodule | 1/1/98 | G0125 |

* NOTE: Carriers must report A4641 for the tracer Rubidium 82 when used with PET scan codes G0030 through G0047 for services performed on or before January 27, 2005 .

** NOTE: Not FDG PET

*** NOTE: For dates of service October 1, 2003, through December 31, 2003, use temporary code Q4078 for billing this radiopharmaceutical.

| Conditions | Coverage Effective Date | ****HCPCS/CPT |
|---|---|---|
| Lung cancer, non-small cell (PET imaging whole body) Diagnosis, Initial Staging, Restaging | 7/1/01 | G0210 G0211 G0212 |
| Colorectal cancer (PET imaging whole body) Diagnosis, Initial Staging, Restaging | 7/1/01 | G0213 G0214 G0215 |
| Melanoma (PET imaging whole body) Diagnosis, Initial Staging, Restaging | 7/1/01 | G0216 G0217 G0218 |
| Melanoma for non-covered indications | 7/1/01 | #G0219 |
| Lymphoma (PET imaging whole body) Diagnosis, Initial Staging, Restaging | 7/1/01 | G0220 G0221 G0222 |
| Head and neck cancer; excluding thyroid and CNS cancers (PET imaging whole body or regional) Diagnosis, Initial Staging, Restaging | 7/1/01 | G0223 G0224 G0225 |
| Esophageal cancer (PET imaging whole body) Diagnosis, Initial Staging, Restaging | 7/1/01 | G0226 G0227 G0228 |
| Metabolic brain imaging for pre-surgical evaluation of refractory seizures | 7/1/01 | G0229 |
| Metabolic assessment for myocardial viability following inconclusive SPECT study | 7/1/01 | G0230 |
| Recurrence of colorectal or colorectal metastatic cancer (PET whole body, gamma cameras only) | 1/1/02 | G0231 |
| Staging and characterization of lymphoma (PET whole body, gamma cameras only) | 1/1/02 | G0232 |
| Recurrence of melanoma or melanoma metastatic cancer (PET whole body, gamma cameras only) | 1/1/02 | G0233 |
| Regional or whole body, for solitary pulmonary nodule following CT, or for initial staging of non-small cell lung cancer (gamma cameras only) | 1/1/02 | G0234 |
| Non-Covered Service PET imaging, any site not otherwise specified | 1/28/05 | #G0235 |
| Non-Covered Service Initial diagnosis of breast cancer and/or surgical planning for breast cancer (e.g., initial staging of axillary lymph nodes), not covered (full- and partial- ring PET scanners only) | 10/1/02 | #G0252 |
| Breast cancer, staging/restaging of local regional recurrence or distant metastases, i.e., staging/restaging after or prior to course of treatment (full- and partial-ring PET scanners only) | 10/1/02 | G0253 |
| Breast cancer, evaluation of responses to treatment, performed during course of treatment (full- and partial-ring PET scanners only) | 10/1/02 | G0254 |

* NOTE: Carriers must report A4641 for the tracer Rubidium 82 when used with PET scan codes G0030 through G0047 for services performed on or before January 27, 2005 .

** NOTE: Not FDG PET

*** NOTE: For dates of service October 1, 2003, through December 31, 2003, use temporary code Q4078 for billing this radiopharmaceutical.

| Conditions | Coverage Effective Date | ****HCPCS/CPT |
|---|---|---|
| Myocardial imaging, positron emission tomography (PET), metabolic evaluation) | 10/1/02 | 78459 |
| Restaging or previously treated thyroid cancer of follicular cell origin following negative I-131 whole body scan (full- and partial-ring PET scanner only) | 10/1/03 | G0296 |
| *Myocardial Perfusion Imaging, (following coronary angiography), 93510-93529); multiple studies, rest or stress (exercise and/or pharmacologic) | 3/14/95 | G0037 |
| *Myocardial Perfusion Imaging (following stress planar myocardial perfusion, 78460); single study, rest or stress (exercise and/or pharmacologic) | 3/14/95 | G0038 |

* NOTE: Carriers must report A4641 for the tracer Rubidium 82 when used with PET scan codes G0030 through G0047 for services performed on or before January 27, 2005 .

** NOTE: Not FDG PET

*** NOTE: For dates of service October 1, 2003, through December 31, 2003, use temporary code Q4078 for billing this radiopharmaceutical.

| Conditions | Coverage Effective Date | ****HCPCS/CPT |
|---|---|---|
| Tracer Rubidium**82 (Supply of Radiopharmaceutical Diagnostic Imaging Agent) (This is only billed through Outpatient Perspective Payment System, OPPS.) (Carriers must use HCPCS Code A4641). | 10/1/03 | Q3000 |
| ***Supply of Radiopharmaceutical Diagnostic Imaging Agent, Ammonia N-13*** | 01/1/04 | A9526 |
| PET imaging, brain imaging for the differential diagnosis of Alzheimer's disease with aberrant features vs. fronto-temporal dementia | 09/15/04 | Appropriate CPT Code from section 60.3.1 |
| PET Cervical Cancer Staging as adjunct to conventional imaging, other staging, diagnosis, restaging, monitoring | 1/28/05 | Appropriate CPT Code from section 60.3.1 |

* NOTE: Carriers must report A4641 for the tracer Rubidium 82 when used with PET scan codes G0030 through G0047 for services performed on or before January 27, 2005 .

** NOTE: Not FDG PET

*** NOTE: For dates of service October 1, 2003, through December 31, 2003, use temporary code Q4078 for billing this radiopharmaceutical.

## APPENDIX 5 — NEW, CHANGED, DELETED, AND REINSTATED HCPCS CODES FOR 2008

### New Codes

| | | | | | | |
|---|---|---|---|---|---|---|
| A4252 | A4648 | A4650 | D2970 | G8351 | G8354 | G8357 |
| G8360 | G8362 | G8365 | G8367 | J0220 | J0400 | J1300 |
| J1561 | | | | | | |

### Changed Codes

| | | | | | | |
|---|---|---|---|---|---|---|
| A4206 | A5105 | A9516 | B4034 | C1716 | C1717 | C1719 |
| C2616 | C2634 | C2635 | C2636 | C2637 | E0630 | E0705 |
| E1801 | E1806 | E1811 | E1816 | E1818 | E1841 | E2205 |
| E2373 | G0380 | G0381 | G0382 | G0383 | G0384 | G8126 |
| G8127 | G8128 | G8196 | G8240 | G8254 | G8271 | G8310 |
| G8326 | G8341 | G8345 | G9012 | G9017 | G9020 | J0702 |
| J1562 | J1566 | J2545 | J3487 | J7187 | J7608 | J7631 |
| J7639 | J9225 | L3806 | L7360 | L7362 | L7364 | L7366 |
| Q4080 | S0161 | S2068 | S5010 | S5013 | S9034 | S9351 |

### Deleted Codes

| | | | | | | |
|---|---|---|---|---|---|---|
| A9565 | B4086 | C1718 | C1720 | C1879 | C2633 | C9232 |
| C9233 | C9234 | C9235 | C9236 | C9350 | C9351 | E2618 |
| G0265 | G0266 | G0267 | G0298 | G0299 | G0375 | G0376 |
| G8158 | G8160 | G8161 | G8163 | G8191 | G8192 | G8194 |
| G8195 | G8197 | G8198 | G8199 | G8201 | G8202 | G8203 |
| G8205 | G8206 | G8207 | G8208 | G8210 | G8211 | G8212 |
| G8213 | G8215 | G8216 | G8218 | G8222 | G8224 | G8225 |
| G8227 | G8228 | G8229 | G8230 | G8232 | G8235 | G8236 |
| G8237 | G8239 | G8241 | G8242 | G8245 | G8247 | G8249 |
| G8250 | G8252 | G8253 | G8255 | G8256 | G8258 | G8259 |
| G8261 | G8262 | G8264 | G8265 | G8267 | G8269 | G8270 |
| G8272 | G8273 | G8275 | G8277 | G8278 | G8280 | G8281 |
| G8283 | G8284 | G8286 | G8287 | G8288 | G8290 | G8291 |
| G8292 | G8294 | G8295 | G8297 | G8300 | G8301 | G8309 |
| G8311 | G8312 | G8313 | G8315 | G8316 | G8317 | G8319 |
| G8320 | G8321 | G8323 | G8324 | G8325 | G8327 | G8328 |
| G8329 | G8331 | G8332 | G8333 | G8335 | G8336 | G8337 |
| G8339 | G8340 | G8342 | G8343 | G8344 | G8346 | G8347 |
| G8348 | G8349 | G8350 | G8352 | G8353 | G8355 | G8356 |
| G8358 | G8359 | G8361 | G8363 | G8364 | G8366 | G8368 |
| J1567 | J7319 | J7345 | J7611 | J7612 | J7613 | J7614 |
| K0553 | K0554 | K0555 | L0960 | L1855 | L1858 | L1870 |
| L1880 | L3800 | L3805 | L3810 | L3815 | L3820 | L3825 |
| L3830 | L3835 | L3840 | L3845 | L3850 | L3855 | L3860 |
| L3907 | L3910 | L3916 | L3918 | L3920 | L3922 | L3924 |
| L3926 | L3928 | L3930 | L3932 | L3934 | L3936 | L3938 |
| L3940 | L3942 | L3944 | L3946 | L3948 | L3950 | L3952 |
| L3954 | L3985 | L3986 | Q4079 | Q4083 | Q4084 | Q4085 |
| Q4086 | Q4087 | Q4088 | Q4089 | Q4090 | Q4091 | Q4092 |
| Q4093 | Q4094 | Q4095 | Q9945 | Q9946 | Q9947 | Q9948 |
| Q9949 | Q9950 | Q9952 | S0147 | S0167 | S0180 | S0820 |
| S1025 | S2078 | S2114 | S2213 | S2250 | S3618 | |

# APPENDIX 6 — PLACE OF SERVICE AND TYPE OF SERVICE

## *Place-of-Service Codes for Professional Claims*

### Database (last updated September 25, 2007)

Listed below are place of service codes and descriptions. These codes should be used on professional claims to specify the entity where service(s) were rendered. Check with individual payers (e.g., Medicare, Medicaid, other private insurance) for reimbursement policies regarding these codes. If you would like to comment on a code(s) or description(s), please send your request to posinfo@cms.hhs.gov.

| Code | Place of Service | Description |
|------|------------------|-------------|
| 01 | Pharmacy | A facility or location where drugs and other medically related items and services are sold, dispensed, or otherwise provided directly to patients. |
| 02 | Unassigned | N/A |
| 03 | School | A facility whose primary purpose is education. |
| 04 | Homeless shelter | A facility or location whose primary purpose is to provide temporary housing to homeless individuals (e.g., emergency shelters, individual or family shelters). |
| 05 | Indian Health Service freestanding facility | A facility or location, owned and operated by the Indian Health Service, which provides diagnostic, therapeutic (surgical and non-surgical), and rehabilitation services to American Indians and Alaska natives who do not require hospitalization. |
| 06 | Indian Health Service provider-based facility | A facility or location, owned and operated by the Indian Health Service, which provides diagnostic, therapeutic (surgical and nonsurgical), and rehabilitation services rendered by, or under the supervision of, physicians to American Indians and Alaska natives admitted as inpatients or outpatients. |
| 07 | Tribal 638 freestanding facility | A facility or location owned and operated by a federally recognized American Indian or Alaska native tribe or tribal organization under a 638 agreement, which provides diagnostic, therapeutic (surgical and nonsurgical), and rehabilitation services to tribal members who do not require hospitalization. |
| 08 | Tribal 638 Provider-based Facility | A facility or location owned and operated by a federally recognized American Indian or Alaska native tribe or tribal organization under a 638 agreement, which provides diagnostic, therapeutic (surgical and nonsurgical), and rehabilitation services to tribal members admitted as inpatients or outpatients. |
| 09 | Prison/correctional facility | A prison, jail, reformatory, work farm, detention center, or any other similar facility maintained by either federal, state or local authorities for the purpose of confinement or rehabilitation of adult or juvenile criminal offenders. (Effective July 1, 2006) |
| 10 | Unassigned | N/A |
| 11 | Office | Location, other than a hospital, skilled nursing facility (SNF), military treatment facility, community health center, State or local public health clinic, or intermediate care facility (ICF), where the health professional routinely provides health examinations, diagnosis, and treatment of illness or injury on an ambulatory basis. |
| 12 | Home | Location, other than a hospital or other facility, where the patient receives care in a private residence. |
| 13 | Assisted living facility | Congregate residential facility with self-contained living units providing assessment of each resident's needs and on-site support 24 hours a day, 7 days a week, with the capacity to deliver or arrange for services including some health care and other services. |
| 14 | Group home | A residence, with shared living areas, where clients receive supervision and other services such as social and/or behavioral services, custodial service, and minimal services (e.g., medication administration). |
| 15 | Mobile unit | A facility/unit that moves from place-to-place equipped to provide preventive, screening, diagnostic, and/or treatment services. |
| 16 | Temporary lodging | A short-term accommodation such as a hotel, campground, hostel, cruise ship or resort where the patient receives care, and which is not identified by any other POS code. (Effective 04/01/08.) |
| 17-19 | Unassigned | N/A |
| 20 | Urgent care facility | Location, distinct from a hospital emergency room, an office, or a clinic, whose purpose is to diagnose and treat illness or injury for unscheduled, ambulatory patients seeking immediate medical attention. |
| 21 | Inpatient hospital | A facility, other than psychiatric, which primarily provides diagnostic, therapeutic (both surgical and nonsurgical), and rehabilitation services by, or under, the supervision of physicians to patients admitted for a variety of medical conditions. |
| 22 | Outpatient hospital | A portion of a hospital which provides diagnostic, therapeutic (both surgical and nonsurgical), and rehabilitation services to sick or injured persons who do not require hospitalization or institutionalization. |
| 23 | Emergency room—hospital | A portion of a hospital where emergency diagnosis and treatment of illness or injury is provided. |
| 24 | Ambulatory surgical center | A freestanding facility, other than a physician's office, where surgical and diagnostic services are provided on an ambulatory basis. |
| 25 | Birthing center | A facility, other than a hospital's maternity facilities or a physician's office, which provides a setting for labor, delivery, and immediate post-partum care as well as immediate care of new born infants. |
| 26 | Military treatment facility | A medical facility operated by one or more of the uniformed services. Military treatment facility (MTF) also refers to certain former U.S. Public Health Service (USPHS) facilities now designated as uniformed service treatment facilities (USTF). |
| 27-30 | Unassigned | N/A |
| 31 | Skilled nursing facility | A facility which primarily provides inpatient skilled nursing care and related services to patients who require medical, nursing, or rehabilitative services but does not provide the level of care or treatment available in a hospital. |
| 32 | Nursing facility | A facility which primarily provides to residents skilled nursing care and related services for the rehabilitation of injured, disabled, or sick persons, or, on a regular basis, health-related care services above the level of custodial care to other than mentally retarded individuals. |

| | | |
|---|---|---|
| 33 | Custodial care facility | A facility which provides room, board, and other personal assistance services, generally on a long-term basis, and which does not include a medical component. |
| 34 | Hospice | A facility, other than a patient's home, in which palliative and supportive care for terminally ill patients and their families are provided. |
| 35-40 | Unassigned | N/A |
| 41 | Ambulance—land | A land vehicle specifically designed, equipped and staffed for lifesaving and transporting the sick or injured. |
| 42 | Ambulance—air or water | An air or water vehicle specifically designed, equipped and staffed for lifesaving and transporting the sick or injured. |
| 43-48 | Unassigned | N/A |
| 49 | Independent clinic | A location, not part of a hospital and not described by any other place-of-service code, that is organized and operated to provide preventive, diagnostic, therapeutic, rehabilitative, or palliative services to outpatients only. |
| 50 | Federally qualified health center | A facility located in a medically underserved area that provides Medicare beneficiaries preventive primary medical care under the general direction of a physician. |
| 51 | Inpatient psychiatric facility | A facility that provides inpatient psychiatric services for the diagnosis and treatment of mental illness on a 24-hour basis, by or under the supervision of a physician. |
| 52 | Psychiatric facility-partial hospitalization | A facility for the diagnosis and treatment of mental illness that provides a planned therapeutic program for patients who do not require full time hospitalization, but who need broader programs than are possible from outpatient visits to a hospital-based or hospital-affiliated facility. |
| 53 | Community mental health center | A facility that provides the following services: outpatient services, including specialized outpatient services for children, the elderly, individuals who are chronically ill, and residents of the CMHC's mental health services area who have been discharged from inpatient treatment at a mental health facility; 24 hour a day emergency care services; day treatment, other partial hospitalization services, or psychosocial rehabilitation services; screening for patients being considered for admission to state mental health facilities to determine the appropriateness of such admission; and consultation and education services. |
| 54 | Intermediate care facility/mentally retarded | A facility which primarily provides health-related care and services above the level of custodial care to mentally retarded individuals but does not provide the level of care or treatment available in a hospital or SNF. |
| 55 | Residential substance abuse treatment facility | A facility which provides treatment for substance (alcohol and drug) abuse to live-in residents who do not require acute medical care. Services include individual and group therapy and counseling, family counseling, laboratory tests, drugs and supplies, psychological testing, and room and board. |
| 56 | Psychiatric residential treatment center | A facility or distinct part of a facility for psychiatric care which provides a total 24-hour therapeutically planned and professionally staffed group living and learning environment. |
| 57 | Non-residential substance abuse treatment facility | A location which provides treatment for substance (alcohol and drug) abuse on an ambulatory basis. Services include individual and group therapy and counseling, family counseling, laboratory tests, drugs and supplies, and psychological testing. |
| 58-59 | Unassigned | N/A |
| 60 | Mass immunization center | A location where providers administer pneumococcal pneumonia and influenza virus vaccinations and submit these services as electronic media claims, paper claims, or using the roster billing method. This generally takes place in a mass immunization setting, such as, a public health center, pharmacy, or mall but may include a physician office setting. |
| 61 | Comprehensive inpatient rehabilitation facility | A facility that provides comprehensive rehabilitation services under the supervision of a physician to inpatients with physical disabilities. Services include physical therapy, occupational therapy, speech pathology, social or psychological services, and orthotics and prosthetics services. |
| 62 | Comprehensive outpatient rehabilitation facility | A facility that provides comprehensive rehabilitation services under the supervision of a physician to outpatients with physical disabilities. Services include physical therapy, occupational therapy, and speech pathology services. |
| 63-64 | Unassigned | N/A |
| 65 | End-stage renal disease treatment facility | A facility other than a hospital, which provides dialysis treatment, maintenance, and/or training to patients or caregivers on an ambulatory or home-care basis. |
| 66-70 | Unassigned | N/A |
| 71 | Public health clinic | A facility maintained by either state or local health departments that provides ambulatory primary medical care under the general direction of a physician. (Effective 10/1/03) |
| 72 | Rural health clinic | A certified facility which is located in a rural medically underserved area that provides ambulatory primary medical care under the general direction of a physician. |
| 73-80 | Unassigned | N/A |
| 81 | Independent laboratory | A laboratory certified to perform diagnostic and/or clinical tests independent of an institution or a physician's office. |
| 82-98 | Unassigned | N/A |
| 99 | Other place of service | Other place of service not identified above. |

## *Type of Service*

### Common Working File Type of Service (TOS) Indicators

For submitting a claim to the Common Working File (CWF), use the following table to assign the proper TOS. Some procedures may have more than one applicable TOS. CWF will reject alerts on codes with incorrect TOS designations. CWF is rejecting codes with incorrect TOS designations.

The only exceptions to this table are:

- Surgical services billed with the ASC facility service modifier SG must be reported as TOS F. The indicator F does not appear on the TOS table because its use is dependent upon the use of the SG modifier.

- Surgical services billed with an assistant-at-surgery modifier (80-82, AS,) must be reported with TOS 8. The 8 indicator does not appear on the TOS table because its use is dependent upon the use of the appropriate modifier. (See Pub. 100-4 *Medicare Claims Processing Manual*, chapter 12, "Physician/Practitioner Billing," for instructions on when assistant-at-surgery is allowable.)

- Psychiatric treatment services that are subject to the outpatient mental health treatment limitation should be reported with TOS T.

- TOS H appears in the list of descriptors. However, it does not appear in the table. In CWF, "H" is used only as an indicator for hospice. The carrier should not submit TOS H to CWF at this time.

- For outpatient services, when a transfusion medicine code appears on a claim that also contains a blood product, the service is paid under reasonable charge at 80 percent; coinsurance and deductible apply. When transfusion medicine codes are paid under the clinical laboratory fee schedule they are paid at 100 percent; coinsurance and deductible do not apply.

Note: For injection codes with more than one possible TOS designation, use the following guidelines when assigning the TOS:

When the choice is L or 1:

- Use TOS L when the drug is used related to ESRD; or
- Use TOS 1 when the drug is not related to ESRD and is administered in the office.

When the choice is G or 1:

- Use TOS G when the drug is an immunosuppressive drug; or
- Use TOS 1 when the drug is used for other than immunosuppression.

When the choice is P or 1:

- Use TOS P if the drug is administered through durable medical equipment (DME); or
- Use TOS 1 if the drug is administered in the office.

The place of service or diagnosis may be considered when determining the appropriate TOS. The descriptors for each of the TOS codes listed in the following table are:

| | |
|---|---|
| 0 | Whole blood |
| 1 | Medical care |
| 2 | Surgery |
| 3 | Consultation |
| 4 | Diagnostic radiology |
| 5 | Diagnostic laboratory |
| 6 | Therapeutic radiology |
| 7 | Anesthesia |
| 8 | Assistant at surgery |
| 9 | Other medical items or services |
| A | Used DME |
| B | High risk screening mammography |
| C | Low risk screening mammography |
| D | Ambulance |
| E | Enteral/parenteral nutrients/supplies |
| F | Ambulatory surgical center (facility usage for surgical services) |
| G | Immunosuppressive drugs |
| H | Hospice |
| J | Diabetic shoes |
| K | Hearing items and services |
| L | ESRD supplies |
| M | Monthly capitation payment for dialysis |
| N | Kidney donor |
| P | Lump sum purchase of DME, prosthetics, orthotics |
| Q | Vision items or services |
| R | Rental of DME |
| S | Surgical dressings or other medical supplies |
| T | Outpatient mental health treatment limitation |
| U | Occupational therapy |
| V | Pneumococcal/flu vaccine |
| W | Physical therapy |

## *Berenson-Eggers Type of Service (BETOS) Codes*

The BETOS coding system was developed primarily for analyzing the growth in Medicare expenditures. The coding system covers all HCPCS codes; assigns a HCPCS code to only one BETOS code; consists of readily understood clinical categories (as opposed to statistical or financial categories); consists of categories that permit objective assignment; is stable over time; and is relatively immune to minor changes in technology or practice patterns.

### BETOS Codes and Descriptions:

1. **Evaluation and Management**

    1. M1A  Office visits—new
    2. M1B  Office visits—established
    3. M2A  Hospital visit—initial
    4. M2B  Hospital visit—subsequent
    5. M2C  Hospital visit—critical care
    6. M3   Emergency room visit
    7. M4A  Home visit
    8. M4B  Nursing home visit
    9. M5A  Specialist—pathology
    10. M5B  Specialist—psychiatry
    11. M5C  Specialist—ophthalmology
    12. M5D  Specialist—other
    13. M6   Consultations

2. **Procedures**

    1. P0   Anesthesia
    2. P1A  Major procedure—breast
    3. P1B  Major procedure—colectomy
    4. P1C  Major procedure—cholecystectomy
    5. P1D  Major procedure—TURP
    6. P1E  Major procedure—hysterectomy
    7. P1F  Major procedure—explor/decompr/excis disc
    8. P1G  Major procedure—other
    9. P2A  Major procedure, cardiovascular—CABG
    10. P2B  Major procedure, cardiovascular—aneurysm repair
    11. P2C  Major procedure, cardiovascular—thromboendarterectomy
    12. P2D  Major procedure, cardiovascular—coronary angioplasty (PTCA)

Appendix 6 — Place of Service and Type of Service

13.  P2E  Major procedure, cardiovascular—pacemaker insertion

14.  P2F  Major procedure, cardiovascular—other

15.  P3A  Major procedure, orthopedic—hip fracture repair

16.  P3B  Major procedure, orthopedic—hip replacement

17.  P3C  Major procedure, orthopedic—knee replacement

18.  P3D  Major procedure, orthopedic—other

19.  P4A  Eye procedure—corneal transplant

20.  P4B  Eye procedure—cataract removal/lens insertion

21.  P4C  Eye procedure—retinal detachment

22.  P4D  Eye procedure—treatment of retinal lesions

23.  P4E  Eye procedure—other

24.  P5A  Ambulatory procedures—skin

25.  P5B  Ambulatory procedures—musculoskeletal

26.  P5C  Ambulatory procedures—groin hernia repair

27.  P5D  Ambulatory procedures—lithotripsy

28.  P5E  Ambulatory procedures—other

29.  P6A  Minor procedures—skin

30.  P6B  Minor procedures—musculoskeletal

31.  P6C  Minor procedures—other (Medicare fee schedule)

32.  P6D  Minor procedures—other (non-Medicare fee schedule)

33.  P7A  Oncology—radiation therapy

34.  P7B  Oncology—other

35.  P8A  Endoscopy—arthroscopy

36.  P8B  Endoscopy—upper gastrointestinal

37.  P8C  Endoscopy—sigmoidoscopy

38.  P8D  Endoscopy—colonoscopy

39.  P8E  Endoscopy—cystoscopy

40.  P8F  Endoscopy—bronchoscopy

41.  P8G  Endoscopy—laparoscopic cholecystectomy

42.  P8H  Endoscopy—laryngoscopy

43.  P8I  Endoscopy—other

44.  P9A  Dialysis services (Medicare fee schedule)

45.  P9B  Dialysis services (non-Medicare fee schedule)

3.  **Imaging**

1.  I1A  Standard imaging—chest

2.  I1B  Standard imaging—musculoskeletal

3.  I1C  Standard imaging—breast

4.  I1D  Standard imaging—contrast gastrointestinal

5.  I1E  Standard imaging—nuclear medicine

6.  I1F  Standard imaging—other

7.  I2A  Advanced imaging—CAT/CT/CTA; brain/head/neck

8.  I2B  Advanced imaging—CAT/CT/CTA; other

9.  I2C  Advanced imaging—MRI/MRA; brain/head/neck

10.  I2D  Advanced imaging—MRI/MRA; other

11.  I3A  Echography—eye

12.  I3B  Echography—abdomen/pelvis

13.  I3C  Echography—heart

14.  I3D  Echography—carotid arteries

15.  I3E  Echography—prostate, transrectal

16.  I3F  Echography—other

17.  I4A  Imaging/procedure—heart, including cardiac catheterization

18.  I4B  Imaging/procedure—other

4.  **Tests**

1.  T1A  Lab tests—routine venipuncture (non-Medicare fee schedule)

2.  T1B  Lab tests—automated general profiles

3.  T1C  Lab tests—urinalysis

4.  T1D  Lab tests—blood counts

5.  T1E  Lab tests—glucose

6.  T1F  Lab tests—bacterial cultures

7.  T1G  Lab tests—other (Medicare fee schedule)

8.  T1H  Lab tests—other (non-Medicare fee schedule)

9.  T2A  Other tests—electrocardiograms

10.  T2B  Other tests—cardiovascular stress tests

11.  T2C  Other tests—EKG monitoring

12.  T2D  Other tests—other

5.  **Durable Medical Equipment**

1.  D1A  Medical/surgical supplies

2.  D1B  Hospital beds

3.  D1C  Oxygen and supplies

4.  D1D  Wheelchairs

5.  D1E  Other DME

6.  D1F  Prosthetic/orthotic devices

7.  D1G  Drugs administered through DME

6.  **Other**

1.  O1A  Ambulance

2.  O1B  Chiropractic

3.  O1C  Enteral and parenteral

4.  O1D  Chemotherapy

5.  O1E  Other drugs

6.  O1F  Hearing and speech services

7.  O1G  Immunizations/vaccinations

7.  **Exceptions/Unclassified**

1.  Y1  Other—Medicare fee schedule

2.  Y2  Other—Non-Medicare fee schedule

3.  Z1  Local codes

4.  Z2  Undefined codes

**NOTES**

**NOTES**